Therapy of Systemic Rheumatic Disorders

Therapy of Systemic Rheumatic Disorders

edited by

Leo B. A. van de Putte
University Hospital Nijmegen
Nijmegen, The Netherlands

Daniel E. Furst
Virginia Mason Medical Center
Seattle, Washington

H. James Williams
University of Utah
Salt Lake City, Utah

Piet L. C. M. van Riel
University Hospital Nijmegen
Nijmegen, The Netherlands

MARCEL DEKKER

MARCEL DEKKER, INC. NEW YORK • BASEL • HONG KONG

Library of Congress Cataloging-in-Publication Data

Therapy of systemic rheumatic disorders/edited by Leo B. A. van de Putte...[et al.]
p. cm.
Includes index.
ISBN 0-8247-9516-4 (alk. paper)
1. Rheumatism—Chemotherapy. 2. Arthritis—Chemotherapy. 3. Musculoskeletal system—Diseases—Chemotherapy. I. Putte, Levinus Boudewijn Abraham van de.
[DNLM: 1. Arthritis, Rheumatoid—drug therapy. 2. Vasculitis—drug therapy. 3. Arthritis—drug therapy. 4. Antirheumatic Agents—therapeutic use. WE 346 T398 1998]
RC927.T498 1998
616.7'23061'dc21
DNLM/DLC for Library of Congress

97-36795
CIP

The publisher offers discounts on this book when ordered in bulk quantities. For more information, write to Special Sales/Professional Marketing at the address below.

This book is printed on acid-free paper.

MARCEL DEKKER, INC.
270 Madison Avenue, New York, New York 10016
http://www.dekker.com

Current printing (last digit):
10 9 8 7 6 5 4 3 2 1

PRINTED IN THE UNITED STATES OF AMERICA

Preface

Treatment of rheumatoid arthritis (RA) and other systemic rheumatic disorders remains a fascinating and rapidly changing field, requiring periodic updates as insights into the pathogenesis of these diseases improve and pharmacotherapeutic possibilities expand. Important improvements in disease assessment have had a profound influence on both the monitoring of various diseases and the timing and use of effective antirheumatic agents.

In terms of total burden of disease on society, rheumatoid arthritis remains a major problem. Recent insights into the pathogenesis of rheumatoid arthritis are beginning to identify new targets for therapy and new therapeutic strategies offer hope for better outcomes.

A major step forward has been the realization that early treatment with second-line agents (also called disease-modifying, remission-inducing, or slow-acting anti-rheumatic drugs) is appropriate, especially in RA. In the past, treatment with second-line agents was often delayed, because few drugs were available and serious side effects were feared. Recently, several observations have led to a more aggressive therapeutic approach in which second-line agents are given at the onset of the disease, often in combination. These observations include data indicating that: rheumatoid arthritis is both a chronic and potentially lethal disease, joint damage occurs in the early phases of the disease, and joint damage is irreversible whereas side effects are almost always reversible, if carefully monitored. In addition, early treatment has now been shown to slow joint damage as assessed by radiographs.

An important new development has been improvement in and standardization of methodology of disease assessment, including better disease activity measurements, response criteria and disease outcome measures. This, in turn, has led to improved disease monitoring, a better definition of drug efficacy and toxicity, and a better understanding of how drugs can be used.

This book deals primarily with those treatments that fundamentally influence the immunoinflammatory processes that underlie the systemic rheumatic disorders. It describes the aforementioned principles as they apply to the second-line agents presently available, from standard medications such as corticosteroids and gold to newer therapeutics such as sulfasalazine, methotrexate, or combination therapy. The text then proceeds into less-studied approaches, such as local therapies and biological agents.

Biological agents deserve particular attention. Advanced molecular biological techniques are now available, not only to unravel the disease process but also to construct agents that interfere with relevant pathogenetic processes. The recent successes with monoclonal antibodies against TNF-α are just one example of what may await us in the future.

Although the emphasis has been on treatment of rheumatoid arthritis, definite and welcome improvements have been made in the treatment of other systemic autoimmune rheumatic disorders. For instance, we now have a new taxonomy of vasculitides, and antibodies like ANCA now allow for better disease classification and monitoring. Also, newer syndromes, such as the antiphospholipid syndrome, have been defined. As in rheumatoid arthritis, there is a growing feeling that adequate treatment as early as possible may prevent or postpone irreversible organ damage.

This book provides a state-of-the-art overview of current therapeutic options, possible treatment dilemmas and recommendations, and how to use currently available drugs. It is hoped that this will be useful to all physicians who treat patients with systemic rheumatic disorders. It is also hoped that progress will be so fast that a new edition will be needed within a few years.

Leo B. A. van de Putte
Daniel E. Furst
H. James Williams
Piet L. C. M. van Riel

Contents

Contributors

Michael Ahern, M.B., B.S., M.D., F.R.A.C.P., F.R.C.P. Flinders University of South Australia, Adelaide, South Australia, Australia

Graciela S. Alarcón, M.D., M.P.H. Division of Clinical Immunology and Rheumatology, Department of Medicine, The University of Alabama at Birmingham, Birmingham, Alabama

Paul A. Bacon, F.R.C.P. Department of Rheumatology, The University of Birmingham, Birmingham, United Kingdom

Howard Bird, M.A., M.D., F.R.C.P. Clinical Pharmacology Unit, University of Leeds, Leeds, United Kingdom

Carol Mary Black, M.D., F.R.C.P. Royal Free Academic Unit of Rheumatology and Connective Tissue Disease, Royal Free Hospital, London, United Kingdom

Maarten Boers, M.D., Ph.D., M.Sc. Department of Internal Medicine and Rheumatology, University Hospital Maastricht, Maastricht, The Netherlands

Ferdinand C. Breedveld, M.D., Ph.D. Department of Rheumatology, Leiden University Hospital, Leiden, The Netherlands

Ken J. Bullpit, M.D. Department of Medicine/Rheumatology, University of California, Los Angeles, School of Medicine, Los Angeles, California

Grant W. Cannon, M.D. Department of Medicine, Veterans Affairs Medical Center, and University of Utah, Salt Lake City, Utah

Hilary A. Capell, M.B., B.C.L., B.A., M.D., F.R.C.P. Centre for Rheumatic Diseases, Royal Infirmary, Glasgow, United Kingdom

Daniel J. Clauw, M.D. Department of Medicine and Orthopedics, Georgetown University Medical Center, Washington, D.C.

Philip J. Clements, M.D. Department of Medicine, University of California, Los Angeles, School of Medicine, Los Angeles, California

Diana Davis, M.B., B.S., M.R.C.P. The Kennedy Institute of Rheumatology, London, United Kingdom

Christopher P. Denton, B.Sc., M.R.C.P. Rheumatology Unit, Royal Free Hospital, London, United Kingdom

B. A. C. Dijkmans, M.D., Ph.D. Rheumatology Department, Free University Hospital, Amsterdam, The Netherlands

Maxime Dougados, M.D. Department of Rheumatology, Hôpital Cochin, Paris, France

John Edmonds, M.B, B.S., F.R.A.C.P. Department of Rheumatology, St. George Hospital, and University of New South Wales, Sydney, New South Wales, Australia

Michael J. Elliott,* M.B., B.S., Ph.D., F.R.A.C.P. Department of Immunology, The Kennedy Institute of Rheumatology, London, United Kingdom

Paul Emery, B.A., M.B., B.Chir., M.R.C.P., M.D., F.R.C.P. Rheumatology and Rehabilitation Research Unit, University of Leeds, Leeds, United Kingdom

Dafna D. Gladman, M.D., F.R.C.P.C. Centre for Prognosis Studies in the Rheumatic Diseases, The University of Toronto, and Toronto Hospital, Toronto, Ontario, Canada

Michael J. Green, M.B. ch B., M.R.C.P. Rheumatology and Rehabilitation Research Unit, University of Leeds, Leeds, United Kingdom

Pierre-André Guerne, M.D., Ph.D. Division of Rheumatology, Department of Medicine, University Hospital of Geneva, Geneva, Switzerland

E. Nigel Harris,[†] M.D. Department of Medicine, University of Louisville, Louisville, Kentucky

Christopher G. Jackson, M.D. Department of Medicine, Division of Rheumatology, School of Medicine, University of Utah, and Veterans Affairs Medical Center, Salt Lake City, Utah

Lawrence Kagen, M.D. Department of Rheumatology, The Hospital for Special Surgery–Cornell University Medical College, New York, New York

C. G. M. Kallenberg, M.D. Department of Clinical Immunology, University Hospital Groningen, Groningen, The Netherlands

Muhammad Asim Khan,[‡] M.D., F.R.C.P., F.A.C.P. Division of Rheumatology, Department of Medicine, Case Western Reserve University, Cleveland, Ohio

John R. Kirwan, B.Sc., M.D., F.R.C.P. Rheumatology Unit, University of Bristol, Bristol, United Kingdom

George D. Kitas, M.D., Ph.D., M.R.C.P. Dudley NHS Trust, and Department of Rheumatology, The University of Birmingham, Birmingham, United Kingdom

Gideon Koren, M.D. Division of Clinical Pharmacology/Toxicology, The University of Toronto, and Mother Risk Program, The Hospital for Sick Children, Toronto, Ontario, Canada

---

Current affiliations:
*ITR Therapeutic Team, SmithKline Beecham Pharmaceuticals, Harlow, United Kingdom.
[†]Office of the Dean, Morehouse School of Medicine, Atlanta, Georgia.
[‡]Department of Medicine/Rheumatology, MetroHealth Medical Center, Cleveland, Ohio.

Keith Lim,* M.B.B.S., M.R.C.P. Rheumatology Unit, University of Bristol, Bristol, United Kingdom

Raashid Luqmani,† D.M., M.R.C.P. Department of Rheumatology, The University of Birmingham, Birmingham, United Kingdom

Ravinder N. Maini, B.A., M.B., B.Chir., F.R.C.P., F.R.C.P. (E) The Kennedy Institute of Rheumatology, London, United Kingdom

Anne McEntegart, B.Sc., M.R.C.P. Centre for Infectious Diseases, Royal Infirmary, Glasgow, United Kingdom

Ann W. Morgan, B.Sc., M.B., Ch.B. (Hon), M.R.C.P. (U.K.) Department of Rheumatology, University of Leeds, Leeds, United Kingdom

Haralampos M. Moutsopoulos, M.D., F.A.C.P., F.R.C.P. Department of Pathophysiology, Medical School, National University of Athens, Athens, Greece

Ann Parke, M.D. Department of Medicine, University of Connecticut Health Center, Farmington, Connecticut

Harold E. Paulus, M.D. Department of Medicine/Rheumatology, University of California, Los Angeles, School of Medicine, Los Angeles, California

Theresa Podrebarac, M.D., F.R.C.P.C. Department of Medicine, University of Ottawa, and Ottawa General Hospital, Ottawa, Ontario, Canada

Anne-Marie Prieur, M.D. Département de Pédiatrie, Rhumatologie Pédiatrique, Hôpital des Enfants-Malades, Paris, France

Michel Revel, M.D. Department of Rehabilitation, Hôpital Cochin, Paris, France

Charles Richardson, M.D. Rheumatology and Rehabilitation Research Unit, University of Leeds, Leeds, United Kingdom

Naomi F. Rothfield, M.D. Division of Rheumatic Diseases, University of Connecticut Health Center, Farmington, Connecticut

David L. Scott, B.Sc., M.D., F.R.C.P. Department of Rheumatology, Kings College Hospital, London, United Kingdom

Robert F. Spiera, M.D. Department of Rheumatology, The Hospital for Special Surgery–Cornell University Medical College, New York, New York

S. ten Wolde, M.D. Department of Rheumatology, Leiden University Hospital, Leiden, The Netherlands

Peter Tugwell, M.D., M.Sc., F.R.C.P.C. Department of Medicine, University of Ottawa, and Ottawa General Hospital, Ottawa, Ontario, Canada

Anke M. van Gestel, M.D. Department of Rheumatology, University Hospital Nijmegen, Nijmegen, The Netherlands

---

Current affiliations:
*Subang Jaya Medical Centre, and University Hospital, Kuala Lumpur, Malaysia
†Department of Rheumatology, Western General Hospital, South Edinburgh, United Kingdom

Piet L. C. M. van Riel, M.D., Ph.D. Department of Rheumatology, University Hospital Nijmegen, Nijmegen, The Netherlands

Panayiotis G. Vlachoyiannopoulos, M.D. Department of Pathophysiology, Medical School, National University of Athens, Athens, Greece

H. James Williams, M.D. Division of Rheumatology, School of Medicine, University of Utah, Salt Lake City, Utah

N. J. Zvaifler, M.D. Department of Rheumatology, University of California, San Diego, La Jolla, California

1

Pathogenic Mechanisms as Targets for Therapy in Rheumatoid Arthritis

N. J. Zvaifler
University of California, San Diego, La Jolla, California

I. INTRODUCTION

Rheumatoid arthritis (RA) is a chronic systemic disorder with its primary manifestations in the joints. The etiology of RA remains obscure, although the pathogenesis is increasingly, becoming well understood. The disease is ubiquitous, occurs in both sexes, favoring women 3:1, and is seen in all parts of the world. Rural populations seem to be less affected with RA than urban dwellers, and the disease may be more severe in developed countries. Variability is not only seen in populations but in individuals. In epidemiological studies, for instance, RA appears to be a mild and often remitting disease, whereas when it is studied in the clinic, it is usually characterized by a relentless, progressive, destructive course. This has led a number of investigators to suggest that RA is not just one disease but rather a common response to a variety of insults. Conversely, patients who have a serological test for an antibody in the blood stream known as rheumatoid factor (RF) and a particular genetic predisposition display all the features of the prototypical disease called RA. These questions cannot be resolved at this time, but in this chapter, RA will be considered a single disease with various phases: (a) those events that initiate the disease (within the first days to weeks after the appearance of clinical symptoms); (b) the chronic inflammatory processes that perpetuate the disease over the ensuing months to years; and (c) and the development of a destructive granulation tissue (pannus) arising from the cells of the intimal lining of the joint that is the major determinant of disability and joint dysfunction. Some emphasis will be given to findings that distinguish RA from other inflammatory forms of synovitis or chronic degenerative joint disease (osteoarthritis, OA). In conclusion, those features of RA that appear to represent targets for therapy will be discussed.

Studies of the synovial membrane in RA suggest that it is a disorder involving immune responses [1,2]. The accumulation of T lymphocytes in the sublining region of the joint, their intimate association with antigen-presenting cells, and the evidence of local immunoglobulin production by B cells and plasma cells support this hypothesis. Simultaneously, the intimal lining of the joint becomes markedly hyperplastic and assumes features of a transformed tissue. The connection between lining hyperplasia and a subintimal immunological reaction is believed to be mediated by factors elaborated by the participating lymphocytes, macrophages, and synovial lining cells (synoviocytes) themselves. Unfortunately, this scheme derives almost exclusively from RA patients with well-established disease, often decades after its inception, and it likely represents the events responsible for the perpetuation of synovitis but may not reflect its initiation.

Joint tissues obtained within a few weeks or months of the onset of RA are limited [3,4]. Grossly, variable amounts of synovial inflammation is observed, and these local macroscopic observations generally correlate with the number and type of infiltrating cells, as determined by conventional histology and immunoperoxidase staining [4]. Unfortunately, the features of vascular proliferation, ingress of mononuclear cells, and increased numbers of synovial lining cells do not distinguish early RA from other forms of acute synovitis or predict the subsequent course of the disease. Based on limited information, the phenotype of the T cells present in the earliest (inductive) phase of RA are similar to those in established disease.

RA usually begins with symptoms of joint pain and swelling, especially in the wrists, second and third metacarpophalangeal joints of the hands, and the fourth and fifth metatarsophalangeal joints of the feet. The knee joint, which is the most accessible source of intra-articular tissues, unfortunately, is not often affected at the beginning of this inflammatory process. Joint inflammation, however, is not unique to RA, and, in fact, studies of early synovitis demonstrate that over time only about 30% of patients will develop typical disease [5]; the remainder develop either another recognizable rheumatic disorder of remit. In this latter group, it may be that the individual has been exposed to an appropriate environmental factor but lacks an appropriate genetic constitution; that is, genes encoding for a specific hypervariable region of the HLA-DR molecule and/or the capacity to make RF. Both are recognized as hallmarks of sustained and severe disease expression. Originally, RF production was considered to be a consequence of the chronic inflammatory process. More recent studies, however, have shown that this autoantibody is in the circulation of patients destined to develop RA on average 5 years before the first clinical disease expression [6]. Even more remarkable is the finding of vascular endothelial abnormalities and lymphocytic infiltration in synovial biopsies from asymptomatic knee joints of patients with established RA [7] or in the noninflamed knee joints of patients with early RA synovitis who have joint involvement elsewhere (N. J. Zvaifler, personal observation). Thus the stage may be set for the development of RA prior to contact with an inciting agent, and it is only the appearance of acute inflammation that calls attention to the joints.

II. GENETIC FACTORS

The strongest evidence in support of an important role for genetic factors comes from an association between RA and certain HLA genes located on the short arm of chromosome 6 in humans. Initially, this was based on reports in Northern Europeans of an association of RA with serologically defined HLA-DR4 specificities (especially, Dw4 and Dw14). Subsequently, there was difficulty explaining the differences in HLA class II association in different populations with different subtypes of HLA-DR4 [8]. For instance, certain native American Indian tribes have a high frequency of RA in the absence of the DR4 haplotype. (They have Dw16—a subtype of DR6.) [9] Similar discrepancies were observed in Japan and in Israeli Jews (DR-1 associated). Conversely, certain DR4 alleles have no association with RA (Dw10, Dw13). These contradictions were reconciled by detailed molecular analysis of the MHC region when it was found that the great majority of affected individuals shared an epitope present in the third allelic hypervariable region (3AHVR) of the HLA-DR β1 chain regardless of the HLA haplotype. This distinctive genetic element is found integrated into a number of alleles, including HLA-DR B1*0401(former Dw4), B1*0404/8 (former Dw14), B1*0101 (former DR1), and B1*1402 (former DRw14/Dw16). The shared amino acid sequence (known as the RA "susceptibility epitope") resides in the α-helical segment of the DR β1 chain between positions 67 and 74 (Fig. 1). This region is a critical binding site for foreign antigens and supports the original notion that specific disease associations likely involve discrete disease-related epitopes immunologically relevant in terms of T-cell recognition. A search of computer-based data banks for peptides analogous to the RA amino acid sequence (QKRAA or QRRAA) have revealed homologies with sequences in bacterial heat shock protein dnaJ [10] and the 110-kD glycoprotein from the capsular antigen of the Epstein-Barr virus [11].

Although it is true that the QKRAA sequence is associated with RA in almost all populations, there is a considerable variation in the strength of the association. In many Europeans, the frequency of the shared epitope approaches 50%, but only 1–2% have the disease. So, clearly, this sequence by itself is insufficient for the development of RA. Furthermore, 15–20% of patients who meet rigid criteria for the diagnosis of RA do not possess this sequence, but usually they have milder forms of RA. An important exception is African-Americans (discussed below).

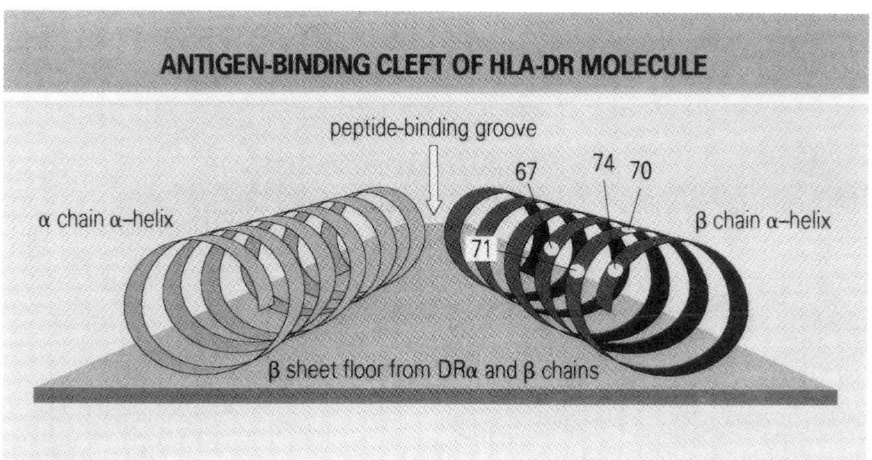

Figure 1 Presumed location of important polymorphic residues within an HLA-DR molecule. Amino acids 67, 70, 71, and 74, the residues noted from sequence comparisons and from site-directed mutagenesis analysis to be critical in the function of DR4, DW14 (*0404) epitope, are shown pointing into or out of the peptide-binding groove as predicted from the three-dimensional structure. The residues pointing into the groove would presumably be important in binding peptide, whereas those pointing out of the α helix would be hypothesized to interact directly with TCR. (From Nepom GT, Nepom B. The major histocompatibility complex. In: Klippel JH, Dieppe PA, eds. Rheumatology. London: Mosby-Year Book Europe, 1994:3:8.5 Fig. 12.9.)

In a susceptibility model, the HLA-DR β1 allele product would be involved in induction of disease, but of late, there has been an increased appreciation of a different role for these genes—namely, their association with persistence and progression of an established pathological immune response. Evidence is accumulating that HLA-DR β1 genes represent severity markers and predict outcome in RA [12]. The development of erosive and seropositive (RF) disease is almost an invariable accompaniment of the disease-associated gene sequences [13]. Patients with extra-articular disease generally carry two disease-linked HLA-DR β1 alleles, whereas those with only moderate disease show one copy of the disease-linked sequence. The proposed hierarchy of allelic HLA-DR β1 combinations in determining severity of rheumatoid arthritis is displayed in Figure 2. As can be seen, homozygous individuals, or those with two alleles, are at the greatest risk for both destructive joint disease and extra-articular manifestations. Patients with Felty's syndrome are almost always homozygous but also show a strong association with a DQ haplotype (DQw7) [8].

A serious reservation concerning the significance of the HLA-DR β1 alleles comes from studies of African-Americans with RA. African-Americans have similar disease severity, frequency and amount of RF, nodules, and radiographic evidence of cartilage and bone erosions as do their white counterparts [14]. Despite this similarity, African-Americans with RA have a low frequency of the rheumatoid epitope, and it is RF positivity, not the presence or the dose of the rheumatoid epitope, that explains disease severity. This suggests that other genes linked to the HLA-DR β1 locus may be more important in either susceptibility to or modulation of RA, and that these are linked to the appropriate alleles in whites but not African-Americans.

Even with the strong evidence of the HLA-DR β1 associations, there is general agreement that RA is genetically homogeneous and its etiology likely to be multifactorial, including both environmental and genetic factors. HLA probably accounts for no more than 30% of the genetic contribution [8]. Other genes of interest are those that code for various immunoglobulin segments, complement components and cytokines, and

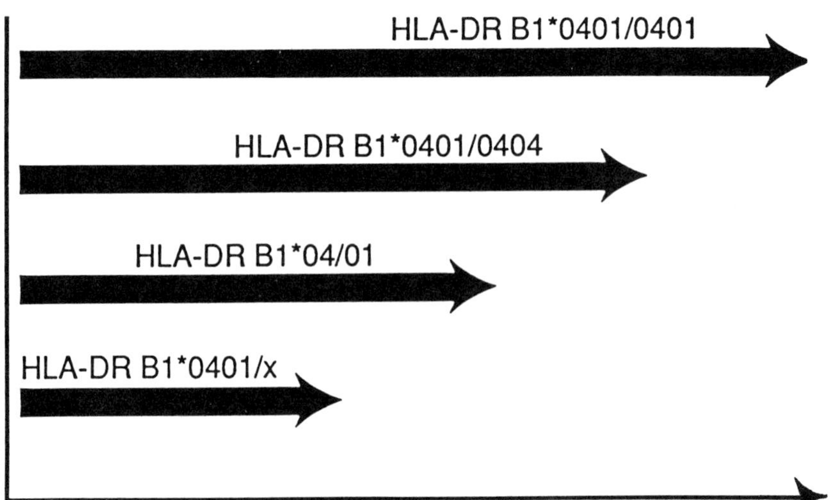

Figure 2 Risk of joint destruction. Risk of extra-articular disease.

both the alpha and beta chains of the T-cell receptor. Because of their involvement in antigen presentation, genes of the HLA-DQ and HLA-DP locus are also candidates for disease susceptibility, but the identification of any genes (other than HLA-DR) intimately involved with RA is lacking.

The essential function of the immune system is the molecular discrimination between self and nonself [15]. This discrimination is the responsibility of T lymphocyte and their ability to detect specific antigen through appropriate cell surface receptors. T cells do not bind to antigens in a native configuration or in soluble form. Rather they recognize antigens as short linear peptides (8–18 amino acids) located within the antigen-binding groove of HLA molecules. Exogenous ("foreign") antigens are internalized by antigen-presenting cells into lysosomal vacuoles where they are hydrolyzed by enzymes and loaded into the binding groove of class II molecules. This complex is transported to the cell surface for recognition by a small population of CD4 lymphocytes bearing discrete T-cell receptors (TCRs) that have been selected to have an affinity for both the antigen and the class II molecules (Fig. 3). For this reason, much work has been done to demonstrate a specific "foreign" RA peptide with affinity for the "shared epitope." The failure to identify an RA arthritogenic peptide does not disprove the model of a specific TCR-MHC–peptide complex, but it has encouraged alternative hypothesis; namely, the role of the disease-associated epitope in RA patients is related to the formation of the TCR repertoire.

The process of education for self-discrimination/nonself-discrimination occurs during T-cell differentiation in the thymus [15]. Early thymocytes, which have rearranged their TCR genes randomly to express either alpha-beta or gamma-delta V regions, encounter an array of self-MHC molecules on the surface of thymic coritcal epithelial cells. The nascent TCR for most thymocytes lacks an appreciable affinity for any available self-MHC molecule, and, in the absence of T-cell activation, these cells undergoes programmed cell death (apoptosis). This initial process of positive selection is followed by the elimination of thymocytes that possess receptors with high affinity for self-MHC plus self-peptide. This negative selections is essential for self-discrimination, since, if such cells were to emigrate to the periphery, they could be the source of an autoimmune attack. In the TCR repertoire hypothesis, the "shared epitope" would be responsible for the elimination of a population of T cells necessary for a protective immune response to an exogenous antigen. Alternatively, the TCR could be molded to have a greater potential for autoreactive responses. It remains to be seen which (if either) of these theories is operative in the pathogenesis of RA.

III. EVENTS IN THE ARTICULAR CAVITY

Except for the pioneering studies of synovial fluids by Ropes and Bauer in the 1930s and 1940s [16], the focus of investigations in RA concentrated on factors present in the blood of patients. Analysis revealed that the substances of interest were globulin molecules and had features of antibodies. Chief among these was a prototypic autoantibody, called RF because of its presence in two-thirds to three-quarters of patients with RA, or antigamma globulin because the responsible immunoglobulins were reacting with the Fc portion of IgG molecules. The initial characterization, based on serological tests, favored the detection of IgM RF, although it was soon established that RF could be found in any of the immunoglobulin subclasses.

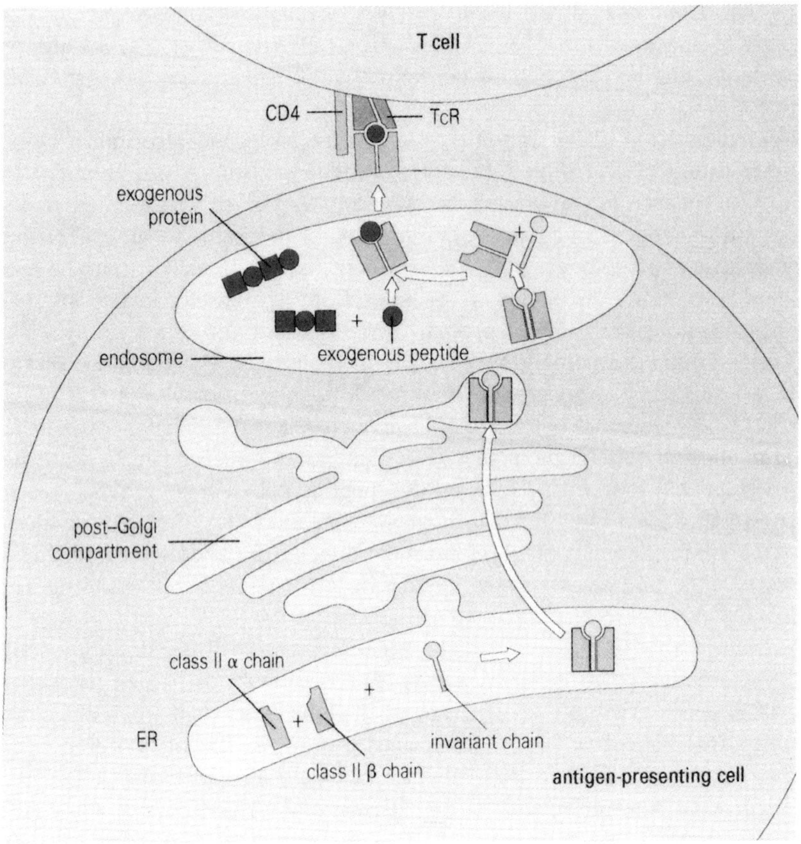

Figure 3 Pathway of HLA class II molecule assembly, antigen processing, and cell surface interactions. Class II α and β chains are assembled in the endoplasmic reticulum (ER) along with the invariant chain, which is thought to interact in such a way that peptide cannot bind to the antigen-binding groove. After transport through the Golgi and post-Golgi compartments, the class II α-β–invariant chain complex moves to an acidic endosome, where the invariant chain is proteolytically cleaved and released from the class II molecule. At this point, exogenously derived peptides which have been brought to the endosome through fusion of phagolysosomes of recycling endosomes may now bind to the class II molecule. This class II molecule–peptide complex then is transported to the cell surface, where it is available to interact with an appropriate T cell. The structure of the class II molecule allows preferential interaction with the CD4 molecule, which facilitates recognition between the class II–peptide complex and an appropriate TcR. (From Nepom GT, Nepom B. The major histocompatibility complex. In: Klippel JH, Dieppe PA, eds. Rheumatology. London: Mosby-Year Book Europe Limited, 1994:3:8.5, Fig. 12.5.)

At the end of the 1950s, attention was redirected to the study of intra-articular events in RA. In a period of less than 5 years, it was shown that (a) the round cells of the rheumatoid synovium produced immunoglobulins and RF; (b) within the membrane were complexes of IgG, IgM, and complement; (c) complement levels in rheumatoid effusions were significantly lower than in comparison serum samples or when compared with synovial fluids from other forms of inflammatory joint disease; and (c) granulocytes from rheumatoid synovial fluids contained intracytoplasmic complexes of immunoglobulins, complement, and anti–gamma globulin. Shortly thereafter, several schemes were proposed to encompass the available information; although differing in emphasis, they were remarkably similar in their conceptualization of the articular inflammatory events in RA [17–19]. The synovial membrane was viewed as an ideal site for an immune response, equipped as it is with a lining layer of phagocytic cells and a vascular stroma adapted for the mobilization and proliferation of lymphocytes. It was proposed that antigens, localized in the articular cavity, stimulate the production of antibody; these combine in the synovial membrane or fluid as immune complexes and activate the complement sequence, thereby generating a variety of biologically active materials, including some with potent chemotactic properties (e.g., C5a, leukotriene B_4, platelet-activating factor, and interleukin-8 [IL-8]). As a consequence, polymorphonuclear leukocytes are drawn into the joint, where they are attracted to and ingest the complexes. During phagocytosis, the neutrophils (and probably also the phagocytic synovial lining cells) release proteinases, prostaglandins, leukotrienes, and reactive oxidants. Any or all of these substances can cause joint inflammation and injury. Simultaneously, there were findings pointing to activation of the kallikrein, coagulation, and fibrinolytic pathways. These too contribute to an intense local inflammatory response.

Support for these ideas solidified in the decade that followed, and thereafter the notion that RA was at least in part an example of an "extravascular immune complex" disease [11] was generally accepted [20]. The nature of the complexes was defined by studies of the synovial tissue B lymphocytes and plasma cells. These were shown to be the source of locally produced immunoglobulins; approximately 50% of which was antibody directed against the Fc portion of IgG (RF). In the blood, the RF tends to occur in all immunoglobulin classes, but the majority is IgM. In contrast, much of the intra-articular RF was of the IgG variety, and its pathogenetic significance was suggested by an ability to form "self-associating complexes" [21]. These IgG–anti-IgG complexes had enhanced complement-fixing activity as compared with IgM RF; the IgG–anti-IgG inclusions could be found in the neutrophils in joint effusions, and their concentration could be correlated with the hypocomplementemia in the inflamed RA synovial fluid [22]. Structural analysis of V gene sequences in the immunoglobulins of RA patients show that almost all of the IgM RF and 50% of IgG derived from B lymphocyte hybridomas or cell lines are encoded in a germline configuration, with very few nucleotide changes. When the same techniques are applied to synovial tissue B lymphocytes, they show nonrandom distribution of replacement mutations in rearranged Ig V genes indicative of an antigen-driven selection of B lymphocytes, and further supporting the notion of local immunological processes in the RA joint [23]. It has also been suggested that the B cells that express RF specificity in the joint can act as antigen-presenting cells. At this site, they could trap and ingest entire immune complexes and present the foreign antigens in the complexes in combination with their own class II molecule to potentially autoreactive T helper cells, thereby avoiding the constraints of immunological tolerance [24].

The significance of RF in the pathogenesis of RA has often been questioned, because it is found in the blood of normal individuals and in many conditions that are not complicated by arthritis. As a "normal" autoantibody, it is likely that RF plays a protective role by identifying circulating immune complexes, binding to them, and enhancing their disposal by phagocytes in the liver and/or spleen. In the articular cavity, these same attributes can be deleterious, because it is an anatomically confined extravascular space with a limited capacity for removing immune reactants. As a result, they languish in the fluid bathing the joint or are taken up by phagocytic cells in the synovial lining [25]. Thus, although RF is not likely to be the cause of RA, it undoubtedly is important for enhancing articular inflammation.

The role of neutrophils in the induction and perpetuation of inflammation is well established, but the events associated with resolution are less understood. At sites of inflammation, senescent neutrophils and their potentially toxic granules are normally recognized by macrophages, engulfed, and transported away before they can lyse and produce tissue injury [26]. Early studies of RA joint effusions showed the presence of small round particles that stained for DNA and which appeared to be derived from dying cells [27]. Subsequently, it was recognized that these morphological features were characteristic of cells undergoing programmed death (or apoptosis) [26].

Any cell can be induced to die by the application of noxious compounds. In acute pathological death, cells tend to swell and lyse. In this process, called necrosis, the cell's contents spill into the extracellular space and elicit inflammation [28,29]. By contrast, apoptosis is a mode of cell death in which single cells are deleted in the midst of living tissues. Apoptosis accounts for the programmed cell death in tissue remodeling and cell loss that accompanies atrophy of adult tissues following withdrawal of endocrine and other growth stimuli. Apoptosis is believed to be responsible for the physiological death of cells in the course of normal tissue turnover (i.e., tissue homeostasis) [30,31]. The morphological changes in apoptosis include plasma membrane blebs, nuclear condensation, and shrinkage in cell volume with a resultant loss of contact with neighboring cells. The nucleus and cytoplasm shrink and often fragment into a series of membrane-bound condensed apoptotic bodies. Following apoptosis, the cells and their nuclear fragments are rapidly phagocytized by their neighbors or by macrophages, thereby protecting them from exposure to the cellular contents.

Examination of the joint aspirates of patients with most forms of inflammatory arthritis show macrophages engulfing intact neutrophils or nuclear particles derived from neutrophils [32]. An exception is RA joint effusions [27]. Recently, this question has been revisited, the original observations confirmed, and the suggestion made that a failure to dispose of apoptotic cells and debris could contribute to chronic inflammation [33]. The defective apoptosis in RA effusions is not absolute, however, because during acute articular inflammation resulting from a local or systemic infection, the disposal of neutrophils by macrophages from the RA joint is easily identified.

Cytokines and their receptors, growth factors, and soluble adhesion molecules have all been measured in synovial fluid and companion serum samples [34–36]. Some are produced in the articular cavity and others appear to have predictive value for progression of RA or response to therapy. Unfortunately, as in most instances with studies of inflammatory synovial effusions, comparisons are primarily made with osteoarthritis joint fluids, not with other—non-RA—chronic inflammatory joint diseases, and their real significance is still a question. However, an appreciation of the cytokine milieu within the RA joint is essential to an understanding of the pathogenesis of RA, and this is discussed below.

IV. HISTOPATHOLOGY OF RHEUMATOID ARTHRITIS

The normal synovium is a delicate structure consisting of an intimal lining and a sublining layer. The former is usually one or two layers deep; the latter comprises occasional small blood vessels, loose stroma, fibroblasts, and fat cells. The lining cells (synoviocytes) can be divided into two populations based on conventional morphology, histochemical staining, and functional capacities. Type A cells (macrophage-like synoviocytes) possess phagocytic vacuoles, macrophages surface markers, surface HLA-DR and Fc receptors, whereas type B cells (fibroblast-like synoviocytes) have features of secretory fibroblasts, including prominent rough endoplasmic reticulum and regular arrays of ribosomes.

Histopathological changes in the RA joint vary considerably. The earliest recorded events include sublining edema and proliferation of blood vessels (Fig. 4a). Fibrin becomes deposited on the surface of the intimal lining facing the joint cavity, and there is a scant interstitial infiltrate with either neutrophils or lymphocytes [37]. Over the ensuing weeks, the intima becomes hyperplastic and the sublining is infiltrated with mononuclear cells and lymphoid aggregates (Fig. 4b). The synoviocytes display high

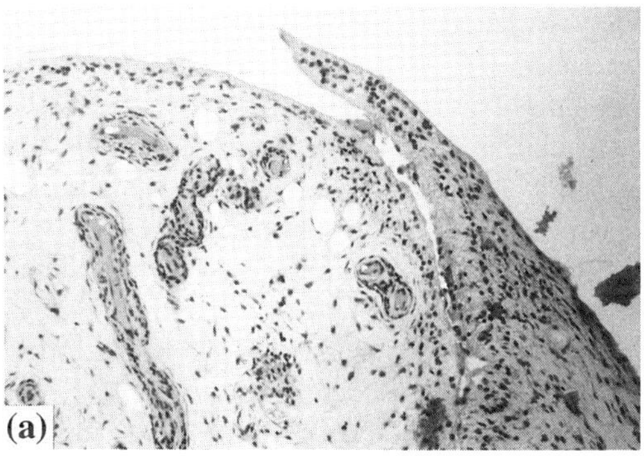

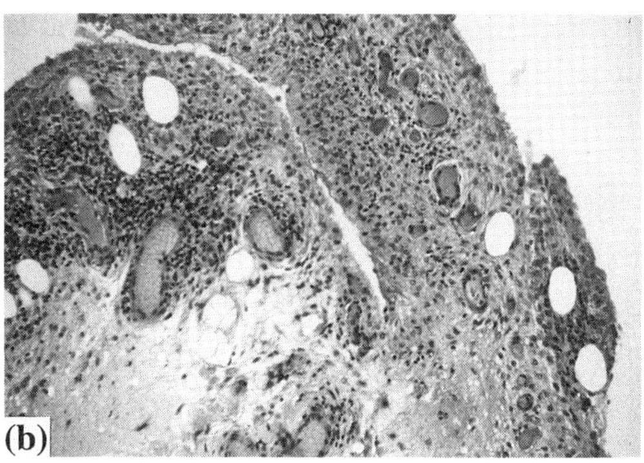

Figure 4 (a) The events in RA during the first days to weeks following initial joint symptoms. A synovial biopsy specimen taken in the third week shows primarily microvascular injury, minimal synovial intimal cell changes, and cellular infiltration. (photomicrograph kindly provided by R. Schumacher.) (b) After several weeks, the inflammation in rheumatoid arthritis resembles an early immune response. A synovial biopsy specimen taken in the third month following in the onset of symptoms shows microvascular injury, early hyperplasia of synovial intimal cells, and collections of mononuclear cells in the subintimal layer, particularly in a perivascular distribution. (Photomicrograph kindly provided by R. Schumacher.) (From Zvaifler NJ. New perspectives on the pathogenesis of rheumatoid arthritis. Am J Med 1988; 85:12–17.)

levels of HLA-DR molecules on their surface (particularly on macrophage-like cells), and large amounts of class II major histocompatibility complex (MHC)mRNA are demonstrable in this region [38]. The lining layer becomes deeper (usually 5–10 cells) as a result of an increase in both type A and B synoviocytes. This many-hundredfold increase in synoviocytes reflects a combination of marked ingress of monocytes/macrophages [39] and a small amount of proliferation in fibroblast-like synoviocytes.

The sublining is often densely infiltrated with lymphocytes. These may be evenly dispersed throughout the tissue or collect into aggregates. T lymphocytes predominate in RA tissue, representing about 40–50% of the total number of synovial cells along with immunoglobulin-producing B cells and plasma cells. Most are $CD4^+$ T helper (TH) cells, with a "memory" phenotype (CD4/29/45RO). The CD4:CD8 ratio ranges from 4:1 to 14:1, unlike synovial fluid where $CD8^+$ T cells equal or outnumber helper cells [40–44]. The CD8 infiltrate in RA tissue is scanty and usually located at the periphery of the lymphoid aggregates. This geography has suggested that within the aggregate, macrophages and/or dendritic cells are presenting antigen to the T helper cells and B cells; and the relative absence of a CD8 population results in an unopposed immunoglobulin production [45].

However, this model is simplistic and not without exceptions. For instance, synovial biopsies from some RA patients show equal numbers of $CD4^+$ and $CD8^+$ T cells in the subintimal region [4,44]. In another study, lymphoid aggregates were identified in only a minority of patients and occasionally the synovium displayed a stromal pattern made up almost exclusively of fibroblasts with only rare T cells. The peripheral blood cells of these RA patients tended to respond briskly to soluble recall antigens (e.g., purified protein derivative [PPD]), whereas blood mononuclear cells from those with intense lymphocytic infiltrates failed to respond [43]. This reciprocal relationship between blood anergy and the degree of inflammatory infiltrate implies a different immunopathogenic mechanism in each subset. Finally, it should be appreciated that even the classic histopathological picture is not unique to RA, for it can be seen in a number of other forms of arthritis, including crystal-induced disease and even osteoarthritis, which are not likely antigen-driven processes.

V. EXPLANATIONS FOR PERSISTENT SYNOVITIS

Three separate (but not mutually exclusive) models have been invoked to explain the histological findings of chronic rheumatoid synovitis (Fig. 5). The first is a classic T-cell–mediated immune response. RA is thought to begin when an "arthrotropic" pathogen enters the joint. No etiological agent has been identified, but it might be a virus or a nonbiodegradable product of bacteria (as in experimental streptococcal cell wall arthritis). Persistence in the synovial tissue would presumably result in a specific T-cell–mediated immune response involving the trimolecular complex of the T-cell receptor, peptide, and the correct class II molecules. Much evidence has been advanced to support this sequence of events [46], and the class II–HLA-DR B1 associations discussed earlier are essential elements in this paradigm. An analogous situation might be the joint lesions of Lyme arthritis, in which spirochetal antigens are likely pathogenic; the histology is similar to RA and persistence of the arthritis is determined by genetic factors [47].

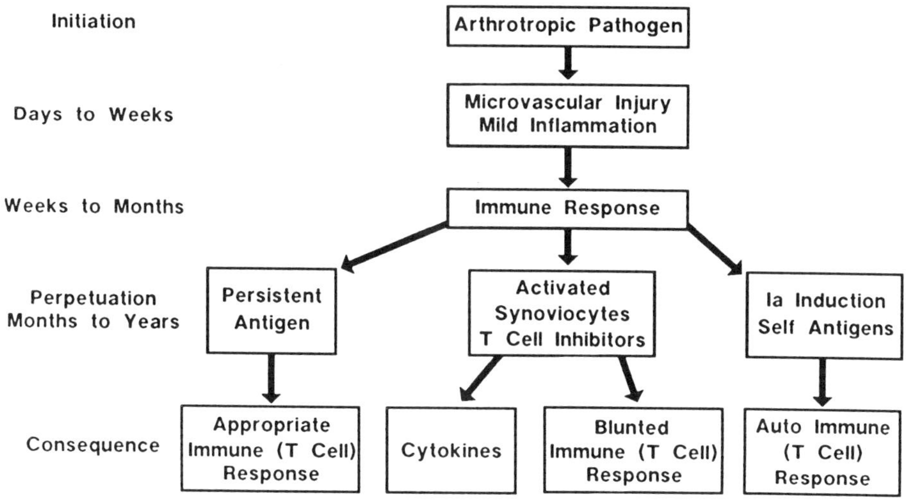

Figure 5 Schematic representation of the several possible pathways involved in the perpetuation of rheumatoid arthritis.

The T cells from RA synovial effusions and subintimal tissues show some evidence of activation, for instance, expression of cell surface markers, such as class II HLA antigens, transferrin receptors, and IL-2 receptors [41,42,48]. Synovial lining cells and interdigitating macrophages also display large amounts of HLA class II molecules. Lymphocytes intimately associated with accessory cells normally produce a variety of lymphokines which, along with macrophage-derived factors, can induce class II antigen expression and promote synoviocyte proliferation and the growth and differentiation of RF-producing B lymphocytes. Additional support for this scenario comes from studies showing that therapies primarily directed at T cells, such as thoracic duct drainage, total nodal irradiation, and cyclosporin A, are modestly effective in RA [46].

Thus, a T-cell–driven specific immune response could explain many of the features of RA, but not all of the data are consistent with this hypothesis. For instance, despite an activation phenotype, most of the lymphocytes in the synovium appear small and quiescent. Little DNA synthesis is demonstrable, and the majority of dividing synovial T cells are $CD8^+$ rather than $CD4^+$ [49]. Also, IL-2 receptor expression, although present, is actually no different than on resting peripheral blood T cells [50]. Even infiltration of the synovium in RA with HLA-DR^+ T cells is nonspecific, since it also occurs in T-cell–independent forms of arthritis (like gout) [51]. More troublesome, however, are two other important facts. The first is the surprising finding that the soluble mediators (i.e., cytokines) produced in the joint are primarily of non–T-cell origin. For instance, important T-cell cytokines, like IL-2 [52], IL-3, IL-4 [53] interferon-γ (IFN-γ) [54], and tumor necrosis factor-α (TNF-α) [52] are barely detectable in synovial fluid or RA tissue. Fewer than 1–2% of lymphocytes in some lymphoid aggregates show IFN-γ [55], whereas in vivo production of these same lymphokines is easily demonstrated in a human T-cell–mediated responses, such as delayed-type hypersensitivity reactions [55] or tuberculous pleuritis [56].

A second factor is the failure consistently to demonstrate restricted T-cell receptor (TCR) V gene usage as would be anticipated in an antigen-driven T-cell response (reviewed in ref. 57). The possible explanations are many; that is, the techniques used to assess TCR abundance, differences in study populations, the point in the disease when tissues are obtained, and the methods for selecting and expanding the cells under study. Early in RA, some restriction of TCR expression in the synovium consistent with a local antigen driven process has been reported [58]. As the disease progresses and the memory T cells enter the inflamed site under the influence of stimuli that are not antigen specific, the TCR repertoire becomes increasingly complex and reflects the make-up of the circulating T cells. Thus, it is likely that the predominance of memory T cells identified in synovial tissue from established RA is not a consequence of in situ expansion of T-cell clones but rather reflects their preferential accumulation and retention [59].

Another limitation is that the majority of TCR gene analyses have concentrated on the beta chain of the TCR, but a few percent of peripheral blood T cells express another TCR. These are gamma/delta T cells, which have membrane CD3 but not the other surface markers associated with functional subsets of alpha/beta T cells, such as CD4 and CD8. In experimental adjuvant arthritis, gamma/delta T cells are expanded in response to mycobacterial antigen, and a similar claim has been made in RA [60–62]. Another analytical problem comes from the increasing appreciation of the several ways that antigens can stimulate T cells. Conventional peptides are presented by MHC molecules to a very small number of T cells that have the appropriate receptor, but there is another class of antigens that stimulate large numbers of T cells and hence are called superantigens [63]. An example is the staphylococcal enterotoxin responsible for the toxic shock syndrome. Superantigens do not require antigen processing, bind avidly to class II molecules, but show only limited HLA-DR restriction, and are recognized by virtually all the T cells that utilize a single or small group of the V-beta gene family of the TCR. Superantigens bridge the antigen-presenting cell and lymphocyte by binding to the external aspect of the beta chain of the class II molecule and the beta chain of the TCR. Up to 10–20% of CD4 and CD8 T cells can be triggered by certain superantigens. In the case of collagen-induced arthritis in the mouse, it has been shown that a mycoplasma superantigen (MAM) can clonally expand autoreactive T cells resulting in an enhancement of triggering of arthritis. Furthermore, in these animals, arthritis that has resolved and been inactive for months will recur following systemic administration of superantigen, perhaps analogous to "flares" of RA thought to be induced by an incidental systemic infection [63]. A superantigen recognized by the V-delta chain of gamma/delta T cells is heat shock protein (HSP) (discussed below). This is of interest because of the reported oligoclonal accumulation of gamma/delta T cells in synovial tissue and the enhanced proliferation of T cells derived from synovial fluid when challenged with HSP. These findings, however, do not explain the known HLA associations with RA.

A. Autoreactive T-Cell Model

Although it is usually assumed that the initiating agent in RA is responsible for both the early changes and the perpetuation of chronic synovitis, this need not be the case. The chronic rheumatoid lesion might be a response to antigens quite distinct from those responsible for starting the process. Such a scenario has been used to explain other chronic inflammatory lesions, like chronic thyroiditis, in which an appropriate response to a presumed viral insult results in the local elaboration of IFN-γ. This cytokine can induce HLA-DR expression on the surface of thyrocytes rendering them targets for immune attack [64]. The reaction between HLA-DR bearing stimulator cells and autologous T lymphocytes is termed the autologous mixed leukocyte reaction (AMLR). Evidence that the synovial lesions in RA represent a localized AMLR is largely circumstantial but of interest [50]. First, the cytokine profile of RA synovitis is similar to an AMLR in that only small amounts of T-cell–derived factors, like IL-2 and IFN-γ, are present [65]. In contrast, allogeneic mixed leukocyte reactions produce high levels of these lymphokines. Also, the cytotoxic T cells present in RA joint effusions are similar to the natural killer (NK)–like cells produced in the AMLR [66]. Finally, the articular cavity and synovium contain an abundance of HLA-DR–rich autologous stimulator cells, including type A synoviocytes, macrophages, and dendritic cells [67].

Autologous stimulation need not be limited to self–HLA-DR molecules. According to theories of molecular mimicry, a foreign antigen can closely resemble a self-antigen and innocent bystanders become targets. This is one of the proposed mechanisms implicating the Epstein-Barr virus (EBV) in the pathogenesis of RA. B lymphocytes are their primary target. Once infected, the B cells carry the EBV viral genome for life. Normal B cells that have been superinfected in vitro spontaneously proliferate and secrete immunoglobulins (including RFs) [68]. In addition, rheumatoid patients are defective in controlling in vitro EBV infection; in part due to deficient IFN-γ secretion by RA T cells [69] and a monocyte-derived IL-1 inhibitor [70]. As noted earlier, there is a homology between the EBV glycoprotein gp110 and the amino acid sequence in the third allelic hypervariable region (3AHVR) of the HLA-DR β1 chain. It has been proposed that immune recognition of the antigens of a pathogen like EBV (or heat shock proteins of gram-negative bacteria) induces a high-affinity cross reaction to the 3AHVR, which would normally be tolerated [11]. Hence, immunity directed against the gp110 of EBV could inadvertently damage normal cells in hosts that express these surface MHC molecules. In the joint, high levels of class II molecules are sustained on a number of cell types, which could explain the perpetuation of synovitis. In a sense, EBV might initiate an AMLR-like reaction in genetically susceptible individuals, with HLA-DR β1 as the target.

Self-molecules, other than HLA-DR, have been proposed as targets for immune attack in arthritis. For instance, type II collagen can cause arthritis in susceptible animals and might contribute to chronic RA, probably as a perpetuating rather than an etiological stimulus. Autoantibodies to proteoglycan, a macromolecule with a protein backbone and large glycosaminoglycan side chains, develop in the course of immune synovitis in rabbits, and the affected joint shows a loss of cartilage proteoglycan. The relevance of this model to human disease is not yet defined, but, as with type II collagen, if immunity to proteoglycan does contribute to cartilage damage, it is likely a secondary phenomenon.

In experimental forms of arthritis (such as adjuvant arthritis), mycobacteria cause chronic inflammatory joint lesions and they have long been implicated in the pathogenesis of RA. Evidence that mycobacteria could provide an important cross-reactive autoantigen comes from the recent recognition that an immunodominant antigen of the mycobacterium is a 65-kD protein with sequence homology to an intracellular stress protein present in all eukaryotic cells [71]. A massive increase in stress proteins was first demonstrated after cells were exposed to heat. Thus, HSPs and stress proteins are interchangeable terms. Because of the ubiquitous nature of these highly conserved proteins, the immune system is likely tolerant to them. Repeated presentation of cross-reactive bacterial HSPs or surface expression of similar proteins on T cells or macrophages might result in loss of tolerance and an autoimmune reaction. Several observations can be cited in support of this hypothesis: RA synovial fluid T cells, which do not proliferate when exposed to certain *Salmonella-Shigella* or *Ureaplasma* organisms, show an augmented reactivity to an acetone-precipitable fraction of *Mycobacterium tuberculosis*. These same fractions of *Mycobacterium* contain antigens that cross react with antibodies to cartilage proteoglycan [60,61]. Mycobacteria have been directly implicated in pathogenesis of adjuvant arthritis, and T-cell clones from affected animals proliferate in the presence of a 65-kD HSP [60]. T-cell clones derived from RA synovial effusions recognize an epitope present in amino acids 1–15 of the HSP-65 molecule [72]. As previously noted, the QKRAA epitope on the HLA-DR4 β1 chain has complete homology with a sequence in an *Escherichia coli* stress protein [10] and could serve as an autoantigen in a manner similar to the EBV molecular mimicry [73]. In both these models (EBV and HSP), the HLA associations would more likely be involved in the progression of RA rather than as a susceptibility or initiating factor. This is consistent with the concept of DR β1 alleles as markers for severity of RA [12,13].

B. Paracrine/Autocrine Model

In the two previous models, T lymphocytes are assigned the major role for the perpetuation of rheumatoid synovitis. Products of these cells theoretically diffuse through the tissues, altering postcapillary venules, inducing the proliferation and differentiation of B cells, and directly influencing macrophages and synoviocytes in the joint lining. Unfortunately, as noted above, this picture is not consistent with much of the data about T-cell activation in the joint.

In contrast to the lymphocytes, synovial macrophage-like and fibroblast-like cells appear highly activated based on their morphology, surface HLA-DR expression, and elaboration of cytokines. Table 1 shows a comparison of cytokine production by various synovial cells. Products of these cells, like IL-1 [74–77], TNF-α [78], IL-6 [79,80], granulocyte-macrophage colony-stimulating factor (GM-CSF) 81, macrophage colony-stimulating factor (M-CSF) (CSF-1) [52], prostaglandins, and collagenase are abundant in synovial fluids and synovial tissues. Recent studies using in situ hybridization to quantify cytokine production at the level of gene expression confirm experiments that detected high levels of secreted cytokines in culture supernatants of synovial tissue cells and in synovial effusions [82]. For instance, IL-1β and TNF-α genes are expressed by large numbers of synovial macrophages. IL-6 probes also hybridized to a high percentage of RA synoviocytes. Although T cells can produce IL-6 under some circumstances, in situ hybridization experiments show most of the IL-6 gene expression in the nonmacrophage, non–T-cell population, and that these cells are located mainly in the intimal lining of the joint. GM-CSF and transforming growth factor (TGF-β) gene expression was observed in a lesser number of cells. As predicted from earlier studies on synovial IFN-γ production [54], the IFN-γ probe did not bind to synovial tissue cells. Interestingly, the failure to detect cytokine mRNA (including IL-1, TNF-α, and IL-6) in mononuclear cells isolated from synovial fluid indicates that the synovium is the source of most articular cytokines.

The cytokine profile of the rheumatoid synovium suggests that chronic articular inflammation is sustained by factors produced by neighboring macrophages and syn-

Table 1 T-Cell and Macrophage/Fibroblast Cytokine Production. Comparison of Cytokines Produced by T Cells and Macrophages/Fibroblasts in the Rheumatoid Arthritis Synovium

Cellular Sources of Synovial Cytokines in Rheumatoid Arthritis	
Cytokines	Detected in RA synovium/synovial fluid[a]
Products of T cells	
IL-2	–
IL-3	–
IL-4	–
IL-6	±
IFN-γ	–
TNF-α	–
TNF-β	–
GM-CSF	–
Products of macrophages/type A synoviocytes	
IL-1	+++
IL-6	+
IL-8	+++
TNF-α	++
M-CSF (CSF-1)	+
IFN-α	±
GM-CSF	+
TGF-β	++
MCP-1	++
Products of fibroblasts/type B synoviocytes	
IL-6	+++
GM-CSF	+
MCP-1	+

[a]Dash indicates negligible or no detection. MCP-1, monocyte chemoattractant protein-1.
Source: Firestein GS. Rheumatoid synovitis and pannus. In: Klippel JH, Dieppe P, eds. Rheumatology. London: Mosby-Year Book, Europe, 1994:1–30.

ovial fibroblasts in a paracrine or autocrine model [59]. This concept of a non–T-cell–driven pathogenesis of synovitis has support in some animal models. For instance, SCID mice lack an immune system, but when infected with *Borrelia* (the agent causing Lyme disease), they develop a severe destructive arthritis that is much worse than seen in normal mouse strains infected with the same organism [83]. Likewise, when RA synovial tissues and normal human cartilage are transplanted into SCID mice, the resident synovial T cells die, but the residual lining cells destroy the articular cartilage [84].

Many factors already identified in the joint could explain lining cell hyperplasia, class II display, and synovial angiogenesis. Figure 6 shows a simplified scheme of the complex cytokine circuits that could exist between synovial cells. For instance, IL-1 and TNF-α (synovial macrophage products) stimulate fibroblast-like synoviocytes pro-

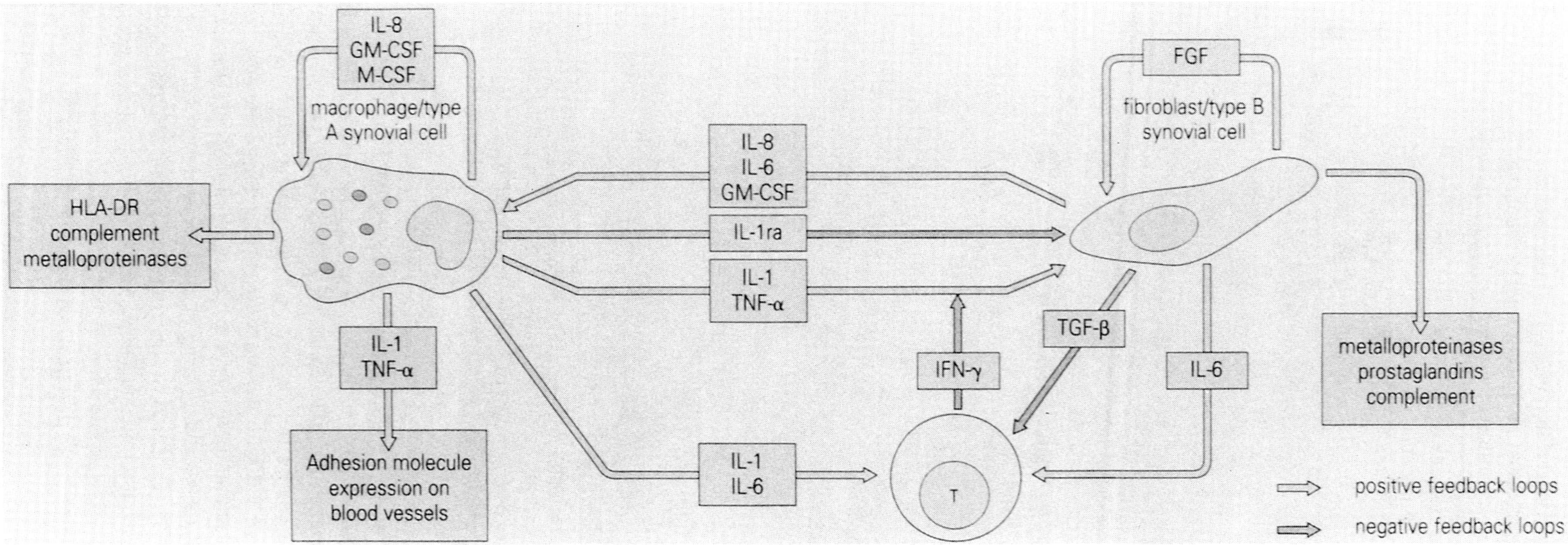

Figure 6 Cytokine networks. Simplified version of the complex cytokine network in rheumatoid arthritis involving macrophages and fibroblasts. The precise T-cell cytokines that might participate are not clear because they are difficult to detect. (From Firestein GS. Rheumatoid synovitis and pannus. In: Klippel JH, Dieppe P, eds. Rheumatology. London: Mosby-Year Book, Europe, 1994:1–30.)

liferation and increase secretion of IL-6, GM-CSF, and collagenase [85,86]. GM-CSF, produced by synovial macrophages, can stimulate fibroblast-like synoviocytes [87] and is a potent inducer of IL-1 secretion and increases DR expression on macrophages [88,89]. TNF-α can synergize with GM-CSF and probably also contributes to macrophage HLA-DR expression [88]. The local production of cytokines by macrophages and fibroblasts could also impact on T cells and contribute to the limited amount of T-cell activation observed. B-cell activation and RF production might result through T-cell–independent mechanisms or as yet undefined cell products.

A prediction of this alternative (paracrine) model is that T cells are not necessarily sequestered in the joint in response to a specific antigen; rather they accumulate under the influence of factors made by synoviocytes [59]. The RA synovium has an over-representation of mature memory helper cells (CD4/29/45RO), whereas naive CD45RA-bearing cells (the suppressor inducer subset) are conspicuously absent [49]. This could be explained by the fact that the movement of lymphocytes from the circulation into the joint is not a random process. Their sites of egress are the postcapillary venules; notably through those with high endothelium (HEV). Transendothelial migration is tightly regulated and involves specific molecules on the surface of the circulating cells and counterreceptors (ligands) for these molecules on the endothelium [90,91]. Three distinct steps account for T-cell adhesion to endothelium. The process begins at sites where narrowing of the vascular bed leads to a diminished flow. Instead of rapidly moving down the center of the blood stream, lymphocytes marginate and begin to roll along the vessel wall. This allows for a loose tethering of lymphocytes to the vascular endothelial cells. The molecules that mediate tethering are members of the family of lectin-binding proteins, called selectins. During its brief roll along the vascular endothelial surface (often less than a few seconds), a lymphocyte must decide whether or not to bind tightly at that site and migrate into tissue. This decision is strongly influenced by factors produced by the vascular endothelium at sites of inflammation or injury, such as cytokines (particularly IFN-γ, IL-1, and TNF-α), platelet-activating factor (PAF), and chemokines. These factors deliver a triggering signal that upregulates the amount or binding avidity of molecules normally present on the surface of the lymphocytes and their counterreceptors on the vascular endothelium. The relevant lymphocyte molecules are members of two integrin families, the alpha 1/beta 2 integrin (LFA-1 or CD11a) and the alpha 4/beta 1 integrin (VLA-4). Engagement by their opposite member on the vascular endothelium (intracellular adhesion molecule [ICAM-1] and vascular cell adhesion molecule [VCAM-1], respectively) results in a dramatic change. Loose tethering becomes a strong adhesion to the endothelium; the lymphocyte spreads and then migrates through the endothelium into the surrounding connective tissues, where additional integrin-matrix interactions occur. Although inflammation is critical to this process, it is noteworthy that, neither antigen nor the T-cell receptor plays any role in tissue localization.

Circulating memory-type lymphocytes express significantly greater amounts of LFA-1 and CD2 (the counterreceptors for ICAM-1 and LFA-3 present on postcapillary venules) than naive lymphocytes [92]. Thus, the preferential accumulation of T cells with a mature phenotype in the inflamed synovium is not surprising. The CD45RO cells also express greater amounts of VLA-4, whose ligands are VCAM-1 and the alternatively spliced form of fibronectin (CS-1), both of which are abundant in the synovial lining and in the endothelium of RA synovial blood vessels [93–95]. Although mature T cells are easily identified in subintimal sites, this information forms the basis for the idea that, they are probably the result—not the cause—of RA synovial inflammation. Currently, there is no knowledge of the fate of memory lymphocytes once they enter into the tissues; whether they are just in transit or retained for long periods of time needs to be defined.

C. Pannus and Joint Destruction

Both joint inflammation and destruction are hallmarks of RA, and one of the major destructive elements is a tissue called pannus. However, a definition of what constitutes pannus, is not unanimous. Some equate pannus with the entire chronically inflamed RA synovium, whereas others consider it a specialized vascular connective tissue at or near the bone/synovium interface. Regardless, synovial lining cells are usually assigned the responsibility for articular bone and cartilage destruction. This paradigm is supported by immunohistochemical analysis and in situ hybridization of biopsy specimens that demonstrate matrix metalloproteinase (MMP) expression as well as the capacities of cultures synoviocytes to respond in vitro to a variety of cytokines and growth factors with the production of MMPs, prostaglandins, growth factors, and cytokines [96–99]. Little is known about when pannus first appears or its initial location, but in established disease, the pannus is usually viewed as an extension of synoviocytes from the joint lining expanding under the influence of an immunologically mediated process. In traditional paradigms of rheumatoid arthritis, T-cell–driven inflammation begets pannus and, hence, articular destruction, but a contrary opinion, namely, that synoviocyte proliferation, pannus formation, and inflammation is an autonomous process independent of T-cell–derived factors, has not been excluded (Fig. 7).

As noted above, the lining of the inflamed joint increases in depth and cell numbers, primarily by accumulation of type A synoviocytes [100]. Concomitantly under the influence of locally produced cytokines and growth factors, otherwise quiescent mesenchymal-derived fibroblasts (type B synoviocytes) change into aggressive, proliferating, invasive cells that express oncogenes, secrete metalloproteinases, and display other features of a "transformed" phenotype (reviewed in refs. 97 and 101). Subsequently, this tumor-like tissue is thought to escape normal constraints and activated synoviocytes,

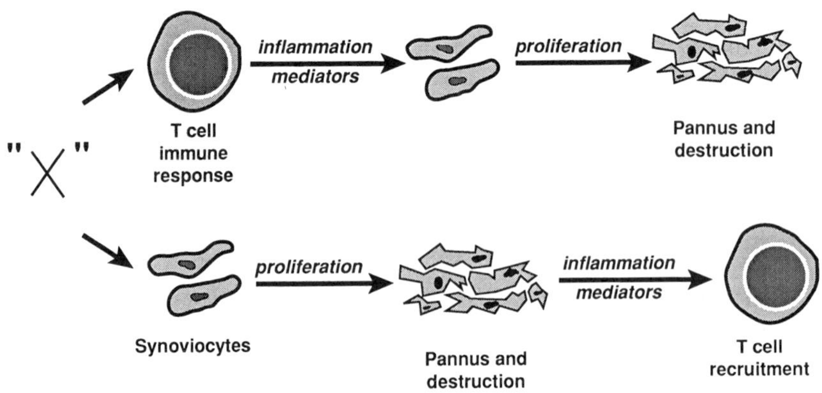

Figure 7 Two alternative pathways by which the unknown inciting factor (X) could induce joint destruction. X can initiate and perpetuate rheumatoid arthritis either by T-cell–dependent or synoviocyte-dependent pathways. (From Ref. 113.)

blood vessels, and mononuclear cells become the pannus that erodes adjacent cartilage and bone.

To understand this process better, in vitro studies have been performed on enzymatically dispersed synovium obtained at joint replacement surgery or synovectomy from RA and osteoarthritis (OA) patients. In primary cultures, especially from RA tissues, lymphocytes, and macrophages comprise approximately 40 and 20% respectively, of the isolated populations, but over time they diminish in number [102]. After three or more passages, the cells that remain are almost exclusively type B fibroblast-like synoviocytes (FLSs). Studies of these FLSs form the basis of numerous publications on synoviocyte proliferation, proteinase production, and HLA-DR expression with exposure to cytokines and growth factors [1,97–99,101,103,104]. In fact, cultured FLSs are often considered in vitro surrogates for pannus. However, since it is likely that the type of isolation techniques and culture condition favor FLS growth, it is possible that cells more relevant to the understanding of pannus might be overlooked.

Information about cartilage destruction comes from detailed morphological studies of the cartilage-pannus junction in well established RA [105–108]. However, the earliest events, are obscure; especially the source of the cells responsible for the initiation of pannus. Normally, in the knee, and perhaps in other joints, an avascular tongue of fibroblast-like cells extends from the synovium onto the cartilage surface. This extension is sometimes referred to as the marginal transitional zone [108]. The initial damage to the rheumatoid cartilage, even before there is ingrowth of blood vessels, occurs when cells of unknown origin arise from the perichondial synovial membrane at the joint margin and dissect under the layer of fibroblast-like cells [106]. Immediately below the invading cells, the matrix of the cartilage is depleted of proteoglycans, and there is a paucity of chondrocytes with many enlarged empty lacunae [107]. Collagenases and other MMPs can be localized in the invasive front [109,110]. Only later do blood vessels proliferate, and the pannus becomes a granulation tissue with a variety of cell types, including monocytes, mast cells, and occasional neutrophils and lymphocytes. Still later a benign-appearing mantle of fibroblast-like cells forms between the cartilage and the overlying synovium [111,112]. At this point, the process appears inactive.

A similar view of pannus formation also divides the process into sequential stages, but emphasize the role of a primitive mesenchymal cell distinct from conventional synoviocytes [107]. The initial invasion of cartilage matrix and subchondral bone occurs at the site of synovial attachment and is mediated by clusters of homogeneous, immature, polyhedral cells with large folded nuclei. This process, which prepares the cartilage for subsequent events, has no associated neovascularization and the responsible cells appear to have a limited life span [107]. Only after the attrition of these primitive cells is there cartilage invasion by a more heterogeneous mixture of fibroblast-like cells, macrophages, and blood vessels. Transition to a permanent fibrous pannus occurs as the fibroblasts become spindle shaped and newly synthesize collagen fibers are deposited.

In the classic model of RA joint destruction, the stimulus to hyperplasia and overgrowth of synoviocytes comes from factors (lymphokines) made by activated lymphocytes. As detailed above, a primary role for T cells, although intellectually appealing, is not proven. An alternative proposal is that the cells responsible for cartilage damage are operating in an autonomous (or semiautonomous) manner under the influence of factors made by the invading cells themselves [113].

One view of joint destruction is based on a malignancy model where synovial lining cells are "transformed" by a proliferation signal that induces them to express oncogenes and their protein products [97,114,115]. This signal could be provided by either a soluble molecule, such as a cytokine or growth factor, or an etiological agent. Thereafter, the cells are induced to grow, produce matrix-degrading enzymes, and alter their display of surface adhesion molecules (integrins), which facilitates migration onto and into solid tissues [116,117]. In this scenario, cartilage and bone are, in effect, innocent bystanders. An alternative scenario makes cartilage the responsible party by facilitating or seducing synoviocytes to leave their normal confines, adhere, and invade. Immune complexes embedded in the cartilage matrix are the historical choice [118], but factors made by chondrocytes or changes in the constituents of the extracellular matrix are other candidates.

Regardless of which view is correct, it is true that fibroblast growth, proliferation, migration, adherence to extracellular matrix, and ability to synthesize extracellular matrix glycoproteins are all under the control of cytokines and growth factors present in abundance in synovial tissues and fluids [97,119]. Type A (monocyte-derived) synoviocytes are in intimate association with fibroblast-like synoviocytes, and the former elaborates a multiplicity of factors that can stimulate the latter; the converse is equally true [103,104]. Under some in vitro conditions, RA synovial fibroblasts constitutively produce cytokines, which is not seen with control synoviocytes derived from osteoarthritis samples [120]. An apparent requirement for prolonged cytokine production by unfractionated RA synovial cells is the presence of other cell types (monocytes and T cells) in the cultures [121]. Presumably, similar cellular cross-talk goes on within an inflammatory environment. As suggested elsewhere [113], these resonating paracrine and autocrine interactions are likely important in the perpetuation of articular tissue destruction and joint inflammation, but it is not clear how they would relate to the initiation of the pannus unless RA synoviocytes have a distinctive susceptibility to a critical soluble factor.

Programmed cell death (apoptosis) is believed to be responsible for the physiological death of cells in the course of normal tissue turnover (i.e., tissue homeostasis) [28]. The relevance of apoptosis to RA is readily apparent when one considers the massive expansion of the synovial lining in the disease. The accumulation of cells in any tissue can be expressed by the following formula: cell number = (cell ingress − cell egress) + (cell proliferation − cell death). Hence, there are two major components to synovial lining expansion. The first, cell trafficking, can account for a significant cellular accumulation if recruitment exceeds the rate that the cells leave the articular cavity. This is likely the case for the macrophage-like synoviocytes (type A) that come to the joint from the bone marrow, terminally differentiate there, and do not proliferate. The increased number of FLSs might reflect excess cell division, although there is not agreement on this subject. In contrast to the synovial T cells, FLSs express a number of protooncogenes which are usually regarded as markers of recent cell activation [114,115,122]. A few cells with morphological features of FLSs stain with antibodies to proliferating cell nuclear antigen (PCNA)–cyclin and nucleolar organizer region. This is taken as evidence that these cells have exited from G0 and are proliferating [123]. The proliferating cells also show evidence of either type I procollagen immunoreactivity or mRNA for collagen but do not display macrophage markers [122–124]. In contrast, thymidine incorporation, evidence of mitosis, or other measures of proliferation are rarely found in synoviocytes [100,124]. Regardless, the fact remains that FLS cell numbers are markedly increased, and, if even a very small percentage were proliferating (<5%), over long periods of time, they would accumulate unless normal mechanisms for disposal were defective.

To date studies of apoptosis in the RA synovium have been limited [125,126]. Conspicuous DNA strand breaks, the hallmark of impending cell death, are present mainly in lining cells (both macrophages and FLSs), but very few cells with the classic morphology of apoptosis can be demonstrated by electronmicroscopy. This may reflect the rapid removal of apoptotic cells seen in normal tissue. Alternatively, some condition in the inflamed joint, either the cytokine environment or hypoxia—reperfusion injury, which are normally strong inducers of programmed cell death, interfere with the apoptotic mechanism, resulting in failure to offset tissue expansion. If this is shown to be the case, then yet another, presumably nonimmunological, process would become an important therapeutic target in RA.

VI. CONCLUSION

This chapter has been designed to familiarize the reader with two separate (but highly integrated) aspects of the pathogenesis of RA. An appreciation of each one is necessary for understanding existing therapeutic strategies or those that are contemplated. The first consideration is the recognition that multiple cells and their products are participating. Lymphocytes—both T cells and B cells—monocytes/macrophages, synoviocytes, vascular endothelial cells, and perhaps polymorphonuclear leukocytes are each potentially important therapeutic targets. For example, using the T cell, current strategies include wholesale elimination of T cells with drugs or monoclonal antibodies; removal or downregulation of "activated" T cells (anti–IL-2 receptor antibody); or elimination of T-cell subsets with anti-CD4 antibody. Future treatments will be aimed at blocking activation of pathogenic T-cell clones through recognition and/or interference with disease-specific MHC alleles, TCR ideotypes, or the entire MHC-peptide-TCR complex. Likewise, the induction of anergy in disease-specific T-cell clones or a switch of the T cells from TH1 to TH2 phenotypes are all plausible strategies. Biochemical manipulations that eliminate or deviate ligand-receptor interactions, intracellular signaling, or gene transcription are all under active investigation. Finally, the cytokines that eventuate from T-cell activation can be neutralized directly or interfered with by occupying cytokine receptors on other cells. Similar approaches have been proposed or are available for the other cellular participants in RA synovitis; for example, anti–IL-1 receptor antagonists and anti-TNF monoclonal antibodies for macrophages or inhibitors of metalloproteinases made by fibroblast-like synoviocytes.

Progress in understanding angiogenesis, vascular permeability, and cellular migration through inflamed blood vessels should lead to important new treatments for RA, because these are fundamental synovial changes in this disease. Strategies that keep circulating cells from gaining access to the joint are attractive. An analogy with warfare is appropriate. It makes little sense to fight the battle in the trenches if it is possible to eliminate reinforcements. Thus, attempts to modify the expression of adhesion molecules on vascular endothelium or interference with their counterreceptors on circulating cells are areas of intense investigation.

The second theme that has been stressed in this chapter is the possibility—indeed the likelihood—that the pathogenetic mechanisms operative at different stages of the disease are distinctive even though the participating cells are the same. Thus the choice of anti-inflammatory therapies, which might be useful early in RA, may not prevent pannus formation or joint destruction at a later stage. Treatments tailored to the events that initiated the disease, or perpetuate it, or eventuate in joint destruction will require an appreciation of those unique aspects of the pathogenesis that are operating over time. Finally, it goes without saying, that should a single etiological agent be found to be responsible for RA, then, hopefully, the disease can be prevented or eradicated so that none of this information becomes critical.

REFERENCES

1. Harris ED Jr. Rheumatoid arthritis. Pathophysiology and implications for therapy. N Engl J Med 1990; 322:1277–1289.
2. Firestein GS. Rheumatoid synovitis and pannus. In: Klippel JH, Dieppe P, eds. Rheumatology. London: Mosby-Year Book, Europe, 1994:1–30.
3. Kulka JP, Bocking D, Ropes MW, Bauer W. Early joint lesions of rheumatoid arthriits. Report of 8 cases with knee biopsies of lesions of less than one year's duration. Arch Pathol 1955; 59:129–139.
4. Lindblad S, Klareskog L, Hedfors E, Forsum U, Sundstrom C. Phenotypic characterization of synovial tissue cells in situ in different types of synovitis. Arthritis Rheum 1983; 26:1321–1332.
5. Devlin J, Gough A, Huissoon A, Jubb R, Emery P. Knee disease in 766 early arthritis patients; relevance to outcome and pathogenesis. Br J Rheumatol 1993; 32(Suppl) Rheumatology's Heberden Round: Abstract #6.
6. Aho K, Heliovaara M, Maatela J, Tuomi T, Palosuo T. Rheumatoid factors antedating clinical rheumatoid arthritis. J Rheumatol 1991; 18:1282–1284.
7. Soden M, Rooney M, Cullen A, Whelan A, Feighery C, Bresnihan B. Immunohistologic features in the synovium obtained from clinical uninvolved knee joints of patients with rheumatoid arthritis. Br J Rheumatol 1989; 28:287–292.
8. Wordsworth BP, Bell JI. The immunogenetics of rheumatoid arthritis. Springer Semin Immunopathol 1992; 14:59–78.
9. Willkens RF, Nepom GT, Marks CR, Nettles JW, Nepom BS. Association of HLA-Dw16 with rheumatoid arthritis in Yakima Indians. Further evidence for the "shared epitope" hypothesis. Arthritis Rheum 1991; 34:43–47.
10. Albani S, Tuckwell JE, Esparza L, Carson DA, Roudier J. The susceptibility sequence to rheumatoid arthritis is a cross-reactive B cell epitope shared by the Escherichia coli heat shock protein dnaJ and the histocompatibility leukocyte antigen DRB1 0401 molecule. J Clin Invest 1992; 89:327–331.
11. Roudier J, Petersen J, Rhodes GH, Luka J, Carson DA. Susceptibility to rheumatoid arthritis maps to a T-cell epitope shared by the HLA-Dw4 DR beta-1 chain and the Epstein-Barr virus glycoprotein gp110. Proc Natl Acad Sci USA 1989; 86:5104–5108.
12. Salmon M. The immunogenetic component of susceptibility to rheumatoid arthritis. Curr Opin Rheumatol 1992; 4:342–347.
13. Weyand CM, Goronzy JJ. HLA-DRB1 alleles as severity markers in RA. Bull Rheum Dis 1994; 43:5–8.
14. McDaniel DO, Alarcon GS, Pratt PW, Reveille JD. Most African-Americans with rheumatoid arthritis do not have the rheumatoid antigenic determinant (epitope). Ann Intern Med 1995; 123:181–187.
15. Rich RR. Human immune response. In: Stein JH, ed. Internal Medicine. 4th ed. St. Louis: Mosby, 1994:2290–2299.

16. Ropes M, Bauer W. Synovial Fluid in Joint Diseases. Boston: Harvard University Press, 1953.
17. Hollander JL, McCarthy DJ, Asorga G, et al. Studies on the immunopathogenesis of rheumatoid joint inflammation: I. The "RA cell" and a working hypothesis. Ann Intern Med 1965; 62:271–280.
18. Ziff M. Heberden Oration: Some immunologic aspects of the connective tissue diseases (1964). Ann Rheum Dis 1995; 24:103–115.
19. Zvaifler NJ. A speculation on the pathogenesis of joint inflammation in rheumatoid arthritis. Arthritis Rheum 1965; 8:289–293.
20. Zvaifler NJ. Rheumatoid synovitis. An extravascular immune complex disease. Arthritis Rheum 1974; 17:297–305.
21. Pope RM, Teller DC, Mannik M. The molecular basis of self-association of antibodies to IgG (rheumatoid factors) in rheumatoid arthritis. Proc Natl Acad Sci USA 1974; 71:517–521.
22. Winchester RJ, Agnello V, Kunkel HG. Gamma globulin complexes of synovial fluids of patients with rheumatoid arthritis. Partial characterization and relationship to lowered complement levels. Clin Exp Immunol 1970; 6:689–706.
23. Mageed RA, Vencovsky J, Maini RN. Rheumatoid factors and germ line genes in rheumatoid arthritis: evidence of an intrinsic B lymphocyte defect. Br J Rheumatol 1994; 33:105–107.
24. Carson DA, Chen PP, Kipps TJ. New roles for rheumatoid factor. J Clin Invest 1991; 87:379–383.
25. Sliwinski AJ, Zvaifler NJ. Removal of aggregated and nonaggregated autologous gamma globulin from rheumatoid joints. Arthritis Rheum 1969; 12:504–514.
26. Savill JI, Wyllie AH, Henson JE, Walport MJ, Henson PM, Haslett C. Macrophage phagocytosis of aging neutrophils in inflammation. Programmed cell death in the neutrophil leads to its recognition by macrophages. J Clin Invest 1989; 83:865–875.
27. Malinin TI, Pekin TJ, Zvaifler NJ. Cytology of synovial fluid in rheumatoid arthritis. Am J Clin Pathol 1967; 47:203–208.
28. Wyllie AH, Kerr JF, Currie AR. Cell death: the significance of apoptosis. Int Rev Cytol 1980; 68:251–306.
29. Kerr JF, Wyllie AH, Currie AR. Apoptosis: a basic biological phenomenon with wide-ranging implications in tissue kinetics. Br J Cancer 1972; 26:239–257.
30. Wyllie AH. Apoptosis (the 1992 Frank Rose Memorial Lecture). Br J Cancer 1993; 67:205–208.
31. Vaux DL. Review: Toward an understanding of the molecular mechanisms of physiological cell death. Proc Natl Acad Sci USA 1993; 90:786–789.
32. Pekin TJ, Malinin TI, Zvaifler NJ. Unusual synovial fluid findings in Reiter's syndrome. Ann Intern Med 1967; 66:677–684.
33. Jones ST, Denton J, Holt PJ, Freemont AJ. Possible clearance of effete polymorphonuclear leukocytes from synovial fluid by cytophagocytic mononuclear cells: implications for pathogenesis and chronicity in inflammatory arthritis. Ann Rheum Dis 1993; 52:121–126.
34. Altomonte L, Zoli A, Mirone L, Scolieri P, Magaro M. Serum levels of interleukin-1b, tumor necrosis factor alpha and interleukin-2 in rheumatoid arthritis. Correlations with disease activity. Clin Rheumatol 1992; 11:202–205.
35. Barrera P, Boerbooms AM, Janssen EM, Sauerwein RW, Gallati H, Mulder J, de Boo T, Demacker PN, van de Putte LB, van der Meer JW. Circulating soluble tumor necrosis factor receptors, interleukin-2 receptors, tumor necrosis factor alpha, and interleukin-6 levels in rheumatoid arthritis. Longitudinal evaluation during methotrexate and azathioprine therapy. Arthritis Rheum 1993; 36:1070–1079.
36. Mason JC, Kapahi P, Haskard DO. Detection of increased levels of circulating intracellular adhesion molecule-1 in some patients with rheumatoid arthritis, but not in patients with

systemic lupus erythematosus. Lack of correlation with levels of vascular cell adhesion molecule-1. Arthritis Rheum 1993; 36:519–527.
37. Schumacher HR, Kitridou RC. Synovitis of recent onset. A clinicopathologic study during the first month of disease. Arthritis Rheum 1972; 15:465–485.
38. Firestein GS, Paine MM, Littman BH. Gene expression (collagenase, tissue inhibitor of metalloproteinases, complement, and HLA-DR) in rheumatoid arthritis and osteoarthritis synovium. Quantitative analysis and effect of intraarticular corticosteroids. Arthritis Rheum 1991; 34:1094–1105.
39. Zvaifler NJ. Macrophages and the synovial lining. Scand J Rheumatol 1995; 24(S101):67–75.
40. Forre O, Thoen J, Lea T, Dobloug JH, Mellbye OJ, Natvig JB, Pahle J, Solheim BG. In situ characterization of mononuclear cells in rheumatoid tissues, using monoclonal antibodies. No reduction of T8-positive cells or augmentation in T4-positive cells. Scand J Immunol 1982; 16:315–319.
41. Klareskog L, Forsum U, Wigren A, Wigzell H. Relationship between HLA-DR–expresssing cells and T lymphocytes of different subsets in rheumatoid synovial tissue. Scand J Immunol 1981; 15:501–507.
42. Konttinen YT, Reitamo S, Ranki A, Hayry P, Kankaanapaa U, Wegelius O. Characterization of the immunocompetent cells of rheumatoid synovium from tissue sections and eluates. Arthritis Rheum 1981; 24:71–79.
43. Malone DG, Wahl SM, Tsokos M, Cattell H, Decker JL, Wilder RL. Immune function in severe, active rheumatoid arthritis. A relationship between peripheral blood mononuclear cell proliferation to soluble antigens and synovial tissue immunohistologic characteristics. J Clin Invest 1984; 74:1173–1185.
44. Young CL, Adamson TC, Vaughan JH, Fox RI. Immunohistologic characterization of synovial membrane lymphocytes in rheumatoid arthritis. Arthritis Rheum 1984; 27:32–39.
45. Janossy G, Panayi G, Duke O, Bofill M, Poulter LW, Goldstein G. Rheumatoid arthritis: a disease of T-lymphocyte/macrophage immunoregulation. Lancet 1981; 2:839–842.
46. Panayi GS, Lanchbury JS, Kingsley GH. The importance of the T cell in initiating and maintaining the chronic synovitis of rheumatoid arthritis [editorial]. Arthritis Rheum 1992; 35:729–735.
47. Lenjassen B, Strauss AF, Steere AC, Kamradt T. The T helper cell response in Lyme arthritis—differential recognition: Borrelia burgdorferi outer surface protein A in patients with treatment-resistant or treatment-responsive Lyme arthritis. J Exp Med 1994; 180:2069–2078.
48. Burmester GR, Jahn B, Gramatzki M, Zacher J, Kalden JR. Activated T cells in vivo and in vitro: divergence in expression of Tac and la antigens in the nonblastoid small T cells of inflammation and normal T cells activated in vivo. J Immunol 1984; 133:1230–1234.
49. Firestein GS, Tsai V, Zvaifler NJ. Cellular immunity in the joints of patients with rheumatoid arthritis and other forms of chronic synovitis. In: Zvaifler NJ, ed. Rheumatic Disease Cinics of North America. Philadelphia: Saunders, 1987:191–213.
50. Firestein GS, Zvaifler NJ. The pathogenesis of rheumatoid arthritis: A critical assessment of the role of autologous stimulation in the perpetuation of rheumatoid synovitis. In: Pisetsky DS, Snyderman R, eds. Rheumatic Disease Clinics of North America. Philadelphia: Saunders, 1987:447–461.
51. Laffon A, Sanchez-Madrid F, Ortiz de Landazuri M, Jimenez Cuesta A, Ariza A, Ossorio C, Sabando P. Very late activation antigen on synovial fluid T cells from patients with rheumatoid arthritis and other rheumatic diseases. Arthritis Rheum 1989; 32:386–392.
52. Firestein GS, Xu WD, Townsend K, Broide D, Alvaro-Gracia J, Glasebrook A, Zvaifler NJ. Cytokines in chronic inflammatory arthritis. I. Failure to detect T cell lymphokines (interleukin 2 and interleukin 3) and presence of macrophage colony-stimulating factor (CSF-

1) and a novel mast cell growth factor in rheumatoid synovitis. J Exp Med 1988; 168:1573–1586.
53. Miossec P, Naviliat M, Dupuy AA, Sany J, Banchereau J. Low levels of interleukin-4 and high levels of transforming growth factor beta in rheumatoid synovitis. Arthritis Rheum 1990; 33:1180–1187.
54. Firestein GS, Zvaifler NJ. Peripheral blood and synovial fluid monocyte activation in inflammatory arthritis. II. Low levels of synovial fluid and synovial tissue interferon suggest that gamma-interferon is not the primary macrophage activating factor. Arthritis Rheum 1987; 30:864–871.
55. Andersson U, Andersson J. Immunolabeling for cytokine-producing cells in tissue and in suspension. In: Fradelizie D, Emelie D, eds. Cytokine-producing Cells. Paris, Atelier de Formatine #63 INSERN, 1995.
56. Barnes PF, Fong SJ, Brennan PJ, Twomey PE, Mazumder A, Modlin RL. Local production of tumor necrosis factor and IFN-γ in tuberculous pleuritis. J Immunol 1990; 145:149–154.
57. Stamenkovic I, Stegagno M, Krane SM, Kurnick JT. T lymphocytes in synovia of patients with rheumatoid arthritis. Springer Semin Immunopathol 1988; 10:169–180.
58. Bucht A, Oksenberg JR, Lindblad S, Gronberg A, Steinman L, Klareskog L. Characterization of T-cell receptor α/β repertoire in synovial tissue from different temporal phases of rheumatoid arthritis. Scand J Immunol 1992; 35:156–165.
59. Firestein GS, Zvaifler NJ. How important are T cells in chronic rheumatoid synovitis? [editorial]. Arthritis Rheum 1990; 33:768–773.
60. van Eden W, Holoshitz J, Nevo Z, Frenkel A, Klajman A, Cohen IR. Arthritis induced by a T-lymphocyte clone that responds to Mycobacterium tuberculosis and to cartilage proteoglycans. Proc Natl Acad Sci USA 1985; 82:5117–5120.
61. Holoshitz J, Klajman A, Drucker I, Lapidot Z, Yaretzky A, Frenkel A, van Eden W, Cohen IR. T lymphocytes of rheumatoid arthritis patients show augmented reactivity to a fraction of mycobacteria cross-reactive with cartilage. Lancet 1986; 2:305–309.
62. Holoshitz J, Matitiau A, Cohen IR. Arthritis induced in rats by cloned T lymphocytes responsive to mycobacteria but not to collagen type II. J Clin Invest 1984; 73:211–215.
63. Friedman SM, Posnett DN, Tumang JR, Cole BC, Crow MK. A potential role for microbial superantigens in the pathogenesis of systemic autoimmune disease. Arthritis Rheum 1991; 34:468–480.
64. Bottazzo GF, Pujol-Borrell R, Hanafusa T, Feldmann M. Role of aberrant HLA-DR expression and antigen presentation in induction of endocrine autoimmunity. Lancet 1983; 2:1115–1119.
65. Suzuki R, Suzuki S, Takahashi T, Kumagai K. Production of a cytokine with interleukin 3-like properties and cytokine-dependent proliferation in human autologous mixed lymphocyte reaction. J Exp Med 1986; 164:1682–1699.
66. Goto M, Zvaifler NJ. Characterization of the killer cell generated in the autologous mixed leukocyte reaction. J Exp Med 1983; 157:1309–1323.
67. Zvaifler NJ, Steinman RM, Kaplan G, Lau LL, Rivelis M. Identification of immunostimulatory dendritic cells in the synovial effusions of patients with rheumatoid arthritis. J Clin Invest 1985; 76:789–800.
68. Slaughter L, Carson DA, Jensen FC, Holbrook TL, Vaughan JH. In vitro effects of Epstein-Barr virus on peripheral blood mononuclear cells from patients with rheumatoid arthritis and normal subjects. J Exp Med 1978; 148:1429–1434.
69. Hasler F, Bluestein HG, Zvaifler NJ, Epstein LB. Analysis of the defects responsible for the impaired regulation of Epstein-Barr virus–induced B cell proliferation by rheumatoid arthritis lymphocytes. I. Diminished gamma interferon production in response to autologous stimulation. J Exp Med 1983; 157:173–188.

70. Lotz M, Tsoukas CD, Robinson CA, Dinarello CA, Carson DA, Vaughan JH. Basis for defective responses of rheumatoid arthritis synovial fluid lymphocytes to anti-CD3 (T3) antibodies. J Clin Invest 1986; 78:713–721.
71. Lamb JR, Bal V, Mendez-Samperio P, Mehlert A, So A, Rothbard J, Jindal S, Young RA, Young DB. Stress proteins may provide a link between the immune response to infection and autoimmunity. Int Immunol 1989; 1:191–196.
72. Gaston JS, Life PF, Bailey LC, Bacon PA. In vitro responses to a 65-kilodalton mycobacterial protein by synovial T cells from inflammatory arthritis patients. J Immunol 1989; 143:2494–2500.
73. Sargent CA, Dunham I, Trowsdale J, Campbell RD. Human major histocompatibility complex contains genes for the major heat shock protein HSP70. Proc Natl Acad Sci USA 1989; 86:1968–1972.
74. Fontana A, Hengartner H, Weber E, Fehr K, Grob PJ, Cohen G. Interleukin 1 activity in the synovial fluid of patients with rheumatoid arthritis. Rheumatol Int 1982; 2:49–53.
75. Wood NC, Symons JA, Duff GW. Serum interleukin-2-receptor in rheumatoid arthritis: a prognostic indicator of disease activity? J Autoimmun 1988; 1:353–361.
76. Nouri AME, Panayi GS, Goodman SM. Cytokines in the chronic inflammation of rheumatic disease. I. The presence of interleukin-1 in synovial fluids. Clin Exp Immunol 1984; 55:295–302.
77. Miossec P, Dinarello CA, Ziff M. Interleukin-1-lymphocyte chemotactic activity in rheumatoid arthritis synovial fluids. Arthritis Rheum 1986; 29:461–470.
78. Saxne T, Palladino J, Heidegard D, Talal N, Wollheim FA. Detection of tumor necrosis factor in rheumatoid arthritis synovial fluid and serum. Arthritis Rheum 1988; 31:1041–1045.
79. Guerne PA, Zuraw BL, Vaughn JH, Carson DA, Lotz M. Synovium as a source of interleukin 6 in vitro. Contribution to local and systemic manifestations of arthritis. J Clin Invest 1989; 83:585–592.
80. Hirano T, Matsuda T, Turner M, Miyasaka N, Buchan G, Tang B, Sato K, Shimizu M, Maini R, Feldmann M. Excessive production of interleukin 6/B cell stimulatory factor-2 in rheumatoid arthritis. Eur J Immunol 1988; 18:1797–1801.
81. Xu WD, Firestein GS, Taetle R, Kaushansky K, Zvaifler NJ. Cytokines in chronic inflammatory arthritis. II. Granulocyte-macrophage colony-stimulating factor in rheumatoid synovial effusions. J Clin Invest 1989; 83:876–882.
82. Firestein GS, Alvaro-Gracia JM, Maki R. Quantitative analysis of cytokine gene expression in rheumatoid arthritis. J Immunol 1990; 144:3347–3353.
83. Schaible UE, Gay S, Museteanu C, Kramer MD, Zimmer G, Eichmann K, Museteanu U, Simon MM. Lyme borreliosis in the severe combined immunodeficiency (scid) mouse manifests predominantly in the joints, heart, and liver. Am J Pathol 1990; 137:811–820.
84. Geiler T, Kriegsmann J, Keyszer GM, Gay RE, Gay S. A new model for rheumatoid arthritis generated by engraftment of rheumatoid synovial tissue and normal human cartilage into SCID mice. Arthritis Rheum 1994; 37:1664–1671.
85. Dayer J-M, Beutler B, Cerami A. Cachectin/tumor necrosis factor stimulates collagenase and prostaglandin E2 production by human synovial cells and dermal fibroblasts. J Exp Med 1985; 162:2163–2168.
86. Dayer JM, de Rochemonteix B, Burrus B, Demczuk S, Dinarello CA. Human recombinant interleukin 1 stimulates collagenase and prostaglandin E2 production by synovial cells. J Clin Invest 1986; 77:645–648.
87. Kaushansky K, Lin N, Adamson JW. Interleukin 1 stimulates fibroblasts to synthesize granulocyte-macrophage and granulocyte colony-stimulating factors. Mechanism for the hematopoietic response to inflammation. J Clin Invest 1988; 81:92–97.
88. Alvaro-Gracia JM, Zvaifler NJ, Firestein GS. Cytokines in chronic inflammatory arthri-

tis. IV. Granulocyte/macrophage colony-stimulating factor-mediated induction of class II MHC antigen on human monocytes: a possible role in rheumatoid arthritis. J Exp Med 1989; 170:865–876.
89. Morrissey PJ, Bressler L, Park LS, Alpert A, Gillis S. Granulocyte-macrophage colony-stimulating factor augments the primary antibody response by enhancing the function of antigen-presenting cells. J Immunol 1987; 139:1113–1119.
90. Kishimoto TK, Anderson DC. The role of integrins in inflammation. In: Gallin JI, Goldstein IM, Synderman R, eds. Inflammation: Basic Principles and Clinical Correlates. 2nd ed. New York: Raven Press, 1992:353–406.
91. Springer TA. Adhesion receptors of the immune system. Nature 1990; 346:425–434.
92. Pietschmann P, Cush JT, Lipsky PE, Oppenheimer-Marks N. Identification of subsets of human T cells capable of enhanced transendothelial migration. J Immunol 1992; 149:1170–1178.
93. Johnson BA, Haines GK, Harlow LA, Koch AE. Adhesion molecule expression in human synovial tissue. Arthritis Rheum 1993; 36:137–146.
94. Elices MJ, Tsai V, Strahl D, Goel AS, Tollefson V, Arrhenius T, Wayner EA, Gaeta FC, Fikes JD, Firestein GS. Expression and functional significance of alternatively spliced CS1 fibronectin in rheumatoid arthritis microvasculature. J Clin Invest 1994; 93:405–416.
95. Morales-Ducret J, Wayner E, Elices MJ, Alvaro-Gracia JM, Zvaifler NJ, Firestein GS. Alpha 4/beta 1 integrin (VLA-4) ligands in arthritis. Vascular cell adhesion molecule-1 expression in synovium and on fibroblast-like synoviocytes. J Immunol 1992; 149:1424–1431.
96. Firestein GS, Zvaifler NJ. Rheumatoid arthritis: A disease of disordered immunity. In: Gallin JI, Goldstein IM, Snyderman R, eds. Inflammation: Basic Principles and Clinical Correlates. 2nd ed. New York: Raven Press, 1992:959–976.
97. Remmers EF, Sano H, Wilder RL. Platelet-derived growth factors and heparin-binding (fibroblast) growth factors in the synovial tissue pathology of rheumatoid arthritis. Semin Arthritis Rheum 1991; 21:191–199.
98. Lafyatis R, Remmers EF, Roberts AB, Yocum DE, Sporn MB, Wilder R. Anchorage-independent growth of synoviocytes from arthritic and normal joints: stimulation by exogenous platelet-derived growth factor and inhibition by transforming growth factor β and retinoids. J Clin Invest 1989; 83:1267–1276.
99. Krane SM, Conca W, Stephenson ML, Amento EP, Goldring MB. Mechanisms of matrix degradation in rheumatoid arthritis. Ann NY Acad Sci 1990; 580:340–354.
100. Revell PA. Synovial lining cells. Rheumatol Int 1989; 9:49–51.
101. Gay S, Gay RE, Koopman WJ. Molecular and cellular mechanisms of joint destruction in rheumatoid arthritis: two cellular mechanisms explain joint destruction? Ann Rheum Dis 1993; 52 Suppl 1:S39–S47.
102. Burmester GR, Dimitriu-Bona A, Waters SJ, Winchester RJ. Identification of three major synovial lining cell populations by monoclonal antibodies directed to la antigens and antigens associated with monocytes/macrophages and fibroblasts. Scand J Immunol 1983; 17:69–82.
103. Alvaro-Gracia JM, Zvaifler NJ, Firestein GS. Cytokines in chronic inflammatory arthritis. V. Mutual antagonism between IFN-γ and TNF-α on HLA-DR expression, proliferation, collagenase production, and GM-CSF production by rheumatoid arthritis synoviocytes. J Clin Invest 1990; 86:1790–1798.
104. Alvaro-Gracia JM, Zvaifler NJ, Brown CB, Kaushansky K, Firestein GS. Cytokines in chronic inflammatory arthritis. VI. Analysis of the synovial cells involved in granulocyte-macrophage colony-stimulating factor production and gene expression in rheumatoid arthritis and its regulation by IL-1 and tumor necrosis factor-alpha. J Immunol 1991; 146:3365–3371.

105. Kobayashi I, Ziff M. Electron microscopic studies on the cartilage-pannus junction in rheumatoid arthritis. Arthritis Rheum 1975; 18:475–483.
106. Shiozawa S, Shiozawa K, Fujita T. Morphologic observations in the early phase of the cartilage-pannus junction: Light and electron microscopic studies of active cellular pannus. Arthritis Rheum 1983; 26:472–478.
107. Fassbender HG. Histomorphological basis of articular cartilage destruction in rheumatoid arthritis. Coll Relat Res 1983; 3:141–155.
108. Allard SA, Bayliss M, Maini RN. The synovium-cartilage junction of the normal human knee. Implications for joint destruction and repair. Arthritis Rheum 1990; 33:1170–1179.
109. Wooley DE, Crossley MJ, Evanson JM. Collagenase at sites of cartilage erosion in the rheumatoid joint. Arthritis Rheum 1977; 20:1231–1239.
110. Okada Y, Takeuchi N, Tomita K, Nakanishi I, Nagase H. Immunolocalization of matrix metalloproteinase 3 (stromelysin) in rheumatoid synovioblasts (B cells): correlation with rheumatoid arthritis. Ann Rheum Dis 1989; 48:645–653.
111. Allard SA, Muirden KD, Maini RN. Correlation of histopathological features of pannus with patterns of damage in different joints in rheumatoid arthritis. Ann Rheum Dis 1991; 50:278–283.
112. Shiozawa S, Tokuhisa T. Contributions of synovial mesenchymal cells to the pathogensis of rheumatoid arthritis. Semin Arthritis Rheum 1992; 21:267–273.
113. Firestein GS, Zvaifler NJ. Pannus and pannocytes: Alternative models of joint destruction in rheumatoid arthritis [editorial]. Arthritis Rheum 1994; 37:783–789.
114. Trabandt A, Aicher WK, Gay RE, Sukhatme VP, Fassbender HG, Gay S. Spontaneous expression of immediately-early response genes c-fos and egr-1 in collagenase-producing rheumatoid synovial fibroblasts. Rheumatol Int 1992; 12:53–59.
115. Trabandt A, Aicher WK, Gay RE, Sukhatme VP, Nilson-Hamilton M, Hamilton RT, McGhee JR, Fassbender HG, Gay S. Expression of the collagenolytic and Ras-induced cysteine proteinase cathepsin L and proliferation-associated oncogenes in synovial cells of MRL/l mice and patients with rheumatoid arthritis. Matrix 1990; 10:349–361.
116. Ruoslahti E, Giancotti FG. Integrins and tumor cell dissemination. Cancer Cells 1989; 1:119–126.
117. Seftor RE, Seftor EA, Gehlsen KR, Stetler-Stevenson WG, Brown PP, Ruoslahti E, Hendrix MJ. Role of the avβ3 integrin in human melanoma cell invasion. Proc Natl Acad Sci USA 1992; 89:1557–1561.
118. Ugai K, Ishikawa H, Hirohata K, Shirane H. Interactions of polymorphonuclear leukocytes with immune complexes trapped in joint collagenous tissues. Arthritis Rheum 1983; 26:1434–1441.
119. Remmers EF, Lafyatis R, Kumkumian GK, Case JP, Roberts AB, Sporn MB, Wilder RL. Cytokines and growth regulation of synoviocytes from patients with rheumatoid arthritis and rats with streptococcal cell wall arthritis. Growth Factors 1990; 2:179–188.
120. Bucala R, Ritchlin C, Winchester R, Cerami A. Constitutive production of inflammatory and mitogenic cytokines by rheumatoid synovial fibroblasts. J Exp Med 1991; 173:569–574.
121. Brennan FM, Maini RN, Feldman M. TNFα—a pivotal role in rheumatoid arthritis? Br J Rheumatol 1992; 31:293–298.
122. Kinne RW, Boehm S, Iftner T, Aigner T, Vornehm S, Weseloh G, Bravo R, Emmrich F, Kroczek RA. Synovial fibroblast-like cells strongly express jun-B and c fos proto-oncogenes in rheumatoid and osteoarthritis. Scand J Rheumatol 1995; 101(Suppl):121–125.
123. Qu Z, Garcia CH, O'Rourke LM, Planck SR, Kohli M, Rosenbaum JT. Local proliferation of fibroblast-like synoviocytes contributes to synovial hyperplasia. Results of proliferating cell nuclear antigen/cyclin, c-myc, and nucleolar organizer region staining. Arthritis Rheum 1994; 37:212–220.

124. Konttinen YT, Nykanen P, Nordstrom D, Saari H, Sandelin J, Santavirta S, Kouri T. DNA synthesis in prolyl 4-hydroxylase positive fibroblasts in situ in synovial tissue. An autoradiography-immunoperoxidase double labeling study. J Rheumatol 1989; 16:339–345.
125. Nakajima T, Aono H, Hasunuma T, Yamamoto K, Shirai T, Hirohata K, Nishioka K. Apoptosis and functional fas antigen in rheumatoid arthritis synoviocytes. Arthritis Rheum 1995; 38:485–491.
126. Firestein GS, Yeo M, Zvaifler NJ. Apoptosis in rheumatoid arthritis synovium. J Clin Invest 1995; 96:1631–1638.

2
Clinical Assessments in Rheumatoid Arthritis

Piet L. C. M. van Riel and Anke M. van Gestel
University Hospital Nijmegen, Nijmegen, The Netherlands

Maarten Boers
University Hospital Maastricht, Maastricht, The Netherlands

David L. Scott
Kings College Hospital, London, United Kingdom

I. INTRODUCTION

As rheumatoid arthritis (RA) is a chronic inflammatory disease primarily affecting the peripheral joints, clinical assessments continue to be of prime importance, both in clinical trials and daily practice. The presentation of RA may vary substantially between patients as well as within the same individual. Some patients experience no pain and have only a few swollen joints, whereas others are disabled by multiple swollen and tender joints. Within an individual patient, periods of active disease can be followed by periods of minor or even no symptoms, which in turn may end in an acute flare of the disease. The progression of the disease process can vary from mild to severely disabling. Clinical assessments are therefore necessary to follow the course of the disease and to evaluate therapeutic interventions.

Measures in rheumatoid arthritis can be classified as process and outcome measures. According to Fries [1], outcome is defined as the end result of the disease, representing variables which are of direct importance to the patient; that is, death, disability, discomfort, iatrogenic events, and economic impact. Process is what happens along the way, and process measures may serve as proxies for outcome [1,2]. Disease activity measures are therefore often process variables.

Numerous measures have been developed to measure aspects of disease activity, including joint counts, laboratory assessments, pain measures, and physical disability or health status measures. Apart from this divergence which is necessary to cover the whole spectrum of "disease activity," there is a need for convergence to reach uniformity among assessors for reasons of comparison and simplicity. In recent years, efforts have been made to reach a consensus about a minimal set of disease activity variables to be measured in clinical trials. In addition, indices have been developed combining several of those disease activity variables into one single score.

Disease activity measures assess a disease state at a certain moment in time. However, to evaluate the course of the disease or the efficacy of treatment, a measure should comprise the dimension time. This can be done by accumulating disease activity measurements or by calculating a change in disease activity over time. In order to evaluate the course of the disease and the effects of a given treatment in an individual patient, response criteria have been developed. The ultimate goal of the treatment of RA is completely to suppress disease activity, often called "remission." Preliminary remission criteria have been developed in the past and have not been adjusted to recent insights in the evaluation of the course of RA. A proposal has been made to define *remission* as the absence of disease symptoms using a validated method during a period of defined minimal duration [3].

When developing or choosing variables or indices to measure disease activity, the aspects of reproducibility and validity are of major importance. Reproducibility (precision) means that repeated measurements under the same circumstances give the same results. Validity means that a measure measures what it is supposed to: Does the measure represents the true state (criterion validity), does it fit with the theory about the process (construct validity), is the measure reasonable (face validity), does it comprise all aspects of the feature to be measured (content validity), and can it detect the smallest important difference between groups or within a group over time (discriminant validity or sensitivity to change) [4]?

In the following paragraphs, the above-mentioned core-sets, indices, response definitions, and remission criteria are discussed.

II. CORE-SET

During the 4th World Health Organization/International League of Associations for Rheumatology (WHO/ILAR) meeting in Geneva (July 1991), it was recognized that further standardization of endpoint measures in clinical trials was necessary. Uniformity of the measured endpoints improves the comparability of different studies. Besides that, minimizing the set of required measures decreases the chance of conflicting results and reduces the probability of reaching significance by chance alone (problem of multiple testing). Potential "core-set" measures should be valid, sensitive to change, reliable, and not redundant. Within EULAR, a core set was agreed on which was based on the statistical evaluation of a large inception cohort of patients with rheumatoid arthritis [5]. This core-set did not include a physician global and recommended the 28-joint count. During the Conference on Outcome Measures in Rheumatoid Arthritis Clinical Trials (OMERACT) in Maastricht, The Netherlands (April 1992), consensus was reached on preliminary core efficacy endpoints [6]. Except for radiographs, the core-set of the American College of Rheumatology (ACR) was conform the OMERACT proposal [7]. During the WHO/ILAR meeting in July 1993, finally agreement was achieved between the different groups on the core-set listed in Table 1. It should be stressed that the core-set is a minimal requirement for each clinical study; in addition, other outcomes such as psychosocial function, patients preferences, treatment dropouts, side effects, and costs should be considered. Further standardization of measurement

Table 1 Core-set of Endpoint Measures in RA Clinical Trials

Joint pain/tenderness: 28 joints
Joint swelling: 28 joints
Acute phase reactants
Pain
Patient global assessment
Physician global assessment
Physical disability
Radiographs (for studies >1 year)

techniques is still required. Recommendations were made by the European League Against Rheumatism (EULAR) [8] and the ACR [7,9].

A. Joint Counts

The most important clinical sign of rheumatoid arthritis activity is joint inflammation. Inflammation is characterized by the symptoms rubor (redness), calor (heat), dolor, tumor, and functio laesa. Joint examination is mainly restricted to the last three areas, that is tenderness, swelling, and limitation of motion/deformity, respectively.

Many different joint counts are available measuring one or more of these aspects. They differ in the number of joints included, whether joints are assessed separetely or combined, whether joints are graded for severity, or weighted for size. In a recent review, Thompson and Kirwan [10] conclude that tenderness and swelling supply different information. Joint tenderness is more sensitive to change and correlates with pain, whereas swollen joint counts predict joint damage. They also conclude that grading for severity improves sensitivity and weighting for joint size improves correlation with the acute phase response, but with both additions, interobserver variation increases [10]. Prevoo et al. [11] conclude that grading of tenderness almost always gives a small improvement in validity and reliability of joint counts, whereas weighting for joint surface area almost always decreases validity and reliability. Both grading and weighting do not improve sensitivity to change and increase interobserver variation [11]. A 28-joint count for tenderness and swelling, not graded and not weighted [12,13], proved to be as valid as more comprehensive joint counts [11,14]. Both the ACR Committee on Outcome Measures in Rheumatoid Arthritis Clinical Trials [15] and the EULAR Standing Committee on International Clinical Studies Including Therapeutic Trials [16] have adapted the use of reduced joint counts for clinical trials. The joints not included in reduced joint counts, however, are of course still of clinical importance in the management of individual patients [15].

B. Acute Phase Reactants

The most frequently used laboratory measures for disease activity are Westergren erythrocyte sedimentation rate (ESR) and C-reactive protein (CRP). They correlate with other measures of disease activity [17], and they are sensitive to change in trials comparing slow-acting antirheumatic drugs [18–20]. There is some evidence that these measures predict x-ray progression [17,21]. Both ESR and CRP are nonspecific measures of inflammation; however, the CRP is more closely related to the inflammatory process and is less susceptible to disturbing factors such as renal function, food intake, and immunoglobulin levels [22]. In some centers, plasma viscosity, as another indirect indicator of the acute phase reaction, is being used instead of ESR [19].

Other laboratory assessments are less valid (platelet count, hemoglobin, [17,18,20,23]) or need further investigation (e.g., cytokines, soluble receptors).

C. Pain

The major problem for patients with active rheumatoid arthritis is pain. Several measurement techniques have been developed, including numerical rating scales, verbal rating scales, visual analog scales (VAS), questionnaires [24,25], and behavioral observation methods [26]. In choosing a measurement, ease of use, reliability, and sensitivity should be considered. The VAS, one of the most frequently used assessments, has been shown to be sensitive to change [18,27,28] but was more difficult for elderly [28] and illiterate patients [29]. Bosi-Ferraz concludes that a numerical rating scale (10 possible scores) proved to be more reliable than a VAS or a verbal rating scale (5 possible scores) in literate and illiterate patients [29]. The Arthritis Impact Measurement Scales pain questions were also sensitive to change [18,27]. It is recommended to use a horizontal VAS of 10 cm with "no pain" at one end and "worst possible pain" at the other end without intervening categories; however, it is also possible to assess pain with a Likert scale (1 = asymptomatic; 2 = mild, 3 = moderate, 4 = severe, 5 = very severe) [9].

D. Global Disease Activity

Although no validation studies are performed, the patient's assessment of global disease activity is generally measured on a VAS using the AIMS question: "Considering all the ways your arthritis affects you, mark 'X' on the scale for how well you are doing." A Likert scale response is also acceptable according to the ACR. The same recommendations as for patient's global assessments apply for the physician's (or assessor's) global assessment of the patient's disease activity; that is, a VAS or a Likert scale [9]. During the OMERACT consensus meeting on endpoints, it appeared that part of the participants felt that the physician's assessment should be included in the core-set, and others felt that it was a redundant measure which should only be used as the overall global criterion against which to compare others [30].

E. Physical/Functional Disability

The available tools to assess disability can be divided into: (a) measures based on clinical judgement, (b) measures based on observed patient performance, and (c) self-reported assessments [31]. Clinical judgment of function will be subject to large interobserver variation and observation of performances is very time consuming. Self-reported questionnaires are the most popular, although there may be discrepancy between the actual performance and the reported performance of patients [32]. Both generic and disease-specific health status questionnaires have been developed [25,33–39]. These questionnaires are often multidimensional assessing physical as well as psychological and social disability. The two most frequently used self-reported questionnaires in the arthritis patient, the Arthritis Impact Measurement Scales (AIMS) and the Health Assessment Questionnaire (HAQ), are sensitive to clinical changes [23,40–42]. The modified HAQ functional disability index predicted increased morbidity and mortality in a study done by Wolfe et al. [36]. Buchbinder compared three quality-of-life measures: a modified McMaster Toronto Arthritis Patient Preference Disability Questionnaire (MACTAR), the HAQ, and the AIMS [27]. The AIMS physical function score appeared to be the least responsive to detect a treatment effect (not statistically significant). The MACTAR questionnaire could detect small clinically important changes in function [37]. Liang (1985) compared efficiency and sensitivity of five health status instruments (HAQ, AIMS, Functional Status Index [FSI], Index of Well Being [IWB], Sickness Impact Profile [SIP]) and concluded that no single instrument consistently outperformed the others [43]. ACR recommendations are: "any patient self-assessment instrument which has been validated, has reliability, has been proven in RA trials to be sensitive to change, and which measures physical function in RA patients is acceptable. Instruments which have been demonstrated to be sensitive in RA trials include the AIMS, the HAQ, the Quality (or Index) of Well Being, the McMaster Health Index Questionnaire (MHIQ), and the MACTAR" [9]. It would be best to choose one of these instrument as the core-set measure for physical function to improve uniformity among trials.

F. Radiographs/Imaging Techniques

In the evaluation of Disease Modifying Anti-Rheumatic Drugs (DMARDs), the assessment of radiographic damage has always been a golden standard. The two most frequently used validated radiographic scoring methods have been developed by Sharp and Larsen [44,45]. Both methods have been modified several times [46–48]. Pincus compared the Steinbrocker radiographic stage, the modified Sharp method, and the Larsen method and concluded that they correlated with each other and showed similar correlations with other clinical measures [49]. A problem using the Sharp or Larsen methods is the so-called "ceiling effect": when the maximum score in a joint is reached, further damage cannot be quantified. According to Sharp, better methods are needed using direct measurements of damage in standard units (mm^2) [44]. Newer imaging techniques, MRI and DEXA, are promising tools for both clinical evaluation and for the testing of new therapies [50–52].

III. INDICES OF DISEASE ACTIVITY

Indices of disease activity combine multiple disease activity measures into a single measure [53]. Advantages of an index are (a) unambiguous interpretation of disease activity, (b) comparability of trial results, and (c) more power in clinical trials. Several indices have been developed using a statistical, pseudostatistical, or heuristic approach. Disadvantages of an index are that it cannot be easily reexpressed into its components and that the calculations involved are more or less intricate. The indices are different with respect to what they measure; that is current disease activity or change, and with respect to their scales: continuous or ordinal (Table 2).

Table 2 Indices of Disease Activity

	Continuous scale	Ordinal scale (n classes)
Current disease activity	Lansbury systemic index Disease activity score	Mallya/mace index (4) Stoke index (4) ARA remission (2)
Improvement criteria: a. change in disease activity b. combination of change and current disease activity	Pooled index	Paulus improvement (2) ACR improvement (2) Simple index (6) EULAR response (3)

A. Current Disease Activity

In the case of following the course of the disease or assessing disease activity at a certain moment in time, a measure assessing current disease activity should be chosen. The advantage of a continuous scale is that no information is lost which increases sensitivity. The Lansbury systemic index is the oldest measure [54], although it has not been thoroughly validated. The Disease Activity Score (DAS) [55,56] is a statistically derived index combining tender joints, swollen joints, ESR, and general health. It has been validated in several studies [17,56,57]. The Mallya/Mace index and its modifications [58–60] is a valid [17,61] ordinal measure of current disease activity. The Stoke index [61] needs further validation. The ARA remission criteria are a special kind of disease activity measures dividing patients in only two categories: remission or no remission [62]. They will be discussed in Section C.

B. Improvement Criteria

For treatment evaluation, a time component should be included in the measure; that is, change in disease activity during a certain period. Response to treatment can be defined for groups; for example, with the pooled index of Smythe [63], or for individual patients, as with the Paulus improvement criteria [64], the preliminary ACR improvement criteria [9], the EULAR response criteria [65], and a simple index to assess disease activity proposed by Scott [66]. Individual response criteria quantify the number of patients actually responding and to what extend they improve, which is an important addition to mean group values as endpoint variables in clinical trials.

1. Improvement Criteria Based on Change in Disease Activity

The pooled Index of Smythe is a linear sum of the weighted mean changes in single measures [63]. The change in a variable is divided by the standard deviation of the difference of that variable. The transformed changes of all variables are summated. Problems with this method are (a) no predefined (number of) single variables to be included, (b) no weights to the relative contribution of single variables, and (c) can only be used to compare groups, because the group standard deviation of the difference has to be calculated.

Ordinal measures for treatment evaluation are the Paulus improvement criteria [64], the preliminary ACR improvement criteria [9], the EULAR response criteria [65], and a simplex index to assess disease activity proposed by Scott [66]. These measures are developed to measure individual treatment response. Paulus arbitrarily selected a group of variables (duration of morning stiffness, ESR, joint pain/tenderness score, joint swelling score, physician's global disease activity, and patient's global disease activity) and studied how many variables had to improve to what extend to discriminate between active drug and placebo. The preliminary ACR improvement criteria [9] are modifications of the Paulus criteria (Table 3). The ACR criteria result from a study investigating ease of use, credibility, and discriminant validity (versus placebo) of improvement criteria [9].

2. *Improvement Criteria Based on Change and Current Disease Activity*

The simplex index [66] and the EULAR response criteria [65] are different because they include not only change in disease activity but also current disease activity. The simple index was proposed by Scott and has some similarities with the American Rheumatism Association criteria for remission in RA [62]. It comprises six variables, four variables reflecting current disease activity (morning stiffness ≤15 min, ≤3 tender joints, ≤3 swollen joints, ≤30 mm/h ESR) and two variables reflecting change from baseline (≥50% pain reduction, ≥40% functional improvement). For every criterion that is met after 6 months of therapy, 1 point is scored. The total score ranged from 0 to 6 and the patients were spread fairly evenly between each of the seven classes of response [66]. Before this simple index can recommended, further validation needs to be done. The EULAR response criteria are based on an index of disease activity (DAS). To be classified as responders patients should have a significant change in DAS and also low current disease activity. Three categories are defined: good, moderate, and non-responders (Table 4).

So far, the EULAR response criteria have been compared with the ACR and the WHO/ILAR response criteria in one double-blind comparative study of two second-line

Table 3 Response Criteria Based on Change in Disease Activity

Improvement in	Paulus (4 of 6) (%)	ACR (5 of 7, first 2 required) (%)
Joint tenderness	≥20	≥20
Joint swelling	≥20	≥20
ESR	≥20	≥20
Physician's global disease activity	≥40	≥20
Patient global disease activity	≥40	≥20
Morning stiffness	≥20	
Patient pain		≥20
Disability		≥20

Table 4 EULAR Response Definition

Current DAS	Decrease in DAS >1.2	>0.6 and ≤1.2	≤0.6
≤2.4	Good		
>2.4 and ≤3.7		Moderate	
>3.7			Non

agents and showed better construct and discriminant validity [60]. The performance of these criteria needs further study in future clinical trials before a uniform measure defining individual treatment response can be selected.

C. Remission Criteria

Complete remission of rheumatoid arthritis means the disappearance of disease activity either spontaneously or with antirheumatic therapy without a relapse of the disease. Although it occurs infrequently, remission is the ultimate goal of therapy and should therefore be defined. Any usable criterion should contain a time component, since follow-up for an indefinite period will not be possible in most clinical settings. The American Rheumatism Association developed preliminary criteria for clinical remission in rheumatoid arthritis [62] (Table 5). The development was based on an optimal discrimination between patients with and without remission according to their rheumatologists.

An arbitrary duration of more than 2 months was chosen because 90% of the patients fulfilled this criterion. There are also several problems with this definition that obstruct clinical usefulness. No specifications are given as to which measurement technique should be used for the different clinical variables, two of the six used variables are not included in the core-set data, and finally the outcome is dichotomous, which implies that a small change in disease activity may have a great impact on the allocated class. Another approach would be to define remission with a continuous variable of disease activity such as the DAS and add the time period that the patient was at a certain level or just calculate the cumulative disease activity over a certain time period. A

Table 5 ARA Remission Criteria 1981

Five or more of the following requirements must be fulfilled for at least 2 consecutive months:
1. Morning stiffness ≤15 minutes
2. No fatigue
3. No joint pain (by history)
4. No joint tenderness or pain on motion
5. No soft tissue swelling in joints or tendon sheaths
6. ESR (Westergren)
X < 30 mm/h
X < 20 mm/h

DAS was calculated for patients who were categorized with the ARA criteria as being in remission or not. At a cutoff value of the DAS of 1.6, the percentage of misclassification for both categories was 10%. The advantage of this method would be that remission can be seen relative to other levels of disease activity [3].

IV. SELF-ADMINISTERED MEASURES

There is an increasing use of self-administered forms in the assessment of disease activity in rheumatoid arthritis. The fact that most of the clinical assessments are very time-consuming procedures might have contributed to this development [67–69]. The validity of several of these variables like the questionnaires to measure function and visual analog scales to assess pain and global functions have been shown reason to include them into the core-set. In recent years, even self-administered forms to measure joint involvement have been developed and evaluated. The reproducibility of one of these self-administered joint counts was satisfactory and comparable to test-retest correlations of other assessments. However, the correlation with the "golden standard," the assessor joint score was too low to be able to replace this one [69]. Further studies are needed to determine the usefulness of these self-administered joint counts in the clinical assessment of rheumatoid arthritis.

V. SUMMARY

Today, agreement exists among rheumatologists that there is a need for uniformity in clinical assessments in rheumatoid arthritis. By consensus, a core-set of variables is selected out of many different variables to be used in clinical trials as a measure of disease activity. This core-set comprises the number of tender joints, number of swollen joints, acute phase reactant, patient's assessment of pain, patient's and physician's assessment of global disease activity, functional disability, and (for studies with a duration of more than 1 year) radiographs. By using this core-set, the comparability of studies will be improved. However, an unambiguous interpretation of disease activity is still not possible with seven or eight variables. Therefore, indices of disease activity have been developed combining disease activity variables into a single measure. These indices can be devided into indices measuring current disease activity, change in disease activity, and a combination of current disease activity and change. The last two categories are called improvement (or response) criteria. Treatment efficacy can be analyzed by comparing mean (change in) disease activity of treatment groups and by comparing the number of responders in each group. This individual treatment response is an addition to mean group response because it indicates whether few patients respond excellently or many patients respond moderately. Remission criteria have been developed to define the absence of disease activity. A usefull measure should define a minimum period of time to satisfy the criteria. Further studies are needed to determine the cutoff point of no disease activity and validate this against the radiographic and functional outcome. Finally, more effort has to be undertaken to standardize the different assessments.

REFERENCES

1. Fries JF. Toward and understanding of patient outcome measurement. Arthritis Rheum 1983; 26:697–704.
2. Fries JF. The hierarchy of outcome assessment. J Rheumatol 1993; 20:546–547.
3. Prevoo MLL, Gestel van AM, Hof van't MA, Rijswijk van MH, Putte van de LBA, Riel van PLCM. Remission in a prospective study of patients with rheumatoid arthritis. ARA preliminary remission criteria in relation to the disease activity score. Br J Rheumatol 1996;
4. Tugwell P, Bombardier C. A methodological framework for developing and selecting endpoints in clinical trials. J Rheumatol 1982; 9:758–762.
5. Riel van PLCM. Provisional guidelines for measuring disease activity in RA clinical trials [editorial]. Br J Rheumatol 1992; 31:793–794.
6. Tugwell P, Boers M, OMERACT COMMITTEE. Developing consensus on preliminary core efficacy endpoints for rheumatoid arthritis clinical trials. J Rheumatol 1993; 20:555–561.
7. Felson DT, Anderson JJ, Boers M, et al. The American College of Rheumatology preliminary core set of disease activity measures for rheumatoid arthritis clinical trials. Arthritis Rheum 1993; 36:729–740.
8. Assessing disease activity in rheumatoid arthritis. The EULAR handbook of standard methods. DL Scott, PL van Riel, D van der Heijde, A Stunicka Benke. 1993.
9. Felson DT, Anderson JJ, Boers M, et al. American College of Rheumatology preliminary definition of improvement in rheumatoid arthritis. Arthritis Rheum 1995; 38:727–35.
10. Thompson PW, Kirwan JR. Joint counts: a review of old and new articular indices of joint inflammation. Br J Rheumatol 1995; 34:1003–1008.
11. Prevoo MLL, van Riel PLCM, van't Hof MA, et al. Validity and reliability of joint indices. A longitudinal study in patients with recent onset rheumatoid arthritis. Br J Rheumatol 1993; 32:589–594.
12. Fuchs HA, Brooks RH, Callahan LF, Pincus T. A simplified twenty-eight-joint quantitative articular index in rheumatoid arthritis. Arthritis Rheum 1989; 32:531–537.
13. Fuchs HA, Pincus T. Reduced joint counts in controlled clinical trials in rheumatoid arthritis. Arthritis Rheum 1994; 37:470–475.
14. Smolen JS, Breedveld FC, Eberl G, et al. Validity and reliability of the twenty-eight-joint count for the assessment of rheumatoid arthritis validity. Arthritis Rheum 1995; 38:38–43.
15. American College of Rheumatology committee on outcome measures in rheumatoid arthritis clinical trials. Reduced joint counts in rheumatoid arthritis clinical trials [editorial]. Arthritis Rheum 1994; 37:463–464.
16. Smolen JS. Report on the EULAR Standing Committee on International Clinical Studies Including Therapeutic Trials. Rheumatol Eur 1994; 23:37–39.
17. van der Heijde DMFM, van't Hof MA, van Riel PLCM, van de Putte LBA. Validity of single variables and indices to measure disease activity in rheumatoid arthritis. J Rheumatol 1993; 20:538–541.
18. Anderson JJ, Chernoff MC. Sensitivity to change of rheumatoid arthritis clinical trial outcome measures. J Rheumatol 1993; 20:535–537.
19. Astbury C, Platt R, Dixon JS, Le Gallex P, Hill J, Bird HA. Optimizing the assessment of disease activity during treatment with anti-rheumatoid drugs. Br J Rheumatol 1993; 32:467–473.
20. Dixon JS. Hayes S, Constable PDL, Bird HA. What are the 'best' measurements for monitoring patients during short-term second-line therapy? Br J Rheumatol 1988; 27:37–43.
21. Leeuwen van MA, Rijswijk van MH, Heijde van der DMFM, et al. The acute-phase response in relation to radiographic progression in early rheumatoid arthritis: a prospective study during the first three years of the disease. Br J Rheumatol 1993; 32:9–13.
22. Leeuwen van MA, Rijswijk van MH. Acute phase proteins in the monitoring of inflammatory disorders. Baillieres Clin Rheumatol 1994; 8:531–552.

23. Ward MW. Clinical measures in rheumatoid arthritis: which are most useful in assessing patients? J Rheumatol 1993; 21:17–21.
24. Melzack R. The McGill pain questionnaire. Pain 1975:1:277–299.
25. Meenan RF, Gertman PM, Mason JM. Measuring health status in arthritis: the arthritis impact measurement scales. Arthritis Rheum 1980; 23:146–152.
26. Anderson K, Bradley LA, McDaniel LK, et al. The assessment of pain in rheumatoid arthritis: disease differentiation and temporal stability of a behavioral observation method. J Rheumatol 1987; 14:700–704.
27. Buchbinder R, Bombardier C, Yeung M, Tugwell P. Which outcome measures should be used in rheumatoid arthritis clinical trials? Clinical and quality-of-life measures' responsiveness to treatment in a randomized controlled trial. Arthritis Rheum 1995; 38:1568–1580.
28. Jensen MP, Karoly P, Braver S. The measurement of clinical pain intensity: a comparison of six methods. Pain 1986; 27:117–126.
29. Bosi Ferraz M, Quaresma MR, Aquino LRL, Atra E, Tugwell P, Goldsmith CH. Reliability of pain scales in the assessment of literate and illiterate patients in rheumatoid arthritis. J Rheumatol 1990; 17:1022–1024.
30. Tugwell P, Boers M, Baker Ph, Wells G, Snider J. Endpoints in rheumatoid arthritis. J Rheumatol 1994; 42(Suppl):21:2–8.
31. Thompson PW. Functional outcome in rheumatoid arthritis. Br J Rheumatol 1988:27(Suppl 1):37–43.
32. Hidding A, Santen van M, Klerk de E, Gielen X, Boers M, Geenen R, Vlayen J, Kester A, Linden van der Sj. Discordance between self-report measures and clinical observations of functional disability in ankylosing spondylitis, rheumatoid arthritis, and fibromyalgia. J Rheumatol 1994; 21:818–823.
33. Ware JE, Donald-Sherbourne C. The MOS 36-item Short-Form Health Survey (SF-36): I. Conceptual framework and item selection. Med Care 1992; 6:473–483.
34. Bergner M, Bobbitt RA, Pollard WE, Martin DP, Gilson BS. The sickness impact profile: validation of a health status measure. Med Care 1976; 14:57–67.
35. Hunt SM, McKenna SP, McEwen J, Williams J, Papp E. The Nottingham Health Profile: subjective health status and medical consultations. Social Sci Med 1981; 15A:221–229.
36. Fries JF, Spitz P, Kraines RG, Holman HR. Measurement of patient outcome in arthritis. Arthritis Rheum 1980; 23:137–145.
37. Tugwell P, Bombardier C, Buchanan WW, Goldsmith CH, Grace E, Hanna B. The MACTAR patient preference disability questionnaire—an individualized functional priority approach for assessing improvement in physical disability in clinical trials in rheumatoid arthritis. J Rheumatol 1987; 14:446–451.
38. Kaplan RM, Bush JW, Berry CC. Health status: types of validity for an index of well-being. Health Serv Res 1976; 11:478–507.
39. Jette AM. Functional status instrument: reliability of a chronic disease evaluation instrument. Arch Phys Med Rehabil 1980; 61:395–401.
40. Meenan RF, Anderson JJ, Kazis LE, et al. Outcome assessment in clinical trials: evidence for the sensitivity of a health status measure. Arthritis Rheum 1984; 27:1344–1352.
41. Anderson JJ, Firschein HE, Meenan RF. Sensitivity of a health status measure to short-term clinical changes in arthritis. Arthritis Rheum 1989; 32:844–850.
42. Potts MK, Brandt KD. Evidence of the validity of the Arthritis Impact Measurement Scales. Arthritis Rheum 1987; 30:93–96.
43. Liang MH, Larson MG, Cullen KE, Schwartz JA. Comparative measurement efficiency and sensitivity of five health status instruments for arthritis research. Arthritis Rheum 1985; 28:542–547.
44. Sharp JT, Lidsky MD, Collins LC, Moreland J. Methods of scoring the progression of radiologic changes in rheumatoid arthritis. Arthritis Rheum 1971; 14:206–220.
45. Larsen A. A Radiologic Method for Grading the Severity of Rheumatoid Arthritis. Thesis, University of Helsinki, Finland, 1974.

46. van der Heijde DM, van Riel PL, Nuver-Zwart HHJ, Gribnau FW, van de Putte LB. Effects of hydroxychloroquine and sulphasalazine on progression of joint damage in rheumatoid arthritis. Lancet 1989; 1:1036–1038.
47. Sharp JT. Assessment of radiographic abnormalities in rheumatoid arthritis: what have we accomplished and where should we go from here? J Rheumatol 1995; 22:1787–1791.
48. Larsen A. How to apply Larsen Score in evaluating radiographs of rheumatoid arthritis in longterm studies? J Rheumatol 1995; 22:1974–1975.
49. Pincus T, Callahan LF, Fuchs HA, Larsen A, Kaye J. Quantitative analysis of hand radiographs in rheumatoid arthritis: time course of radiographic changes, relation to joint examination measures, and comparison of different scoring methods. J Rheumatol 1995; 22:1983–1989.
50. Weissman BNW. Imaging techniques in RA. J Rheumatol 1994; 21(Suppl 42):14–19.
51. Gough AKS, Lilley J, Eyre S, Holder RL, Emery P. Generalised bone loss in patients with early rheumatoid arthritis. Lancet 1994; 334:23–27.
52. Deodhar AA, Brabyn J, Jones PW, Davis MJ, Woolf AD. Measurement of hand bone mineral content by dual energy x-ray absorptiometry: development of the method, and its application in normal volunteers and in patients with rheumatoid arthritis. Ann Rheum Dis 1994; 53:685–690.
53. Boers M, Tugwell P. The validity of pooled outcome measures (indices) in rheumatoid arthritis clinical trials. J Rheumatol 1993; 20:568–574.
54. Lansbury A. A method for summation of the systemic indices of rheumatoid activity. Am J Med Sci 1956; 232:300–310.
55. van der Heijde DMFM, van 't Hof MA, van Riel PLCM, van de Putte LBA. Development of a disease activity score based on judgment in clinical practice by rheumatologists. J Rheumatol 1993; 20:579–581.
56. Prevoo MLL, van 't Hof MA, Kuper HH, van Leeuwen MA, van de Putte LBA, van Riel PLCM. Modified disease activity scores that include twenty-eight-joint counts. Arthritis Rheum 1995; 38:44–48.
57. Fuchs HA. The use of the disease activity score in the analysis of clinical trials in rheumatoid arthritis. J Rheumatol 1993; 20:1863–1866.
58. Mallya RK, Mace BEW. The assessment of disease activity in rheumatoid arthritis using a multivariate analysis. Rheumatol Rehab 1981; 20:14–17.
59. van Riel PLCM, Reekers P, van de Putte LBA, Gribnau FWJ. Association of HLA antigens, toxic reactions and therapeutic response to auranofin and aurothioglucose in patients with rheumatoid arthritis. Tissue Antigens 1983; 22:194–199.
60. Corkill M, Kirkham BW, Chikanza IC, Gibson T, Panayi GS. Intramuscular depot methylprednisolone induction of chrysotherapy in rheumatoid arthritis: a 24-week randomized controlled trial. Br J rheumatol 1990; 29:274–279.
61. Davis MJ, Dawes PT, Fowler PD, et al. Comparison and evaluation of a disease activity index for use in patients with rheumatoid arthritis. Br J Rheumatol 1990; 29:111–115.
62. Pinals RS, Masi AT, Larsen RA. Preliminary criteria for remission in rheumatoid arthritis. Arthritis Rheum 1981; 24:1308–1315.
63. Smythe HA, Helewa A, Goldsmith CH. "Independent assessor" and "pooled index" as techniques for measuring treatment effects in rheumatoid arthritis. J Rheumatol 1977; 4:144–152.
64. Paulus HE, Egger MJ, Ward JR, Williams HJ, CSSRD. Analysis of improvement in individual rheumatoid arthritis patients treated with disease-modifying antirheumatic drugs, based on the findings in patients treated with placebo. Arthritis Rheum 1990; 33:477–484.
65. van Gestel AM, Prevoo MLL, van 't Hof MA, van Rijswijk MH, van de Putte LBA, van Riel PLCM. Development and validation of the European League Against Rheumatism response criteria for rheumatoid arthritis. Comparison with the preliminary American College

of Rheumatology and theWorld Health Organization/International League of Associations for Rheumatology criteria. Arthritis Rheum 1996; 39:34–40.
66. Scott DL. A simple index to assess disease activity in RA. J Rheumatol 1993; 20:582–584.
67. Stucki G, Liang MH, Stucki S, Bruhlmann P, Michel BA. A self-administered Rheumatoid Arthritis Disease Activity Index (RADAI) for epidemiological research: psychometric properties and correlatiobn with parameters of disease activity. Arthritis Rheum 1995; 38:795–798.
68. Stucki G, Stucki S, Bruhlmann P, Maus S, Michel BA. Comparison of the validity and reliability of self-reported articular indices. Br J Rheumatol 1995; 34:760–766.
69. Prevoo MLL, Kuper HH, Hof van 't MA, Leeuwen van MA, Putte van de LBA, Riel van PLCM. Validity and reproducibility of self-administered joint counts. A large prospective longitudinal followup study in patients with rheumatoid arthritis. J Rheumatol 1996; 23:841–845.

SELECTED READING

Proceedings 5th Joint World Health Organization and International League of Associations for Rheumatology Task Force Meeting on Rheumatic Diseases. J Rheumatol 1994; 21(Suppl 41).

Conference on Outcome Measures in Rheumatoid Arthritis Clinical Trials. J Rheumatol 1993; 20:525–591.

Outcome measures in rheumatoid arthritis. Proceedings of a Satellite Symposium 57th American College on Rheumatology National Symposium. J Rheumatol 1994; 21(suppl 42).

3

Prognostic Markers for Rheumatoid Arthritis

Michael J. Green, Charles Richardson, and Paul Emery
University of Leeds, Leeds, United Kingdom

I. INTRODUCTION

A. Disease Outcome

The disease course of patients with rheumatoid arthritis (RA) is a variable one with a wide spectrum of clinical features and differences in the rates of progression. It has proven difficult to define accurately the outcome in patients with RA, and consequently the task of evaluating potential prognostic markers is complicated.

Radiological assessments are frequently used as a "gold standard" against which other outcome measures are compared. The endpoint is usually the progression of radiological erosions which themselves are relatively easy to see and diagnose and do not fluctuate with disease activity. As such, they provide a permanent record for the serial evaluation of disease progression. A number of scoring systems have been developed for the assessment of radiological erosions and cartilage loss, but it is important to note that the extent of change in the individual does not always correlate with patient function or current disease activity (i.e., the changes are historical and may not give an accurate description of what is happening at that particular moment).

The presence of erosions has been used as a prognostic marker, but there are a number of objections to this. First, erosions are a relatively late phenomenon in the disease process and are seen in less than 40% of cases of "early RA." Second, there are problems in their quantification, as demonstrated by the large interobserver and intraobserver variability in the measurement erosions. It may be possible to overcome some of these problems by using ultrasound and MRI imaging to identify erosions, but these techniques must currently be regarded as experimental. Finally, it must not be forgotten that erosions are an interpretation of the two-dimensional appearance of a three-dimensional event (essentially one is trying to identify holes in the bony cortex viewed two dimensionally).

The presence of erosions at onset of the disease has been associated with a poor outcome. This is hardly surprising, as they are an endproduct of joint damage brought about by established invasive pannus. The presence of such erosive damage can be quite asymptomatic. As the major costs of arthritis are associated with a loss of function, there is greater logic for using functional changes as the primary outcome measure. With time, it is likely that quality of life measures will partly replace the functional scores. Currently, these last two assessments have not been adequately used in long-term studies. Although after many years, in patients with severe disease, poor function and radiological change are correlated. In early disease, there may be a divergence between radiological change and functional loss. As will be seen later, the functional status is determined much more by subjective factors, whereas the radiological erosions correlate with the inflammatory markers. A further distinction has been made between process measures and outcome measures, with the difference being that the former reflects acute changes, whereas the latter represents the effect of cumulative damage. Thus, commonly employed measures of outcome used in clinical practice are joint counts (which is also a process measure), measurements of functional capacity, assessments of morbidity (e.g., admissions to hospital), health economic assessments, laboratory markers of the acute phase response; and the progression of radiological change.

B. Why Measure Prognostic Markers?

Untreated RA has a bad prognosis. Currently employed therapies have demonstrated evidence of short-term benefit but long-term data are lacking. The tendency to introduce disease-modifying drugs only in established (erosive) disease, which is much less likely to produce a profound effect on outcome, may have been contributory to this poor long-term result. Prognostic markers present at the disease onset which can correctly identify patients at risk of progressive destructive disease would have enormous clinical value, enabling the targeting of intensive therapy to those at most risk, whereas avoiding potentially toxic therapy for those patients with a good prognosis. At present, there is no prognostic marker capable of performing this function perfectly. In this chapter, we discuss the markers currently used to give prognostic information, and we have chosen to address the problem from a pathogenic point of view. A major problem in predicting prognosis relates to the early diagnosis of RA. The essential features of RA which one needs to diagnose early are its chronicity and progression; clearly on clinical grounds this is not possible without predictive indicators. A realistic analogy of this situation is with that in oncology where one has to diagnose a malignant potential usually by a mixture of physical signs and histology. In our experience of early arthritis patients, we have found it more helpful to establish initially whether disease will be persistent (equivalent to RA) and then subsequently stage the patient for the severity markers, and it is for this latter function that the prognostic markers are currently used.

C. Currently Employed Prognostic Markers

Rheumatoid arthritis is associated with an array of abnormalities measurable in the laboratory. Correlations between clinical features and several of these abnormalities have been demonstrated. Some appear to act as markers of disease activity only and others give prognostic information.

In general, prognostic markers can be divided into *quantitative* and *qualitative*. The former are more suitable for monitoring disease activity and are a consequence of systemic disease which itself is attributable to proinflammatory cytokines, whereas the latter are independent of disease activity and as such can be employed in early disease. The markers most commonly used are summarized in Tables 1–4.

An ideal prognostic marker would have the following characteristics:

1. Present at onset
2. Independent of disease stage and activity
3. Sensitive and specific
4. Straightforward and inexpensive to assay

II. QUANTITATIVE PROGNOSTIC MARKERS

Quantitative markers are present in *all* patients with sufficiently extensive RA. Quantitative markers cannot routinely be used for prognostic purposes in early disease, and they are frequently not of prognostic use, because they are not present in the majority of patients at presentation, probably because of insufficient disease mass. These quantitative markers are believed to be secondary to the effect of elevated systemic concentrations of proinflammatory cytokines which themselves are produced in the synovium and released into the circulation with effects on the liver, bone marrow, and brain. As a consequence, these markers are a reflection of disease activity and/or process. The systemic concentrations of these markers can be profoundly and rapidly altered by factors such as steroids and, more specifically, anticytokines. This potential variation in their concentration must be considered when such markers are being used for prognosis. Serial measurements may provide more reliable prognostic information, but the time taken to acquire them is an obvious disadvantage.

A. The Acute Phase Response

The term *acute phase response* is used to describe the complex series of local and systemic events which accompany tissue inflammation. The local events consist of vasodilatation, cellular infiltration, and generation of lysosomal enzymes, kinins, and oxygen free radicals. The systemic events consist of fever, alterations of "middle 66" metabolism, activation of the hypothalamo-pituitary-adrenal axis, and the hepatic synthesis of the acute phase proteins. The proinflammatory cytokines interleukin 1 (IL-1), interleukin 6 (IL-6), and tumor necrosis factor-α (TNF-α) are central to the development of the acute phase response. The cytokines (IL-6 in particular) stimulate the hepatic synthesis of the acute phase proteins, the measurement of which can be used to quantify the acute phase response [1,2] and hence the magnitude of synovial inflammation. The acute phase proteins most commonly measured are the C-reactive protein (CRP) and fibrinogen levels (measured indirectly as the erythrocyte sedimentation rate [ESR], and plasma viscosity). The measurement of cytokines themselves provides no significant advantage over the measurement of CRP, which as a cumulative measure has proven to be more sensitive and more accurate.

1. C-Reactive Protein

The precise physiological role of CRP is not known, although based on the results of in vitro experiments, it probably has a role in host defense. It binds to C-polysaccha-

Table 1 Four Star Cohort Studies

Study	Sample size	Disease duration	Study duration	Outcome measure	Prognostic factors examined	Conclusions
Van Leeuwen et al., (a) 1993 (8) and (b) 1995 (45)	(a)149 (b) 110	<1 year	3 years	(a) Radiographs every 6 months (b) Radiographs initially and at 3 years	(a) Serial CRP monthly (stratified for HLA, RF, age, and sex) (b) RF isotypes initially and throughout 3 years HLA	(a) Serial CRP level correlates well with outcome. (b) Each isotype titer at entry correlated with radiological progression. Serial level of IgM titer is predictor of outcome. No added significance of IgG or IgA serial titers. HLA-DR4 not predictive.
Gough et al., 1994 (29)	120 (ACR criteria) and healthy controls	Mean 7.4 months	1 year	Radiographs at 0 abd 12 months	HLA status	HLA-DR4 and particularly Dw4/Dw14 predicts the development of erosive disease.
van der Heijde, 1992 (46)	147	<1 year	2 years	Disability Radiographs 6 monthly	Clinical and laboratory markers of disease, including RF, CRP, HLA, JC, nods	Disability: No relevant predictor. Radiographs: damage predicted by APR combined with DR2/DR4 and RF.
Young et al. 1988 (23)	149	<1 year	3 years	Radiographs initially and then 12 monthly	Clinical and laboratory markers of disease, including DD, JC, RF, CRP, HLA	RF is strongest predictor of radiographic progression. HLA Dw2 and B7 linked to subluxation of the cervical spine.
Kaarela, 1985 (47)	200	<6 months	6–9 years Mean 7.6 years	Radiographs Function Clinical	Clinical and lab markers, including DO, D of J, Age, Sex, JC, CRP, RF, HLA	Symmetrical, peripheral joint disease strongest predictors.

Table 2 Three Star Cohort Studies

Study	Sample size	Disease duration	Study duration	Outcome measure	Prognostic factors	Conclusions
van der Heide, 1995 (48)	128	< 1 year	12 months	Radiographs at 0 and 12 months	Clinical and lab markers	Radiographic damage, RF at baseline and persistent high JC are predictive factors.
van Zeben et al. 1991 (49)	222	< 5 years Mean of 1.4 years	2 years	Clinical function and radiograph	HLA status	HLA-DR4 predictive of more severe disease and radiographic damage.
van Zeben et al. 1993 (50)	132	< 5 years Mean 1.4 years	Mean 6 years	Clinical function and radiograph	Clinical and lab markers, including RF isotypes, HLA, agalact	JC, RF, HAQ, IgG or IgM HLA-DR4 and elevated agalact best predictors of some of the outcome measures.
Luukkainen et al. 1983 (51)	107	6 months	3 years	Radiographs initially and 3 years	Clinical and lab markers, including orosmucoid, ANA, RF, function, radiographs	Early radiographic changes best predictive factor. Grip, ESR, serum iron, C1 esterase level, RF, and old age also had prognostic value.
Mottonen, 1988 (52)	58	< 2 years Mean 8 months	2 years	Radiographs initially and 6 monthly	Clinical and lab markers	Swelling better than tenderness in predicting erosions. Tenosynovitis predicted erosion extent. ESR better than CRP or Hb. HLA DR4 and RF were not predictive.
Combe et al., 1995 (53)	94	< 12 months Mean of 7.8 months	Mean 8.1 years	Radiographs initially and at the study end	Clinical and lab markers, including syst disease, CRP, ESR, HLA, Anti-ker, Anti-RA33	ESR, CRP, plts, and low Hb at onset were predictors of severe disease progress. RF titer and IgG isotype were predictive. HLA-DR4/1 strongly linked to severity.

(*continued*)

Table 2 Continued

Study	Sample size	Disease duration	Study duration	Outcome measure	Prognostic factors	Conclusions
Emery et al. 1992 (54)	49 with early symmetrical arthritis (i.e., RA like)	Mean 12.9 weeks	48 weeks	Clinical lab raiographs at 0, 3, 6, 12, and 48 weeks	HLA and DRB1, hypervariable region, Sulf capacity and RF	Individually all predicted progression of disease. Together they demonstrated a strong relative risk of disease persistence.
de Vries et al. 1993 (55)	118	<1 year	3 years	Radiographs initially and at 3 years	TCR-Vβ8	Allele polymorphism is NOT associated with prevalence. BUT is predictive of disease progression.
Flemming et al., 1976 (56)	102	<1 year	4.5 years	Radiographs annually clinical, function	Distribution of involved joints, age, type of onset, radiographic and lab markers	Initial large joint and 1–3 MTP involvement insidious onset, rapid progression to symmetrical disease, older age, RF, and erosions predictive of more severe disease.
Desiree et al. 1991 (57)	147	<1 year	2 years	Clinical, radiographs, and lab	Age <60 years	More severe disease course in the older age group.

Table 3 Two Star Cohort Studies

Study	Sample size	Disease duration	Study duration	Outcome measure	Prognostic factors	Conclusions
Fleming et al., 1976 (58)	102	< 1 year	Mean 4.5 years	Function, clinical	Clinical and lab	Age, grip, JC, wrist/MTP involvement, function, number of ARA criteria, ESR, Hb, urea, RF, erosions at presentation were predictive.
Dawes et al., 1994 (59)	65	Mean 11.7 months	8 years	Radiographs	Erosions at presentation	Progression of erosions over first year is moderate predictor.
Salmon et al., 1992 (60)	65 Symmetrical polyarthritis	< 5 months	4 years	ARA criteria at outcome.	HLA-DR status	DR4 and DR1 predict persistence but not disease initiation
Sjoblom et al., 1984 (61)	103	Median 12 years	2 years	Radiographs	Clinical and lab, including A1-AT, Cer, oroso, and IgG's	CRP, haptoglobins were predictive. IgM negatively correlated. Early deterioration correlated with IgM, hapt, JC, Hb.
van Zeben, 1993 (26)	135 (Women only)	< 5 years	Mean of 6 years	Clinical, radiographs yearly	Original and serial RF isotypes	Persistent RF and titer in the first 3 years (particularly the IgA level) predicted severity.
Teittsson et al., 1984 (30)	33	< 1 year	2–4 years	Radiographs yearly	RF isotype at presentation	IgA RF in early disease predicts severity.
van Schaardenburg et al., 1993 (27)	130	Not stated	Mean 5.6 years	Function, mortality, radiographs	RF age > 60	Age predicted function. RF predicted severity and mortality. RF more significant in older age group.

(continued)

Table 3 Continued

Study	Sample size	Disease duration	Study duration	Outcome measure	Prognostic factors	Conclusions
Mau et al., 1996 (62)	109 ARA > 5	12 months	Mean 6 years	Work and function	Sex, RF, radiographs, employment, status, function, JC, ESR,	Age >50 and ESR > 60 or longest DD and function predict employment prospect at 3 years.
Eberhadt et al., 1995 (63)	63	1 year	5 years	HAQ initially and at 5 years	HAQ at presentation	No significant change in HAQ at 5 years.
J Devlin et al 1996 (9)	109	<1 year	2 years	HAQ 6 monthly	Suppression of CRP over 2 years	Suppression of CRP predicts improvement.
Corbett et al., 1993 (25)	102	Not stated	Mean 15.2 years	Mortality, disability	Nods, RF, erosions, cervical subluxation, body mass	Age, Hb, body mass, ESR, urea predict mortality. Grip, cervical subluxation JC > 12, erosions at 2 years predict disability.
Pincus et al., 1994 (64)	75	Mean 11.2 years	15 years	Mortality	Clinical and questionnaires on activities of daily living	Simple questionnaires and joint counts can predict mortality.
Michel et al., 1991 (65)	395	Not stated	Mean 6.7 years	Time lapse to first fracture.	Sex, previous osteo-porosis, HAQ, steroid dose	Female sex, previous history of osteoporosis >5 mg prednisolone predict early fracture.
Silman et al., 1986 (41)	59	<18 months	3 years	Function, VAS, wrist extension	HLA-DR4 status, RF	RF predicts severity. DR4 status does not predict poor prognosis.

Table 4 One Star Plus Miscellaneous Studies

Predictive measure	Study	Sample size	Disease duration	Study duration	Outcome measure	Prognostic factors	Conclusions
One star	Eberhardt et al., 1988 (R66)	71	<2 years	At least 2 years	Radiographs, clinical	RF isotypes	No significant correlations.
	Westedt et al., 1985 (67)	57	30 <1 year; 25 >2 years	1 year	Radiographs, clinical, systemic disease	RF isotypes, immune complexes	No significant correlation. Early patients with a raised serum IgA IC developed erosions earlier.
	Leigh et al., 1992 (68)	330	Not stated	8 years	HAQ at 0 + 8 years	HAQ at presentation	HAQ predicts future disease and function.
Cross-sectional	Reeback et al., 1984 (69)	72	18 months	2 years	HAQ, wrist extension	Clinical and lab	HAQ and JC predict poor outcome.
	Brennan et al., 1996 (70)	175	6 months	Assessed after 12 months	Radiograph	Clinical and lab B1	RF, DD>3 months, male sex, >2 large joints
	Toda et al., 1994 (71)	160	Median 8 years	5 years	Radiograph	HLA-DR β1 allele	Homozygous state predicts poor prognosis. Alleles appear to act recessively.
	Moreno et al., 1996 (72)	90 patients	At least 3 years	Cross sectional	Radiograph, clinical	HLA DR4 and DR1	Shared epitope is strong predictor.
	Wollheim et al., 1988 (73)	96	Median 12 years	Cross sectional	One off radiographs	Clinical and lab	DD strongest predictive factor. Also CRP and IgM RF. Sex, IgG, IgA, RF not predictive.
	de Carvalho et al., 1980 (74)	188	Not stated	3–12 years cross sectional	Radiograph taken at varying points of disease duration	Clinical such as nods. Laboratory markers such as ANA, RF, ESR	Nodules not linked to more severe disease progression. ESR, ANA and ESR appear to be indicators of more advanced disease

(*continued*)

Table 4 Continued

Predictive measure	Study	Sample size	Disease duration	Study duration	Outcome measure	Prognostic factors	Conclusions
Sulphoxidation	Emery et al., 1992 (28)	54	Not stated	1 and 4 years	Clinical	Sulf status	Poor sulf. status predicts persistence
Bone	Gough et al., 1994 (19)	62	<1 year	1 year	Clinical, lab BMD	Pyridinoline and deoxypyridinolone	Collagen cross links correlate with disease activity, loss of BMD but not function.
Cartilage	Wollheim et al., 1995 (17)	18	<2 years	6 years	Hip replacements	COMP level	Early COMP level predicts joint destruction.
	Mansson et al., 1994 (75)	18	"Early RA"	Up to 4 years	Early hip erosions	COMP, CPII, BSP, 846	Cartilage-derived macromolecules may be of value in predicting disease progression.
Agalactosyl IgG	van Zeben et al., 1992 (32)	127 females	<5 years	2 years	Clinical, radiographs yearly	Agalactolysation of IgG	Agalactolysation of IgG elevated in RA at diagnosis and predicts severity.
	Young et al., 1991 (33)	60 early synovitis	<12 months	2 years	Clinical, function	Agalactolysation of IgG, RF	RF and level of agalactolysation of IgG at presentation predicts development of RA.
Antikeratin antibodies	Paimela et al., 1992 (76)	71	<1 year	2 years	Clinical, laboratory, radiographs	Antikeratin antibodies	Fluctuance anti-ker related to disease activity. It may have prognostic significance.
Bone marrow stromal cell	Lee et al., 1996 (77)	143	Not stated	Cross sectional	Clinical	Serum level of BST-1	All patients with a high level of BST-1 had severe disease. May be prognostic.

Abbreviations: A1-AT, alpha$_1$-antitrypsin level; agalact IgG, % agalactolization of IgG; Alb, albumin; ANA, antinuclear factor; Anti-ker, anti-keratin antiboides; anti-peri, antiperinuclear antibodies; Anti- RA33, antirheumatoid arthritis antibody 33; ASM, anti–smooth muscle antibodies; BSP, bone sialoprotein; BST-1, bone marrow stromal cell antigen - 1; C, propeptide; Cer, ceruloplasmin; COMP, cartilage oligomeric matrix; CPII, type II procollagen; CRP, C-reactive protein; Cu, serum copper; D of J, distribution of joints; DD, duration of disease; DO, disease onset; educ; education; EMS, early morning stiffness; ESR, erythrocyte sedimentation rate; FH, family history; HAQ, Health Assessment Questionnaire; Hb, hemoglobin; H/crit, hematocrit; HLA, human lymphocyte antigen; IgG, immunoglbulin; JC, joint counts; Jsurg, joint surgery; nods, subcutaneous nodules; oroso, orosomucoid; RF, rheumatoid factor; sulf, sulfoxidation; syst, systemic; Syst, systemic symptoms; teno, tenosynovitis; VAS, visual analogue scale; WS, walking speed; 846, the chondroitin sulfate epitope.

rides in the cell wall of many bacteria, fungi, and parasites evoking a number of secondary effects, including precipitation and complement fixation. Serum amyloid A protein, a similar acute phase protein, is of interest because it is the precursor of type AA amyloid fibrils. However, it is poorly immunogenic and assays are less readily available.

The CRP level is generally accepted as the most accurate measure of the acute phase response and hence of tissue inflammation. In the normal individual, the basal concentration is extremely low or undetectable. In response to inflammation, CRP can rapidly increase up to 1000-fold. Importantly, even at these high concentrations, CRP can still be accurately quantified and the rate of catabolism remains constant. Therefore, the major determinant of the plasma concentration is the rate of synthesis. The CRP level is not affected by any of the confounding factors which influence the ESR and viscosity (see below). These features make it the best measurement available for the monitoring of therapy in the rheumatic diseases.

As a prognostic marker, CRP has the following limitations: elevation in the CRP level (and the acute phase response in general) is nonspecific and can only be interpreted in the light of appropriate clinical information; the CRP is rapidly suppressed in response to steroid therapy when given intra-articularly [2a]; there is a significant interpatient variation in the CRP response to a given stimulus, as such isolated values must be interpreted with caution; a patient's CRP concentration can increase many times from the basal level and still lie within the normal range while being markedly abnormal for that individual. These factors make it a good marker of disease activity but limit its suitability as a prognostic marker.

2. *ESR*

The ESR is an indirect measure of the acute phase response. It is a measure of the rate of sedimentation of erythrocytes in a vertical tube over a standard period of 1 hr. The rate of erythrocyte sedimentation is determined by the negative electrical charge on the erythrocyte surface which prevents aggregation. Certain plasma proteins (in particular fibrinogen) decrease this negative charge and hence increase aggregation and sedimentation. The approximate contribution of the plasma proteins to the ESR are fibrinogen, 55%; α_2-macroglobulin, 27%; immunogobulin, 11%; and albumin, 7% [2]. The aggregation of erythrocytes is also influenced by their number, shape, and deformibility, such that the ESR has an inverse relationship with hematocrit. Because the ESR predominantly reflects changes in the fibrinogen concentration, there is a lag phase between the onset (or resolution) of *any* inflammatory stimuli and a change in the ESR. As the ESR reflects changes in several acute phase reactants (as well as immunoglobulins), it provides a wider screen for the detection of inflammatory disease than the CRP level. The advantages of the ESR are its sensitivity, ease of performance, low cost, and familiarity. Its disadvantages of the low specificity, interobserver variation in measurement, and the wide range of other factors which will affect it. It can be seen that the ESR, with its sensitivity, is an ideal screening test for inflammatory disease, whereas the CRP level is well suited for monitoring, although both have similar limitations as prognostic markers.

3. *Plasma Viscosity*

The plasma viscosity, like the ESR, is predominantly determined by the fibrinogen concentration. It has the same kinetics in response to inflammation as the ESR but has the advantage of being independent of age and RBC concentration and morphology. In addition, the test can be automated and performed on stored samples. However, by not being affected by anemia, it is less sensitive than the ESR as a screening test for inflammatory disease.

4. Use of the Acute Phase Response in the Management/Outcome of RA

The acute phase proteins have been used clinically for the assessment of disease activity and the response to therapy for many years with isolated readings reflecting the current state of disease activity. It should be remembered that the acute phase response is a dynamic process, and a single CRP or ESR reading provides only a "snapshot" of ongoing systemic inflammatory processes. Serial measurements provide a better indication about the true magnitude of "systemic disease/inflammation."

A number of studies have reported that a persistently elevated acute phase response is associated with an increased rate of radiological progression compared with those with a normal ESR and CRP level [3–5]. In addition, a fall in the CRP level in response to second line therapy represents the first objective sign of clinical improvement [6]. Furthermore, the development of generalized osteoporosis in early RA was shown to be significantly correlated with a persistently elevated CRP level [7]. It has been argued that using time-integrated values of serial CRP measurements (i.e., area under the curve) is the most accurate method to quantify the fluctuating activity of the acute phase response.

In a study of 110 patients with RA, van Leeuwen et al., (8) reported a significant correlation between the time-integrated CRP and the rate of radiological progression over 3 years and used this relationship to predict subsequent radiological progression. Indeed it has been shown that with a line time-shift analysis that the best correlation has been the CRP values 3 months earlier. Thus, the reason a quantitative measure is predictive of outcome is because the outcome measure provides a delayed readout. It can be argued that a limitation to the use of CRP as a predictive factor is that it represents a "self-fulfilling" prognosis; that is, patients with a large disease bulk have an elevated acute phase response, and therefore it is not surprising that their outcome is poor. In the future, serial CRP values may prove to be a marker of "change in prognosis"; however, this needs to be established in clinical practice.

Recent data have shown that in early disease there is a good correlation between acute phase response and functional outcome in that over 100 patients followed from onset with elevated CRP levels have shown a close correlation between initial changes in the CRP levels and improvement in function. Furthermore, in patients who normalized their CRP levels, there was no further functional deterioration for the next 2 years (9).

B. Hematology Investigations

1. Hemoglobin

Anemia is the most common extra-articular manifestation of RA. The causes of the anemia in RA are multiple, although the most important is the anemia of chronic disease (ACD) [10,11]. In RA, the ACD develops within 1–2 months of the onset of systemic disease. The anemia is generally mild, with the hemoglobin concentration rarely falling below 10 g/dL, and it fluctuates with the disease course and correlates with the magnitude of the acute phase response. The etiology of the anemia of chronic disease is multifactorial and not fully understood. The proinflammatory cytokines IL-1, IL-6, and TNF-α appear central in its pathogenesis. The following mechanisms may be relevant to the development of anemia: inhibition of erythropoietin production [12], inhibition of erythropoiesis [13,14], shortened RBC survival [15], and enhanced reticuloendothelial retention of iron.

There is a correlation between the CRP level and the percentage of patients with anemia, but the degree of anemia does not become severe until the CRP is markedly elevated. The erythrocyte half-life of 120 days and the many other causes of anemia in RA make the Hb value too difficult to interpret in an individual patient for it to be used as a disease activity or prognostic marker. Indeed in clinical practice, rather than the Hb being used to monitor disease, activity, the more common problems encountered is whether the magnitude of the patient's acute phase response (measured by CRP level) is sufficient to account for their anemia or are others causes responsible.

A low hemoglobin level at presentation has been associated with a poor prognosis in a number of clinical series, but again it does not provide a good prognostic marker, because it is a product of "disease bulk" and arguably has more limitations than using the acute phase response as a predictive marker.

C. Bone and Cartilage

There are a number of direct and indirect measures of the effect of rheumatoid disease on bone which can be used quantitatively. The most direct measure is the biochemical assessment of the products of cartilage and bone metabolism as found in the synovial fluid, serum, and urine. A second measure, the radiological erosion, represents the consequence of established severe rheumatoid disease. Finally, the development of accurate bone densitometry has provided a method to assess bone loss both locally, at the disease site, and systematically from the axial and apendicular skeleton.

1. Markers of Bone and Collagen Breakdown

An accurate quantitative marker of bone and cartilage breakdown should be a useful tool for monitoring disease activity and prognosis in RA. The primary pathological event in RA is probably an inflammatory synovitis, therefore, it is only with disease extension that bone and cartilage become involved. Recent advances in the understanding of bone and cartilage physiology and composition have opened up a new field of research evaluating the use of tests for tissue-derived molecules in body fluids as markers of diseased joint structures.

Cartilage and bone components appearing in the synovial fluid are cleared by lymphatic drainage. In the circulation, they are taken up by the liver and excreted in the urine and feces. Therefore, the serum concentration may be only a small percentage of that seen in the synovial fluid. Interpretation of serum levels is further complicated by an inability to distinguish between the influence of catabolic and synthetic changes. Elevated levels may result from either "overflow" from increased synthesis or increased release due to accelerated tissue catabolism. The ideal marker should be tissue specific, not metabolized before its measurement in the serum or urine, and specific for anabolic or catabolic processes.

2. Markers of Cartilage Breakdown

Cartilage Collagen-derived Fragments. At least 16 genetically distinct collagens are recognized, but 4 alone (types II, IX, X, and XI) are cartilage specific and thus potentially useful markers of cartilage damage [16]. The most widely available measurement of collagen II breakdown has been the urinary hydroxyproline concentration. Hydroxypropline is an amino acid mainly found in collagen where it stabilizes the triple helix of the collagen molecule. However, it lacks specificity, being found in many tissues, complement factor C1q, and food.

Aggrecan and Aggrecan Epitopes. Aggrecans are tissue specific, abundant, and have a rapid turnover, and theoretically they should be excellent markers of cartilage damage. However, serum concentrations of aggrecans are of limited value owing to their rapid clearance from the circulation and lymph node metabolism. Levels of aggrecans in synovial fluid correlate with cartilage destruction but have the inherent disadvantage of requiring joint aspiration [17].

Noncollagenous Cartilage Proteins. Many matrix proteins have been characterized within cartilage. Of these, cartilage oligomeric matrix protein (COMP) appears to be a promising marker of cartilage damage. The physiological role of COMP is not known, although it is believed to be involved in cartilage repair. High COMP release in early disease predicts rapidly progressive destruction in RA. [17].

3. Markers of Bone Turnover

Bone loss occurs in two forms in RA. Periarticular osteoporosis represents local disease, whereas axial and appendicular osteoporosis is a consequence of systemic inflammatory disease.

Osteocalcin. The concentration of osteocalcin has been shown to correlate with the rate of bone formation [17]. In addition, it is reduced in steroid-induced osteoporosis [18]. However, in RA, it has not been possible to demonstrate a consistent level of osteocalcin either in the synovium or serum and any value as a disease marker has yet to be defined.

Collagen Cross Links (Pyridinolines). The 3-hydroxypyridinium compounds (pyridinoline and deoxypyridinoline) are the maturation products of intermediate ketoamine cross links formed between mature collagen fibrils. Cross links form between mature collagen fibrils, and on breakdown of the collagen, are released in peptides which can be further broken down to the free pyridinolines. Pyridinoline is found in both types I (bone) and II (cartilage) collagen, whereas deoxypyridinoline is found mainly in type I collagen and consequently provides a better marker of bone breakdown. However, the relationship between the two cross links in urine is similar, indicating that the major contributor is probably bone [18].

A timed urine collection is required for accurate quantification of 3-hydroxypyridium compound production, because there is considerable variation in their rate of excretion. In early RA, an increased rate of cross link excretion has been reported that correlated with the development of axial skeleton osteoporosis [19].

Collagen Synthesis. Collagen synthesis can be measured by assaying its C-terminal propeptide (PIICP or chondrocalcin) in serum or synovial fluid [20]. This has not been established as a disease marker in RA.

4. *Markers of Synovitis*

The N-terminal collagen III propeptide and serum hyaluronan have been used to quantify the amount of synovitis present in early disease. The value of this as a marker of disease activity is not known.

In summary, these bone markers appear to be reflections of disease activity. Their role as markers of disease activity have not yet been fully defined much less their potential role as prognostic markers.

III. QUALITATIVE PROGNOSTIC MARKERS

A. Antibody-Related Abnormalities

There are three major antibody-related abnormalities that have been thought to be of etiological importance in rheumatoid arthritis.

1. *Rheumatoid Factors*

Rheumatoid factors (RFs) are antibodies directed against antigenic components on the Fc fragment of immunoglobulin G (IgG). In RA, the rheumatoid factor is polyclonal, reacting with a wide range of determinants on both the CH_2 and CH_3 domains of IgG. It is found in all classes of immunoglobulin. The classic RF is an IgM molecule detected by the agglutination or flocculation of IgG-coated cells or particles. Of all the tests described, it is the one that comes closest to being diagnostic, although it is not specific for RA, being found in other connective tissue diseases, transiently during some infections, and in up to 15% of the population aged more than 65 years [21]. It is present in 75% of patients with RA using a cutoff level for positivity which excludes 95% of the normal population.

A number of investigators have reported that RF either alone or in combination with other predictive markers is a clinically useful method of identifying patients with a poor prognosis. Woolf et al. [22] followed up a cohort of 100 patients with early RA for 5 years. They reported that RF positivity at onset of symptoms was associated with a more severe disease course. As a predictive marker of persistent disease, it had a specificity and sensitivity of 83 and 24%, respectively.

In a prospective study of 133 patients presenting with early RA, Young et al. [23] reported that a high RF, low Hb, and elevated platelet count were the most powerful predictors for the development of erosive change during a 3-year follow-up, with these same factors being preditive of the severity of erosions at 10 years [24]. After a further 5-year follow-up, RF positivity (within 2 years of presentation) was the best serological predictor of functional outcome [25]. Other investigators have reported similar results [26]. Van Schardenburg et al. [27] performed a retrospective study to investigate the effect of age (under age 60 vs over age 60) on outcome after 5 years of disease. At final evaluation, seropositive patients (of both age groups) had suffered significantly more disease activity and radiographic damage than those who were seronegative for RF. The amount of radiological progression was similar in seropositive patients in both age groups, although the functional outcome was worse in the over age 60 group indicating reduced functional reserves. The mortality of the seropositive patients (but not seronegative) was higher than in the general population. Strikingly, the relative risk of dying was six times greater in the seropositive patients than the seronegative patients.

Emery et al. [28] investigated the role of genetic factors in the development of erosions in RA to see if they could be used to predict outcome in early disease. They reported that of 49 patients presenting to an early arthritis clinic, 25 had developed erosions at 4 years. The relative risk of erosion development was 1.8 for RF seropositivity. Gough et al. [29] reported that RF seropositivity in early RA was associated with a relative risk for the development of erosions at 1 year of 13.49 (sensitivity 95%, specificity 39%).

These studies indicate that RF seropositivity at the onset of RA is associated with a more progressive disease course resulting in increased disability and radiological progression. In addition, it was possible to increase the predictive value of the RF by combining it with genetic markers (see below).

Since the introduction of isotype-specific assays for RF, a number of studies have been published concerning the clinical value of isotype analysis. All isotypes of RF have been shown to be associated with a more progressive disease course. However, IgA RF appears to be more specifically associated with the development of erosions in early disease and a persistent disease course [26,30,31].

In summary, the presence of rheumatoid factor in a patient with symmetrical small joint disease indicates persistent disease and poor prognosis, the essential hallmarks of RA; indeed it is one of the diagnostic criteria for the disease. However, the label of RA is perhaps less important than an accurate prognosis of future disability allowing accurate targeting of treatment. The major value of RF has been in the predicting of outcome and its association with a high frequency of systemic and extra-articular manifestations.

2. *Agalactosyl IgG*

Serum IgG from patients with RA contains an increased number of oligosaccharide moieties with outer arms which lack galactose (termed agalactosyl IgG) and terminate in N-acetylglucosamine. These imunoglobulins may be functionally deficient in their ability to bind to macrophage receptors and when a part of an immune complex may not be cleared fully. In a cohort of 127 female patients with RA followed up for 6 years, it was reported that those who had increased levels of agalactosyl IgG had significantly more disease activity and bony erosions and were treated with more second-line agents than those who did not [32]. In addition, it was reported that the combination of RF positivity and increased agalactosyl IgG levels gave a positive predictive value for the diagnosis of RA in 94% of patients presenting to an early synovitis clinic (33). Its disadvantage is that it is clearly a product of the overall disease activity and correlates with activity measures.

3. *Collagen Antibodies*

Antibodies directed against denatured and mature collagen type II are found in up to 30% of the rheumatoid patients in cross-sectional studies. This is a low frequency compared with disease-specific autoantibodies seen in other autoimmune diseases. However, inducing an immune response to type II collagen can produce arthritis in susceptible rats. Interestingly, a recent study has shown that the highest levels of native type II collagen antibodies were detected earliest in disease and there was an association with early erosive disease and the major histocompatibility complex (MHC)–associated disease epitope, suggesting that these antibodies may not be present merely as a result of cartilage destruction (34).

B. Sulfoxidation

Certain diseases involving specific tissue destruction, such as Parkinson's disease, are thought to be inducible by environmental contaminants. Such compounds, traditionally called xenobiotics, are normally metabolized in the liver by a range of detoxification enzymes. A failure or abnormality of one of these enzyme systems may predispose to disease. These detoxification enzymes are often polymorphic. Thus within a population, a subgroup will exist who have different enzyme activity from the rest: this difference may be tested for using a probe drug.

For sulfoxidation (S-oxidation), the probe drug S-carboxymethyl-L-cysteine was found to be handled in a defective fashion by about 33% of the population, whereas 2% showed no S-oxidation capacity at all [35]. Using this probe drug, a sulfur oxidation index (SI) was calculated defined as the percentage of sulfides divided by the percentage of sulfoxides in the urinary metabolites. The majority of the population have an SI ≥6. An original study demonstrated that 65% of RA patients have an impaired SI, 18% of whom were non–sulfur oxidizers. Interestingly, poor S oxidation is also associated with increased susceptibility to toxicity with D-pencillamine, and aurothiomalate therapy. The risk of toxicity to D-penicillamine was further increased in those patients who were HLA DR3 positive [36]. Thus, for D-penicillamine, the majority of severe reactions could be accounted for by the presence of either defective sulfur oxidation or HLA DR3. S oxidation status has been monitored before and after the introduction of second-line drugs and has been shown to be independent of disease activity and drug therapy [37].

It is now recognized that the probe drug is probably measuring the activity of the enzyme cysteine dioxygenase. This enzyme catalyses the rate-limiting conversion of cysteine to sulfate. Consistent with the defective S oxidation present seen in RA, the serum cysteine levels are significantly higher, and sulfate levels are consistently lower with a correlation between the cysteine to sulfate ratio and the SI index (38).

An association between poor S oxidation and erosive disease has been consistently demonstrated and represents a small but definite effect. This may be because a defective enzyme restricts the amount of sulfate available for repair of glycoaminoglycans. The availability of the purified enzyme and the identification of two enzyme isoforms should lead to a informative probe in the near future.

C. MHC

The association between rheumatoid arthritis and the HLA-DR locus has been long demonstrated [39]. Comparison of the amino acid sequences of RA associated and nonassociated subtypes of HLA-DR4 has revealed important differences. Those DR4 subtypes associated with RA show a striking conservation of the amino acid sequence in the third hypervariable region of the β chain. In addition, this highly conserved region has been demonstrated in non-DR4 alleles associated with RA and is termed the *disease epitope*.

In general terms, the prevalence of RA in the white population is 1%, and the disease epitope is found in 95% of patients with the disease and 45% of the total population. If the disease epitope is to be used simply as a marker in establishing the diagnosis of RA, it has a specificity of 56%, sensitivity of 95%, and a positive predictive value of 2.1%. Clearly, if used in isolation as a diagnostic test, it does not add greatly to the clinician's assessment. It should also be recognized that the so-called disease epitope represents MHC class II alleles (susceptibility genes) that have been positively selected by evolution. As such, they are physiological and not truly "disease genes." Therefore, it is not surprising that the penetrance of the rheumatoid phenotype is low.

In the heterozygous state, the disease epitope confers susceptibility, indicating that it has a dominant mode of action. However, when two disease epitopes are inherited together, this greatly increases the penetrance and severity of the ensuing disease.

Salmon [40] noted that, in some series, patients with early disease show little or no association with any HLA alleles. In addition, patients with severe forms of RA frequently possessed a double dose of the disease eptiopes, with a disproportionate tendency toward posession of different forms of the disease epitopes. Salmon argued that the shared epitope was only a marker for severity and chronicity of the disease process and not a marker of susceptibility. This important issue cannot be properly addressed until the diagnosis of RA becomes more than an application of syndromic criteria. In practical terms, what really matters is the identification of patients at risk of a destructive arthritis. The actual label that is attached to their disease is often of lesser importance. A number of reports have looked at the influence of the disease epitope on disease outcome and have given conflicting results.

Silman et al. [41] followed the progress of 59 patients with RA for 3 years. They found no evidence that the HLA status provided an indication of subsequent outcome nor that it predicted the response to therapy. Moens et al. [42] reported that HLA status was not useful in predicting the outcome of 111 consecutive rheumatoid patients treated with penicillamine and followed up for 7 to 9 years. Finally, Paimela et al. [43] found similar clinical improvements in HLA-DR4 positive and negative rheumatoid subjects followed for 3 years.

A number of more recent studies have not supported such a negative view. van Zeben [44] examined prognostic factors in a longitudinal study. She studied 132 females with RA of less than 60 months' duration and followed for 6 years. The variables most predictive of a poor outcome included RF, DR4 status, swollen joint count and erosion scores. The accuracy of predicting the outcome erosions using combinations of these markers varied between 70 and 80% [44]. For 12 months, Gough et al. [29] prospectively followed 120 patients presenting to an early arthritis clinic who fulfilled the ACR criteria for RA. Of these patients, 64% possessed the conserved epitope as opposed to 45% of a control population. The prevalence of the conserved epitope was lower than that quoted in several previous studies. However, with follow-up a much stronger association developed with persistent erosive disease. One interpretation of this is that the milder forms of RA are not as strongly associated with the disease epitope, although the two conditions are clinically indistinguishable at an early stage. The presence of either the disease epitope or RF provided a relative risk for the development of radiological erosions of 13.49 (sensitivity, 95%; specificity, 39%), whereas the presence of both the disease epitope and RF produced a relative risk of 8.13 (sensitivity, 53%; specificity, 88%). Finally, within the rheumatoid population, the frequency of compound heterozygotes (Dw4/Dw14) was found to be disproportionately increased compared with that expected. The compound heterozygote group accounted for 9.2% of the rheumatoid patients. With one exception, all of these patients developed radiological erosions at 1 year, indicating that they have a particularly poor prognosis.

Earlier work from the same group of investigators [54] reported the use of genetic factors as predictors of outcome in patients presenting with a persistent symmetrical arthritis (rheumatoid-like but not fulfilling ACR criteria for the diagnosis). They reported on 49 patients presenting with a persistent inflammatory arthritis to an early arthritis clinic. At presentation, none of these patients had radiological erosions, but 25 developed them after 4 years of follow-up. Patients with the disease epitope had a relative risk for the development of erosions of 1.9. Other risk factors for the development of erosions in these patients were poor sulfoxidation status (relative risk 2.5) and RF positivity (relative risk 1.8). The possession of two or three of these risk factors increased the relative risk to 11.6.

In summary, it is now believed that the strongest association with the conserved epitope is with the more severe forms of disease. There is a much weaker association with mild disease. The disease epitope may not in itself appear to predispose to the development of the disease but may contribute to the degree of severity in patients who develop an inflammatory synovitis. It shows promise as a marker to differentiate between self-limiting and persistent disease. The possession of a double dose of the disease-associated alleles appears to be associated with a particularly bad prognosis.

IV. COHORT STUDIES OF DISEASE PROGNOSIS—REVIEW

The above discussion represents a summary of the currently used clinical, laboratory and radiological markers employed to predict severity in rheumatoid arthritis. Prospective cohort studies to investigate these variables are difficult to design and laborious to undertake. Previous studies have varied in design, duration, number of patients, length of disease, patient selection, and the choice of outcome measures. This leads to difficulty in comparison, which makes interpretation hazardous. Results of studies have often been contradictory and conclusions variable. If the natural history of RA is to be improved by therapeutic intervention, the ability to predict accurately the prognosis is important early in the disease. Prospective studies should include patients with a similar disease duration that is accurately calculated and at an early stage (e.g., <1 year).

Inconsistencies in previous studies have resulted from comparison between cohorts of patients of varying sizes, investigating different markers, and using a range of outcome measures. There must therefore be a sufficient number of patients to allow precise interpretation of results. Radiological damage has repeatedly been shown to be an indicator of poor functional outcome and disease severity and is a necessary part of the final assessment.

One of the wide-ranging markers discussed above has consistently shown a strong correlation with clinical, laboratory, and radiological outcome measures. This is the presence of the so-called shared epitope. Many of the most informative studies have used the measurement of genetic markers to predict a more severe disease course.

As exhaustive coverage of all previous cohort studies on prognostic markers of disease progression would be difficult to interpret. A selection of the better-designed studies on prognostic markers have been reviewed and ranked by quality in a table format for ease of comparison (see Tables 1–4). The studies with a cohort of greater than 100, disease duration less than 1 year, the incorporation of HLA status as a predictive measure, and radiographs to assess outcome at the head of the table and are given four stars. Proceeding down the table, other studies are included which do not fully satisfy these criteria, and these have been ranked from three to one stars, depending on how many of the four variables mentioned above apply to the paper. At the end of the table, we have included cross-sectional and miscellaneous studies investigating some of the more novel prognostic markers for disease progression.

V. SUMMARY

There are a wide range of investigations that can be used as prognostic markers in rheumatoid arthritis. They can be divided into quantitative and qualitative markers. The most commonly used quantitative markers are the CRP and ESR. The former can be used to monitor disease activity and extent. A limitation to their usefulness is the fact that they are a reflection of disease activity and fluctuate with this. As such, isolated values must be interpreted in the light of clinical information. Serial measurements may provide more accurate prognostic information but are inconvenient and still have the limitation of being self-fulfilling. They may be valuable for determining a "change in prognosis".

Markers of cartilage and bone breakdown have promise as clinical markers of disease activity but are not yet established in routine practice and must be regarded as a research tool at present. In established disease, quantitative markers give adequate prognostic information for the clinician. But in the pre-erosive, presystemic phase of the disease, the qualitative markers are crucial. In addition, genetic markers do provide confirmation of the homogeneity of the patient populations.

The most commonly used qualitative factor used is the RF. This and the disease epitope have an additive predictive value in the prediction of progressive destructive joint disease. Genetic markers have yet to be established in routine clinical practice but have the great advantage of being independent of disease stage and therefore applicable to early nonerosive disease.

REFERENCES

1. Thompson D, Whicher JT, Banks RE. Acute phase reactants in predicting disease outcome. Bailleres Clin Rheumatol 1992; 6(2):393–404.
2. Stuart J, Whicher JT. Tests for detecting and monitoring the acute phase response. Arch Dis Child 1988; 63:115–117.
2a. Sheeran TP, Robobottom CA, Wanklin PD, Winkles J, Richardson K, Gordon C, Emery P. Clinical and Experimental Rheumatology 1993; 11:49–52.
3. Amos RS, constable TJ, Crockson RA, Crockson AP, McConkey B. Rheumatoid arthritis: relation of serum C-reactive protein and erythrocyte sedimentation rates to radiographic changes. Br Med J 1977; I:195–197.
4. Scott DL, Coulton BL, Symmons DPL, Poppert AJ. Long term outcome of treating rheumatoid arthritis: results after 20 years. Lancet 1987; 1(8542)1108–1111.
5. Dawes PT, Fowler PD, Clarke S, Fisher J, Lawton A, Shadforth MF. Rheumatoid arthritis: treatment which controls the C-reactive protein and erythrocyte sedimentation rate reduces radiological progression. Br J Rheumatol 1986; 25:44–49.
6. Luqmani RA, Sheeran TP, Winkles J, Richardson M, Robinson M, Emery P. Cytokines and the acute phase response in rheumatoid arthritis. Br J Rheumatol 1991; 30(Suppl 2):6.
7. Gough AKS, Lilley J, Eyre S, Emery P: Generalised bone loss in patients with early rheumatoid arthritis. Lancet 1994; (8914) 344:23–27.

8. van Leeuwen MA, van Rijswijk MH, van der Jeijde DFM, te Meerman GJ, van Riel PLCM, Houtman PM, van de Putte LB, Limburg PC. The acute phase response in relation to radiographic progression in early rheumatoid arthritis: a prospective study during the first three years of treatment. Br J Rheumatol 1993; 329 (suppl 3):9–13.
9. Devlin J, Gough A, Huissoon A, Perkins P, Holder R, Reece R, Arthur V, Emery P. The actue phase and function in early rheumatoid arthritis. CRP levels correlate with functional outcome. J Rheumatol 1997; 24:9–13.
10. VreugdenhilG, Wognum AW, van Eijk HG, Swaak AJD. Anaemia in rheumatoid arthritis: the role of iron, vitamin B12, and folic acid deficiency, and erythropoietin responsiveness. Ann Rheum Dis 1990; 49:93–98.
11. Baer AN, Dessypris EN, Krantz SB. The pathogenesis of anaemia in rheumatoid arthritis: A clinical and laboratory analysis. Semin Arthritis Rheum 1990; 19(4):209–223.
12. Faquin WC, Schneider TJ, Goldberg MA. Effect of inflammatory cytokines on hypoxia-induced erythropoietin production. Blood 1992; 79(8):1987–1984.
13. Johnson RA, Waddelow TA, Caro J, Oliff A, Roodman GD. Chronic exposure to tumour necrosis factor in vivo preferentially inhibits erythropoiesis in nude mice. Blood 1989; 74(1):130–138.
14. Johnson CS, Chang MJ, Furmanski P. In vitro effects of tumour necrosis factor in normal and erythroluekemic mice: Characterisation and Therapeutic applications. Blood 1988; 76(6):1875–1883.
15. Dinant HJ, DeMaat CEM. Erythropoiesis and mean red cell lifespan in normal subjects and patients with the anaemia of active rheumatoid arthritis. British J Haematol 1978; 39:437–444.
16. Thomas JT, Ayad S, Grant ME. Cartilage collagens: strategies for the study of their organisation and expression in the extra-cellular matrix. Ann Rheum Dis 1994; 53:488–496.
17. Wolheim FA: Biochemical markers of joint tissue destruction in rheumatoid arthritis. Rheumatol Eur 1995;2(Suppl 2):173–175.
18. Taylor AK, Lueken SA, Libanati C, Baylink DJ. Biochemical markers of bone turnover for the clinical assessment of bone metabolism. Rheum Dis Clin North Am 1994; 20:589.
19. Gough AKS, Peel NFA, Eastall R, Holder R, Lilley J, Emery P. Excretion of pyridinium crosslinks correlates with disease activity and appendicular bone loss in early rheuamtoid arthritis. Ann Rheum Dis 1994; 53:14–17.
20. Poole AR. Biological markers in rheumatoid arthrits. Semin Arthritis Rheum 1994; 23(Suppl 2):17–31.
21. Maddison PJ. Autoantibody profile. In: The Oxford Textbook of Rheumatology. Oxford University Press: 1993:394–395.
22. Woolf AD, Hall ND, Goulding NJ, Kantharia B, Maymo J, Evison G, Maddison PJ. Predictors of the long term outcome of early synovitis: a 5 year follow up study. Br J Rheumatol 1991; 30:251–254.
23. Young A, Corbett M, Winfield J, et al. A prognostic index for erosive changes in the hands, feet and cervical spines in early rheumatoid arthritis. Br J Rheumatol 1988; 27:94–101.
24. Corbett M, Young A. The Middlesex Hospital prospective study of early rheumatoid disease. Br J Rheumatol 1988; 27(Suppl 2):171–172.
25. Corbett M, Dalton S, Young A, Silman A, Shipley M. Factors predicting death, survival and functional outcme in a prospective study of early rheumatoid disease over fifteen years. Br J Rheumatol 1993; 32:717–723.
26. van Zeben D, Hazes JMW, Zwinderman AH, Cats A, van der Voort, Breedveld FC. Clinical significance of rheumatoid factors in early rheumatoid arthritis: results of a follow up study. Ann Rheum Dis 1992; 51:1029–1035.
27. Van Schaardenburg D, Hazes DM, de Boer A, Zwinderman AH, Meijers KA, Breedveld FC. Outcome of rheumatoid arthritis in relation to age and rheumatoid factor at diagnosis. J Rheumatol 1993; 20(1):45–52.

28. Emery P, Bradley H, Arthur V, Tunn E, Waring RH. Genetic factors influencing the outcome of early arthritis-the role of sulphoxidation status. Br J Rheumatol 1992; 31:449–451.
29. Gough A, Faint J, Salmon M, Hassell A, Wordsworth P, Pilling S, Birdley A, Emery P. Genetic typing of patients with inflammatory arthritis at presentation can be used to predict outcome. Arthritis Rheum 1994; 37:1166–1170.
30. Teitsson I, Withrington RH, Seiffert MH, Valdimarsson HI. Prognostic value of Ig A rheumatoid fatctor. Ann Rheum Dis 1984; 43:673–678.
31. Eberhart KB, Trusdsson L, Petterson H, Svensson B, Stigsson L, Eberhart JL, Wollheim FA. Disease activity and joint damage progression in early rheumatoid arthritis and relation to IgG, IgA, and Ig M rheumatoid factor. Ann Rheum Dis 1990; 49:906–909.
32. Van Zeben D, Rook GAW, Hazes JMW, Zwinderman AH, Zhang Y, Ghelani S, Rademacher TW, Breedveld F. Early agalactosylation of IgG is associated with a more progressive disease course in patients with rheumatoid arthritis: Results of a follow up study. Br J Rheumatol 1994; 33:36–43.
33. Young A, Smuar N, Bodman K, Goyal S, Sinclair H, Roitt I, Isenberg D. Agalctosyl IgG: An aid to differential diagnosis in early synovitis. Arthritis Rheum 1991; 34(11):1425–1429.
34. Cook A, Rowley JM, Mackay IR, Gough A, Emery P. Antibodies to type II collagen in early rheumatoid arthritis: correlation with disease progression. Arthritis Rheum 1996; 39(10):1720–1727.
35. Mitchell SC, Waring RH, Haley CS, Idle JR, Smith RI. Genetic aspects of the polymodally distributed sulphoxidation of S-Carboxymethyl-L-Cysteine in man. Br J Pharmacol 1984; 18:507–521.
36. Emery P, Panayi GS, Huston G. D-penicillamine induced toxicity in rheumatoid arthritis: the role of sulphoxidation status and HLA-DR3. J Rheumatol 1984; 11(5):626–632.
37. Emery P, Bradley H, Arthur V, Jubb R, Waring RH. Increased prevalence of poor sulphoxidation in patients with rheumatoid arthritis. Ann Rheum Dis 1991; 51:318–320.
38. Bradley H, Gough AK, Sokhi RS, Hassell A, Waring R, Emery P. Sulphate metabolism is abnormal in patients with rheumatoid arthritis. J Rheumatol 1994; 21:1192–1116.
39. Wordsworth BP, Salmon M. The HLA class II component of susceptibility to rheumatoid arthrits. Baillieres Clin Rheumatol 1992; 6(2):325–357.
40. Salmon M: The immunogenetic component of susceptibility to rheumatoid arthritis. Curr Opin Rheumatol 1992; 4(3):342–347.
41. Silman AJ, Reeback J, Jaraquemada D. HLA-DR4 as a predictor of outcome three years after onest of rheumatoid arthritis. Rheumatol Int 1986; 6:233–235.
42. Moens Hj, Ament BJ, Felkamp BW. Longterm follow up of treatment with D-penicillamine for rheumatoid arthritis; effectivity and toxicity in relation to HLA antigens. J Rheumatol 1987; 14:1115–1119.
43. Paimela L, Leirsalo-Repo M, Helve T: The prognostic value of HLA DR4 and B27 antigens in early rheumatoid arthritis. Scand J Rheumatol 1993; 220–224.
44. van Zeben D. Factors predicting outcome of rheumatoid arthritis, results of a followup study: J Rheumatol 1993; 20:8:1288–1296.
45. van Leeuwen MA, Westra J, van Riel PLCM, Limburg PC, van Rijswijk MH. IgM, IgA and IgG rheumatoid factors in early rheumatoid arthritis predictive of radiological progression? Scand J Rheumatol 1995; 24:146–153.
46. van der Heijde DMFM, van Riel PLCM, van Leeuwen MA, van't Hof MA, van Rijswijk MH, van de Putte LBA. Prognostic factors for radiographic damage and physical disability in early rheumatid arthritis. A prospective follow-up study of 147 patients. Br J Rheumatol 1992; 31:519–525.
47. Kaarela K. Prognostic factors and diagnostic criteria in early rheumatoid arthritis. Scand J Rheumatol 1985; 57(Suppl):1–54.
48. van der Heide Agnes, Remme C A, Hofman D K, Jacobs JWG, Bijsma JWJ. Prediction of progression of radiologic damage in newly diagnosed rheumatoid arthritis. Arthritis Rheum 1995; 38(10):1466–1474.

49. van Zeben D, Hazes J M W, Zwinderman A H, Cats A, Schreuder G M T, D'Amaro J, Breedveld F C. Association of HLA-DR4 with a more progressive disease course in patients with rheumatoid arthritis. Arthritis Rheum 1991; 34:822–830.
50. van Zeben D, Hazes J M W, Zwinderman A H, Vandenbroucke J P, Breedveld F C. Factors predicting outcome of rheumatoid arthritis: results of a follow-up study. J Rheumatol 1993; 20:1288–1296.
51. Luukkainen R, Kaarela K, Isomaki H, Martio J, Kiviniemi P, Rasanen J and Sarna S. The prediction of radiological destruction during the early stage of rheumatoid arthritis. Clin Exp Rheumatol 1983; 1:295–298.
52. Mottonen T T. Prediction of erosiveness and rate of development of new erosions in early rheumatoid arthritis. Ann Rheum Dis 1988; 47:648–653.
53. Combe B, Eliaou J F, Daures J P, Meyer O, Clot J, Sany. J Prognostic factors in rheumatoid arthritis comparative study of two subsets of patients according to severity of articular damage. Br J Rheumatol 1995; 34:529–534.
54. Emery P, Salmon M, Bradley H, Wordsworth P, Tunn E, Bacon P A, Waring R. Genetically determined factors as predictors of radiological change in patients with early symmetrical arthritis. Br Med J 1992; 305:1387–1389.
55. Vries N de, Prinsen CFM, Mensink EBJM, van Riel PLCM, van't Hof MA, van de Putte LBA. A T cell receptor β chain variable region polymorphism associated with radiographic progression in rheumatoid arthritis. Ann Rheum Dis 1993; 52:327–331.
56. Fleming A, Benn R T, Corbett M, Wood PHN. Early rheumatoid diseases II. Patterns of joint involvement. Ann Rheum Dis 1976; 35:361–364.
57. van der Heij de DMFM, van Riel PLCM, Miek A, et al. Older versus younger onset rheumatoid arthritis: Results at onset and after 2 years of a prospective follow up study of early rheumatoid arthritis. J Rheumatol 1991; 18:1285–1289.
58. Flemming A, Crown J M, Corbett M:Prognostic value of early features in rheumatoid disease. Br Med J 1976; 1:1243–1245.
59. Dawes PT, Plant MJ, Jones PW, et al. Measurement and prediction of radiological progression of early RA. J Rheumatol 1994; 21(10):1808–1813.
60. Salmon M, Wordsworth P, Emery P, Tunn E, Bacon PA, Bell JI. The association of HLA DR β alleles with self-limiting and persistent forms of early symmetrical polyarthritis. Br J Rheumatol 1993; 32:628–630.
61. Sjoblom KG, Saxne T, Pettersson H, Wollheim FA. Factors related to the progression of joint destruction in rheumatoid arthritis. Scand J Rheumatol 1984; 13:21–27.
62. Mau W, Bornmann M, Weber H, Weidemann HF, Hecker H, Raspe HH. Prediction of permanent work disability in a follow-up study of early rheumatoid Arthritis: Results of a tree structured analysis using RECPAM. Br J Rheumatol 1996; 35:652–659.
63. Eberhardt KB, Fex E. Functional impairment and disability in early rheumatoid arthritis—development over 5 years. J Rheumatol 1995; 22(6):1037–1042.
64. Pincus T, Brooks RH, Callahan LF. Prediction of long-term mortality in patients with rheumatoid arthritis according to simple questionnaires and joint count measures. Ann Intern Med 1994; 120:26–34.
65. Michel BA, Bloch DA, Fries JF. Predictors of fractures in early rheumatoid arthritis. J Rheumatol 1991; 18:804–808.
66. Eberhardt KB, Svensson Bjorn, Treudsson L, Wollheim FA. The Occurrence of rheumatoid factor iIsotypes in eEarly definite rheumatoid arthritis—no relationship with erosions or disease activity. J Rheumatol 1988; 15:1070–1074.
67. Westedt ML, Daha MR, Baldwin WM, Stijnen T, Cats A. Serum immune complexes IgA appear to predict erosive arthritis in a longitudinal study in rheumatoid arthritis. Ann Rheum Dis 1986; 45:809–815.
68. Leigh JP, Fries JF. Predictors of disability in a longitudinal sample of patients with rheumatoid arthritis. Ann Rheum Dis 1992; 51(5):581–587.

69. Reeback J, Silman A. Predictors of outcome at two years in patients with rheumatoid arthritis. J R Soc Med 1984; 1002–1005.
70. Brennan P, Silman A. Simple algorithm to predict radiological erosions. Br Med J 1996; 313:471–476.
71. Toda Y, Minamikawa Y, Akagi S, Sugano H, Mori Y, Nishimura H, Arita S, Sugino Y, Ogawa R. Rheumatoid-susceptible alleles of HLA-DRB1 are genetically recessive to nonsusceptible alleles in the progression of bone destruction in the wrists and fingers of patients with RA. Ann Rheum Dis 1994; 53:587–592.
72. Moreno I, Valenzuela A, Garcia A, Yelamos J, Sanchez B, Hernanz W. Association of the shared epitope with radiological severity of rheumatoid arthritis. J Rheumatol 1996; 23:6–9.
73. Wollheim FA, Pettersson H, Saxne T, Sjoblom KG. Radiographic assessment in relation to clinical and biochemical variables in rheumatoid arthritis. Scand J Rheumatol 1988; 17:445–453.
74. de Carvalho AH. Graudal radiographic progression of rheumatoid arthritis related to some clinical and laboratory parameters. Radiol Diagn 1980; 21:551–555.
75. Mansson, Garey D, Alini M, Lonescu M, Rosenburg L C, Poole A R, Saxne T: Bone metabolism in rheumatoid arthritis. Skeletal Markers in Rheumatoid Arthritis 1995: 1071–1077.
76. L Paimela, M Gripenberg, P Kurki, Leirisalo-Repo M. Antikeratin antibodies: diagnostic and prognostic markers for early rheumatoid arthritis. Ann Rheum Dis 1992; 51:743–746.
77. Lee BO, Ishihara K, Denno K, Kobune Y, Itoh M, Muraoka O, Kaisho T, Sasaki T, Ochi T, Hirano T. Elevated levels of the soluble form of bone marrow stromal cell antigen 1 in the sera of patients with severe rheumatoid arthritis. Arthritis Rheum 1996; 39:629–637.

4

Clinical Trials Revisited

Harold E. Paulus and Ken J. Bulpitt
University of California, Los Angeles, Los Angeles, California

I. INTRODUCTION

In this chapter, we briefly review the use of clinical trials in rheumatoid arthritis, and then we present personal opinions regarding some of the key factors required to demonstrate efficiently the benefits achieved with several classes of drugs used to treat this chronic irregularly progressive disease.

II. HISTORY OF CLINICAL TRIALS IN RHEUMATOID ARTHRITIS

Physicians responsible for the care of patients with rheumatoid arthritis (RA) have aggressively sought and adopted new treatments, attempting to help patients whose RA continued to progress despite the use of standard therapies. The presence of a large reservoir of inadequately treated, chronically symptomatic patients exhibiting measurable signs of inflammation and functional incapacity has made rheumatoid arthritis an excellent vehicle for therapeutic experimentation. The background of individual fluctuations of disease activity and the relatively modest impact of most therapies mandates the use of control groups and the application of statistical methods to clinical studies of RA.

Many of the standard drugs for RA were initially developed for other purposes and adopted for RA when astute clinicians noted improvement of some of their patients in "n of one" clinical trials. These were reported as case reports or accumulated clinical experience without the benefit of control groups or sophisticated statistical analysis. Examples include Forrestier's report in 1935 of a favorable response in 70–80% of 550 patients treated with gold salts [1]. Other seminal early reports include chloroquine, 1951 [2], d-penicillamine, 1964 [3], nitrogen mustard, 1951 [4], methotrexate, 1951 [5], cyclophosphamide, 1968 [6], and sulfasalazine, 1948 [7]. Phenylbutazone was marketed in 1949 but no controlled clinical trial was published until 1956 [8]. Indeed awarding of the Nobel Prize in medicine for the use of cortisone in RA was based on simple clinical observations that were reported in 1949 [9].

These early observations were not fully accepted, however, until they were later confirmed by controlled clinical trials, and rheumatologists have been in the forefront in the design and application of controlled clinical trials for a chronic, nonlethal disease. Fraser reported the first comparison of gold sodium thiomalate against placebo in 1945 [10], but the first carefully controlled double-blind classic trial of gold therapy was not reported until 1960 by the Empire Rheumatism Council [11]. Early controlled trials in RA were reported for chloroquine in 1956 [12], d-penicillamine in 1973 [13], methotrexate in 1985 [14,15], cyclophosphamide in 1970 [16], sulfasalazine in 1983 [17], aspirin in 1965 [18,19], phenylbutazone in 1956 [8], and cortisone in 1955 [20].

Ad hoc clinical measures for outcomes assessment were used in the early clinical trials. In addition to a global impression of the patient's response, they often attempted to quantitate various aspects of the cardinal signs of inflammation: pain, swelling, heat, redness, and loss of function. Examples include pain scales, dolorimeter readings, tender joint counts, duration of morning stiffness, time to onset of fatigue, swollen joint counts, ring sizing, grip strength, walking time, and quantitation of acute phase reactants. The first composite index for clinical assessment of RA was published in 1958 by Lansbury [21]. The Empire Rheumatism Council gold trial [11] in 1960 used a sophisticated double-blind pseudo–placebo-controlled trial design and standardized prespecified clinical outcome measures. The seven-day variability study by the Cooperating Clinics in 1965 [22], as refined by Mainland in 1967 [23], and the Ritchie articular index in 1968 [24] documented the reproducibility and variability of the measures that became standard in RA clinical trials and established the central role of joint counts in these trials. These measures were adopted by the U.S. Food and Drug Administration (FDA), and they were used in numerous pharmaceutical industry clinical trials of new nonsteroidal anti-inflammatory drugs (NSAIDs) during the 1970s and 1980s [25].

"Loss of function" was estimated using the American Rheumatism Association Functional Classification, first published in 1949 [26], but its four functional classes were too broad to measure the modest responses to most therapeutic interventions. Self-report functional questionnaires such as the HAQ (Health Assessment Questionnaire) and the AIMS (Arthritis Impact Measurement Scales), introduced in 1980 [27,28], and the MACTAR in 1987 [29] were able to detect much smaller changes in function.

Grading of radiographic evidence of joint damage began with Steinbrocker's four anatomical stages [26] in 1949. Sharp developed a system for quantitative scoring of articular radiographic changes in 1971 [30]; the Larson system followed in 1977 [31].

The multitude of outcome measures used, and selectively reported, made it difficult to compare the published results of RA clinical trials. The FDA has placed primary emphasis on four measures: the tender and swollen joint counts and the patient and physician global assessments. Independent committees of the American College of Rheumatology (ACR) and the European League Against Rheumatism (EULAR) began to evaluate RA outcome measures in about 1990. In 1992, an international working group met in Maastrich, The Netherlands, as OMERACT (Outcome Measures in Rheumatoid Arthritis Clinical Trials) and recommended a limited "core" set of preferred measures that should be included in every clinical trial [32]. The selected measures are (a) painful joint count; (b) swollen joint count; (c) patient global assessment of RA activity; (d) physician global assessment of RA activity; (e) patient assessment of pain; (f) index of self-reported physical function by a validated instrument such as the HAQ; (g) acute phase reactants (ESR or CRP); and (h) for studies longer than 1 year, joint radiographs are recommended. These core outcome measures are now generally accepted and should be used in all RA clinical trials. Other measures may be added to individual trials if desired.

A composite index to analyze and report improvement of individual patients in RA clinical trials was proposed in 1990 based on reanalysis of a number of reported CSSRD (Cooperative Systematic Studies of Rheumatic Diseases) placebo-controlled DMARD (disease-modifying antirheumatic drug, also described as second-line agents and slowly acting antirheumatic drugs) studies [33]. Although it preceded and thus did not use all of the core-set measures, this approach was applied and modified in numerous clinical trials, because it is well suited to intent-to-treat analysis and increases the power of statistical analyses. The next step was the incorporation of the core measures into a composite index of individual improvement. In 1994, an ACR committee with international representation, after extensive discussion, testing in existing RA data bases, and case by case comparisons with the clinical judgment of experienced rheumatologists, recommended the following criteria for improvement in an RA patient. There must be ≥20% improvement in both the number of painful/tender joints and the number of swollen joints; in addition, three of the remaining five core measures also must improve by ≥20% (pain, physical function, erythrocyte sedimentation rate [ESR] or C-reactive protein [CRP], patient global, physician global) [34]. Use of this composite index markedly increases the discriminatory power of clinical trials and permits enumeration of the outcomes of individual patients with calculation of the probability that a patient starting the treatment will improve with it.

In an attempt to emphasize the importance of long-term cumulative joint damage in assessing the benefits of RA treatments, a World Health Organization conference in 1993 recommended a new therapeutic classification, D-CART (disease-controlling antirheumatic therapy), which requires the treatment both to improve and sustain function in association with decreased inflammatory synovitis and to prevent or significantly decrease the rate of progression of joint damage for at least 1 year [35]. Clinical trials designed to support a D-CART claim have not yet been reported, and it remains a desired target for future therapies. A 1994 review of published clinical trials of at least 1-year duration that included serial joint radiographs suggests that such studies are possible, but large numbers of subjects will be needed to demonstrate D-CART effects with available disease-modifying antirheumatic drugs (DMARDs) [36].

Currently, health services researchers and health policy planners are returning to the initial emphasis on patient opinion. However, patient opinion is now segmented and quantitated using validated instruments that permit one to draw conclusions about concepts such as patient satisfaction, health-related quality of life, utility scores, economic cost-utility analysis, and cost per quality adjusted life-year gained (QUALY) [37,38]. In some countries, cost-effectiveness analyses are required before drugs are approved for use. These analyses are based in social sciences research methods, and they have been used in rheumatology to study the effects of total joint arthroplasty on the quality of well-being of osteoarthritis patients [39], the cost effectiveness of auranofin [40,41], and the cost-utility of misoprostil [42]. These studies must be interpreted with caution, however, because the many methodological and data selection decisions that must be made by the authors of cost-effectiveness studies make them susceptible to influence by unintentional or intentional bias, and small changes in the assumptions may markedly change the results of a study [43,44].

III. FACTORS IN TRIAL DESIGNS FOR NSAIDS

Untreated patients with active RA almost immediately recognize the benefit of effective doses of an NSAID; conversely, the benefits rapidly disappear when the drug is excreted, producing an NSAID-withdrawal flare of the symptoms and signs of joint inflammation. Because of this rapid onset and offset of NSAID effects, it is easy to design a controlled clinical trial in suitable patients using core-set outcome measures.

Patient selection is crucial. Patients must have easily measurable symptoms and signs of joint inflammation (activity criteria) that gets worse when their pretrial NSAID is withdrawn. NSAID-withdrawal flare criteria must be met; these criteria specify the minimum degree of worsening required for entry into the trial and guarantee that only NSAID-responsive patients are studied. The duration of the pretrial NSAID withdrawal should be flexible and will depend on the half-life of the NSAID being withdrawn. If a patient does not flare within 7 to 10 days, NSAIDs are not needed and the patient is excluded; in RA patients, the usual cause is concurrent corticosteroid therapy. Even small doses of prednisone can obscure an NSAID effect, and initial NSAID trials generally should exclude patients taking corticosteroids. However, because of their delayed and incomplete effects, background DMARDs may be continued in short-term NSAID trials provided the patients satisfy activity and flare criteria at entry.

NSAID trials must be double blind and randomized. Initial trials should be placebo controlled and may be of short duration; benefit is easily detectable in 2–4 week trials. Because placebo treatment of an NSAID-withdrawal flare is ineffective, patients should be allowed to withdraw if they do not perceive sufficient benefit after the first week of double-blind therapy. Outcome measurements at the time of withdrawal can be carried forward for statistical comparison with other end-of-treatment observations, and dropout rates for the different treatment groups are compared. Note that this powerful study design will not work if patients are discouraged in any way from dropping out. NSAIDs and NSAID-containing analgesics and corticosteroids are readily available and patients will use them surreptitiously if necessary to please their physician by remaining in the trial. Ideally, rescue analgesics should not be permitted in a placebo-controlled NSAID trial. Because the patients randomized to placebo receive no benefit and endure additional discomfort, they should be offered inclusion in subsequent open "clinical experience" trials.

Although it is easy to differentiate NSAID from placebo, it has been difficult to differentiate reliably one NSAID from another and to differentiate statistically between different doses of the same NSAID. Dose-finding clinical trials should be anchored with a placebo group, and the doses chosen should be as widely separated as possible; 10-fold differences in doses should be detectable, but 2- or 3-fold dosage differences often are not significantly different in reasonable size trials. For this reason, early dose-finding trials often fail to determine clearly the most effective dose, although they are also needed to demonstrate tolerability.

After the effective dose range has been determined in short placebo-controlled trials, longer studies are needed to establish tolerability. These may be 6 months or longer in duration, and should use active control NSAIDs to help to position the new NSAID vis-à-vis its probable competition. The statistical methodology for equivalence trial designs should be used to determine sample sizes, which will be much larger than those for placebo-controlled studies.

IV. FACTORS IN TRIAL DESIGN FOR DMARDS

If a patient continues to have active RA despite treatment with NSAIDs (and often low-dose prednisone), the addition of a DMARD such as gold or methotrexate usually results in measurable additional benefit when compared with the addition of a placebo, but it may take weeks or months before the additional benefit is detected. When a DMARD is discontinued, weeks (for methotrexate) to months (for gold) may elapse before the benefit is lost and a DMARD-withdrawal flare occurs. In terms of study design, DMARDs are differentiated from NSAIDs because they produce additional benefit when added to continuing background NSAID and/or corticosteroid therapy (and they are not corticosteroids). Delayed onset of benefit is not required, and it is possible that a biological product or other future DMARD may act rapidly.

Patients for DMARD clinical trials must satisfy predefined disease activity criteria despite stable NSAID and/or corticosteroid background therapy for a specified period of time—usually 4–8 weeks. The background therapy is continued unchanged throughout the trial; it is particularly important that the dose of background corticosteroids be constant. Prior DMARDs must be discontinued for a substantial time before trial entry—usually at least 1 month for methotrexate and 3 months for other DMARDs, although patients are often unstable 1 month after methotrexate withdrawal, and their disease activity may increase for several months thereafter. Placebo controls are ethical in DMARD trials because background therapy is continued unchanged. Early studies of a new DMARD are usually done in patients who have tried and failed several other DMARDs and thus are not being deprived of the opportunity to take a standard DMARD.

The standard comparator in DMARD clinical trials is placebo. Significant advantage to the DMARD should be evident with sample sizes of 75–150 per group. It is much more difficult to find significant differences between two DMARDs or between different doses of the same drug. This causes problems in dose finding studies; consequently, the initial recommended dose may be selected because of a side effect such as diarrhea with auranofin, or for cost considerations, with some of the biological agents.

Partly because of their longer duration, withdrawals are a problem in DMARD trials. After a 6- to 9-month placebo-controlled trial, the patients remaining are those who have done reasonably well, although fewer placebo patients will complete the trial; thus "completer" analyses tend to underestimate the differences between drug and placebo. Analysis based on the last recorded value includes the dropouts and more accurately reflect the true differences between drug and placebo. Intent-to-treat analysis of the proportions of patients satisfying the ACR individual improvement criteria [34] are very helpful for clinicians who would like to know the probability of successful treatment for a patient who is starting treatment.

For new DMARDs, comparison with standard DMARDs is useful. However, DMARD clinical trials that use an active DMARD control should use equivalence designs for sample size and power calculations, because the true differences may be so small that huge sample sizes would be required.

Clinical trials evaluating combinations of DMARDs have been difficult. The ideal design compares DMARD I versus DMARD II versus the combination, with a placebo control group to anchor the study, in patients not previously treated with either DMARD. This design allows one to evaluate additive and synergistic effects. Unfortunately, combination studies with a balanced design have failed to show significant advantage for the combination therapies [45–48]. An alternative design studies patients who have tolerated but have had incomplete responses to a DMARD. The patients continue this DMARD at the same dose and add either placebo or a second DMARD to see if the second DMARD produces more benefit than placebo. This design minimizes withdrawals for toxicity to the first DMARD, and it has successfully demonstrated additional benefit (compared with placebo) when cyclosporin was added in methotrexate-treated patients with continued active RA [48]. In addition, this design corresponds to clinical practice, as physicians who are searching for ways to help patients who have not responded sufficiently to standard therapies often prefer to add new treatments without stopping the previous therapy.

Many biological products are being evaluated as potential DMARDs. Trial design for a biological agent is similar to that for a DMARD, but with a few caveats. Since biologicals are designed to affect a specific physiological (immunological) process, a marker should be used to demonstrate that the product produces the desired biological effect regardless of its clinical impact. This guarantees the presence of drug activity. Most biologicals must be administered parenterally, which complicates the logistics of the clinical trial but does not really change its design. Great care must be taken to be certain that the biological product does not change when its manufacturing procedures are "scaled-up" for commercial production. Since the biological agent may be active in picogram or nanogram amounts and may be only a tiny fraction of the final extract that is administered, expression of the dose as milligrams of protein in the extract may be inaccurate if the concentration of the active component is not rigorously controlled. The ultimate role of biological products in the management of RA is not yet clear, but their high cost may relegate them to an adjunct role as bridge therapy when a DMARD is started or as crisis therapy for patients whose disease activity is out of control. Specific studies will have to be designed to evaluate these uses.

V. FACTORS IN TRIAL DESIGN FOR D-CART

D-CART trials differ from DMARD trials in their emphasis on the long-term effects of the treated RA on the patient's joint structure and functional capacity. They require a study duration of at least 1 year and use joint radiographs and measures of physical function such as the HAQ as the primary outcome measures. Improvement in disease activity measures is assumed, and is a secondary measure in D-CART trials. The tested therapy must be shown to decrease the progression of structural damage and prevent functional deterioration.

The most efficient population for D-CART studies are those patients with early RA who have a high probability of rapidly progressive erosive disease; that is, patients with positive rheumatoid factor, generalized active disease, and perhaps with the genetic susceptibility epitope that has been associated with erosive disease [50–52]. These patients should have minimal radiographic joint damage at entry, but have considerable functional limitation due to active RA. With effective treatment, measures of physical function should improve as disease activity is suppressed, and joint erosions should develop more slowly than in a control group.

The choice of a control group is difficult because of the long duration of the trial. It is not ethical to withhold treatment from a placebo group while their joints are progressively eroding; even if a placebo patient group is used, they will be withdrawn if their RA progresses rapidly; thus limiting the magnitude of the cumulative structural changes from baseline in this important outcome measure. Use of an active control treatment will decrease the differences between the treatment and control groups, but will probably be necessary for ethical reasons. Sample sizes will be large, although studies of 2–3 years' duration may allow smaller samples than those of 1 year.

Joint radiographic techniques should be standardized; both hands and feet should be assessed. A standardized scoring system should be used by experienced readers [30,31]. Dropouts should be followed at protocol-specified intervals to see whether any advantage or disadvantage from the initial treatment persists after it is stopped.

Attempts at D-CART clinical trials are just beginning, with many methodological problems still to be solved. Despite their difficulty, they should be pursued because they more closely approach the ideal goal of lifetime control of RA with maintenance of normal function.

REFERENCES

1. Forrestier J. Rheumatoid arthritis and its treatment with gold salts. J Lab Clin Med 1935; 20:837.
2. Brennecke FE, Alving AS, Arnold J, et al. A preliminary report on the effects of certain aminoquinolines in the treatment of rheumatoid arthritis. J Lab Clin Med 1951; 38:798–799.
3. Jaffe IA. Rheumatoid arthritis and arteritis. Report of a case treated with penicillamine. Ann Intern Med 1964; 61:556-564.
4. Jiminez-Diaz L, Lopez-Garcia E, Merchante A, Perianes J. Treatment of rheumatoid arthritis with nitrogen mustard. Preliminary report. JAMA 1951; 147:1418–1419.
5. Gubner R, August S, Ginsberg V. Therapeutic suppression of tissue reactivity. II. Effects of aminopterin in rheumatoid arthritis and psoriasis. Am J Med Sci 1951; 221:176–182.
6. Fosdick WM, Parsons JL, Hill DF. Long-term cyclophosphamide therapy in rheumatoid arthritis. Arthritis Rheum 1968; 11:151–160.
7. Svartz N. The treatment of rheumatoid arthritis with acid azo compounds. Rheumatism 1948; 4:56–60.
8. Fjellstrom KE, Goldberg L, Lindgren G, Nilsson F. Therapeutic effect of phenylbutazone in active periods of rheumatoid arthritis. Acta Med Scand 1956:154(Suppl 312):425 -428.
9. Hench PS, Kendall EC, Slocumb CH, Polley HF. The effect of a hormone of the adrenal cortex (17-hydroxy-11-dehydrocortisone: compound E) and of pituitary adrenocorticotropic hormone on rheumatoid arthritis: preliminary reoprt. Mayo Clin Proc 1949; 24:181–197.
10. Fraser TN. Gold therapy in rheumatoid arthritis. Ann Rheum Dis 1945; 4:71–75.
11. Research Subcommittee of the Empire Rheumatism Council. Gold therapy in rheumatoid arthritis. Report of a multicentre controlled trial. Ann Rheum Dis 1960; 19:95–119.
12. Freedman A. Chloroquine and rheumatoid arthritis: a short-term controlled trial. Ann Rheum Dis 1956; 15:251–256.
13. Multicentre Trial Group. Controlled trial of d(-)penicillamine in severe rheumatoid arthritis. Lancet 1973; 1:275–280.
14. Weinblatt ME, Coblyn JS, Fax DN, et al. Efficacy of low-dose methotrextate in rheumatoid arthritis. N Engl J Med 1985; 312:815–822.
15. Williams HJ, Wilkens RF, Samuelson CO Jr, et al. Comparison of low dose oral pulse methotrexate and placebo in the treatment of rheumatoid arthritis. A controlled clinical trial. Arthritis Rheum 1985; 28:721–730.
16. Cooperating Clinics Committee of the American Rheumatism Association. A controlled trial of cyclophosphamide in rheumatoid arthritis. N Engl J Med 1970; 283:883–889.
17. Pullar T, Hunter JA, Capell HA. Sulphasalazine in rheumatoid arthritis. A double-blind

comparison of sulphasalazine with placebo and sodium aurothiomolate. Br Med J 1983; 287:1102–1104.
18. Fremont-Smith K, Bayles TB. Salicylate therapy in rheumatoid arthritis. JAMA 1965; 192:1133–1136.
19. American Rheumatism Association Cooperative Clinics Committee. Aspirin in rheumatoid arthritis, a seven-day, double-blind trial—preliminary report. Bull Rheum Dis 1965; 16:388–391.
20. Empire Rheumatism Council. Multicentre controlled trial comparing cortisone acetate and acetylsalicylic acid in the long-term treatment of rheumatoid arthritis. Ann Rheum Dis 1955; 14:353–370.
21. Lansbury J. Report of a three-year study on the systemic and articular indexes of rheumatoid arthritis: theoretical and clinical considerations. Arthritis Rheum 1958; 1:505–522.
22. Cooperating Clinics Committee of the American Rheumatism Association. A seven-day variability study of 499 patients with peripheral rheumatoid arthritis. Arthritis Rheum 1965; 8:302–334.
23. Mainland D. The estimation of inflammatory activity in rheumatoid arthritis: role of composite indices. Arthritis Rheum 1967; 10:712–777.
24. Ritchie DM, Boyle JA, McInnes JM, et al. Clinical studies with an articular index for the assessment of joint tenderness in patients with rheumatoid arthritis. Q J Med 1968; 37:393–406.
25. McMillen J, Leer JA, Ridolfo A, et al. Guidelines for clinical evaluation of nonsteroidal antiinflammatory drugs. Drug Res Rep 1971; 15:S-2 to S-26.
26. Steinbrocker D, Traeger CH, Batterman C. Therapeutic criteria in rheumatoid arthritis. JAMA 1949; 140:659–662.
27. Fries JF, Spitz P, Kraines RG, Holman HR. Measurement of patient outcome in arthritis. Arthritis Rheum 1980; 23:137–145.
28. Meenan RF, Gertman PM, Mason JH. Measuring health status in arthritis: the arthritis impact measurement scales. Arthritis Rheum 1980; 23:146–152.
29. Tugwell P, Bombardier C, Buchanan WW, et al. The MACTAR patient preference disability questionnaire—an individualized functional priority approach for assessing improvement in physical disability in clinical trials in rheumatoid arthritis. J Rheumatol 1987; 14:446–451.
30. Sharp JT, Lidsky MD, Collins LC, Moreland J. Methods of scoring the progression of radiologic changes in rheumatoid arthritis. Arthritis Rheum 1971; 14:706–720.
31. Larson A, Dale K, Eek M. Radiographic evaluation of rheumatoid arthritis and related conditions by standard reference films. Acta Radiol Diagn 1977; 18:481–491.
32. Felson DT, Anderson JJ, Boers M, et al. The American College of Rheumatology preliminary core set of disease activity measures for rheumatoid arthritis clinical trials. Arthritis Rheum 1993; 36:729–740.
33. Paulus HE, Egger MJ, Ward JR, Williams HJ. Analysis of improvement in individual rheumatoid arthritis patients treated with disease-modifying antirheumatic drugs, based on findings in patients treated with placebo. Arthritis Rheum 1990; 33:477–484.
34. Felson DT, Anderson JJ, Boers M, et al. American College of Rheumatology. Preliminary definition of improvement in rheumatoid arthritis. Arthritis Rheum 1995; 38:727–735.
35. Edmonds JP, Scott DL, Furst DE, Brooks P, Paulus HE. Antirheumatic drugs: a proposed new classification. Arthritis Rheum 1993; 36:336–339.
36. Paulus HE, Bulpitt KJ. DC-ART Classification. Review of relevant clinical studies. J Rheumatol 1994; 21(Suppl 41):8–20.
37. Guyatt GH, Feeny DH, Patrick DL. Measuring health-related quality of life. Ann Intern Med 1993; 118:622–629.
38. Stoddard GL, Drummond MF. How to read clinical journals: VII. To understand an economic evaluation (Part A). (Department of Clinical Epidemiology and Biostatistics, McMaster University Health Sciences Center) Can Med Assoc J 1984; 130:1428–1434.

39. Liang MH, Cullen KE, Larson MG, et al. Cost-effectiveness of total joint arthroplasty in osteoarthritis. Arthritis Rheum 1986; 29:937–943.
40. Thompson MS, Read JL, Hutchings C, Paterson M, Harris ED Jr. The cost-effectiveness of auranofin: results of a randomized clinical trial. J Rheumatol 1988; 15:35–42.
41. Bombardier C, Ware J, Russell IJ, et al. Auranofin therapy and quality of life in patients with rheumatoid arthritis. Results of a multicenter trial. Am J Med 1986; 81:565–578.
42. Gabriel SE, Campion ME, O'Fallon WM. A cost-utility analysis of misoprostil prophylaxis for rheumatoid arthritis patients receiving nonsteroidal antiinflammatory drugs. Arthritis Rheum 1994; 37:333–341.
43. Kassirer JP, Angell M. The Journal's policy on cost-effectiveness analyses. N Engl J Med 1994; 331:669–670.
44. Stucki G, Johannesson M, Liang MH. Is misoprostil cost-effective in the prevention of non-steroidal anti-inflammatory drug-induced gastropathy in patients with chronic arthritis? A review of conflicting economic evaluations. Arch Intern Med 1994; 154:2020–2025.
45. Bunch TW, O'Duffy JD, Tompkins RB, et al. Controlled trial of hydroxychloroquine and d-penicillamine singly and in combination in the treatment of rheumatoid arthritis. Arthritis Rheum 1984; 27:267–276.
46. Williams HJ, Ward JR, Reading JC, et al. Comparison of auranofin, methotrexate, and the combination of both in the treatment of rheumatoid arthritis: a controlled clinical trial. Arthritis Rheum 1992; 35:259–269.
47. Willkens RF, Urowitz MB, Stablein DM, et al. Comparison of azathioprine, methotrexate and the combination of both in the treatment of rheumatoid arthritis: a controlled clinical trial. Arthritis Rheum 1992; 35:849–856.
48. Faarvang KL, Egsmose C, Kryger P, et al. Hydroxychloroquine and sulfasalazine alone and in combination in rheumatoid arthritis: a randomized double blind trial. Ann Rheum Dis 1993; 52:711–715.
49. Tugwell P, Pincus T, Yocum D, et al. Combination therapy with cyclosporine and methotrexate in severe rheumatoid arthritis. N Engl J Med 1995; 333:137–141.
50. Nepom GT, Byers P, Seyfried C, et al. HLA genes associated with rheumatoid arthritis: identification of susceptibility alleles using specific oligonucleotide probes. Arthritis Rheum 1989; 32:15–21.
51. Weyand CM, Hicok KC, Conn DL, et al. The influence of HLA-DRB1 genes on disease severity in rheumatoid arthritis. J Clin Invest 1992; 89:2033–2039.
52. Stockman A, Emery P, Doyle T, et al. Relationship of progression of radiographic changes in hands and wrists, clinical features and HLA-DR antigens in rheumatoid arthritis. J Rheumatol 1991; 18:1001–1007.

5
Second-line Agent Treatment: When and Whom

David L. Scott
Kings College Hospital, London, United Kingdom

I. INTRODUCTION

Selecting which drugs to give to which patients is at the center of clinical practice. In rheumatoid arthritis (RA), the question is especially complex. The main issue is which patients to give slow-acting antirheumatic drugs (SAARDs) such as gold, sulfasalazine, and methotrexate. There will never be a single correct answer for an individual patient. Clinical judgment will remain a complex matter which cannot readily be reduced to a simple formula. But there are broad issues which can be easily dissected. Relevant questions include which RA patients should be given SAARDs, when should they be given SAARDs, and is it best to give single agents or combinations. I have approached the issues involved in selecting antirheumatic therapy by considering therapeutic strategies using single SAARDs, the assessment of disease activity, and the effects of SAARDs. I have based my views on when and whom to treat from an analysis of these issues.

II. WHAT IS A SLOW-ACTING ANTIRHEUMATIC DRUG?

It is accepted most patients with RA require nonsteroidal anti-inflammatory drugs (NSAIDs) for symptomatic control of pain and stiffness, which are often given together with an analgesic for this purpose. Although chemically diverse and capable of a variety of different effects, the NSAIDs have similar effects on arachidonic acid metabolism.

The grouping together of SAARDs is more controversial. As a group, these drugs are chemically diverse, probably have quite different modes of action, and aside from being slow-acting, are unique only in providing symptomatic relief in RA. Confusion especially arises when the term *disease-modifying antirheumatic drug* (DMARD) is used in the belief that these agents affect the course of RA. Extensive international discus-

Table 1 Conventional Classification for Antirheumatic Drugs

Class	Examples
Nonsteroidal anti-inflammatory drugs (NSAIDs)	Indomethacin Ibuprofen
Corticosteroids	Prednisolone
Slow-acting antirheumatic drugs (SAARDs)	Gold Sulfasalazine Methotrexate

sions led by the WHO/ILAR task forces have led to a reassessment of the situation (Edmonds et al., 1993a and 1993b).

The conventional classification of these drugs is given in Table 1. The proposed revised classification is shown in Table 2. In essence, it is proposed that current SAARDs all have the ability to modify the symptoms of RA. They meet the criteria for classification as symptom-modifying antirheumatic drugs (SMARDs). They may also be disease modifying and make the criteria for disease-controlling antirheumatic therapy (DCART) status, but at present, this is unproven and must not be a major need for their clinical use. Thus, SAARDs should mainly be used because they improve patients' symptoms.

The drugs used as SAARDs vary slightly from country to country and also with time. The main drugs consist of injectable gold, oral gold, sulfasalzaine, methotrexate, penicillamine, antimalarials (chloroquine and hydroxychloroquine), azathioprine, cyclosporin, and occasionally cytotoxic drugs (cyclophosphamide and chlorambucil).

III. WHEN TO GIVE SAARDS

The balance of evidence favors using SAARDs in three clinical situations: (a) early disease; (b) erosive disease (defined radiologically); (c) active disease assessed clinically and by laboratory markers of disease activity such as erythrocyte sedimentation

Table 2 Revised Classification for Antirheumatic Drugs

Class of drug	Features
1. Symptom-modifying antirheumatic drugs (SMARDs)	Improve symptoms and clinical features of synovitis nonsteroidal anti-inflammatory drugs corticosteroids slower-acting drugs (e.g., gold)
2. Disease-controlling anti-rheumatic therapy (D-CART)	Change the course of rheumatoid arthritis by: improve and sustain function in association with decreased inflammatory synovitis prevent or significantly decrease the rate of progression of structural joint damage Changes must be sustained for a minimum period of 1 year

Source: After Edmonds et al. (1993).

rate (ESR), C-reactive protein (CRP), and anemia. The aim in early disease is to control symptoms and to prevent erosions. The aim in erosive disease is to reduce the progression of damage in a strategy of secondary prevention. The aim in active disease is to control symptoms. The balance of evidence shows that SAARDs can be used at most stages of RA for symptomatic relief and are effective in both early and late RA. In terms of their symptomatic response, SAARDs reduce symptoms of joint pain and swelling. They decrease the elevated acute phase response. They also make patients feel generally better.

There is good experience from using SAARDs in early RA (Donnely et al., 1992). In this context, early means within the first year of the onset of symptoms, and it may even be considered to be within 3 to 6 months of the onset of RA. Studies by Emery (1993 and 1994) strongly suggest there are benefits in early RA, especially when used in conjunction with markers to predict disease outcome. For example, those patients who are seropositive for the rheumatoid factor possess HLA Dw4/14 and are slow acetylators. There is also good recent experience using SAARDs in late disease (Houssein et al., 1994). Indirect evidence suggests the early use of SAARDs improves function (Comer et al., 1994) and a review of clinical practice suggested patients are being started on SAARDs at an earlier stage in the course of their disease (Spector et al., 1988). Taken together, there is an overwhelming balance of specialist opinion in favor of the early use of SAARDs.

Should SAARDs be used before NSAIDs or in preference to these drugs? Although this seems an illogical question, and that a reasonable assumption is that SAARDs should always be given after NSAIDs, there is no clear reason for making such a conjecture. At the present time, it is reasonable to use SAARDs after NSAIDs. But there is an eed to keep an open mind on this question. There is increasing evidence that the toxicity of NSAIDs is higher than previously thought and that SAARDs may be less toxic.

Guidelines from the United Kingdom (Report of Joint Working Group, 1992) and North America (American College of Rheumatology Ad Hoc Committee on Guidelines, 1996) indicate the problems of deciding when to initiate SAARDs. Both guidelines agree that initial drug treatment of RA usually involves NSAIDs to reduce joint pain and swelling and improve function, and that through these have analgesic and anti-inflammatory properties they neither alter the course of the disease nor prevent joint destruction. The guidelines stress that the exact place of SAARDs is less clear cut with various schools of thought about their use. Although aggressive disease or the early onset of erosions indicates the need for rapid treatment with a SAARD (Van der Heijde et al., 1989), a minority opinion advocates the earliest possible introduction of a SAARD (Wilske and Healey, 1989). This is controversial subject (Hess and Luggen, 1989); it has the drawback of giving potentially toxic drugs without adequate justification to many patients who might do well without needing them or who only have a transient synovitis. It may also exhaust the limited number of drug options at an early stage, with subsequent difficulties in controlling aggressive disease later. But early treatment with SAARDs may control the disease before erosions develop and limit its progression. Many prefer a traditional approach in which initial treatment to control symptoms with a nonsteroidal anti-inflammatory drug is followed by treatment with a SAARD in patients who have persistently active disease.

Patients with active RA should receive SAARDs. There is no absolute definition of active disease, but clinical trials usually involve giving SAARDs to patients with six or more active joints, six or more tender joints, 45 min or more morning stiffness, and an ESR of 30 mm/h or more. The selection of these criteria for SAARD treatment is derived from the classic studies of therapy such as the Empire Rheumatism Council (Research Committee of the Empire Rheumatism Council, 1960) study of injectable gold.

There are two problems with using these criteria. First, most rheumatologists do not follow them. I have reanalyzed data from 282 RA patients started on therapy with a SAARD as part of a European collaborative study (Table 3). Many patients had relatively mild disease when started on therapy, and yet these responded equally well. Second, there is limited evidence that patients with different degrees of disease activity have been studied adequately even in recently introduced drugs such as methotrexate. This agent provides a good example for the overall problem. Although methotrexate is a widely used SAARD, there are no special criteria concerning which patients should be given this drug (Bannwarth et al., 1994). Schnabel and Gross (1994) have highlighted its favorable profile of safety and tolerability. Seideman (1993) pointed out that despite its frequent use, the relationship between different methotrexate doses and clinical effects remains unclear. Methotrexate doses should probably be adjusted individually for each patient in order to improve efficacy and decrease dose-dependent side effects, but the optimal methods are uncertain. Thus, methotrexate illustrates the complexity of trying to select the best SAARD and optimal dose for an RA patient.

IV. RELEVANT ENDPOINTS AND CLINICAL INDICATIONS

Defining optimal SAARD therapy involves having at least a partial ideal of the main endpoints it should affect and the extent of changes which should be anticipated. The three characteristics of D-CART therapy can be used to define this issue: These are beneficial changes in the clinical features of synovitis, function, and progressive joint damage. The long-term effects of SAARDs on these endpoints were reported by Capell et al. (1991) in a cohort of 123 RA patients followed for 10 years from the time of prescription of their initial SAARD. At 10 years, 24 patients had died and 7 were not traced. Analysis of the results in the 92 patients evaluated at 10 years showed improvement in articular index, pain score, and ESR. The functional index showed a trend toward deterioration which did not reach significance. Sixty-seven of the 92 patients remained on a SAARD at 10 years with a median duration of treatment of 107 months.

Table 3 Disease Duration and Activity in 282 Patients Started on a Slow-acting Drug

Disease duration (years)		ESR (mm/h)		Morning stiffness (minutes)		No. swollen joints	
Group	% patients	Group	% patients	Group	% patients	Group	% patients
>5	39	<30	18	<30	12	>5	37
2–5	25	30–60	49	30–59	20	6–8	36
<2	35	>60	33	>60	68	>9	28

Source: Taken from information collected as part of the Concerted Action Programme of the European Workshop for Rheumatology Research (Scott et al., 1992).

There was a correlation between area under the curve for ESR over 10 years and radiological progression of disease in hands, knees, and hips. Radiographic scores correlated well with the functional index at the outset and at 10 years and also with the change in the radiographic score over the 10-year period.

A. Symptoms

The main features of active synovitis are many tender and/or swollen joints, articular pain, high patient/physician assessments of disease activity, and an elevated acute phase response shown by elevated ESR and CRP. There is good evidence that if patients with active RA do not receive SAARDs, their disease is poorly controlled. Porter and Capell (1993) evaluated the natural history of such untreated RA over 6 months in 142 RA patients randomized to receive placebo in five double blind, placebo-controlled trials of possible SAARDs conducted in their unit. There was no significant change in ESR or most clinical features during that time. The mean ESR actually increased at 3 months by 2 mm/h. Only 5% of patients more than halved their ESR over the 6 months. However, there was a small significant fall in articular index over 6 months of placebo treatment.

There is some evidence that small joint synovitis in the hands and feet has a different clinical course to large joint involvement. Hassell et al. (1995) showed small joint synovitis often occurs in the absence of an abnormal acute phase response (ESR or CRP), and it is possible for disease activity measures to appear controlled while inflammation continues in small joints causing radiographic damage. This may explain the paradox of improving disease activity but not outcome. They suggest that small joint inflammation and damage are separate from large joint damage and should be assessed independently.

B. Function

Function can be assessed by disease specific instruments such as the Health Assessment Questionnaire (HAQ) or generic instruments such as the Nottingham Health Profile or SF-36. There is good evidence that slow-acting drugs improve function. One key study was reported by Porter et al. (1994). They analyzed functional outcome in 190 RA patients who had tolerated SAARD therapy with injectable gold, sulfasalazine, or penicillamine for 5 years. Function was measured using the modified HAQ. Patient function improved significantly compared with baseline. Its improvement was maximal by 1–2 years; thereafter it declined slowly. However, after 5 years of treatment, function was still significantly better than before treatment had started. There were highly significant improvements in all variables measured to assess disease activity, which remained well controlled throughout the 5-year period.

A recent report by Fries et al. (1996) has described associations between consistent SAARD use and long-term functional outcomes in 2888 RA patients followed up prospectively for up to 20 years (average 9 years) at eight specialist centers. Increased SAARD use was strongly associated with better long-term Disability Index values. The association was strengthened when restricted to more seriously affected Rheumatoid factor–positive patients. Their results suggest up to a 30% reduction in long-term disability with consistent SAARD use.

C. Radiographs

Progressive joint damage is accompanied by increasing radiographic abnormalities. These do not reflect disease activity at the time the radiograph is taken but indicate overall damage to the joints (Dacre and Buckland-Wright, 1992). Radiology gives a good indication of the progression of arthritis and its related functional outcome. As radiographic changes do not necessarily have direct effects on patient's health status, they lie between process and outcome variables. Radiographic erosions are a relatively late phenomenon; they are seen in less than 40% of cases of early RA. Erosion scores are quantitative, but the development of a first erosion is a qualitative change from the nonerosive state. Many methods of scoring radiographs have been devised, but two are in common usage: the Sharp method (Sharp et al., 1984) used predominantly in the United States, in which each a number of joints in the hand and wrist are graded for erosions and narrowing, and the method of Larsen (Larsen et al., 1987), in which radiographic appearances are compared with those in reference films. Van der Heije et al. (1995) examined early radiographic damage in RA and its prediction by joint inflammation. They found progressive radiographic damage in newly diagnosed RA is independently associated with the presence of rheumatoid factor and damage at baseline and with cumulative joint inflammation. Preventing joint damage is most likely to be achieved in RA patients with active synovitis who are rheumatoid factor positive. There is also good evidence that patients with a high CRP level, especially in early RA, are more likely to have progressive joint damage (van Leeuwen et al., 1993).

D. The Limitations of Selection

Although SAARD therapy is often focused on 'ideal' patients with many active joints, a high ESR and short disease duration, many other patients may benefit. Pullar and Capell (1986) studied 150 RA patients treated with sulfasalazine and found clinical improvement in all subgroups, including patients with an initial low ESR. Thus, patients of all ages, sex, disease durations, rheumatoid factor status, radiographic grading, and ESR levels can benefit from a SAARD.

E. The Consequences of RA

Pincus and Callahan (1993) pointed out that most patients with RA experience disease progression over periods longer than 5 years characterized by radiographic joint destruction, declines in functional capacity to perform activities of daily living, and frequent work disability. Such long-term consequences may be viewed as "side effects" of disease, which must be balanced against possible side effects of drugs in planning treatment. Aggressive approaches, which may include acceptance of mild and even moderate side effects of drugs, may be appropriate in efforts to prevent side effects of RA. Pincus (1994) suggested that the traditional approach to RA therapy, from less toxic to more toxic drugs, is inadequate owing to this progression and suggested it should be viewed as an urgent medical problem—a "medical emergency"—in order to control the long-term consequences of the disease process.

V. WHICH PATIENTS SHOULD RECEIVE SAARDS?

Patients with active RA should usually have SAARDs. Age, sex, rheumatoid factor positivity, genetic background, and race are all factors which could potentially alter a response to SAARDs. The most well-evaluated issue is age, and several studies have looked at its effects together with the effects of sex in some cases. Several studies showed no important effects of age or sex. Bologna et al. (1996) assessed whether age influences the efficacy and toxicity of one SAARD, methotrexate, in 469 RA patients who were divided into those aged above and those below 65 years. There were no difference in clinical and biological variables. The number of patients in remission and the frequency and type of side effects were similar. The implication is that age has little effect on SAARD therapy. A similar finding was reported by Capell et al. (1993); an analysis of experience in 1140 RA patients during the first year of SAARD therapy showed neither age nor sex had an influence on the response to treatment, although patients with a longer disease duration showed a greater tendency to stop treatment. The same group reported on the effects of sulfasalazine in relation to age (Wilkieson et al., 1993). They studied the risk: benefit ratio in relation to age, retrospectively combining five prospective studies of enteric-coated sulfasalazine therapy in 352 patients. Sulfasalazine was equally effective in all age groups and the toxicity profile was also similar in all age groups.

By contrast, other studies showed a potential effect of both age and sex. De La Mata et al. (1995) reported an observational study of 629 patients treated with SAARDs between 1979 and 1991; they noted that there were some sex differences with penicillamine with greater toxicity in female and elderly patients. The other SAARDs did not show such an effect. Wijnands et al. (1993) examined those factors which influence the discontinuation of SAARDs in a prospective study of 245 patients with recently diagnosed RA. There were statistically significant influences of both age and sex on the discontinuation rate of chrysotherapy because of toxicity. The discontinuation of sulfasalazine was also increased by advanced age. Overall elderly patients have a greater risk of stopping therapy owing to toxicity, although its efficacy seems similar.

As seropositive patients have more severe disease and a worse prognosis, it is sensible to consider all seropositive cases for therapy with a SAARD. However, there is no need to restrict therapy to such cases. Although RA patients who are seropositive for rheumatoid factor have more severe disease and are more likely to need SAARDs, there is evidence that seronegative cases respond well to SAARDs. An example is the study of Farr et al. (1995); they found that seronegative patients respond positively to sulfasalazine. It is therefore important not to exclude seronegative cases from therapy.

The effects of race and genetic background can only be considered indirectly through studies of disease activity. There is good evidence that RA is less severe in nonwhite patients. For example, Chikanza et al. (1994) compared the clinical, serological, and radiographic expression of RA in UK white and ethnic black patients from Zimbabwe. Articular manifestations of RA were less severe in the black patients with RA from Zimbabwe with less early morning stiffness, fewer active joints, fewer joint deformities, and better grip strength. White patients had a higher frequency of extra-articular manifestations. The radiographic changes in the black patients were less severe than those in the white patients. Thus, patients with RA who are nonwhite may have less to gain from using a SAARD.

Other genetic factors are involved. Wijnands et al. (1993) found HLA-DR3 was related to discontinuation of chrysotherapy because of toxicity, whereas stopping hydroxychloroquine because of lack of efficacy occurred less frequently in HLA-DR3-positive cases.

VI. STRATEGIES FOR USING SINGLE SAARDS

Aggressive rheumatoid disease or the early onset of erosions indicate a need for rapid treatment with a SAARD. The early use of potentially toxic drugs without adequate justification to many patients who might do well without them or who only have a transient synovitis is possibly unjustified. Most rheumatologists use SAARDs in patients with persistent active disease whose symptoms have not been adequately controlled by nonsteroidal drugs alone.

Meta-analysis of clinical trials of slow-acting drugs (Felson et al., 1990) has shown that the antimalarials, hydroxychloroquine and chloroquine, and auranofin are less active, especially in erosive disease; sulfasalazine, penicillamine, methotrexate, and gold injections are appropriate for patients with erosions, and especially those who are seropositive and have a high ESR; but gold injections give more adverse reactions than other drugs. The degree of anticipated change associated with these drugs is only modest (McDuffie, 1990; Capell et al., 1990), although they undoubtedly produce short-term changes. Wolfe (1990) has argued that although all markers of outcome—mortality, functional ability, cumulative pain, economic costs, and adverse drug reactions—are unfavourably affected in rheumatoid disease, therapy alters the slope of RA decrement either permanently or intermittently. As such changes are difficult to measure in short-term cross-sectional studies, the effects of treatment are often underestimated.

But not all meta-analyses show such distinctions between SAARDs. Capell et al. (1993) evaluated the comparative merits of commonly used SAARDs. They use a collected analysis on results obtained during the first year of treatment in 1140 patients with RA treated with gold, penicillamine, sulfasalazine, or auranofin from a single center. The drugs performed similarly, with about 60% of patients continuing to receive each of these drugs for at least 1 year. Neither gender nor age had an influence on the response to treatment. Patients with a longer disease duration showed a greater tendency to stop treatment. The median percentage improvement was 33% in visual analogue pain score and 50% in ESR.

Gotzsche et al. (1992) also undertook a meta-analysis of placebo-controlled trials of methotrexate, auranofin, penicillamine, azathioprine, sulfasalazine, gold sodium thiomalate, and chloroquines. They noted that the difference between drugs and placebo in the ESR was only 8.8 mm/h. In multiple linear regression analyses, with the physician's global evaluation and relative change in joint tenderness count as outcome variables, a substantial sample size bias was demonstrated. The effect decreased with increasing sample size. The risk of dropping out from any cause was larger on drug than on placebo. Of the 3439 patients, 4 went into complete remission on drug. They concluded that the benefits of SAARDs remained uncertain.

Fries (1990) suggested that a new approach is needed with SAARDs and termed this the "saw tooth" strategy. His recommended new approach is based on six principles: early use of these drugs; continual serial use of different agents; regular qualitative monitoring of disability to detect progression; includes progression; setting a disability ceiling for the individual patient; sequential change in slow-acting drug therapy when that ceiling is reached; and the deployment of analgesics and nonsteroidal anti-inflammatory drugs as adjunctive rather than first-line therapy. Whether such an approach will be used in clinical practise remains to be seen.

Pincus (1994) has highlighted the limitations of randomized controlled clinical trials which include excessive attention to group data rather than individual patient responses, the exclusion of many cases, small study numbers with insufficient statistical power to identify clinically important trends, and a time frame too short to recognize clinically meaningful differences between treatment regimens.

VII. TOXICITY PROFILES

Side effects can limit the use of SAARDs and they cause potential life-threatening adverse reactions such as marrow depression. This has led to the concept of toxicity profiles for these drugs by Singh et al. (1991), who developed profiles for seven SAARDs from 2479 RA patients consecutively enrolled at five specialist centers. Close similarities were found between toxicity profiles of parenteral gold and D-penicillamine, and between azathioprine and methotrexate. Rash was frequently seen with gold compounds and D-penicillamine, whereas upper gastrointestinal toxicity was common with immunosuppressive agents such as methotrexate. Further work in this area by Fries et al. (1993) showed the least toxic SAARD was hydroxychloroquine followed by intramuscular gold and then penicillamine, methotrexate, and azathioprine. Oral gold (auranofin) was most toxic, but this resulted from a high frequency of minor complications. The toxicity of methotrexate and azathioprine was similar to that of the most toxic nonsteroidal anti-inflammatory drugs such as indomethacin. The current SAARDs seem closely clustered by their toxicity with the only surprise being the relative safety of parenteral gold.

VIII. WHEN TO GIVE INDIVIDUAL SLOW-ACTING DRUGS

The choice of SAARDs must be based on evidence of their efficacy, the needs of individual patients, and the experience of the clinician. My own first choices are parenteral gold, methotexate, or sulfasalazine, although not in any particular order. I use cyclosporine as a "first reserve" and give other drugs such as antimalarials, penicillamine, azathioprine, and oral gold to selected cases. Kay and Pullar (1992) found large variations among UK rheumatologists in prescribing SAARDs. In a survey of 75 specialists, they found sulfasalazine was the most popular first-choice drug. There was marked variation in what was accepted as an adequate trial of therapy. The main SAARDs are listed in Table 4. All the drugs have shown efficacy in one or more randomized controlled trials. Some, such as penicillamine, azathioprine, and oral gold (auranofin) are either used infrequently or their use is declining; I will not consider them in detail. The main question is whether to prescribe parenteral gold, methotrexate, or sulfasalazine as first choice drug, with antimalarials and cyclosporin in reserve.

A. Parenteral Gold

Parental gold has been used for over 50 years. Its value was established by the Empire Rheumatism Council trial (1960). Since then many studies have confirmed its efficacy (Butler, 1984). Its use is limited by its slow onset of action, and it may take over 3 months for any appreciable improvement. A more rapid response can be achieved by using intramuscular steroids when starting gold therapy. Choy et al. (1993) showed intramuscular methylprednisolone was effective over 2–12 weeks of treatment at the

Table 4 Slow-acting Drugs for Rheumatoid Arthritis

Drug	Usual dose	Effectiveness	Personal assessment
Injectable gold (myocrysin)	50 mg weekly to 50 mg monthly	Good	Valuable but toxic
Penicillamine	250–500 mg daily	Good	Little used
Sulfasalazine	0.5–2.0 g daily	Good	Standard first choice
Methotrexate	7.5–15.0 mg weekly	Good	Standard first choice
Azathioprine	50–150 mg daily	Good	Reserve drug
Oral gold (auranofin)	6–9 mg daily	Moderate	Little used
Chloroquine	125–250 mg daily	Moderate	Little used
Hydroxychloroquine	200–400 mg daily	Moderate	Reserve drug
Cyclosporin	2.0–3.5 mg/kg	Moderate	Reserve drug (role still being defined)

initiation of gold treatment. Recent work involving my unit (data in preparation) has shown that 120 mg IM methylprednisolone monthly is more effective than 80 mg. Heytman et al. (1994) followed RA patients treated with methylprednisolone in the induction of chrysotherapy for over 3 years. There had significant decreases in mean disability measured by HAQ but not other clinical or laboratory measures.

There is evidence parenteral gold reduces radiographic progression. Iannuzzi et al. (1983) reviewed 60 published studies employing gold and other SAARDs to evaluate the evidence therapy slows radiographic progression; 17 studies included radiographic assessment of treated and control groups. They found evidence suggesting both gold and cyclophosphamide can retard radiographic progression of joint destruction. More recently, Buckland-Wright et al. (1993) used microfocal radiology to evaluate the effect of IM gold on erosion area in early RA. After 6 months, gold halted disease progression and 23% of cases showed erosion repair.

Despite these advantages, long-term observational studies question the continuing benefits of chrysotherapy. Epstein et al. (1991) studied 822 RA patients reviewing their sociodemographic and clinical characteristics, course, and therapy. There were no changes in the course of RA over 5 years. The use of parenteral gold for at least 2 consecutive years at the start of the observation period produced, on average, no change in the course over 5 years. They interpreted these data as showing gold had limited value. Graudal et al. (1994) studied 93 RA patients treated with gold for 3–13 years. Joint swelling, ESR, and radiographic assessments improved in the first year of therapy, with good clinical responses for up to 10 years but associated progressive joint damage and loss of range of joint movement.

There is good overall evidence for short-term efficacy of gold, although this cannot be extrapolated to a long-term effect on outcome. For example, an observational study of the clinical effects of gold evaluated 98 patients over 12 months; all clinical outcome measures improved (Wolfe et al., 1993). The toxicity of gold, wihch limits its initial value, becomes a less frequent problem with increasing duration of therapy. Direct comparisons of gold and methotexate show no clear-cut differences, although the studies are small and lack statistical power (Wolfe, 1993; Harth, 1993).

B. Methotrexate

The use of methotrexate in RA has been a major advance from the 1980s. Its initial use in psoriatic arthritis because of skin disease induced improvements in synovitis, and subsequent placebo-controlled trials in RA confirmed its efficacy. The main important advantage of methotrexate is its long-term effect. In one study, where patients received weekly oral methotrexate for up to 90 months, there were significant, maintained improvements from baseline in most clinical parameters (Kremer and Phelps, 1992). Weinblatt et al. (1992) assessed efficacy and safety over 84 months in 26 cases; there were continuing improvements after 36 months of therapy, and 12 patients treated for 84 months maintained improvements in painful joints, swollen joints, pain, and global assessments, Tischler et al. (1993) reported 126 RA patients treated for 3 years or more. The probability of continuing therapy was 72% at 2–3 years, 45% had marked improvements, and 6% achieved clinical remission.

Most rheumatologists prescribe methotrexate as a weekly dose, but the optimal dosage regimen is not known. A study of 47 RA patients taking methotrexate for at least 8 months with stable disease were randomly assigned to receive usual therapy or second-weekly dosing (Kremer et al., 1995). Only 12 of 23 patients receiving alternate-weekly methotrexate did not have a disease flare over the 6 months study period. However, some patients will tolerate a lengthened dosage interval, and this may be used as an alternative to dose reduction. There is debate about the optimal dose. I rarely exceed 15 mg weekly, but many other rheumatologists give far higher doses.

Alarcon et al. (1992) reviewed clinical and radiographic effects of methotrexate and suggested its effects on radiographic progression were open to question. They performed a meta-analysis of 353 methotrexate-treated cases and 205 controls to compute monthly rates of disease progression; these were similar for methotrexate-treated cases and controls. However, Lopez-Mendez et al. (1993) reported a randomized study of radiographic progression in 211 RA patients given auranofin, methotrexate, or a combination of the two. Worsening erosion and joint space narrowing scores occurred in all three treatment groups but were only significant in those treated with auranofin, showing radiographic progression may be slowed with methotrexate. Finally, Rau et al. (1991) studied 31 patients in whom parenteral gold therapy had failed treated with methotrexate for at least 24 months. The rate of progression was less during methotrexate therapy.

A meta-analysis of 66 randomized controlled trials involving 3957 patients with RA treated for 3 months to 2 years (Felson et al., 1990) showed methotrexate in doses of at least 7.5 mg weekly was as effective as intramuscular gold, sulfasalazine, and penicillamine in reducing joint pain, tenderness, and ESR. In four other trials (totalling 371 patients), methotrexate was at least as effective as azathioprine (Hamdy et al., 1987; Arnold et al., 1990; Jeurissen et al., 1991; Wilkens et al., 1992). Improvement begins earlier with methotrexate (within 4 to 6 weeks) than with other antirheumatic drugs (e.g., within 2 to 3 months after sulfasalazine and probably 6 months with gold).

C. Sulfasalazine

The efficacy sulfasalazine has been established by randomized controlled trials in the UK (Neumann et al., 1983; Pullar et al., 1983). It has favorable effects on clinical, functional, and radiographic measures (Capell,1995). An analysis by Pullar et al. (1987)

provided indirect evidence that sulfasalazine reduced radiographic progression over 2 years. This was later confirmed in a 1-year randomized controlled trial comparing it with hydroxychloroquine (van der Heijde et al., 1989). More recent studies have continued to confirm its efficacy; for example, the Australian Multicentre Trial Group (1992) showed, in early RA, there are significant improvements in clinical and biochemical variables. Another study by Hannonen et al. (1993) evaluated 80 patients with symptomatic disease for less than 12 months. Sulfasalazine was superior to placebo in reducing laboratory features of inflammation and clinical parameters of disease activity; fewer erosive changes developed in with receiving active treatment. In a retrospective survey of 352 cases, sulfasalazine was equally effective in young and old patients (Wilkieson et al., 1993). It had a relatively rapid onset of action (Porter et al., 1992). A study of its long-term use by van Riel et al. (1995) reported experience in The Netherlands in a cohort of patients with early RA where it was mainly given as a first-choice SAARD. There was a better survival with sulfasalazine than either hydroxychloroquine or parenteral gold. In 9% of the patients, it was withdrawn as a complete remission was obtained. The evidence shows that sulfasalazine is widely used in RA and may be best employed in early disease.

D. Hydroxychloroquine and Chloroquine

Hydroxychloroquine and chloroquine drugs have similarities; both have been shown to be effective in randomized controlled trials, and my personal preference favors hydroxychloroquine. It may have an optimal role in mild RA. A study of 104 patients with mild disease (Davis et al., 1991) who had synovitis limited to their hands and feet with low ESRs and CRP levels showed significant improvements in clinical and laboratory features with hydroxychloroquine. Another large randomized trial by Clark et al. (1993) in 126 patients with early RA showed hydroxychloroquine gave significant improvements in clinical variables but not in the ESR. Side effects were uncommon. The balance of evidence favors hydroxychloroquine in milder cases of early RA (Harris, 1993).

E. Cyclosporin

There is strong evidence from randomized trials that cyclosporin A can control the symptoms of early and late RA. Wells and Tugwell (1993) reviewed its use in five prospective clinical trials. A composite effect score for efficacy and the rates of drop out due to toxicity were each compared with earlier meta-analyses evaluating the relative efficacy and toxicity of second-line drugs for RA; cyclosporin was better than placebo. Forre (1994) showed cyclosporin reduced radiographic progression in advanced disease. More recently, Pasero et al. (1996) have provided evidence that cyclosporin reduces radiographic progression in early disease. Their study has one unusual feature in that it compared cyclosporin therapy to a panel of other slow-acting drugs. They enrolled 361 patients with RA under 4 years' duration. By 12 months radiographic progression was significantly reduced in patients given cyclosporin. Finally, a new microemulsion oral formulation of cyclosporin has been tested in RA; it has better bioavailability and appears preferable for routine clinical use (van den Borne et al., 1995). The main disadvantage of cyclosporin is the high incidence of renal toxicity, which limits its therapeutic value in RA. Regular monitoring of blood pressure and renal function is needed.

IX. COMBINATION THERAPY

The use of several SAARDs in RA is controversial. McCarty (1993) presents an elegant case for this approach. He considers that single agents often fail to control synovial inflammation adequately. Combination therapy with relatively small doses of several agents shown to be effective in controlled trials when used alone can produce sustained and marked therapeutic control. As in the treatment of malignancy or tuberculosis, the use of potent drugs in combination may prevent or delay the clonal expansion of resistant cells. If this is indeed the case in the treatment of RA, then consideration should be given to the routine use of drug combinations. It is conceivable that we do patients a disservice by using potentially valuable drugs sequentially rather than in tandem. Whatever its merits, combination drug therapy for seropositive RA is clearly a stop-gap measure whose usefulness will end as more specific means of controlling joint inflammation become available.

Paulus (1993) has provided a different perspective. He noted that, to date, it has been exceptionally difficult to prove that any combination of disease-modifying antirheumatic drugs is more effective than its components used one at a time. However, only a few of many possible combinations have been evaluated in clinical trials. Careful attention to the details of patient selection, study design and duration, and choice of primary outcome measures is essential. A logical strategy for protocol development emphasizes the use of multiple small pilot studies to screen series of combinations and doses to identify a few that appear to show clinical benefit. The most promising combinations can then be evaluated in large, double-blind, randomized, pivotal studies with a higher probability of success.

Wilke et al. (1993) made a more complex case. They argued that long-term outcome of sequential monotherapy based on the therapeutic pyramid has been disappointing. A review of prognostic factors, acute disease activity measures, functional measures, and the results of preliminary trials with combination therapy suggests that specific goals of treatment can be established and that logical, aggressive treatment in early disease can be accomplished. These goals should include prompt control and continuous reduction of the active joint count to less than or equal to 4 and normalization of acute phase reactants. The "graduated-step paradigm" of treatment designed with these goals in mind is described, and a retrospective series that gives an estimate of outcome with its use is reported.

In a review of monotherapy in RA, Emery (1993) suggested that there is an underlying assumption that current therapy is inadequate and that the whole therapeutic approach to RA needs rethinking. But even if combination therapy is adopted, we need a more discriminating approach using prognostic indicators to identify the minority of patients with persistent unresponsive disease and poor outcomes for whom more aggressive therapy should be reserved. The role of combination therapy will be defined in the next decade.

X. CONCLUSIONS

The balance of evidence favors the increased use of SAARDs. They should invariably be used in patients with early, active RA. However their use should also extend to milder disease and late RA. The most effective SAARDs are parenteral gold, methotrexate, and sulfasalazine with antimalarials having a role in mild disease and cyclosporin being of value as a "first-reserve" agent. Combination therapy is the likely direction of future research.

REFERENCES

Alarcon GS, Lopez-Mendez A, Walter J, Boerbooms AM, Russell AS, Furst DE, Rau R, Drosos AA, Bartolucci AA. Radiographic evidence of disease progression in methotrexate treated and non methotrexate disease modifying antirheumatic drug treated rheumatoid arthritis patients: a meta-analysis. J Rheumatol 1992; 19:1868–1873.

Alarcón GS, López-Méndez A, Walter J, et al. Radiographic evidence of disease progression in methotexate treated and nonmethotrexate disease modifying anti rheumatic drug treated rheumatoid arthritis patients. J Rheumatol 1992; 19:1868–1873.

American College of Rheumatology Ad Hoc Committee on clinical guidelines. Guidelines for the management of rheumatoid arthritis. Arthritis Rheum 1996; 39:713–722.

Arnold MH, O'Callagham J, McCredie M, et al. Comparative controlled trial of low-dose weekly methotrexate versus azathioprine in rheumatoid arthritis. Br J Rheumatol 1990; 29:120–125.

Australian Multicentre Clinical Trial Group: sulphsalazine in early rheumatoid arthritis. J Rheumatol 1992; 19:1672–1677.

Bannwarth B, Labat L, Moride Y, Schaeverbeke T. Methotrexate in rheumatoid arthritis. An update. Drugs 1994; 47:25–50.

Bologna C, Viu P, Jorgensen C, Sany J. Effect of age on the efficacy and tolerance of methotrexate in rheumatoid arthritis. Br J Rheumatol 1996; 35:453–457.

Buckland-Wright J, Graham S, Chikanza I, Grahame R. Quantitative microfocal radiography detects changes in erosion area in patients with early rheumatoid arthritis treated with myocrisin. J Rheumatol 1993; 20:243–247.

Butler RC. Gold in the treatment of rheumatoid arthritis. In: Rheumatoid Arthritis. The Treatment Controversy. Goddard DH, Butler RC, eds. Bath, UK: Pitman Press, Bath, 1984:8–36.

Capell HA, Marabani M, Madhok R, Torley H, Hunter JA. Degrees and extent of response to sulphasalazine or penicillamine therapy for rheumatoid arthritis: results from a routine clinical environment over a two year period. Q J Med 1990; 75:335–344.

Capell HA, Murphy EA, Hunter JA. Rheumatoid arthritis: workload and outcome over 10 years. Q J Med 1991; 79:461–476.

Capell HA, Porter DR, Madhok R, Hunter JA. Second line (disease modifying) treatment in rheumatoid arthritis: which drug for which patient? Ann Rheum Dis 1993; 52:423–428.

Capell HA. Clinical efficacy of sulphasalazine—a review. Br J Rheumatol 1995; 34(Suppl)2:35–39.

Chikanza IC, Stein M, Lutalo S, Gibson T. The clinical, serologic and radiologic features of rheumatoid arthritis in ethnic black Zimbabwean and British Caucasian patients. J Rheumatol 1994; 21:2011–2015.

Choy EHS, Kingsley GH, Corkhill MM, Panayi GS. Intramuscular methylprednisolone is superior to pulse oral methylprednisolone during the induction of chrysotherapy. Br J Rheumatol 1993; 32:734–739.

Clark P, Casas E, Tugwell P, Medina C, Gheno C, Tenorio G, Orozco JA. Hydroxychloroquine compared with placebo in rheumatoid arthritis: a randomised trial. Ann Intern Med 1993; 119:1067–1071.

Co-operating Clinics Committee of the American Rheumatism Association. A controlled trial of gold salt therapy in rheumatoid arthritis. Arthritis Rheum 1973; 16:353–358.

Comer M, Scott DL, Doyle DV, Huskisson EC, Hopkins A. Clinical guidelines and the outcome of rheumatoid arthritis. Br J Rheumatol 1994; 33(Suppl 1):139.

Dacre JE, Buckland-Wright JC. The course and outcome of rheumatoid arthritis. Radiological measures of outcome. Baillieres Clin Rheumatol 1992; 6:39–67.

Davis MJ, Dawes PT, Fowler PD, Clarke S, Fisher J, Shadforth MF. Should disease modifying drugs be used in mild rheumatoid arthritis? Br J Rheumatol 1991; 30:451–454.

De La Mata J, Blanco FJ, Gomez-Reino JJ. Survival analysis of disease modifying antirheumatic drugs in Spanish rheumatoid arthritis patients. Ann Rheum Dis 1995; 54:881–885.

Donnelly S, Scott DL, Emery P. The long term outcome and justification for early treatment. Clin Rheumatol: Int Pract Res 1992; 6:251–260.

Edmonds JP, Scott DL, Furst DE, Brooks PM, Paulus HE. Anti-rheumatic drugs: a proposed new classification. Arthritis Rheum 1993a; 36:336–339.

Edmonds JP, Scott DL, Furst DE, Paulus HE. New classification of anti-rheumatic drugs. The evolution of a concept. J Rheumatol 1993b; 20:585–587.

Emery P. Monotherapy in rheumatoid arthritis. Br J Rheumatol, 1993; 32:21–23.

Emery P. The optimal management of early rheumatoid disease: the key to preventing disability. Br J Rheumatol 1994 33:765–768.

Epstein WV, Henke CJ, Yelin EH, Katz PP. Effect of parenterally administered gold therapy on the course of adult rheumatoid arthritis. Ann Intern Med 1991; 114:437–444.

Farr M, Waterhouse L, Johnson AE, Kitas GD, Jubb RW, Bacon PA. A double-blind controlled study comparing sulphasalazine with placebo in rheumatoid factor (RF)–negative rheumatoid arthritis. Clin Rheumatol 1995; 14:531–536.

Felson DT, Anderson JJ, Meenan R. The comparative efficacy and toxicity of second line drugs in rheumatoid arthritis. Results of two meta-analyses. Arthritis Rheum 1990; 33:1449–1461.

Forre O, the Norwegian Arthritis Study Group. Radiologic evidence of disease modification in rheumatoid arthritis patients treated with cyclosporin: results of a 48-week multicentre study comparing low dose cyclosporin with placebo. Arthritis Rheum 1994; 37:1506–1512.

Fries JF, Williams CA, Morfeld D, Singh G, Sibley J. Reduction in long-term disability in patients with rheumatoid arthritis by disease-modifying antirheumatic drug-based treatment strategies. Arthritis Rheum 1996; 39:616–622.

Fries JF, Wiliams CA, Ramey D, Bloch DA. The relative toxicity of disease-modifying antirheumatic drugs. Arthritis Rheum 1993; 36:297–306.

Fries JF. Re-evaluating the therapeutic approach to rheumatoid arthritis: the 'sawtooth' strategy. J Rheumatol 1990; 22(Suppl):12–15.

Gotzsche PC, Podenphant J, Olesen M, Halberg P. Meta-analysis of second-line antirheumatic drugs: sample size bias and uncertain benefit. J Clin Epidemiol 1992; 45:587–594.

Graudal HK, Graudal N, Jurik AG. On the course of seropositive arthritis during and after long-term gold therapy. Scand J Rheumatol 1994; 23:223–230.

Hamdy H, McKenndry RJR, Mierins E, Liver JA. Low-dose methotrexate compared with azathioprine in the treatment of rheumatoid arthritis. Arthritis Rheum 1987; 30:361–368.

Hannonen P, Mottonen T, Hakola M, Oka M. Sulfasalazine in early rheumatoid arthritis. A 48-week double-blind, prospective, placebo-controlled study. Arthritis Rheum 1993; 36:1501–1509.

Harris ED. Hydroxychloroquine is safe and probably useful in rheumatoid arthritis. Ann Intern Med 1993; 119:1146–1147.

Harth M. Gold in rheumatoid arthritis: standard, substitute of sham? J Rheumatol 1993; 20:771–773.

Hassell AB, Plant MJ, Clarke S, Fisher J, Jones PW, Saklatvala J, Fowler PD, Shadforth MF, Dawes PT. Small joint synovitis in rheumatoid arthritis: should it be assessed separately? Br J Rheumatol 1995; 34:51–55.

Hess EV, Luggen ME. Remodelling the pyramid—a concept whose time has not yet come. J Rheumatol 1989; 16:1175–1176.

Heytman M, Ahern MJ, Smith MD, Roberts-Thompson PJ. The long-term effect of pulsed corticosteroids on the efficacy and toxicity of chrysotherapy in rheumatoid arthritis. J Rheumatol 1994; 21:425–444.

Houssien DA, Smith EC, Berry H, Scott DL. Cyclosporin therapy and the radiological progression of established rheumatoid arthritis. Br J Rheumatol 1994; 33(Suppl 2):25.

Iannuzzi L, Dawson N, Zein N, Kushner I. Does drug therapy slow radiographic deterioration in rheumatoid arthritis? New Engl J Med 1983; 309:1023–1028.

Jeurissen MEC, Boerbooms AMTh, van de Putte LBA, et al. Methotrexate versus azathioprine in the treatment of rheumatoid arthritis. Arthritis Rheum 1991; 34:961–972.

Kay EA, Pullar T. Variations among rheumatologists in prescribing and monitoring of disease modifying antirheumatoid drugs. Br J Rheumatol 1992; 31:477–483.

Kremer JM, Phelps CT. Long-term prospective study of the use of methotrexate in the treatment of rheumatoid arthritis. Update after a mean of 90 months. Arthritis Rheum 1992; 35:138–145.

Kremer JM, Davies JMS, Rynes RI, Fink S, Lawrence DA, Petrillo GF, Mullaly PM. Every other week methotrexate in patients with rheumatoid arthritis: a double blind, placebo controlled prospective study. Arthritis Rheum 1995; 38:601–607.

Larsen A, Dale K, Eek M. Radiographic evaluation of rheumatoid arthritis and related conditions.

Lopez-Mendez A, Daniel WW, Reading JC, Ward JR, Alarcon GS. Radiographic assessment of disease progression in rheumatoid arthritis patients enrolled in the cooperative systematic studies of the rheumatic diesease program randomized clinical trial of methotrexate, auranofin, or a combination of the two. Arthritis Rheum 1993; 36:1364–1369.

McCarty DJ. Personal experience in the treatment of seropositive rheumatoid arthritis with drugs used in combinations. Semin Arthritis Rheum 1993; 23(Suppl 1):42–49.

McDuffie FC. How we got in to be where we are. J Rheumatol 1990; 17(Suppl 23):1–3.

Neumann VC, Grindulis KA, Hubball S, et al. Comparison between penicillamine and sulphasalazine in rheumatoid arthritis: Leeds-Birmingham trial. Br Med J 1983; 287:1099–1102.

Pasero G, Prioli F, Marubini E, et al. Slow progression of joint damage in early rheumatoid arthritis treated with cyclosporin A. Arthritis Rheum 1996;

Paulus HE, Egger MJ, Ward JR, Williams HJ. Analysis of improvement in individual rheumatoid arthritis patients treated with disease-modifying anti-rheumatic drugs, based on the findings in patients treated with placebo. Arthritis Rheum 1990; 33:477–484.

Paulus HE. Protocol development for combination therapy with disease-modifying antirheumatic drugs. Sem Arthritis Rheum 1993; 23(Suppl 1):19–25.

Pincus T, Callahan LF. The 'side effects' of rheumatoid arthritis: joint destruction, disability and early mortality. Br J Rheumatol 1993; 32 (Suppl 1):28–37.

Pincus T. Rheumatoid arthritis: a medical emergency? Scand J Rheumatol 1994; 100(Suppl):21–30.

Porter D, Madhok R, Hunter JA, Capell HA. Prospective trial comparing the use of sulphasalazine and auranofin in patients with rheumatoid arthritis. Ann Rheum Dis 1992; 51:461–464.

Porter DR, Capell HA. The 'natural' history of active rheumatoid arthritis over 3-6 months—an analysis of patients enrolled into trials of potential disease-modifying anti-rheumatic drugs, and treated with placebo. Br J Rheumatol 1993; 32:463–466.

Porter DR, McInnes I, Hunter J, Capell HA. Outcome of second line therapy in rheumatoid arthritis. Ann Rheum Dis 1994; 53:812–815.

Pullar T, Capell HA. Selection of suitable patients for second-line therapy in rheumatoid arthritis. Br J Rheumatol 1986; 25:276–281.

Pullar T, Hunter JA, Capell HA. Sulphasalazine in rheumatoid arthritis: a double lind comparison of sulphasalazine with placebo and sodium aurothiomalate. Br Med J 1983; 287:1102–1104.

Pullar T, Hunter JA, Capell HA. Effect of sulphasalazine on the radiological progression of rheumatoid arthritis. Ann Rheum Dis 1987; 46:398–402.

Rau R, Herborn G, Karger T, Werdier D. Retardation of radiologic progression in rheumatoid arthritis with methotrexate therapy: a controlled study. Arthritis Rheum 1991; 34:1236–1244.

Report of a joint working group. Guidelines and audit measures for the specialist supervision of patients with rheumatoid arthritis. J R Coll Physicians Lond 1992; 26:76–82.

Research Sub-committee of the Empire Rheumatism Council. Gold therapy in rheumatoid arthritis. Report of a multi-centre controlled trial. Ann Rheum Dis 1960; 34:416–421.

Schnabel A, Gross WL. Low-dose methotrexate in rheumatic diseases—efficacy, side effects, and risk factors for side effects. Semin Arthritis Rheum 1994; 23:310–327.

Seideman P. Methotrexate—the relationship between dose and clinical effect. Br J Rheumatol 1993; 32:751–753.

Sharp JT, Lidsky MD, Collins LC et al. Methods of scoring the progression of radiological changes in rheumatoid arthritis. Arthritis Rheum 1971; 14:706–720.

Singh G, Fries JF, Williams CA, Zatarain E, Spitz P, Bloch DA. Toxicity profiles of disease modifying antirheumatic drugs in rheumatoid arthritis. J Rheumatol 1991; 18:188–194.

Spector TD, Thompson PW, Evans SJW, Scott DL. Are slow-acting anti-rheumatic drugs being given earlier in rheumatoid arthritis? Br J Rheumatol 1988; 27:498–499.

Tishler M, Caspi D, Yaron M. Long-term experience with low dose methotrexate in rheumatoid arthritis. Rheumatol Int 1993; 13:103–106.

van den Borne BE, Landewe RB, Goei The HS, Mattie H, Breedveld FC, Dijkmans BA. Relative bioavailability of a new oral form of cyclosporin A in patients with rheumatoid arthritis. Br J Clin Pharmacol 1995; 39:172–175.

Van der Heide A, Remme CA, Hofman DM, Jacobs JW, Bijlsma JW. Prediction of progression of radiologic damage in newly diagnosed rheumatoid arthritis. Arthritis Rheum 1995; 38:1466–1474.

Van der Heijde DM, Van Riel PL, Nuver-Zwart JH, Gribnau FW, Van de Putte LB. Effects of hydroxychloroquine and sulphasalazine on progression of joint damage in rheumatoid arthritis. Lancet 1989; I1:1036–1038.

van Leeuwen MA, van Rijswijk MH, van der Heijde DM, Te Meerman GJ, van, Riel PL, Houtman PM, van De Putte LB, Limburg PC. The acute-phase response in relation to radiographic progression in early rheumatoid arthritis: a propsective study during the first three years of the disease. Br J Rheumatol 1993; 32(Suppl 3):9–13.

van Riel PL, van Gestel AM, van de Putte LB. Long-term usage and side-effect profile of sulphasalazine in rheumatoid arthritis. Br J Rheumatol 1995; 34(Suppl 2):40–42.

Weinblatt ME, Weissman BN, Holdsworth DE, Fraser PA, Maier AL, Falchuk KR, Coblyn JS. Long-term prospective study of methotrexate in the treatment of rheumatoid arthritis. 84-month update. Arthritis Rheum 1992; 35(2):129–137.

Wells G, Tugwell P. Cyclosporin A in rheumatoid arthritis: overview of efficacy. Br J Rheumatol 1993; 32(Suppl 1):51–56.

Wijnands MJ, Van 't Hof MA, van Leeuwen MA, van Rijswijk MH, van de, Putte LB, van Riel PL. A prospective analysis of risk factors for the discontinuation of second-line antirheumatic drugs. Pharm World Sci 1993; 15:203–207.

Wilke WS, Sweeney TJ, Calabrese LH. Early, aggressive therapy for rheumatoid arthritis: concerns, descriptions, and estimate of outcome. Semin Arthritis Rheum 1993; 23(Suppl 1):26–41.

Wilkens RF, Urowitz MB, Stablein DM, et al. Comparison of azathioprine, methotrexate, and the combination of both in the treatment of rheumatoid arthritis. Arthritis Rheum 1992; 35:849–856.

Wilkieson CA, Madhok R, Hunter JA, Capell HA. Toleration, side-effects and efficacy of sulphasalazine in rheumatoid arthritis patients of differing agents. Q J Med 1993; 86:501–505.

Wilske KR,Healey LA. Remodelling the pyramid - a concept whose time has come. J Rheumatol 1989; 16:565–567.

Wolfe F, Hawley DJ, Cathey MA. Measurement of gold treatment effect in clinical practice: evidence for effectiveness of intramuscular gold therapy. J Rheumatol 1993; 20:797–802.

Wolfe F. 50 years of anti-rheumatic therapy: the prognosis of rheumatoid arthritis. J Rheumatol 1990; 22(Suppl):24–32.

Wolfe F. The curious case of intramuscular gold. Rheum Dis Clin North Am 1993; 19:173–187.

6

Aggressive Treatment of Rheumatoid Arthritis: When, Whom, and How

Graciela S. Alarcón
The University of Alabama at Birmingham, Birmingham, Alabama

I. INTRODUCTION

Over the last years, significant advances have been made toward understanding the etiopathogenesis of rheumatoid arthritis (RA), while at the same time, it has become evident that the disease results in significant functional losses, persistent pain, added comorbidities, financial difficulties, and reduced life expectancy [1–4]. Rheumatologists have become disenchanted with the traditional treatment approach of gradual escalation of pharmacological agents based on the assumption that nonsteroid anti-inflammatory drugs (NSAIDs) should be used early in the disease course, whereas drugs considered to be potentially more toxic should be reserved for later on [5–7]. Detractors of this approach have pointed out the need to intervene early if the ravages caused by persistent synovitis are to be prevented [7–10]. Unfortunately, it is not prudent to be aggressive early with all patients, since some patients may actually either not have RA but another disorder (e.g., Lyme polyarthritis, a systemic connective tissue disease), have a self-limited course, or may have a benign form (nondestructive) of RA. Restricting RA to those patients who may meet the American Rheumatism Association (ARA; now the American College of Rheumatology, ACR) criteria for the classification of this disorder does not guarantee that syndromes that have a prognosis different from that of RA may not be included [11]. Thus, as important as early aggressive treatment for patients with RA may be, equally important is the ability to identify those patients who are likely to develop destructive disease.

II. IDENTIFICATION OF PATIENTS LIKELY TO DEVELOP A DESTRUCTIVE ARTHROPATHY

As noted by Harris [12], once cartilage damage has occurred and erosions are observed in plain radiographs, the disease is well established and may run its course independently of the pharmacological agent(s) used. There are emerging clues for identifying those patients at risk for developing erosive disease, who should be therefore subjected to aggressive and potentially toxic treatment. Using these clues, can we identify these patterns in a relatively inexpensive way so that a staging strategy can be implemented at most secondary and tertiary care facilities around the world?

Several clinical features have been recognized over time to predict the course of RA. Those consistently found to be associated with destructive RA include insidious rather than acute disease onset, persistent synovitis, elevated C-reactive protein (CRP) levels (or other indicators of persistent inflammation), rheumatoid factor positivity, and the early appearance of erosions [13–17]. Extra-articular features such as subcutaneous nodules, vasculitis, or organ system involvement have also been recognized as being associated with destructive disease.

More recently, it has been postulated that there is a gene-dose effect accounting not only for disease susceptibility but more importantly for disease severity, including destructive arthropathy, the presence of subcutaneous nodules, and the occurrence of extra-articular manifestations in individuals with RA. Thus patients carrying a double dose of the so-called rheumatoid epitope (QKRAA or QRRAA in positions 67–74 of the third hypervariable region [HVR3] of the HLA-DRB1 allele) in an HLA-DR4 allele (DRB1* 0401, *0404, *0405, *0408 *0409, *0410) have been shown to have worse disease than those carrying a single dose or carrying it in non-DR4 alleles (DRB1 *0101, *0102, *1001, *1402, *1406) [18–20]. These data have been obtained in different white populations in North America and Europe [21–25]. Favoring the importance of the rheumatoid epitope are the data obtained in monozygotic twins, as well as that in patients with early RA. A high degree of concordance for the rheumatoid epitope among a group of 91 twins has been reported by Jawaheer et al. [26], whereas Gough et al. [25] reported the presence of the epitope in a large proportion of patients with early symmetrical polyarthritis who evolved into a destructive arthropathy. Finally, in white populations in whom RA is known to be of mild or moderate severity, the rheumatoid epitope has been found to be less frequent and/or to be carried in non-DR4 alleles and/or not be associated with disease severity [27–30]. Similar findings have been reported in Asians from China [31].

In contrast, it has been found that nearly two-thirds of African-American RA patients do not carry the rheumatoid epitope in either an HLA-DR4 or a non-DR4 allele [32, 33], and there is neither an overrepresentation of other DR specificities in these X/X individuals nor the sequence of interest is present in a non-DR4 allele not previously recognized as carrying the rheumatoid epitope [34]. Disease severity in this ethnic group appeared to be unrelated to the presence and the dose of the rheumatoid epitope [34]. Overall, however, African-Americans exhibit clinical and radiographic disease characteristics comparable to the white individuals, suggesting that there is a lot more to destructive arthropathy than the rheumatoid epitope. Finally, the frequency distribution of the alleles encoding for the rheumatoid epitope and the epitope itself appears to be very different in patients with early RA [20].

It thus appears premature to rely solely on DR typing using oligonucleotide probes to identify the presence (and dose) of the rheumatoid epitope or HVR3 and thus determine the probability that a patient with RA of relative recent onset will or will not develop destructive arthropathy over time even if the cost of oligotyping is made affordable and available to the majority of patients with RA [35]. Studies in populations from other ethnic groups, in patients with early disease, and in those with disease of variable severity are needed before oligotyping can be recommended as a screening tool in patients with early RA. These data are being gathered by investigators around the world and valuable information should be available soon. In the meantime, the presence of other known risks factors (such as seropositivity for IgM-rheumatoid factor) needs to be considered. In fact, Gough et al. found that the rheumatoid epitope and seropositivity have a relative risk (RR) for the occurrence of erosions of ~13 but an unacceptable low specificity; when both the rheumatoid epitope and seropositivity were combined, the RR dropped to ~8 and the specificity improved considerably, but the sensitivity became unacceptably low [25]. Whether HLA-DQB1 typing may allow a better identification of subjects prone to develop destructive RA has been proposed by some investigators [36] but has not been uniformly substantiated. The sentiment is that the HLA-DQB1* alleles associated with RA are linked to the "rheumatoid epitope"-bearing DRB1 alleles (specifically HLA-DQB1 *0301, *0302, and *0501). Whether HLA-DPB1* alleles may play a role in disease severity has not been established to date [37].

An alternative for identifying patients who may develop rapidly progressive disease is to detect preerosive disease with sufficient accuracy and reproducibility and at a reasonable cost, with a different imaging technique than plain radiography, given the fact that when erosions are visualized with conventional radiographs, the disease is already destructive. Over the years, several imaging techniques have been considered, but none has been found to be adequate in detecting preerosive or erosive disease not otherwise established by plain radiographs; the possible exception is magnetic resonance imaging (MRI) [38–42]. This technique, in contrast with plain radiography, offers the unique opportunity of visualizing soft tissues of different densities and thus synovial pannus, synovial effusion, tenosynovitis, and early erosions can be identified. However, there are only a few studies comparing MRI and conventional radiographs, with some showing consistently better visualization of the articular structures with MRI and others showing inconsistent advantages of one method over the other [38, 40–42]. With regard to the hand/wrist joints in particular, there is not a standard protocol to obtain the images (e.g., sequences, use of contrast), the table time is still too long (~45 minutes), and there is no consensus on how to score the images obtained. If over and above these uncertainties the issues of availability and affordability are considered, it can be safely stated that at the present time, it is not possible to use MRI as a screening imaging technique for the identification of patients destined to have rapidly progressive destructive RA.

Two other imaging techniques have been proposed as predictive of the later occurrence of a destructive arthropathy; scintigraphy using labeled polyclonal human IgG (HIG) and the use of bone densitometry [43, 44]. Increased uptake of HIG has been found to correlate with the clinical and laboratory features of active disease [43], whereas decreased periarticular bone mass has been found to correlate with disease severity rather than with disease activity [44]. Experience with these techniques is limited to some

European centers; they need to be independently evaluated by other investigators before they are accepted as the techniques of choice for predicting destructive arthropathy in patients with early RA.

Going back to the basics, the rheumatologist is confronted with the need to identify the "at risk" patient using indicators different from those provided by the history and physical examination. As a result, there is a renewed interest in the utilization of laboratory parameters associated with inflammation [15, 16]. Some investigators have proposed to measure serum and synovial fluid levels of interleukin-6 (1L-6) [45], whereas others have emphasized the importance of measuring CRP or the erythrocyte sedimentation rate (ESR) as indicators of active disease; CRP has been shown closely to parallel changes in disease activity and to correlate with the later occurrence of destructive arthropathy [14, 15]; it can be measured in most commercial laboratories in a valid and reliable manner on fresh or frozen (and thawed) sera and thus offer distinctive advantage over either 1L-6 or the ESR.

Thus, the identification of RA patients that could benefit from early and aggressive treatment modalities is still based on clinical parameters known to be associated with progressive and destructive disease. Laboratory features associated with inflammation may, however, be very helpful in following RA patients over time as demonstrated by van der Heijde et al., who were able to predict radiographic damage with 83% of accuracy in 147 patients with early RA. These investigators used either the ESR or CRP, HLA-DR4 (or DR2 as a protective marker), and rheumatoid factor positivity as predictors [46]. DR oligotyping, if used in conjunction with other parameters (e.g., rheumatoid factor positivity), may be very valuable in some patients, but, as already noted, relying solely on it to prognosticate outcome in patients with undiagnosed early polyarthritis or early RA appears to be somewhat premature at the present time.

III. WHEN TO TREAT

The appropriate time to initiate an aggressive treatment program will thus be the time at which the rheumatologist regards the RA patient prone to develop a destructive arthropathy. As discussed, this does not necessarily imply that radiographic evidence of erosions and/or joint space narrowing has occurred, but merely that it may occur. The longer a patient exhibits no evidence of erosive disease, the less likely the patient is of developing a rapidly progressive course later on. Thus persistently active disease within a few months of disease onset and the detection of capsular distention, ligamentous laxity, and/or joint instability [5] should be the appropriate time to initiate an aggressive treatment program. It should be noted, however, that some patients may appear to have a benign course early on, only to manifest severe and persistent proliferative synovitis later. Constructing a time-oriented graph, where joint counts for pain/tenderness and swelling, as well as laboratory parameters associated with inflammation are plotted, may help the clinician determine the point in time at which aggressive treatment modalities should be implemented.

Some rheumatologists have favored staging RA in much the same way as oncologists do with different neoplastic disorders. More than one method to stage the disease has been proposed; the simplest one includes only joint counts [47], whereas other methods include more than one parameter [48–50]. In one of these methods, disease staging is done based on the activity of the disease and the presence or absence of "bad" prognostic factors [48]; activity is a composite of pain, morning stiffness, joint counts for pain/tenderness, and/or swelling, and either CRP or ESR and is graded as absent, mild, moderate, or severe. For this grading system, deteriorating function, persistently elevated ESR or CRP, rheumatoid factor positivity at high titer, and the presence of extra articular manifestations (to include rheumatoid nodules, eye involvement, sicca, vasculitis, and/or pleuro/pulmonary or pericardial involvement) and of erosive disease are considered "bad" prognostic factors [48].

Another method which has been used in some of our studies includes different permutations of the following parameters: the ARA/ACR functional class, the presence (and number) of extra articular manifestations (as noted before), and the presence (and magnitude) of erosive disease [49]; according to this method, a patient with ARA/ACR functional class 1, no radiographic demonstrable disease by plain radiography, and no extra-articular manifestations will have a score of one, whereas a patient with significant functional impairment, erosions, and several extra-articular manifestations, most commonly subcutaneous nodules, sicca, and anemia, will have a score of four.

Another scoring method is the one developed by van der Heijde et al., referred to as the "disease activity score" (DAS), consists of the following variables: the Ritchie index, swollen joints, ESR, and general health [50]. The DAS has been used by other investigators and has been found to be simple and effective, and thus it is recommended particularly for RA clinical trials [51]. Finally, the ERAS (early rheumatoid arthritis study) group from England is currently using the following individual parameters to identify patients at risk of developing destructive disease: female gender, early erosions, persistent synovitis, positive rheumatoid factor, and the presence of the rheumatoid epitope [35, 52, 53]. In most situations, however, the clinician is left to make an individualized decision based on her or his own experience of whether the patient is "destined" to have destructive disease and proceed accordingly.

IV. HOW TO TREAT

A. Combination Therapy

Aggressive treatment for RA does not necessarily have the same meaning to all clinicians. *Aggressive* may be viewed by some as the early initiation of a disease-modifying antirheumatic drug (DMARD), whereas for others, it may mean the initiation of more than one DMARD simultaneously or sequentially. The rationality for combined treatment regimens is sound from the pharmacological and biological point of view. It is well known that synergism (i.e., the beneficial effect of two drugs being more than the sum of their effects) may occur. Ideally, the drugs to be combined should have different mechanism of action and a different toxicity profile; this may allow the use of lower doses of two (or more) compounds with a possible decrease in their side effects. From the biological point of view, the use of drugs that may exert their antirheumatic properties at different target points in the pathogenic process is also appealing; such rationality has been used for years by oncologists and infectologists for the treatment of neoplastic disorders and infections diseases. Combination DMARD therapy is discussed in Chapter 14.

From the design point of view, several methods of "combination therapy" have been proposed; the most conventional or traditional method to prove that two drugs are better than either one alone is to conduct a three-arm double-blind, randomized clinical trial where treatment with drug A (and placebo B), treatment with drug B (and placebo A), and treatment with both drugs A and B are compared; the sample size for such a study will, by necessity, be large, since it is hard to document differences between two potentially active treatments. Other less conservative approaches include the addition of a second DMARD to patients that are considered partial responders/failures to a given DMARD. For such a design, the first DMARD is considered "the anchor" drug, and the second drug is added to achieve maximal response in all study subjects. The other two approaches are the step-down approach proposed by Wilske, in which patients are started simultaneously on several DMARDs shortly after disease onset [10], and the step-up approach, or the overlapping use of different DMARDs in patients failing one or more DMARDs.

Whatever the method chosen for the use of combination therapy in RA, it is of utmost importance that all drugs have adequate antirheumatic properties, and different toxicity profiles. The proper conduct of combination studies in RA involves an estimation of the sample size needed to demonstrate that the combination is better than monotherapy and that improvement be clearly defined. The use of composite indices and of global measures rather than individual measures of improvement to identify responders and nonresponders may allow the conduct of studies in a smaller number of subjects. Finally, the outcome measures should be clearly established and have adequate metric properties [54–59]. Many of the published studies are methodologically flawed (e.g., inadequate sample size, nonblinded, multiple outcome measurements); from these studies, it has become clear, however, that there are some combination drug regimens that should be avoided either because they use compounds which are antagonic (e.g., D-penicillamine and antimalarials) [60] or have unacceptable toxicity (e.g., cyclophosphamide and azathioprine) [61,62].

Several combination regimens have been studied in the recent past, including chloroquine/D-penicillamine and either drug alone (72 patients [63]); oral gold salts and methotrexate (335 patients [64]), oral gold salts and antimalarials (229 patients [65]), hydroxychloroquine and sulfasalazine (91 patients [66]), azathioprine and methotrexate (209 patients [67]), antimalarials and methotrexate (40 patients [68]), sulfasalazine and D-penicillamine (32 patients [69]) methotrexate and cyclosporine A (148 patients [70]), and methotrexate, sulfasalazine; and antimalarials (102 patients [71]).

A review of different combination regimens [72] as well as a formal meta-analysis (which excludes those trials reported after 1993) have been published [73]. Despite the fact that the overall tone of these reviews is clearly not in favor of combination therapies, rheumatologists continue to explore different combination modalities as they continue to witness only occasional remissions and sustained improvement using single-drug therapies. It should be noted that a favorable response was more rapidly observed in the combination drug regimen of methotrexate and oral gold salts than with either drug alone [64]; in addition, disease progression over the duration of the trial occurred in the three treatment groups, but it was only statistically significant in the oral gold salt–treated group (which does not necessarily imply that the combination is better but that methotrexate is better than oral gold salts) [74].

The combination of antimalarials and methotrexate has been reported to be more efficacious than antimalarials alone, and it has been hypothesized that hydroxychloroquine may provide a liver protective effect when methotrexate is used (i.e., overall lower serum levels of transaminases than when methotrexate was combined with other drugs). The evidence for this protective effect is, however, circumstantial at best [75], although it has been recently postulated that the protective effect of chloroquine (and likely of hydroxychloroquine) may be due to a decrease in the bioavailability of methotrexate [76].

Another combination which is receiving attention is that of methotrexate and sulfasalazine [77–79]; despite the fact that both compounds are antifolates, their combined use appears to be well tolerated even without folate supplementation except in patients with preexistent folate deficiency [80]. Sulfasalazine, in contrast to methotrexate, is only a weak antifolate, and it is unclear whether its antirheumatic effect is mediated by either the proximal or the distal enzymes of the folate pathway; nevertheless, this combination should be used with caution. For unclear reasons, the addition of sulfasalazine to patients who develop peripheral nodulosis on methotrexate may result in a reduction in the size and number of these nodules [81].

Of interest is the work of the RAIN (rheumatoid arthritis investigational network) American group that has recently published their data using triple DMARD therapy [71]; the regimen includes sulfasalazine, methotrexate, and hydroxycholoquine. The study did not include sulfasalazine nor hydroxychloroquine alone groups, and neither did it include these two drugs together. The study included 102 patients and demonstrated a significant advantage of the triple DMARD combination over methotrexate alone or methotrexate and sulfasalazine; furthermore, the toxicity profile of the three arms of the study were comparable even though the patients were not supplemented with either folic or folinic acid. Not surprisingly, this therapeutic modality has been embraced by rheumatologists (in the United States at least), but the exact proportion of patients being offered this regimen as their first option is unknown. Finally, the beneficial effect of adding cyclosporin A to patients with RA considered to be only partial responders to methotrexate has recently been reported by Tugwell et al. in a study that included 148 patients. The limiting factor in adopting this regimen relates to the potential nephrotoxicity of cyclosporine [82].

It has been postulated by more than one rheumatologist that a randomized double-blind clinical trial, even if its duration is adequate, may not be large enough or long enough to demonstrate the value of these combined regimens. Also, observational studies of a large number of patients with RA in whom disease activity, disease severity, and prognostic factors are carefully documented and in whom different treatment regimens (e.g., early monotherapy, early combined therapy, traditional therapy) are used, may not only provide information which better reflects the course of a disease like RA, which spans several years, but also reflects more accurately what happens in actual clinical practice. Thus observational studies, rather than randomized clinical trials, may permit the determination of the value of different treatment approaches, and as in other rheumatic diseases, combined treatment regimens may prove to be better than single-drug regimens in controlling the inflammatory process which will, if left unchecked, lead to a destructive articular process [83–88].

In short, after careful review of the literature, the combinations that may be superior to single-drug regimens and that appear to be based on adequate data are those of oral gold salts and methotrexate, antimalarials and methotrexate, cyclosporin A and methotrexate, and antimalarials, methotrexate, and sulfasalazine, but whether any of the combined regimens are superior to single-drug therapy in halting disease progression, as determined radiographically, is still a matter of controversy. The combination of hydroxychloroquine, sulfasalazine, and methotrexate appear to be excellent, but it is premature to endorse these regimens until a larger database becomes available.

B. Monotherapy

If monotherapy is chosen for the aggressive treatment of RA, methotrexate is still preferred in the Americas because of its proven efficacy, its known toxicity profile [89, 90], the availability of measures aimed at reducing these toxicities [91, 92], its potential for halting disease progression (as determined radiographically) [74], specially if used as the first DMARD [93], and the experience of the rheumatology community with this compound for well over 15 years. It is beyond the scope of this chapter to describe in detail the specifics of how to use this drug. The frequency with which laboratory tests should be performed is not canonical, but general guidelines, including when and in whom to obtain liver biopsies, have been recently published [94] and are being adopted throughout the world. Of interest is the fact that methotrexate competes with sulfasalazine as the preferred drug for monotherapy in RA in Europe [95]. These divergent preferences across continents do not necessarily reflect differences in disease severity, but suggest that practice patterns are influenced by a number of other factors which are not necessarily disease related (and which have not been examined to date) [95–97].

C. Corticosteroids

Corticosteroids were first introduced into medical practice in the early 1950s and were thought at the time to be curative of RA. But once the devastating effects of their prolonged use in moderate to high dose became evident, rheumatologists generally have tried to use them only in small doses (≤7.5 mg of prednisone or equivalent) with increases being made only during periods of disease exacerbation, with higher doses being reserved for patients with serious extra-articular disease manifestations [95, 96, 98–100]. Although some rheumatologists clearly prefer not to use corticosteroids at all in patients with RA, the fact of the matter is that they are used in the large majority of patients in whom data have been gathered and published in the rheumatology literature (e.g., baseline data for randomized clinical trials). However, even at small doses, their use is not devoid of side effects, as demonstrated by Saag et al., who found an increase in the occurrence of fractures, serious infections, and gastrointestinal events in RA patients using corticosteroids [90]. More recently, the use of up to 7 mg of prednisone (or equivalent) for any 24-h period and at the discretion of the patient has been advocated by Wilder [101]. The advantage of this regimen over the traditional fixed dose is that the patient may use a much lower dose in the "good" days, minimizing the cumulative exposure to the compound; as a consequence, a less degree of adrenal suppression and fewer side effects may ensue.

Parenteral corticosteroids are used as temporizing measures during period of intense disease activity but should be avoided, if at all possible. However, larger or "pulse" doses of methylprednisolone (i.e., 600–1000 mg) are still used by some rheumatologists, but their effect is short lived. The reported rebound in disease activity within days of the pulse and the occurrence of serious arrhythmias are sufficient reasons, in my view, not to use them. Intra-articular corticosteroids, whether or not followed by joint rest, are used to control disease activity when one or a few joints are disproportionately involved in relation to most others (assuming they are not infected) [102–105].

D. Other Treatment Modalities

There has been a renewed interest in the antirheumatic properties of some antimicrobials of the tetracycline family (minocycline in particular), but when and how to use minocycline (or other antibiotics) remains to be defined [106–109]. The possible mechanisms of action invoked range from a purely anti-inflammatory effect to a purely antimicrobial one, but definite data to support either mechanism, or both, are not available. At any rate, minocycline appears to be a reasonable alternative for patients with moderately active RA, but not for those in desperate need of more aggressive therapy. The role of other antibiotics (tetracycline and nontetracycline derivatives), their route of administration (oral vs parenteral), and their efficacy/toxicity in comparison with current DMARDs has yet to be determined.

A number of biological products directed at specific mediators of the inflammatory-immune process are undergoing phase I and II clinical trials [110–114]; of them, the most promising compound is the antibodies against tumor necrosis factor (TNF or soluble[s] TNF) receptor [115, 116].

V. HOW TO EVALUATE TREATMENT RESPONSE

Realistic goals should be established a priori when a treatment plan is outlined. Ideally, these goals should include preservation of articular/nonarticular structures and the ability to perform leisure and nonleisure daily activities; freedom from pain; the ability to tolerate any side effects that may result from the medications used; and no decrease in life expectancy. With the available drugs, however, it may not be possible to accomplish these goals, but others may be within reach; for example, to suppress (halt) disease activity and therefore increase the duration of quality life years by delaying the onset of articular damage.

Of the many parameters used over the years by rheumatologists to assess disease activity in RA, such as the duration of morning stiffness, grip strength, walking time, ring size, joint counts, some have proven to have poor metric properties and others to provide redundant information; recently, this subject has been extensively reviewed, with the specific purpose of determining the measures that should be obtained to establish the benefits of a given therapeutic maneuver for patients with RA enrolled in randomized clinical trials [117–119]. As noted, a core set of criteria has been established and endorsed by different rheumatology professional organizations around the world, but how to use these criteria (individually or jointly as a composite measure or index and what magnitude of change should be considered acceptable) is being currently examined [118, 119]. These criteria may not prove to be particularly useful for the long-term follow-up of individual patients. They omit, for example, side effects from pharmacological agent(s) which may render a treatment useless even if synovitis is apparently under control [120–124]. These criteria are also not patient oriented but are clinician oriented. For a given patient, being able to perform specific activities (e.g., playing golf, dancing, swimming) may be more relevant than being able to perform other activities usually assessed on most functional instruments currently in use (e.g., walking, getting in and out of a car).

In short, whereas the core set of criteria are very likely to be useful in the setting of clinical trials, for the long-term follow-up of individual patients, the rheumatologist should in conjunction with the patient establish goals that are valid to both, relatively simple to use and understand, and are likely to be informative over time.

VI. CONCLUSIONS

Advances in the basic understanding of the etiopathogenesis of RA will more likely lead to better therapeutic interventions. Advances in trial design and drug testing may allow rheumatologists to rapidly discard products of limited efficacy or undue toxicity. In the meantime, rheumatologists should follow the literature carefully if advances in both basic sciences, clinical trials, and observational studies are going to have any impact on the care of patients afflicted with RA. Aggressive and early therapy in patients with RA is recommended for those patients "destined" to have a destructive arthropathy, but how to identify these subjects in a reliable and cost-effective way remains to be determined.

REFERENCES

1. Pincus T. Rheumatoid arthritis: disappointing long-term outcomes despite successful short-term clinical trials. J Clin Epidemiol 1988; 41:1037–1041.
2. Kushner I. Does aggressive therapy of rheumatoid arthritis affect outcome? J Rheumatol 1989; 16:1-4.
3. Wolfe F, Hawley DJ, Cathey MA. Clinical and health status measures over time: prognosis and outcome assessment in rheumatoid arthritis. J Rheumatol 1991; 18:1290–1297.
4. Sherrer YS, Bloch DA, Mitchell DM, et al. The development of disability in rheumatoid arthritis. Arthritis Rheum 1986; 29:494-500.
5. McCarty DJ. Personal experience in the treatment of seropositive rheumatoid arthritis with drugs used in combination. Semin Arthritis Rheum 1993; 23:42–49.
6. Wolfe F, Mitchell DM, Sibley JT, et al. The mortality of rheumatoid arthritis. Arthritis Rheum 1994; 37:481–494.
7. Hess EV, Luggen ME. Remodeling the pyramid--A concept whose time has not yet come. J Rheumatol 1989; 16:1175–1176.
8. Wilke WS, Sweeney TJ, Calabrese LH. Early, aggressive therapy for rheumatoid arthritis: concerns, descriptions, and estimate of outcome. Semin Arthritis Rheum 1993; 23:26–41.
9. Bensen WG, Bensen W, Adachi JD, Tugwell P. Remodeling the pyramid: the therapeutic target of rheumatoid arthritis. J Rheumatol 1990; 17:987–989.
10. Wilske KR. Inverting the therapeutic pyramid: observations and recommendations on new directions in rheumatoid arthritis therapy based on the author's experience. Semin Arthritis Rheum 1993; 23:11–18.
11. McCarty DJ, O'Duffy JD, Pearson L, Hunter JB. Remitting seronegative symmetrical synovitis with pitting edema. RS_3PE Syndrome. JAMA 1985; 254:2763–2767.
12. Harris ED Jr. Rheumatoid arthritis: pathophysiology and implications for therapy. N Engl J Med 1990; 322:1277–1289.
13. Fuchs HA, Kaye JJ, Callahan LF, et al. Evidence of significant radiographic damage in rheumatoid arthritis within the first 2 years of disease. J Rheumatol 1989; 16:585–591.
14. Davies MJ, Dawes PT, Fowler PD, et al. Comparison and evaluation of a disease activity index for use in patients with rheumatoid arthritis. Br J Rheumatol 1990; 29:111–115.
15. Blackburn WDJ. Validity of acute phase proteins as markers of disease activity. J Rheumatol 1985; 21:9–13.

16. van Leeuwen MA, van Rijswijk MH, van der Heijde DM, et al. The acute-phase response in relation to radiographic progression in early rheumatoid arthritis: a prospective study during the first three years of the disease. Br J Rheumatol 1993; 32(Suppl 3):9–13.
17. Choy EH, Scott DL. Prognostic markers in rheumatoid arthritis and classification of antirheumatic therapies. Drugs 1995; 1:15–25.
18. Weyand CM, Hicok KC, Conn DL, Goronzy JJ. The influence of HLA-DRB1 genes on disease severity in rheumatoid arthritis. Ann Intern Med 1992; 117:801–806.
19. Weyand CM, Xie C, Goronzy JJ. Homozygosity for the HLA-DRB1 allele selects for extraarticular manifestations in rheumatoid arthritis. J Clin Invest 1992; 89:2033–2039.
20. Weyand CM, Goronzy JJ. HLA-DRB1 alleles as severity markers in rheumatoid arthritis. Bull Rheum Dis 1994; 43:5–8.
21. Wordsworth BP, Lanchbury JSS, Sakkas LL, et al. HLA-DR4 subtype frequencies in rheumatoid arthritis indicate that DRB1 is the major susceptibility locus within the HLA class II region. Proc Natl Acad Sci 1989; 86:10049–10053.
22. Nepom GT, Nepom BS. Prediction of susceptibility to rheumatoid arthritis by human leukocyte antigen genotyping. Rheum Dis Clin North Am 1992; 18:785–792.
23. Watanabe Y, Tokunaga K, Mutsuki K, et al. Putative amino acid sequence of HLA-DRB chain contributing to rheumatoid arthritis susceptibility. J Exp Med 1989; 169:2263–2268.
24. Gao X, Olsen NJ, Pincus T, Stastny P. HLA-DR alleles with naturally occurring amino acid substitutions and risk for the development of rheumatoid arthritis. Arthritis Rheum 1990; 33:939–946.
25. Gough A, Faint J, Salmon M, et al. Genetic typing of patients with inflammatory arthritis at presentation can be used to predict outcome. Arthritis Rheum 1994; 37:1166–1170.
26. Jawaheer D, Thomson W, MacGregor AJ, et al. Homozygosity: for the HLA-DR shared epitope contributes the highest risk for rheumatoid arthritis concordance in identical twins. Arthritis Rheum 1994; 37:681–686.
27. Benazet JF, Reviron D, Mercier P, et al. HLA-DRB1 alleles associated with rheumatoid arthritis in Southern France. Absence of extraarticular disease despite expression of the shared epitope. J Rheumatol 1995; 22:607–610.
28. Yelamos J, García-Lozano JR, Moreno I, et al. Association of HLA-DR4-Dw15 (DRB1*0405) and DR10 with rheumatoid arthritis in Spanish population. Arthritis Rheum 1993; 36:811–814.
29. Massardo L, Aguirre V, Garcia ME, et al. Clinical expression of rheumatoid arthritis in Chilean patients. Semin Arthritis Rheum 1995; 25:203–213.
30. Boki KA, Drosos AA, Tzioufas AG, et al. Examination of HLA-DR4 as a severity marker for rheumatoid arthritis in Greek patients. Ann Rheum Dis 1993; 52:517–519.
31. Seglias J, Li EK, Cohen MG, et al. Linkage between rheumatoid arthritis susceptibility and the presence of HLA-DR4 and DRB allelic third hypervariable region sequences in Southern Chinese persons. Arthritis Rheum 1992; 35:163–167.
32. McDaniel DO, Alarcón GS, Pratt PW, Reveille JD. Most African-American patients with rheumatoid arthritis do not have the rheumatoid antigenic determinant (epitope). Ann Intern Med 1995; 123:181–187
33. Reveille JD, Alarcón GS, Fowler SE, et al. HLA-DRB1 genes and disease severity in rheumatoid arthritis. Arthritis Rheum 1996; 39:1802–1807.
34. López-Méndez A, Paul WA, Alarcón GS. Rheumatoid arthritis in American blacks: a clinical and radiological study. J Rheumatol 1989; 16:1197–2000.
35. Emery P, Salmon M. Early rheumatoid arthritis: time to aim for remission? Ann Rheum Dis 1995; 54:944–947.
36. Lanchbury JSS, Sakkas LI, Marsh SGE, et al. HLA-DQ B1 allele is determinant of susceptibility to DR-4 associated rheumatoid arthritis. Human Immunol 1989; 26:59–71.
37. Morozzi G, Galeazzi M, Delfino L, et al. Allelic variations of DPB1, DQA1, DQB1 and DRB1 and rheumatoid arthritis: further genetic and statistical considerations [Varianti

alleliche dei DPB1, DQA1, DQB1, DRB1 e artrite reumatoide: ulteriori considerazioni genetiche e statistiche]. Ann Intern Med Ital 1995; 10:171–174.
38. Jevtic V, Watt I, Rozman B, et al. Pre-contrast and postcontrast (Gd-DTPA). Magnetic resonance imaging of hand joints in patients with rheumatoid arthritis. Clin Radiol 1993; 48:176–181.
39. Murakami DM, Bassett LW, Seeger LL. Advances in imaging of rheumatoid arthritis. Clin Orthop Related Res 1991; 265:83–95.
40. Rubens DJ, Blebea JS, Totterman SMS, Hooper MM. Rheumatoid arthritis: evaluation of wrist extensor tendons with clinical examination versus MR Imaging—a preliminary report. Radiology 1993; 187:831–838.
41. Foley-Nolan D, Stack JP, Ryan M, et al. Magnetic resonance imaging in the assessment of rheumatoid arthritis—a comparison with plain film radiographs. Br J Rheumatol 1991; 30:101–106.
42. Poleksic L, Zdravkovic D, Jablanovic D, et al. Magnetic resonance imaging of bone destruction in rheumatoid arthritis: Comparison with radiography. Skeletal Radiol 1993; 22:577–580.
43. Etherington J, Coleman M, Phillips C, et al. HIG isotope bone scanning shows specificity for rheumatoid arthritis against seronegative arthritis. Arthritis Rheum 1993; 37:S250.
44. Deodhar AA, Brabyn J, Jones PW, et al. Measurement of hand bone mineral content by dual energy x-ray absorptiometry: development of the method, and its application in normal volunteers and in patients with rheumatoid arthritis. Ann Rheum Dis 1994; 53:685–690.
45. Everson MP, McDuffie DS, Bowden J, Blackburn WD Jr. Correlation of serum and synovial fludi IL-6 levels with disease activityin RA patients. Arthritis Rheum 1990; 33:S148.
46. van der Heijde DM, van Riel PL, van Leeuwen MA, et al. Prognostic factors for radiographic damage and physical disability in early rheumatoid arthritis. A prospective follow up study of 147 patients. Br J Rheumatol 1992; 31:519–525.
47. Pincus T, Brooks RH, Callahan LF. Prediction of long-term mortality in patients with rheumatoid arthritis according to simple questionnaire and joint count measures. Ann Intern Med 1994; 120:26–34.
48. Willkens RF. Prognostic staging for therapy of rheumatoid arthritis. Semin Arthritis Rheum 1991; 21:40–43.
49. Alarcón GS, Tracy IC, Blackburn WD. Toxicity as the main limiting factor in the use of methotrexate in rheumatoid arthritis. Arthritis Rheum 1989; 32:671–676.
50. van der Heijde DM, van't Hof M, Theunisse L et al. Judging disease activity in clinical practice in heumatoid arthritis: first step in the development of a disease activity score. Ann Rheum Dis 1990; 49:916–920.
51. Fuchs HA. The use of the disease activity score in the analysis of clinical trials in rheumatoid arthritis. J Rheumatol 1993; 20:579–581.
52. Richardson C, Emery P. Laboratory markers of disease activity. J Rheumatol 1996; 23:23–30.
53. Emery P. Therapeutic approaches for early rheumatoid arthritis. How early? How aggressive? Br J Rheumatol 1995; 2:87–90.
54. Scott DL, Spector TD, Pullar T. What should we hope to achieve when treating rheumatoid arthritis? Ann Rheum Dis 1989; 48:256–261.
55. Scott DL, Dacre JE, Greenwood A. Can we develop simple response criteria for slow-acting antirheumatic drugs? Ann Rheum Dis 4995; 49:196–198.
56. Mottonen TT. Prediction of erosiveness and rate of development of new erosions in early rheumatoid arthritis. Ann Rheum Dis 1988; 47:648–653.
57. Paulus HE. Protocol development for combination therapy with disease-modifying antirheumatic drugs. Semin Arthritis Rheum 1993; 23:19–25.

58. Jaffe I. New approaches to the management of rheumatoid arthritis. J Rheumatol 1992; 19:2–8.
59. Tugwell P, Boers M, Baker P, et al. Endpoints in rheumatoid arthritis. J Rheumatol 1994; 21:2–8.
60. Bunch TW, O'Duffy JD, Tompkins RB, O'Fallon WM. Controlled trial of hydroxychloroquine and d-pencillamine singly and in combination in the treatment of rheumatoid arthritis. Arthritis Rheum 1984; 27:267-276.
61. McCarty DJ, Carrera GF. Intractable rheumatoid arthritis. Treatment with combined cyclophosphamide, azathioprine, and hydroxychloroquine. JAMA 1982; 248:1718–1723.
62. Csuka ME, Carrera GF, McCarty DJ. Treatment of intractable rheumatoid arthritis with combined cyclophosphamide, azathioprine, and hydroxychloroquine: A follow-up study. JAMA 1986; 255:2315–2319.
63. Gibson T, Emery P, Armstrong RD, et al. Combined d-penicillamine and chloroquine treatment of rheumatoid arthritis: a comparative study. Br J Rheumatol 1987; 26:279–284.
64. Williams HJ, Ward JR, Reading JC, et al. Comparison of auranofin, methotrexate, and the combination of both the treatment of rheumatoid arthritis. A controlled clinical trial. Arthritis Rheum 1992; 35:259–269.
65. Luthra HS. Midwest Cooperative Rheumatoid Disease Study Group: double-blind study comparing auranofin and hydroxychloroquine alone and in combination in rheumatoid arthritis. Arthritis Rheum 1990; 33:S25.
66. Faarvang KL, Egsmose C, Kryger P, Podenphant J, et al. Hydroxychloroquine and suylphasalazine alone and in combination in rheumatoid arthritis: a randomised double blind trial. Ann Rheum Dis 1993; 52:711–715.
67. Willkens RF, Urowitz MB, Stablein DM, et al. Comparison of azathioprine, methotrexate, and the combination of both in the treatment of rheumatoid arthritis. A controlled clinical trial. Arthritis Rheum 1992; 35:849–856.
68. Trnavsky K, Gatterová J, Linduskovà M, Pelísková Z. Combination therapy with hydroxychloroquine and methotrexate in rheumatoid arthritis. Z Rheumatol 1993; 52:292–296.
69. Taggart AJ, Hill J, Astbury C, et al. Sulphasalazine alone or in combination with d-penicillamine in rheumatoid arthritis. Br J Rheumatol 1987; 26:32–36.
70. Bensen W, Tugwell P, Roberts RM. Combination therapy of cyclosporine with MTX and gold in RA (2 pilot studies). J Rheumatol 1994; 21:2034-2038.
71. O'Dell JR, Haire CE, Erikson N, et al. Treatment of rheumatoid arthritis with methotrexate alone, sulfasalazine and hydroxychloroquine, or a combination of all three medications. N Engl J Med 1996; 334:1287–1291.
72. Brooks PM. Combination therapy in rheumatoid arthritis. Agents Actions 1993; 44:95–103.
73. Felson DT, Anderson JJ, Meenan RF. The efficacy and toxicity of combination therapy in rheumatoid arthritis: A meta-analysis. Arthritis Rheum 1994; 37:1487–1491.
74. Alarcón GS, López-Méndez A, Walter J, et al. Radiographic evidence of disease progression in methotrexate treated and nonmethotrexate disease modifying antirheumatic drug treated rheumatoid arthritis patients: a meta-analysis. J Rheumatol 1992; 19:1868–1873.
75. Fries JF, Singh G, Lenert L, Furst DE. Aspirin, hydroxychloroquine, and hepatic enzyme abnormalities with methotrexate in rheumatoid arthritis. Arthritis Rheum 1990; 33:1611–1619.
76. Seideman P, Albertioni F, Beck O, et al. Chloroquine reduces the bioavailability of methotrexate in patients with rheumatoid arthritis. A possible mechanism of reduced hepatotoxicity. Arthritis Rheum 1994; 37:830–833.
77. Shiroky JB. Combination sulfasalazine and methotrexate in the management of rheumatoid arthritis. J Rheumatol 1996; 23:72–74.

78. Shiroky JB. Unsubstantiated "risk" of antifolate toxicity with combination methotrexate and sulfasalazine therapy. Arthritis Rheum 1993; 36:1757–1758.
79. Nisar M, Carlisle L, Amos RS. Methotrexate and sulphasalazine as combination therapy in rheumatoid arthritis. Br J Rheumatol 1994; 33:651–654.
80. Morgan SL, Baggott JE, Alarcón GS. Methotrexate and sulfasalazine combination therapy: is it worth the risk? Arthritis Rheum 1993; 36:281–282.
81. Chatham WW. Methotrexate associated rheumatoid nodulosis-improvement with addition of sulfasalazine [abstract]. Arthritis Rheum 1992; 35:R15.
82. Tugwell P, Pincus T, Yocum D, et al. Combination therapy with cyclosporine and methotrexate in severe rheumatoid arthritis. N Engl J Med 1995; 333:137–141.
83. Edworthy SM, Bloch DA, Brant RF, Fries JF. Detecting treatment effects in patients with rheumatoid arthritis: the advantage of longitudinal data. J Rheumatol 1993; 20:40–44.
84. Hawley DJ, Wolfe R. Are the results of controlled clinical trials and observational studies of second-line therapy in rheumatoid arthritis valid and generalizable as measures of rheumatoid arthritis outcomes? An analysis of 122 studies. J Rheumatol 1991; 18:1008–1014.
85. Weinblatt ME, Maier AL. Disease-modifying agents and experimental treatments of rheumatoid arthritis. Clin Orthop Related Res 1991; 265:103–115.
86. Pincus T. Limitations of randomized clinical trials to recognize possible advantages of combination therapies in rheumatic diseases. Semin Arthritis Rheum 1993; 23:2–10.
87. Feinstein AR. An additional basic science for clinical medicine: II. The limitations of randomized trials. Ann Intern Med 1983; 99:544–550.
88. Felson DT. Clinical trials in rheumatoid arthritis under attack: are practice-based observational studies the answer? J Rheumatol 1991; 18:951–953.
89. Tugwell P, Bennett K, Gent M. Methotrexate in rheumatoid arthritis. Indications, contraindications, efficacy, and safety. Ann Intern Med 1987; 107:358–366.
90. Willkens RF. Resolve: Methotrexate is the drug of choice after NSAIDs in rheumatoid arthritis. Semin Arthritis Rheum 1990; 20:76–80.
91. Morgan SL, Baggott JE, Vaughn WH, et al. The effect of folic acid supplementation on the toxicity of low-dose methotrexate in patients with rheumatoid arthritis. Arthritis Rheum 1990; 33:9–18.
92. Morgan SL, Baggott JE, Vaughn WH, et al. Supplementation with folic acid during methotrexate therapy for rheumatoid arthritis. A double-blind, placebo-controlled trial. Ann Intern Med 1994; 121:833–841.
93. Rich E, Moreland LW, Walker SL, et al. Alarcón GS. Lack of radiographic progression in seropositive RA patients treated with methotrexate as the first DMARD [abstr]. Arthritis Rheum 1996; 39:S320.
94. Kremer JM, Alarcón GS, Lightfoot RW Jr., et al. Methotrexate for rheumatoid arthritis. Suggested guidelines for monitoring liver toxicity. Arthritis Rheum 1994; 37:316–328.
95. Kay EA, Pullar T. Variations among rheumatologists in prescribing and monitoring of disease modifying antirheumatoid drugs. Br J Rheumatol 1992; 31:477–483.
96. Criswell LA, Redfearn WJ. Variation among rheumatologists in the use of prednisone and second-line agents for the treatment of rheumatoid arthritis. Arthritis Rheum 1994; 37:475–480.
97. Baum SK, Tracy IC, Henderson EH, Alarcón GS. Combination of disease-modifying antirheumatic drugs in the treatment of rheumatoid. A survey of Alabama rheumatologists. Arthritis Care Res 1991; 4:48–51.
98. Weiss MM. Corticosteroids in rheumatoid arthritis. Semin Arthritis Rheum 1989; 19:9–21.
99. Sternberg EM, Wilder RL. Neuroendocrine humoral factors in rheumatoid arthritis. In: McCarty DJ, Koopman WJ, eds. Arthritis and Allied Conditions. London: Lea & Febiger, 1993:665–682.

100. Saag KG, Koehnke R, Caldwell JR, et al. Low dose long-term corticosteroid therapy in rheumatoid arthritis: an analysis of serious adverse events. Am J Med 1994; 96:115–123.
101. Wilder RL, Sternberg FM. Neuroendocrine humoral factors in rheumatoid arthritis and related conditions. Curr Opin Rheumatol 1990; 2:436–440.
102. McCarty DJ, Harman JG, Grassanovich JL, Qian C. Treatment of rheumatoid joint inflammation with intrasynovial triamcinolone hexacetonide. J Rheumatol 1995; 22:1631-1635.
103. Chatham W, Williams G, Moreland L, et al. Intraarticular corticosteroid injections: should we rest the joints? Arthritis Care Res 1989; 2:70–74.
104. McCarty GM, McCarty DJ. Intrasynovial corticosteroid therapy. Bull Rheum Dis 1994; 43:2–4.
105. Neustadt DH. Intra-articular therapy for rheumatoid synovitis of the knee: Effects of the postinjection rest regimen. Clin Rheumatol Prac 1996; 3:65–68.
106. Skinner M, Cathcart ES, Mills JA, Pinals RS. Tetracycline in the treatment of rheumatoid arthritis. A double blind controlled study. Arthritis Rheum 1971; 14:727-732.
107. Breedveld FC, Dijkmans BAC, Mattie H. Minocycline treatment for rheumatoid arthritis: an open dose finding study. J Rheumatol 1990; 17:43–46.
108. Kloppenburg M, Breedveld FC, Terwiel JP, et al. Minocycline in active rheumatoid arthritis. A double-blind, placebo-controlled trial. Arthritis Rheum 1994; 37:629-636.
109. Tilley BC, Alarcón GS, Heyse SP, et al. Minocycline in rheumatoid arthritis: A 48 week, double-blind, placebo-controlled trial. Ann Intern Med 1995; 122:81–89.
110. Moreland LW, Bucy RP, Tilden A, et al. Use of a chimeric monoclonal anti-CD4 antibody in patients with refractory rheumatoid arthritis. Arthritis Rheum 1993; 36:307–318.
111. Moreland LW, Pratt PW, Bucy RP, et al. Treatment of refractory rheumatoid arthritis with a chimeric anti-CD4 monoclonal antibody. Long-term follow-up of CD4+ T cell counts. Arthritis Rheum 1994; 37:834–838.
112. Moreland LW, Sewell KL, Sullivan WF, et al. Treatment of refractory rheumatoid arthritis with DAB_{486} IL-1 fusion toxin: double-blind, placebo-controlled study. Arthritis Rheum 1993; 36:R24.
113. Roux-Lombard P, Punzi L, Hasler F, et al. Soluble tumor necrosis factor receptors in human inflammatory synovial fluids. Arthritis Rheum 1993; 36:485–489.
114. Wooley PH, Dutcher J, Widmer MB, Gillis S. Influence of a recombinant human soluble tumor necrosis factor receptor FC fusion protein on type II collagen-induced arthritis in mice. J Immunol 1993; 151:6602-6607.
115. Elliott MJ, Feldmann M, Maini RN. TNF alpha blockade in rheumatoid arthritis: rationale, clinical outcomes and mechanisms of action. Intern J Immunopharmacol 1995; 17:141–145.
116. Fox DA. Biological therapies: a novel approach to the treatment of autoimmune disease. Am J Med 1995; 99:82–88.
117. Felson DT, Anderson JJ, Boers M, et al. The American College of Rheumatology preliminary core set of disease activity measures for rheumatoid arthritis clinical trials. Arthritis Rheum 1993; 36:729–740.
118. Felson DT, Anderson JJ, Boers M, et al. American College of Rheumatology preliminary definition of improvement in rheumatoid arthritis. Arthritis Rheum 1995; 38:727–735.
119. Paulus HE, Egger MJ, Ward JR, et al. Analyses of improvement in individual rheumatoid arthritis patients treated with disease-modifying antirheumatic drugs, based on the findings in patients treated with placebo. Arthritis Rheum 1990; 33:477–484.
120. Fries JF. Effectiveness and toxicity considerations in outcome directed therapy in rheumatoid arthritis. J Rheumatol 1996; 23:102–106.
121. Fries JF, Williams CA, Ramey DR, Bloch DA. The relative toxicity of alternative therapies for rheumatoid arthritis: Implications for the therapeutic progression. Semin Arthritis Rheum 1993; 23:68–73.

122. Fries JF, Williams CA, Ramey D, Bloch DA. The relative toxicity of disease-modifying antirheumatic drugs. Arthritis Rheum 1993; 36:297–306.
123. Fries WF, Williams CA, Bloch DA. The relative toxicity of nonsteroidal antiinflammatory drugs. Arthritis Rheum 1991; 34:1353–1360.
124. Singh G, Fries JF, Williams CA, et al. Toxicity profiles of disease modifying antirheumatic drugs in rheumatoid arthritis. J Rheumatol 1991; 18:188–194.

7
Hydroxychloroquine

Howard Bird and Ann W. Morgan
University of Leeds, Leeds, United Kingdom

I. INTRODUCTION

Payne first reported the use of antimalarials in the treatment of rheumatological conditions in 1894 when quinine was used in the treatment of discoid lupus erythematosus [1]. In 1951, Page reported improvement in the arthritis and skin lesions of two patients with rheumatoid arthritis and discoid lupus erythematosus using the antimalarial mepocrine [2]. Over the next 12 years, several studies confirmed that antimalarials resulted in an improvement in the systemic features and subjective and objective evidence of joint inflammation in 60–80% of subjects with rheumatoid arthritis, although their effects may be delayed for up to 1 year [3].

Hydroxychloroquine is now the most frequently used antimalarial in rheumatology, as it has the lowest toxicity. Initially its efficacy was inferred from the more numerous studies on chloroquine. Early reports of retinal toxicity threatened the use of antimalarials 25 years ago, but with the use of lower doses and regular ophthalmological assessments, these drugs now have one of the lowest toxicity profiles among the disease-modifying antirheumatic drugs (DMARDs) currently available. Hydroxychloroquine has maintained a role in the treatment of slowly progressive or early rheumatoid disease and the rheumatic complications of lupus. However, there is little radiographic evidence available to suggest hydroxychloroquine is able to slow the progression of joint damage.

The mechanism of action remains to be fully elucidated but appears to be different to other antirheumatic drugs. This has given rise to a renewed interest in hydroxychloroquine and its use in combination therapy.

II. PHARMACOLOGY

A. Chemistry

Hydroxychloroquine was first synthetized in 1946 in the attempt to produce a drug that was less toxic, but which retained the efficacy of chloroquine. The only structural dif-

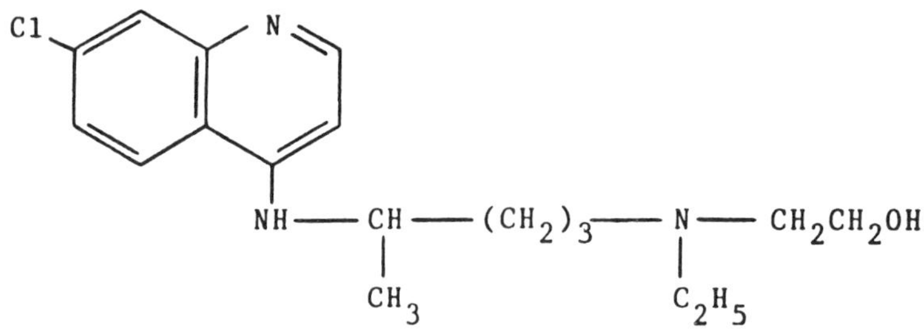

ference is the presence of a hydroxyethyl group in place of an ethyl group on the -4-N atom [4]. It's pharmacological properties are thus very similar to chloroquine, although with significantly less toxicity at comparable doses [5].

B. Pharmacokinetics

The drug is estimated by gas liquid chromatography [5]. Pharmacokinetic properties of all antimalarials are similar. They are rapidly absorbed almost completely [6], and in the plasma, about 50% of the drug is bound to plasma proteins.

After distribution, fat, bone, and brain contain the lowest amounts of these 4-aminoquinolines. Spleen, lungs, and adrenals contain more than kidney and liver, but the highest concentrations are found in melanin-containing tissue, particularly the choroid and ciliary body of the eye [6].

Hydroxychloroquine is particularly eliminated in the feces; chloroquine particularly in the urine. Elimination is in two stages, the first with a half-life of 3 days and the second with a half-life of 18 days [7]. Although the drug is excreted in human milk, the amount is too small to be harmful [8].

C. Mechanism of Action

Antimalarials are known to exert antirheumatic and immunosuppressive actions making them effective in many rheumatological conditions. There has been a wide range of reports on their potential mechanism of action with no single pathway apparent. One of the criticisms of earlier research is that the doses used in vitro were far higher than those achieved in vivo.

Early studies in the 1960s demonstrated chloroquine's ability to bind strongly to double-stranded DNA, thus stabilizing the double helix [9, 10]. Chloroquine inhibits DNA polymerase and, albeit less effectively, RNA polymerase [11]. With the advent of mefloquine, these actions are no longer felt to be responsible for the antiplasmodial effects [12] but may still have a minor role in their antirheumatic actions.

One of the central mechanisms of antimalarial action is now thought to be secondary to the drug's accumulation within the intracellular acid—vesicles, lysosomes, endosomes, phagolysosoms, transport vesicles, and Golgi complex [13] resulting in an increased pH. These acidic cytoplasmic compartments are present in all nucleated mammalian cells and participate in endocytic and exocytic pathways. Briefly, phagocytosed material passes through a series of vesicles which progressively become more acidic on the way to the lysosome. This acidic environment allows dissociation of extracellular receptors from their attached ligand so that the receptor may be processed and returned to the cell surface, with the ingested protein undergoing enzymic degradation. An acidic environment is needed for many enzymic reactions as well as for macromolecule assembly in the endosomes and posttranslation modification of newly synthesized proteins within the Golgi apparatus. The accumulation of the basic antimalarial drugs within these organelles causes the pH to shift toward normal, which is then outside the optimal range for many acid protease enzymes. This also includes some phospholipase enzymes, particularly phospholipase A_2, which is an important regulatory enzyme in the production of arachidonic acid and its metabolites [14].

Fox has recently proposed a model to explain the selective alteration of certain autoimmune functions by antimalarials which leaves other immune functions intact [14]. This action is typified by the absence of opportunistic infections and lack of significant hemopoietic toxicity. Models also need to explain the slow onset of action. His model proposes that self-peptides bind with either high- or low-affinity to self-histocompatibility antigens. During the process of thymic maturation, T cells will react to those autoantigens with a high affinity for the major histocompatibility complex (MHC) with subsequent removal from the circulation allowing only the T cells reactive to low-affinity autoantigen to remain into adult life. A critical step in regulating the immune response in the ingestion and "processing" of antigens by cells of the macrophage cell lines. This is followed by presentation of small high immunogenic peptides, in association with the MHC class II molecules, to immunocompetent cells. The increased lysosomal pH caused by antimalarials also interferes with the processing of these antigens and the formation of stable complexes with the MHC class II proteins [15,16]. This effect is most noticeable for those with a low affinity for MHC proteins. Increasing intravesicle pH may consequently downregulate the immune response selectively against the remaining autoantigenic peptides; given Fox's assumptions are correct [16]. The mechanism of action is different to other antirheumatic drugs making it well suited for use in combination therapy.

Hydroxychloroquine may also exert direct effects on the immune system with the inhibition of production of interleukin-1α (IL-1α) from monocytes and IL-6 from T cells and monocytes, although with no effect on IL-2, IL-4, tumor necrosis factor-α (TNF-α) and interferon-γ (IFN-γ) [17]. Chloroquine may directly inhibit T-cell proliferation by selectively interfering with IL-1 production by monocytes in doses achievable in vivo [18]. It has also been proposed that many slow-acting antirheumatic drugs accelerate differentiation of monocytes to macrophages which have a reduced capacity to secrete IL-1β. However, the levels of chloroquine required to induce differentiation in vitro seems high compared with therapeutic levels achieved in vivo [19]. As well as interfering with other phagocytic functions listed above, hydroxychloroquine has also been shown to partially inhibit superoxide anion production in doses that can be achieved therapeutically [20].

III. CLINICAL USE

A. Indications

Hydroxychloroquine sulfate may be used in the treatment of:

1. Rheumatoid arthritis
2. Juvenile chronic arthritis

3. Discoid and systemic lupus erythematosus
4. Dermatological conditions caused or aggravated by sunlight

B. Contraindications

1. Preexisting maculopathy
2. Previous sensitivity to 4-aminoquinolone compounds
3. Pregnancy

Caution should be used in the following situations:

1. Patients taking medications which may cause adverse ocular or skin reactions
2. Hepatic disease which may need estimation
3. Renal disease of HCQ levels
4. Simultaneous use of hepatotoxic or nephrotoxic drugs
5. Severe gastrointestinal disorders
6. Neurological disorders
7. Blood disorders
8. Porphyria cutanea tarda
9. Quinine sensitivity
10. Glucose-6-phosphate dehydrogenase deficiency
11. Psoriasis

IV. CLINICAL EFFICACY OF HYDROXYCHLOROQUINE

A. Rheumatoid Arthritis

As stated previously, hydroxychloroquine has been shown to be an effective treatment of rheumatoid arthritis in a number of controlled studies. Until recently there had only been two double-blind placebo-controlled studies using hydroxychloroquine. The first by Hamilton and Scott [21] was a 24-week crossover trial using 600 mg of hydroxychloroquine and a placebo of 3 mg of hydroxychloroquine. The results favored hydroxychloroquine in terms of joint swelling and tenderness, grip strength, erythrocyte sedimentation rate (ESR), and patient assessment of symptoms in the 41 patients studied. Statistical significance was only reached in terms of a reduction in the number of analgesics taken [21]. The treatment period of 3 months was probably too short for maximal benefit to have been achieved. One further 6-month double-blind placebo-controlled study included 103 patients and used 800 mg of hydroxychloroquine daily. Hydroxychloroquine was reported to be superior to placebo by 15–40% in a number of ways, including the American Rheumatism Association functional class, a clinical index, and patient assessment [22]. These early studies used higher doses of hydroxychloroquine than that of the maximum of 400 mg or 6.5 mg/kg/day currently recommended. Clark et al. have recently published a 24-week randomized placebo-controlled double-blind parallel trial using 400 mg of hydroxychloroquine [23]. They enrolled 126 consecutive patients, with confirmed rheumatoid arthritis of less than 5 years' duration into two matched groups. They showed a clinical and statistically significant improvement over placebo in joint score (20% mean improvement with 19% by more than 50%), grip strength (22% mean improvement with 21% more than 50%), patient global assessment (16%), and physician global assessment (12%). Side effects were mild with no patients requiring discontinuation of treatment. The investigators concluded that hydroxychloroquine is moderately effective in early rheumatoid arthritis [23]. Davis specifically designed a 12-month double-blind placebo-controlled study in a group of 104 patients with mild RA, where accepted clinical practice would be to use a nonsteroidal anti-inflammatory agent alone. In those patients who tolerated nonsteroidals, a stable dose was maintained in both groups throughout the treatment period. Mild rheumatoid arthritis was defined as synovitis limited to the hands and feet, an ESR <30 mm/h, and C-reaction protein (CRP) <20 mg/L. There was a significant improvement in clinical and laboratory parameters in the hydroxychloroquine-treated group by 6 months when compared with pretreatment levels and the control group, which was maintained at 12 months. Toxicity was low and fewer patients withdrew owing to lack of efficacy in the treatment group (8 vs 18). The effect on radiographic progression was not clear, as there was no difference in erosions between the two groups, but progression may be expected to be slower in this group with mild disease. The investigators suggest further studies over longer periods are needed to establish whether treatment of mild disease influences long-term outcome but would recommend that treatment of this group should be more aggressive than with NSAIDs alone [24].

A controlled double-blind study compared 200 with 400 mg of hydroxychloroquine sulfate in 54 patients. The two groups were considered homogeneous and both dose regimens were effective with a significant reduction in disease activity at 12 months. Of the 9 laboratory and 11 clinical indices used, no statistically significant differences were found in efficacy between the two doses, but the incidence of side effects was three times greater when the higher dose was used [25].

Similar results were found in another small double-blind study that compared chloroquine 250 mg with 200 mg and 400 mg of hydroxychloroquine. All three treatment groups showed a significant clinical improvement from baseline, especially using the Ritchie Articular Index. There was no statistically significant difference between the groups, but the results tended to be more favorable toward chloroquine with a slower onset of improvement using 200 mg of hydroxychloroquine [26].

Larger controlled trials are clearly needed to establish the lowest effective dose so the incidence of retinotoxicity may be reduced further. The advantages of using high initial doses to shorten the onset of clinical improvement with a lower maintenance doses needs to be determined.

1. Comparison with Other Disease-Modifying Antirheumatic Drugs

There have only been a small number of double-blind trials comparing hydroxychloroquine with other disease-modifying antirheumatic drugs (DMARDs) with larger numbers of open studies which have provided additional information.

An early double-blind study was performed at the Mayo clinic, which randomly allocated 56 patients into three groups receiving D-penicillamine, hydroxychloroquine, and a continuation of the two. D-penicillamine alone was found to be statistically superior to the other two groups in achieving a general response (69 vs 44% at 2 years). However, when the subgroups that demonstrated a marked improvement or induction of remission were analyzed, those on hydroxychloroquine fared better (25 vs 11%) compared with penicillamine alone [27]. This was a very well-designed study, but the results need to be interpreted with caution in view of the small sample size.

Two retrospective chart review studies were performed by the same center and compared hydroxychloroquine with intramuscular gold using life table analysis. In the first study, intramuscular gold was discontinued less frequently than hydroxychloroquine for lack of benefit (18 vs 40%). At this time, drugs were discontinued within 3 to 6 months for lack of efficacy [28]. The second study which continued the treatment for longer before withdrawing owing to lack of efficacy showed hydroxychloroquine, intramuscular gold, and D-penicillamine were all withdrawn for lack of efficacy in 6% of patients [29]. A prospective single-blind study randomized 40 patients into two groups receiving 400 mg of hydroxychloroquine or 6 mg of auranofin. A statistically significant improvement in all parameters of clinical efficacy was seen in the hydroxychloroquine group over baseline, which was not the case for all parameters, especially pain, morning stiffness, and time to onset of fatigue in the auranofin groups. However, there was no overall statistically significant difference between both treatment groups [30]. A study comparing chloroquine with intramuscular gold and azathioprine in 33 patients showed no statistically significant difference between the three treatment groups [31].

A 48-week randomized double-blind study compared hydroxychloroquine (400 mg daily for 24 weeks followed by 200 mg daily for 24 weeks) with 2 g of sulphasalazine daily. Sixty patients with classic or definite rheumatoid arthritis were evenly allocated to the two groups. The sulfasalazine group demonstrated statistically significant improvement in disease activity variables from the baseline by three months with all but 1 of the 13 variables improving by 48 weeks. No improvement was found within the hydroxychloroquine group by 3 months, but 8 of the 13 variables had improved by 48 weeks. More subjects receiving hydroxychloroquine withdrew for lack of efficacy (9 vs 3), whereas there were fewer side effects in the group receiving hydroxychloroquine with one subject being withdrawn for lack of efficacy compared with four in the sulfasalazine group. At the end of the study, there was no statistical difference between the two groups. The investigators included that sulfasalazine was slightly more effective but had greater adverse effects [32]. These patients also had radiographs taken of their hands and feet at the start of the study and after 24 and 48 weeks of treatment. At the onset, there were no significant differences in the number of erosions between the two groups, whereas both after 24 and 48 week, there was a significant increase in the number of erosions in the hydroxychloroquine-treated group ($P < .02$) [33]. A more recent study compared hydroxychloroquine and sulfasalazine alone and in combination but did not find a statistically significant difference between combination treatment on sulfasalazine or between both drugs given alone [34].

There have been suggestions that other disease-modifying drugs may be slightly more effective than hydroxychloroquine, but these have not always reached statistical significance or small numbers of patients have been studied. Hydroxychloroquine, however, has consistantly demonstrated reduced toxicity when compared with these other drugs. It is therefore clear that few large prospective double-blind studies comparing hydroxychloroquine with other DMARDs and placebo are needed to establish efficacies.

2. *Use of Hydroxychloroquine in Combination Therapy*

There are many good theoretical reasons to justify the use of hydroxychloroquine in combination therapy. Its low toxicity when compared with other disease-modifying agents has already been discussed, as has its proposed mechanism of action, which appears to be different from the other agents, suggesting potential greater efficacy when used in combination. The use of drugs with different toxicity profiles may again avoid the additive risks of bone marrow suppression or renal and respiratory impairment when other drugs are used in combination. Again, it may be possible to use lower doses of drugs in combination to reduce toxicity while maintaining efficacy [3]. Combination therapy is used by many rheumatologists usually in refractory cases, but to date there have been only a few well-designed prospective double-blind studies showing any advantage, although the preliminary reports of some open nonrandomized studies have suggested it may be useful.

There are three prospective double-blind trials to date. The first, performed at the Mayo Clinic, has already been discussed. Here a combination of D-penicillamine and hydroxychloroquine was less effective than D-penicillamine alone [29]. Dawes compared intramuscular gold plus hydroxychloroquine with intramuscular gold plus placebo in 101 patients over 1 year. Although both regimens were effective, the disease activity index favored combination therapy ($P < .05$) [35]. More recently, Porter [36] randomized 142 patients with a suboptimal response to intramuscular gold after 6 months of treatment to receive hydroxychloroquine 400 mg daily or placebo. The investigators found no difference in outcome in terms of efficacy or toxicity and felt there was no justification for adding hydroxychloroquine to those patients with suboptimal response to gold [36].

One of the largest studies to date was performed by Sievers and Hurri [37]. This open nonrandomized study compared 240 patients treated with antimalarials alone (400 mg hydroxychloroquine or 200–400 mg chloroquine) during 1957–1959 to 249 patients receiving a combination of antimalarials and intramuscular gold during 1960–1961. Patients with stage I and II disease using Steinbrocker's criteria had better results with a 49% remission or major improvement with antimalarials alone compared with 66% receiving combination therapy. Hospitalized patients receiving antimalarials alone achieved a 36% remission or major improvement compared with 43% showing the same degree of improvement on combination therapy [37]. Unfortunately, there was no comparator group of patients receiving only intramuscular gold.

Combinations using low-dose cytotoxic agents have been described. A recent abstract compared the efficacy of 200 mg of hydroxychloroquine with hydroxychloroquine plus methotrexate 7.5 mg weekly. All six clinical variables and two laboratory variables improved favorably with combination therapy within the 6 months, whereas hydroxychloroquine only influenced three clinical and no laboratory variables [38]. Although the combination proved more potent than hydroxychloroquine alone, the lack of a group taking methotrexate only prevents all the difference being attributed to methotrexate. Biro published a small study in abstract form on 20 patients with active rheumatoid arthritis who were taking hydroxychloroquine. Equal numbers were then given additional methotrexate or azathioprine for at least 12 weeks. All had continued disease activity when the third drug was added to the regimen, so that all patients were taking an average of 270 mg hydroxychloroquine, 1.43 mg/kg/day azathioprine, and 0.117 mg/kg/day methotrexate. They remained on all three drugs for an average of 14.7 months, after which 2 were lost to follow up, 1 withdrew owing to stomatitis, and the remaining 17 showed a marked improvement in disease activity with little toxicity [39].

McCarty and associates [40] reported a combination study of hydroxychloroquine, cyclophosphamide, and azathioprine in 31 patients with intractable rheumatoid arthritis. All subjects had failed to respond to a combination or oral gold and hydroxychloroquine with an additional nine patients also taking azathioprine. The gold preparation was substituted for cyclophosphamide in this open and uncontrolled study. The efficacy of this combination proved to be very good, with 16 achieving complete remission, 7 near remission, and the remaining 7 having completed the study a partial clinical response. However, the toxicity was unacceptably high, with 25 developing some side effects; most importantly, 4 patients developed infections and 4 others developed unrelated malignancies (colon carcinoma, endometrial carcinoma and previous colon carcinoma, erythroleukemia, and carcinoma of the lung). Although it is difficult to attribute the malignancies directly to the treatment, it was concluded that cyclophosphamide was too toxic for routine use [40].

One alternative view proposed by Bitter is that rheumatoid arthritis should be considered a "nonmalignant B-lymphoproliferative disorder and as such requires the use of high doses of toxic drugs with different mechanisms of action to eradicate the disease" [41].

Although the theoretical reasons for the use of hydroxychloroquine in combination therapy remain attractive, definite conclusions cannot be drawn from the small sample size and preliminary nature of many of these reports. More studies are needed before large double-blind studies may begin.

B. Other Indications

1. Juvenile Chronic Polyarthritis

There have been many varied reports on the effectiveness of hydroxychloroquine in the treatment of juvenile chronic polyarthritis in the literature. A number of open and retrospective trials have suggested remission rates of 5–45% with improvement in 16–75% of children [42–45]. A large placebo-controlled trial compared the efficacy of hydroxychloroquine and D-penicillamine in children with severe active juvenile polyarthritis. All three groups, including placebo, demonstrated a dramatic improvement at 1 year. The only index that was significantly better in the hydroxychloroquine group was pain on movement with no significant difference between D-penicillamine and placebo [46]. This trial was also recently included in a meta-analysis of three double-blind randomized placebo-controlled trials which included D-penicillamine, hydroxychloroquine, and methotrexate 5 and 10 mg. A total of 520 children were included, and only 10 mg methotrexate showed significantly greater improvement than placebo [47]. These previous studies have demonstrated that hydroxychloroquine has the lowest number of side effects with only small numbers requiring discontinuation of the drug [42]. Keratopathy was felt to be the major toxic feature by Laaksonen. This occurred with high serum levels, and a maximum dose of 5–7 mg/kg/day was recommended as in adults [48]. Retinopathy does not appear to have been reported.

2. Systemic Lupus Erythematosus

Antimalarials were first shown to be effective in discoid lupus in 1894 [1]. Renewed interest occurred in the 1950s when Christianson and Nielson demonstrated a 70% initial response in patients with discoid lupus erythematosus treated with mepacrine. On withdrawing the drug, 46% relapsed within 6 months and 80% by 1 year [49]. Similar results were obtained by Buchanan, with an initial response in 30 of 32 patients with discoid lupus with 7 of the 13 discontinuing the drug relapsing [50]. It is now well established that hydroxychloroquine has a 50% response rate in cutaneous lupus erythematosus with side effects and similar efficacy to many of the other agents used [51]. An early open study by Dubois in 1954 demonstrated 75% of patients with mild systemic lupus erythematosus (SLE) benefited from therapy with a number of antimalarials with less improvement in those judged to have severe lupus [52]. He followed this up by a larger study of 175 patients, suggesting a good response to antimalarials in 75–85% [53]. The use of antimalarials has also been suggested to reduce the dose of corticosteroids needed to control SLE [54]; whether this is sufficient enough to be clinically meaningful has been questioned [55].

Surprisingly, despite the widespread use of hydroxychloroquine in SLE, there have been no placebo-controlled trials for initiating therapy. The majority of the evidence advocating the use of hydroxychloroquine is from the open and placebo-controlled trials withdrawing therapy. In 1976, Rudnicki et al. reported an increased incidence of cutaneous manifestations and undefined flares in disease activity on stopping hydroxychloroquine [56]. A placebo-controlled study withdrawing hydroxychloroquine in patients with stable SLE was associated with a relative risk of 2.5 for new or worsening lupus manifestations and 6.1 for "severe" flares over 24 weeks [57].

Hydroxychloroquine has been reported to be effective in relieving such features as polyarthragia, polyarthritis, pleuritis, skin manifestations, and constitutional symptoms. It is not generally advocated for treatment of major systemic features such as renal or central nervous system (CNS) involvement [58]. Morand has recently reviewed the use of hydroxychloroquine within a single rheumatology practice retrospectively using life table methods. A total of 403 patients were isolated (366 with rheumatoid arthritis and 37 with SLE). They demonstrated that hydroxychloroquine was continued for significantly longer ($p < 0.001$) with a cumulative probability of 8% discontinuing within 24 months. This shows a significant trend to continued efficacy of hydroxychloroquine for long periods with this group of patients [58] in spite of little supporting evidence from large placebo-controlled trials.

3. *Primary Sjögren's Syndrome*

A small study comprising three patients suggested a positive effect of hydroxychloroquine in the treatment of primary Sjögren's syndrome with a reduction in ESR and gamma globulin levels and an increased hemoglobin concentration [59]. An open study was then performed on 20 patients comparing hydroxychloroquine and placebo. The 10 patients receiving hydroxychloroquine demonstrated a significant reduction in ESR and immunoglobulin (IgG) levels, but subjective clinical benefits were not reported [60].

These early promising trials led to a 2-year double-blind prospective placebo-controlled crossover trial using 400 mg hydroxychloroquine and involving 19 patients. Again a significant reduction in immunoglobulins (IgG and IgM) occurred with a trend for reduction in ESR. Disappointingly, no beneficial effects in signs and symptoms were shown or any change in tear gland activity [61] despite the favorable immunological response.

4. *Psoriatic Arthritis*

The use of antimalarial drugs in psoriatic arthritis is controversial owing to anxiety that they may precipitate an exacerbation of psoriasis. The suggestion of a flare up in psoriasis came from a number of case reports documenting exacerbations, some of which led to exfoliative dermatitis [62–64]. Many others have not been able to substantiate these claims and would not consider psoriasis as a contraindication to antimalarial therapy [65–67]. There have, therefore, been few studies to establish the efficacy of antimalarials in this condition. Recently, a retrospective analysis was made of 32 patients treated with chloroquine for psoriatic arthritis. A total of 24 patients received chloroquine for a minimum of 6 months and 75% of these had a 30% reduction in the actively inflamed joint count with a significant reduction in the number of actively inflamed joints. Only six patients developed an exacerbation of psoriasis and only one was severe enough to discontinue therapy. No cases of exfoliative dermatitis occurred. A control group of 24 patients was identified from the same database. Here 58% showed a 30% reduction in actively inflamed joint count. Six patients experienced a flare up of their psoriasis. Although the results were not statistically significant, they suggest prospective randomized double-blind control trials are warranted [67].

V. SIDE EFFECTS

Hydroxychloroquine has an excellent overall toxicity record, especially when it is compared with other DMARDs. In recommended doses, it has a similar side effect profile to chloroquine but the incidence is at least 50% less [68]. As many as half of the patients may develop some side effects, but these usually resolve spontaneously or with dose reduction [69]. The most serious potential side effect is retinopathy, which initially threatened to prevent the use of antimalarials for the long-term treatment of rheumatoid arthritis 25 years ago [70].

A. Gastrointestinal

Many gastrointestinal disturbances such as nausea, diarrhea, anorexia, abdominal cramps, and rarely vomiting may occur. These usually resolve immediately on dose reduction or on stopping treatment [71].

B. Dermatological

Skin rashes sometimes occur with pigmentous changes in skin and mucous membranes. Bleaching of hair and hair loss have all been reported. These also usually resolve readily on stopping treatment [71].

C. Neuromuscular

Less frequently, muscle weakness, vertigo, tinnitus, nerve deafness, headaches, nervousness, and emotional upsets have been reported. Rarely have there been reports of neuromyotoxicity and toxic psychosis.

D. Ophthalmological

These side effects threatened the long-term use of antimalarials, but with low daily doses and regular ophthalmological examination, these problems can be minimized. The most appropriate methods for monitoring these complications remain a topical issue as hydroxychloroquine is now becoming increasingly popular both alone and in combination therapy.

Corneal deposits of presumed antimalarial salts occur within the basic epithelium and were first described in 1958 [72]. They may occur in up to 90% of patients taking chloroquine, but an incidence of <5% was found using hydroxychloroquine in doses of 500 mg/day. These deposits are largely asymptomatic [73] and are reportedly reversible on stopping treatment [71].

True hydroxychloroquine retinopathy has recently been defined as the presence of bilateral reproducible, positive field defects that can be demonstrated by two different tests of visual field examination [73]. This definition, however, it not currently used by all ophthalmologists. Early changes such as premaculopathy classically result in fine pigmentary stripping of the macula with loss of the foveal reflex, although the latter is extremely uncommon [73]. Detection of visual field loss to red test objects reportedly detects early retinal scotomata and a loss with white test objects implies absolute scotomata and more advanced retinopathy.

Visual symptoms such as spots and the fall out of letters occur late and are rarely present in the early stages. The significance of premaculopathy is unclear, as no patient with premaculopathy secondary to hydroxychloroquine has progressed on to develop true retinopathy [74]. However, in patients with less than 20/20 vision, absolute scotomata, abnormal color vision (Ishihara testing), and positive fluorescein findings, visual deterioration may continue after antimalarial therapy has been stopped. This is assuming hydroxychloroquine retinopathy behaves in a similar way to that from chloroquine [73].

The incidence of hydroxychloroquine retinopathy appears to be low. MacKenzie retrospectively reviewed 900 patients and found that the development of retinopathy occurred when a daily dose of greater than 6.5 mg/kg/day of hydroxychloroquine was used [74]. This was confirmed by Bernstein, whose extensive reviews of the world literature found only 18 patients with true retinopathy. Four of these had received doses less than 6.5 mg/kg/day, three of whom had taken hydroxychloroquine for 10, 19, and 20 years, and the fourth had also taken chloroquine for 8.75 years [75]. Further analysis of all published cases from the U.S. Food and Drug Administration (FDA) reports of retinopathy attributed to hydroxychloroquine did not reveal any evidence of permanent visual field scotomata occurring when a daily dose of less than 6.5 mg/kg/day was used [76]. This has led Bernstein to conclude that hydroxychloroquine does not cause any risk of retinopathy when used at a maintenance dosage of no more than 6.5 mg/kg body weight, or when the duration of treatment is less than 10 years, or when there is no evidence of renal insufficiency (60% renal excretion). The latter two features merely indicate the need for more frequent ophthalmological examinations [76]. Easterbrook's [73] prospective study of 2000 patients treated with antimalarials found only three patients with definite maculopathy associated with hydroxychloroquine and all were overdosed. A fourth patient developed classic retinopathy after 2 months, which returned to normal despite continuing with a reduced dose of the medication [73]. Johnson and Vine [75] believe patients can tolerate high cumulative doses with little evidence of retinopathy providing the daily dose did not exceed 6.5 mg/kg/day [77]. The manufacturers now recommended pretreatment and 6-monthly ophthalmological examinations (previously 3-monthly). They state that examination should include testing of visual activity, careful ophthalmoscopy, and central visual testing with a red target. Many ophthalmologists now feel patients should take some responsibility for their screening and would give them an Amsler grid after the first consultation [76]. Many also recommend that the patient should examine their eyes monthly using a white Amsler grid and to report back if they notice any fading of the squares [73, 76]. In a reliable patient, this will readily pick up shallow paracentral scotomata which can be confirmed using Humphrey perimeters [73]. Easterbrook did not find any advantage in using red Amsler grids rather than white ones [73]. Color vision should also be tested and the Ishihara plates, which are readily available, may pick up early relative scotomata, especially in the elderly whose visual fields may be in question. Color vision may be normal with relative scotomata, with the loss of color recognition usually indicating the presence of absolute scotomata and a more ominous prognosis even if medication is discontinued [73]. Easterbrook believes macular dazzle testing, fluorescein angiography, electroretinography, electroculography, and dark adaption testing are either too variable or may be normal in well-established cases of retinopathy and consequently not suitable for routine examinations. Interestingly, the manufacturers recommend careful ophthalmoscopy by an expert for the detection of maculopathy. In one study by an ophthalmologist, the vast majority of patients with bilateral reproducible relative scotomata showed no fundal abnormalities. The development of an abnormal fundus with increased macula pigmentation or classic bullseye retinopathy is usually associated with absolute scotomata and thus advanced retinopathy [73].

The frequency of ophthalmological examinations after the initial assessment is controversial. The manufacturers recommend 3-monthly examinations, whereas many ophthalmologists feel annual assessments may be more appropriate, especially with monthly Amsler grid testing at home [73, 76, 78]. Others believe retinopathy occurs so rarely if appropriate doses of antimalarials are used and that there is no longer an indication for routine screening [79].

E. Miscellaneous

Bone marrow depression is rare, but periodic blood counts are advisable with the discontinuation of hydroxychloroquine if abnormalities develop. Porphyria cutanea tarda may be exacerbated and caution is also advised if those with glucose-6-phosphate dehydrogenase deficiency [73].

F. Overdosage

Children, especially infants, are particularly sensitive to 4-aminoquinolones and as little as 1–2 g has proved fatal. An adult male is reported to have survived an overdose of 36 tablets with an estimated dose of 54 tablets proving rapidly fatal. Symptoms in overdose include headache, visual disturbance, cardiovascular collapse, and convulsions followed by sudden early respiratory and cardiac arrest. Treatment should, therefore, be prompt and symptomatic, with emptying of the stomach by emesis or gastric lavage followed by finely powdered charcoal in a dose of at least five times that of the overdose via a nasogastric tube within 30 min of ingestion. Parenteral diazepam should be given in all cases, as it has been shown to reverse chloroquine cardiotoxicity. Respiratory support may be needed and shock treated by appropriate use of fluids and doparine depending on central venous pressures. Anyone surviving the acute phase will need careful monitoring for at least 6 hours [73].

VI. SPECIAL CIRCUMSTANCES

Hydroxychloroquine is not recommended for use in neonates and should be used cautiously in small children who are particularly sensitive to the toxic effects of 4-

aminoquinolones. Use in pregnancy should be avoided, as it crosses the placenta and may cause fetal abnormalities. A chemically related compound, chloroquine phosphate, has been found to cause fetal cochlear damage when used in high doses during pregnancy [71]. However, those possible teratogenic effects must be balanced against the dangers of a flare up in disease activity during pregnancy. This is particularly important in lupus with the possible increased risk of losing the pregnancy [80]. Although hydroxychloroquine has been detected in human breast milk, the amount is felt to be too small to be harmful [81]. No special precautions are necessary in the elderly providing they have normal renal function.

A. Concurrent Disease

1. Epilepsy

Chloroquine has been shown to induce convulsions in known epileptics.

2. Renal Failure

The dose of hydroxychloroquine needs to be reduced in renal impairment according to the glomerular fibration rate (GFR):

GFR 20–50 mL/min max 75 mg daily
10-20 mL/min max 50 mg daily
< 10 mL/min contraindicated

B. Drug Interactions

Many drug interactions have been inferred from the more widespread use of chloroquine.

Aminoglycosides: Chloroquine blocks transmission at the neuromuscular junction which is potentiated by aminoglycosides [82].

Antacids: They may reduce the bioavailability of hydroxychloroquine and should be given four hours apart [83].

Cimetidine: This inhibits the metabolism of hydroxychloroquine increasing its plasma concentrations.

Digoxin: Hydroxychloroquine may increase plasma digoxin levels [84].

Neostigmine, pyridostigmine: Their effects may be antagonized by hydroxychloroquine [81].

REFERENCES

1. Payne JF. A postgraduate lecture on lupus erythematosus. Clin J 1894; 4:223–229.
2. Page F. Treatment of lupus erythematosus with mepacrine. Lancet 1951; ii:755–758.
3. Paulus HE. Antimalarial agents compared with or in combination with other disease-modifying antirheumatic drugs. Am J Med 1988; 85 Suppl.4A:45–52.
4. Surrey AR, Hammer HF. Preparation of 7-chloro-4-(4-N-ethyl, N-2-hydroxyethylamino)-1-methyl-butlarino)-quinoline and related compounds. J Am Chem Soc 1950; 72:1814.
5. McChesney EW, Fitch CD. 4-aminoquiolones. In: Peters W, Richards WHG eds. Handbook of Experimental Pharmacology: Antimalarial drugs II. Berlin: Springer Verlag 1984; 68/II:3–60.

6. McChesney EW. Animal toxicity and pharmacokinetics of hydroxychloroquine sulphate. Proceedings of a symposium: a reassessment of Plaquenil in the treatment of rheumatoid arthritis. Am J Med 1983; suppl 75:11–18.
7. McKenzie AII. Pharmacologic actions of 4-aminoquinoline compounds. Proceedings of a symposium: a reassessment of Plaquenil in the treatment of rheumatoid arthritis. Am J Med suppl 75:5–10.
8. Anon. British National Formulary. British Medical Association and the Drug Pharmaceutical Society of Great Britain, 1990.
9. Stollar D, Levine L. Antibodies to denatured deoxyribonucleic acid in lupus erythematosus serum. V. Mechanism of DNA-anti-DNA inhibition by chloroquine. Arch Biochem Biophys 1963; 101:335–341.
10. Cohen SN, Yielding JL. Spectrophotometric studies of the interaction of chloroquine with deoxyribonucleic acid. J Biol Chem 1965; 240:3123–3131.
11. Gabourel JD. Effects of hydroxychloroquine on the growth of mammalian cells in vitro. J Pharmacol Exp Ther 1963; 141:122–141.
12. Ginsburg H, Geary TG. Current concepts and new ideas on the mechanism of action of quinoline-containing antimalarials. Biochem Pharmacol 1987; 36:1567–1576.
13. Krogstad DJ, Schlesinger MD. Acid-vesicle function, intracellular pathogens and the action of chloroquine against plasmodium falciparum. New Engl J Med 1987; 317:542–559.
14. Fox RI. Mechanism of action of hydroxychloroquine as an antirheumatic drug. Semin Arthritis Rheum 1993; 23(Suppl. 1):82–91.
15. Grey HM, Chesnut R. Antigen processing and presentation to T cells. Immunol Today 1985; 6:101–110.
16. Guidos C, Wong M, Lee KC. A comparison of the stimulatory activities of lymphoid dendritic cells and macrophages in T cell proliferative respones to various antigens. J Immunol 1984; 133:1179–1185.
17. Sperber K, Quraishi H, Kalb TH, Panja A, Stecher V, Mayer L. Selective regulation of cytokine secretion by hydroxychloroquine: Inhibition of interleukin 1 alpha (IL-1α) and IL-6 in human monocytes and T cells. J Rheumatol 1993; 20:803–808.
18. Salmeron G, Lipsky PE. Immunosuppressive potential of antimalarials. Am J Med 1983; 75(Suppl. 1A):19–24.
19. Allison AC, Waters RV. Long-acting antirheumatic drugs incude differentiation of cells of the monocyte-macrophage lineage and alter the expression of cytokines and IL-1 receptor antagonist. Agents Actions 1993; (Suppl. 44):113–127.
20. Hurst NP, French JK, Bell AL, Nuki G, O'Donnell ML, Betts WH, Cleland LG. Differential effects of mepacrine, chloroquine and hydroxychloroquine on superoxide anion generation, phospholipid methylation and arachidonic acid releases by human blood monocytes. Biochem Pharmacol 1986; 35:3083–3089.
21. Hamilton EBD, Scott JT. Hydroxychloroquine sulphate (Plaquenil) in treatment of rheumatoid arthritis. Arthritis Rheum 1962; 5:502–512.
22. Mainland D, Sutcliffe MI. Hydroxychloroquine sulphate in rheumatoid arthritis, a six month, double-blind trial. Bull Rheum Dis 1957; 13:287–290.
23. Clark P, Casas E, Tugwell P, Medina C, Gheno C, Tenorio G, Orozco JA. Hydroxychloroquine compared with placebo in rheumatoid arthritis: A randomised controlled trial. Ann Intern Med 1993; 119:1067–1071.
24. Davis MJ, Dawes PT, Fowler PD, Clarke S, Fisher J, Shadforth MF. Should disease-modifying agents be used in mild rheumatoid arthritis? Br J Rheumatol 1991; 30:451–454.
25. Pavelka K jr, Pavelka K sen, Peliskova Z, Vacha J, Trnavsky K. Hydroxychloroquine sulphate in the treatment of rheumatoid arthritis: a double blind comparison of two dose regimens. Ann Rheum Dis 1989; 48:542–546.
26. le Gallez P, Bird HA, Smith RPS, Greenwood M, Nicol CG, Cox GA, Wright V. A comparison of two dose levels of hydroxychloroquine with chloroquine in rheumatoid. Br J Clin Pract 1987; 41Supp. (52):16–23.

27. Bunch TW, O'Duffy JD, Tompkins RB, O'Fallon WM. Controlled trial of hydroxychloroquine and D-penicillamine singly and in combination in the treatment of rheumatoid arthritis. Arthritis Rheum 1984; 27:267–276.
28. Richter JA, Runge LA, Pinals RS, Oates RP. Analysis of treatment terminations with gold and antimalarial compounds in rheumatoid arthritis. J Rheumatol 1980; 7:153–159.
29. Husain Z, Runge LA. Treatment complications of rheumatoid arthritis with gold, hydroxychloroquine, D-penicillamine and levamisole. J Rheumatol 1980; 7:825–830.
30. Bird HA, le Gallez P, Dixon JS, Surrall KE, Cole DS, Goldman MH, Wright V. A single blind comparative study of auranofin and hydroxychloroquine in patients with rheumatoid arthritis. Clin Rheumatol 1984; 3(Suppl. 1):57–66.
31. Dwosh IL, Stein HB, Urowitz MB, Smythe HA, Hunter T, Orgyzlo MA. Azathioprine in early rheumatoid arthritis compare with gold and chloroquine. Arthritis Rheum 1977; 20:685–592.
32. Nuver-Zwart IH, van Riel PLCM, van de Putte LBA, Gribnau FWJ. A double blind comparative study of sulphasalazine and hydroxychloroquine in rheumatoid arthritis: evidence of an earlier effect of sulphasalazine. Ann Rheum Dis 1989; 48:389–395.
33. van der Heijde DM, van Reil PL, Nuver-Zwart IH, Gribnau FW, van de Putte LB. Effects of hydroxychloroquine and sulphasalazine on progression of joint damage in rheumatoid arthritis. Lancet 1989; 2:1036–1038.
34. Faarvang KL, Egsmose C, Kryger P, Podenphant J, Ingeman-Nielson M, Hansen TM. Hydroxychloroquine and sulphasalazine and in combination in rheumatoid arthritis: a randomised double-blind trial. Ann Rheum Dis 1993; 52:711–715.
35. Dawes PT, Fowler PD, Shadforth MF, et al. Combined gold and hydroxychloroquine in rheumatoid arthritis. Clin Rheumatol 1984; 3(Suppl. 1):S7–66.
36. Porter DR, Campbell HA, Hunter J. Combination therapy in rheumatoid arthritis—no benefit of addition of hydroxychloroquine to patients with a suboptimal response to intramuscular gold therapy. J Rheumatol 1993; 20:645–649.
37. Sievers K, Hurri L. Combined therapy of rheumatoid arthritis with gold and chloroquine. Acta Rheum Scand 1963; 9:48–55.
38. Trnavsky, Gatterova J, Linduskova, Peliskova Z. Combination therapy with methotrexate and hydroxychloroquine in rheumatoid arthritis. Rev Esp Reumatol 1993; 20(Suppl. 1):140.
39. Biro J, Segal AM, MacKenzie AH, Mazanec DJ, Wilke WS. The combination of methotrexate (MTX) and azathioprine (AZA) for resistant rheumatoid arthritis (RA). Arthritis Rheum 1987; 30:S18.
40. McCarty DJ, Carrera GF. Intractable rheumatoid arthritis. Treatment with combined cyclophosphamide, azathioprine and hydroxychloroquine. JAMA 1982; 248:1718–1723.
41. Bitter T. Combined disease-modifying demotherapy for intractable rheumatoid arthritis. Clin Rheum Dis 1984; 10:413–428.
42. Grondin C, Malleson P, Petty RE. Slow-acting antirheumatic drugs in chronic arthritis of childhood. Semin Arthritis Rheum 1988; 18:38–47.
43. Kvien TK, Hoyeraal HM, Sandstad B. Slow acting antirheumatic drugs in patients with juvenile rheumatoid arthritis—evaluated in a randomised, parallel 50 week clinical trial. J Rheumatol 1985; 12:533–539.
44. Manners PJ, Ansell BM. Slow acting antirheumatic drug use in systemic onset juvenile chronic arthritis. Paediatrics 1986; 77:99–103.
45. Stillman JS. Antimalarials in the treatment of juvenile rheumatoid arthritis. In: Moore TD, ed. Arthritis in Childhood. Columbus, OH: Ross Laboratories, 1981:125–127.
46. Brewer EJ, Giannini EIT, Kuzmina N, Alkseev L. Penicillamine and hydroxychloroquine in the treatment of severe juvenile rheumatoid arthritis. Results of the USA-USSR double-blind placebo-controlled trial. New Engl J Med 1986; 314:1269–1276.
47. Giannini EH, Cassidy JT, Brewer EJ, Shaikov A, Maximov A, Kuzmina N. Comparative

efficacy and safety of advanced drug therapy in children with juvenile rheumatoid arthritis. Semin Arthritis Rheum 1993; 23:34–46.
48. Laaksonen AL, Koshiahde V, Juva K. Dosage of antimalarial drugs for children with juvenile rheumatoid arthritis and systemic lupus erythematosus. Scand J Rheumatol 1974; 3:103–108.
49. Christiansen JV, Nielsen JP. Treatment of lupus erythematosus with mepacrine. Br J Dermatol 1956; 68:73–87.
50. Buchanan RN. Quinacrine in the treatment of discoid lupus erythematosus: a five year follow up survey. Results and evaluation. South Med J 1959; 52:978–983.
51. Ruzicka T, Sommerburg C, Goerz G, Kind P, Mensing H. Treatment of cutaneous lupus erythematosus with acitretin and hydroxychloroquine. Br J Dermatol 1992; 127:513–518.
52. Dubois EL. Effect of quinacrine (Atabrine) in treatment of systemic and discoid lupus erythematosus. Arch Intern Med 1954; 94:131–141.
53. Dubois EL. Antimalarials in management of discoid and systemic lupus erythematosus. Semin Arthritis Rheum 1978; 8:33–51.
54. Ziff M, Esserman P, McEwen C. Observations on the course and treatment of systemic lupus erythematosus. Arthritis Rheum 1956; 1:332–350.
55. Rothfield N. Efficacy of antimalarials in systemic lupus erythematosus. Am J Med 1988; 85(Suppl. 4A):53–56.
56. Rudnicki RD, Gresham GE, Rothfield NF. The efficacy of antimalarials in systemic lupus erythematosus. J Rheumatol 1975; 2:323–330.
57. Lockshin MD. Therapy for systemic lupus erythematosus. New Engl J Med 1991; 324:189–191.
58. Morand EF, McCloud PI, Littlejohn GO. Continuation of long-term treatment with hydroxychloroquine in systemic lupus erythematosus and rheumatoid arthritis. Ann Rheum Dis 1992; 51:1318–1321.
59. Lakhanpal S, Duffy J, Griffing WL, Conn DL, Luthra HS. Sjögrens syndrome: treatment with D-penicillamine and hydroxychloroquine. J Rheumatol 1985; 12:1028–1029.
60. Fox FI, Chan E, Benton L, Fong S, Friedlaender M, Howell FV. Treatment of primary Sjögren's syndrome with hydroxychloroquine. Am J Med 1988; 85(Suppl. 4A):62–67.
61. Kruize AA, Hené RJ, Kallenberg CGM, van Bijsterveld OP, van der Heide A, Kater L, Bijlsma JW. Hydroxychloroquine treatment for primary Sjögrens syndrome: a two year double blind crossover trial. Ann Rheum Dis 1993; 52:360–364.
62. Cornblett T. Action of synthetic antimalarial drugs on psoriasis. J Invest Dermatol 1956; 26:435–436.
63. Olsen TG. Chloroquine and psoriasis. Ann Intern Med 1981; 94:546.
64. Luzar MJ. Hydroxychloroquine in psoriatic arthropathy exacerbations of psoriatic skin lesions. J Rheumatol 1982; 9:462–464.
65. Kammer GM, Soter NA, Gibson DJ, Schur PH. Psoriatic arthritis: a clinical immunologic and HLA study of 100 patients. Sem Arthritis Rheum 1979; 9:75–97.
66. Sayers ME. Use of antimalarial drugs for the treatment of psoriatic arthritis. Am J Med 1992; 93:474–475.
67. Gladman DD, Blake R, Brubacher B, Farewell VT. Chloroquine therapy in psoriatic arthritis. J Rheumatol 1992; 19:1724–6.
68. Scherbel AL, Schuter SL, Harrison JW. Comparison of effects of two antimalarial agents, hydroxychloroquine sulphate and chloroquine phosphate in patients with rheumatoid arthritis. Clev Clin Q 1957; 24:98–104.
69. Scherbal AL, Harrison JW, Atdjium M. Further observations on the use of 4-aminoquinoline compounds in patients with rheumatoid arthritis or related diseases. Clev Clin Q 1958; 25:95–111.
70. Rynes RI. Toxicity of antimalarial drugs in rheumatoid arthritis. Agents Actions 1993; 44(Suppl):151–157.

71. Anon. ABPI Data Sheet Compendium, Datapharm Publications Ltd (London), 1994–95:1445–1446.
72. Hobbs H, Calnan C. The ocular complications of chloroquine retinopathy. Lancet 1958; 1:1207–1209.
73. Easterbrook M. The ocular safety of hydroxychloroquine. Semin Arthritis Rheum 1993; 23(Suppl 1):62–67.
74. MacKenzie AH. Dose refinements in long-term therapy of rheumatoid arthritis with antimalarials. Am J Med 1983; 75(Suppl 1A):40–45.
75. Bernstein HN. Ocular safety of hydroxychloroquine. Ann Ophthalmol 1991; 23:292–296.
76. Bernstein HN. Ocular safety of hydroxychloroquine sulfate (Plaquenil). South Med J 1992; 82:274–279.
77. Johnson MW, Vine AK. Hydroxychloroquine therapy in massive total doses without retinal toxicity. Am J Ophthalmol 1987; 104:139–144.
78. Maksymowych W, Russell AS. Antimalarials in rheumatology: efficacy and safety. Semin Arthritis Rheum 1987; 16:206–221.
79. Morsman CDG, Livesey SJ, Richards IM, Jessop JD, Mills PV. Screening for hydroxychloroquine retinal toxicity: Is it necessary? Eye 1990; 4:572–576.
80. Parke A. Antimalarial drugs and pregnancy. Am J Med 1988; 85(Suppl. 4A):30–33.
81. Anon. Hydroxychloroquine (sulphate). In: Dollery C. ed. Therapeutic Drugs, Vol. 1. London: Churchill Livingstone, 1991:H72–H76.
82. Tseng J. Clinical and experimental studies on the mechanism of neuromuscular blockade by chloroquine diarotate. Jpn J Anesth 1971; 20:441–503.
83. Mc Elnay JC, Mukhtar HA, D'Arcy PF, Temple DJ, Collier PS. The effect of magnesium bisilicate and kaolin in the in vivo absorption of chloroquine. J Trop Med Hyg 1982; 85:159–163.
84. Leden I. Digoxin-hydroxychloroquine interaction. Acta Med Scand 1982; 211:411–412.

8
D-Penicillamine

Howard Bird and Ann W. Morgan
University of Leeds, Leeds, United Kingdom

I. INTRODUCTION

Dimethyl-D-cysteine was discovered among the hydrolysis products of penicillin by Abraham et al. [1] and named penicillamine. The cupruretic effect of penicillamine was noted by Walse, who subsequently successfully used this drug in the treatment of Wilson's disease [2]. The drug was also successfully used in cystinuria [3] and heavy metal poisoning. Reactive thiol agents were subsequently demonstrated to dissociate certain macroglobulins in vitro [4] and in vivo in Waldenström's macroglobulinaemia [4, 5]. Subsequently, D-penicillamine was shown to reduce titers of rheumatoid factor in vitro and in vivo [6,7,8]. Jaffe then demonstrated the clinical improvement it produced in rheumatoid arthritis [9], which was then confirmed by others [10,11].

Although a nonpatented "orphan" drug, clinical support for its likely benefit in rheumatoid disease was strong. By 1973 [12], its clinical use in this condition was accepted and subsequent studies over a period of 10 years demonstrated that it remained effective at lower doses. Although D-penicillamine was pharmacologically the most effective of several sulfide compounds used to dissociate rheumatoid factor by Jaffe, other analogues continue to be developed by different drug companies, since the basic structure is not subject to patent. Bucillamine, for example, is one of the most popular disease-modifying drugs currently used in Japan.

II. PHARMACOLOGY

A. Chemistry

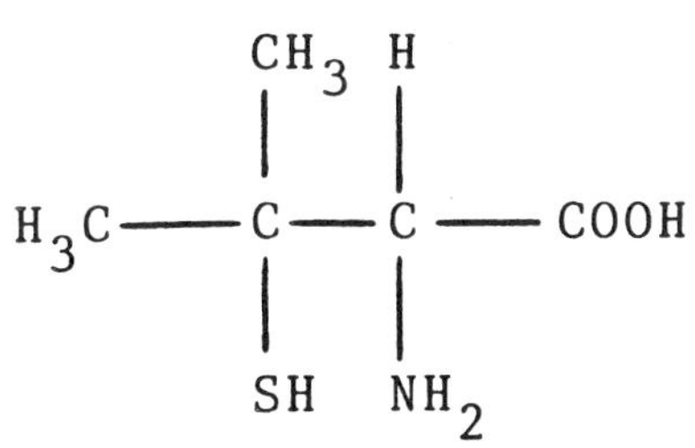

Penicillamine may exist as the D- or L-stereoisomer, but when it is derived from the controlled hydrolysis of penicillin, it is in the D-form only. This is the form available for therapeutic use, which is optically laevorotatory in aqueous solution.

B. Pharmacokinetics

The drug can be assayed by high-performance liquid chromatography using an electrochemical detector and a fluorescent derivitization [13]. It is rapidly but incompletely absorbed from the gastrointestinal tract. The fraction of absorption (40% in normal fasting subjects) is reduced by food [14,15]. Peak plasma concentrations after oral administration occur after 2 h. The plasma half-life is approximately 60 min [16]. This is biphasic with a short early elimination phase (about 1 hr). Dose-dependent kinetics have been suggested [17]. The volume of distribution is 57 L in normal individuals, and protein and tissue binding is extensive (in excess of 80%).

Oxidation, methylation, and formation of stable complexes with protein have all been demonstrated in vivo or in vitro. Metabolism to a sulfoxide may occur and may be relevant to toxicity [18]. Poor sulfoxidation has been linked to an increased risk of toxicity [19], particularly in the presence of HLA-DR3 or HLA-B8.

C. Mechanism of Action

The mechanism of action of D-penicillamine is still not known, but it is presumed that the drug modulates the immune system via sulfydryl exchange. The activity of many cells in the immune system are modulated according to whether cell surface receptor sulfydryl groups are oxidized or reduced. The latter results from D-penicillamine therapy. 5-Thiopyridoxine, with a reactive sulfydryl group, suppresses rheumatoid disease in a manner similar to D-penicillamine with similar side effects, although this compound has no effects on copper disposition or dermal collagen [20,21]. Captopril, structurally similar to D-penicillamine with an active sulfydryl group, is also effective in rheumatoid arthritis [22]. It seems the metal chelation properties are therefore not important. Indeed triene, a metal chelator, is ineffective in rheumatoid arthritis. Penicillamine's effects on collagen, with its ability to react with aldehyde groups, reversibly thinning the skin [23,24], may account for its action in systemic sclerosis. The ratio of soluble poorly polymerized collagen to insoluble polymerized collagen is increased in the skin [25] but not in the rheumatoid synovium [26]. The action of the drug on a variety of enzymes probably results from its interference with sulfydryl/disulphide interchange and its reaction with carboxy and aldehyde groups.

D-penicillamine drugs has been shown to have various actions on inflammation and immunological mechanisms. Present evidence does not support a major effect on neutrophils in vivo [27], although there are effects on oxidative metabolism with depression of myelopyroxidase in vitro. No changes in the numbers or functions of T and B lymphocytes have been identified [28,29], although there is a dose-related inhibitory effect on transformation of lympocytes [30,31]. In the presence of copper or caeruloplasmin, D-penicillamine generates hydrogen peroxide, which inhibits a number of T-lymphocyte functions [32], although this does not necessarily explain the action in vivo.

D-penicillamine is associated with limited suppression of the synthesis of immunoglobulin (Ig) M, A, and E antibodies. This may be mediated by the effects of D-penicillamine/copper sulfate complexes on helper T cells [33]. The drug may enhance clearance of immune complexes or interefer with intracellular synthesis or release of components of these complexes [34]. It also has antiviral activity [5].

III. Clinical Use

A. Indications

D-penicillamine may be used in the treatment of:

1. Rheumatoid arthritis
2. Juvenile chronic polyarthritis
3. Psoriatic arthritis and spondyloarthropathies
4. Progressive systemic sclerosis and morphea
5. Wilson's disease
6. Cystinuria

B. Contraindications

1. Hypersensitivity to penicillamine except in life-threatening situations
2. Previous serious adverse reactions to penicillamine (sensitivity to penicillin is not a contraindication to a trial of D-penicillamine)
3. Agranulocytosis or severe thrombocytopenia due to penicillamine
4. Lupus erythematosus

IV. CLINICAL EFFICACY OF D-PENICILLAMINE

A. Rheumatoid Arthritis

Most published studies of penicillamine in rheumatoid arthritis have been based on the original dosage of 250-mg increments increasing at 2-week intervals to a maintenance dose of up to 1500 mg. All have produced broadly similar results, although the more recent trend has been to reduce dosing, with most patients nowadays aiming for a maintenance level of 500 mg/day, with some climbing to 750–1000 mg/day.

A controlled trial in 1973 from the multicenter trial group [35] showed 1.5 g D-penicillamine a day to be superior to placebo over a 12-month period in 105 patients with severe rheumatoid arthritis. All measurements of disease activity except radiographic change in the small joints of the hand showed greater improvement on D-penicillamine, although the proportion of patients experiencing side effects at this dose (60%) was substantial. A 1975 study [36] compared lower doses of 600 and 1200 mg/day with placebo over a 6-month period in 121 patients with rheumatoid arthritis. Both regimens were superior to placebo, with there being no significant difference in efficacy between them. Thereafter standard dosing was established at around 500 mg/day. The first major American study [37] compared penicillamine 500 and 125 mg/day with placebo over 36 weeks in 225 patients. The 500-mg group showed statistically significant improvement over the placebo group. Surprisingly, there was little difference in efficacy between 125 and 500 mg/day.

D-penicillamine is effective both in seronegative and seropositive rheumatoid disease [38]. Improvement usually commences 12–16 weeks after the commencement of dosing. Synovial swelling and tendon and rheumatoid nodules decrease. Some have even suggested radiographic improvement [39]. The drug is also helpful in the treatment of rheumatoid vasculitis [40,41], secondary amyloid disease [42], and rheumatoid lung disease [43].

1. Comparison with Other Disease-Modifying Antirheumatic Drugs

In 1976, gold and D-penicillamine were compared in 87 rheumatoid arthritis patients over 2 years [44]. The dose of penicillamine was high. There was no significant difference between the drugs. Nowadays, gold injections are often given more frequently than the monthly injections used in this evaluation and the dose of penicillamine would be lower.

D-penicillamine is as effective as azathioprine at 2.5 mg/kg/day, which is a little higher dose than conventionally used now, over one year [45]. Penicillamine has been claimed to be more effective than hydroxychloroquine at a dose of 2.2 mg/kg/day in a small but well-controlled double-blind study in 41 patients over 2 years [46].

A 1987, life table analysis comparison of rheumatoid arthritis treated with sulfasalazine, sodium aurothiomalate, and penicillamine suggested that penicillamine and sulfasalazine were withdrawn slightly more frequently on the grounds of inefficacy compared with gold, which was more frequently withdrawn because of side effects [47]. Subsequently, definitive comparison of sulfasalazine and penicillamine over 2 years in 200 patients showed no clinically relevant difference between the two drugs. Fifty-one percent of the patients on sulfasalazine were able to continue treatment for 2 years compared with 40% of patients receiving penicillamine [48].

2. Use of D-penicillamine in Combination Therapy

The recent vogue for combination therapy has to be balanced against the tendency to use even lower doses of penicillamine. A Japanese paper has demonstrated fewer withdrawals from side effects from an initial dose of 300 mg three times a week even though this was in a different genetic group [49]. A further study from Japan, also on Japanese patients, added either bucillamine (a close penicillamine analogue) or placebo to patients who had not experienced adequate benefit from injectable gold alone. Bucillamine was shown to be more effective than placebo in this context, although the group size was small [50]. Other studies are in progress comparing combinations of disease-modifying drugs either in series or in parallel.

B. Other Indications

1. Juvenile Chronic Polyarthritis

D-penicillamine is also effective in juvenile chronic polyarthritis. The incidence of adverse effects is probably less than that seen in adults [51,52]. The drug does not interfere with growth, and healing of bone lesions has been reported in a single study in seropositive juvenile chronic polyarthritis [53].

2. Psoriatic Arthritis and Spondyloarthropathies

No large-scale studies have been performed. The small studies available suggest that the drug is not effective in psoriatic arthritis, ankylosing spondylitis, or associated seronegative spondarthropathies except in exceptional cases [54–56]. If the clinical picture resembles rheumatoid disease, however, the chances of improvement are greater.

3. Systemic Sclerosis and Morphea

Initial claims suggest benefit in combating early skin involvement in both progressive systemic sclerosis and morphea [57].

A retrospective analysis supported an increased 5-year survival rate (88 vs 66%) and a decrease in the rate of new visceral organ involvement if D-penicillamine was used [58]. Efficacy has also been claimed in localized scleroderma (morphea) [59]. Striking claims have been made for penicillamine in patients with early diffuse systemic sclerosis [60], with the drug producing apparently better results than those achieved in earlier controlled studies with different agents such as 5-Fluorouracil [61] or clorambucil [62]. Further controlled studies of penicillamine in this condition are eagerly awaited.

V. SIDE EFFECTS

A. Mucocutaneous

An itchy maculopapular rash occurring during the first few weeks of therapy is the commonest side effect associated with D-penicillamine [63]. An eczematous rash may occur idiosyncratically at any stage of therapy. A late rash, itchy and associated with irregular plaques that resemble psoriasis, which is often misdiagnosed as seborrhoeic dermatitis, tends to occur after at least 6 months of therapy. It has been suggested that this lesion is a type of pemphigoid [64–66].

B. Renal

Complicated proteinuria is a well-recognised adverse events [9, 67]. It is seem less frequently in patients taking D-penicillamine for Wilson's disease. Rheumatoid arthritis patients taking a 750-mg daily dose for more than 6 months have a 30% incidence [68]. Lower dosing schedules, for example, 250 mg/day, are less likely to be associated [69,70]. Other studies have suggested no correlation between dose and proteinuria [71–73].

Proteinuria usually commences between 4 and 18 months and a relationship to HLA-B8 and HLA-DRW3 has been described. Some subjects become frankly nephrotic. Hematuria indicates deterioration of glomerular function and gross haematuria warns of the rare rapidly progressive glomerular nephritis [74–76].

Electron micrograph examination reveals changes similar to those of minimal change membranous glomerular nephritis [77,78]. Immunofluorescent studies have indicated the existence of granular deposition along the basement membrane, with IgG and complement comprising the most frequently components. The pathogenesis of this adverse event is though to be immune complex mediated [79].

There is controversy over treatment. Providing proteinuria does not exceed 2.0 g/day, most physicians continue D-penicillamine with close monitoring [80]. If proteinuria becomes excessive or hematuria complicates it, cessation of therapy is recommended with the many alternative and perhaps more potent disease-modifying drugs available.

C. Hematological

Thrombocytopenia is the commonest and first adverse effect (a platelet count of $<100{,}000/mL^3$) [76]. The effect is likely to be dose related [81,82] and is more commonly seen in patients who have previously received gold therapy. It is usually rapidly reversable on stopping D-penicillamine [70]. It is sensible to discontinue therapy if the platelet counts drop to $<100{,}000/mL^3$. For a drop below $150{,}000/mL^3$, a reduction in dose should be instituted.

Agranulocytosis has also been described [83], with neutropenia occurring in less than 2% of patients on low-dose D-penicillamine regimens [84]. The rare bone marrow aplasia may be fatal, although idiosyncratic. The mean dose at the time of marrow depression has been recorded as 615 mg/day, the event occurring between 3 and 60 months after the start of therapy [85]. In some cases, a gradual downward trend in leukocyte and platelet counts precedes the event. In general, the onset is less precipitous than the marrow aplasia seen with injectable gold.

D. Gastrointestinal

Dysguesis and hypoguesis (total or partial loss of taste) has occurred in up to 25% of patients starting on higher doses of D-penicillamine (1500 mg/day), although this complication is less frequently seen when treatment is instituted at a lower dose [9,80]. A metallic or salty taste in the mouth is sometimes described. Copper or zinc supplementation does not appear to improve things [34,80]. Anorexia, nausea, and vomiting occasionally occur [86], and an exceptional fatal cholestatic hepatitis has been described [87].

E. Lung

Hemorrhagic pneumonitis has been described in six patients exhibiting rapidly progressive crescentic glomerular nephritis. Gross hematuria may warn of this complication [88,89,40]. For the syndrome resembling idiopathic Goodpasture's syndrome, aggressive plasma pheresis with rescue by steroids may be the most effective treatment. Occasionally, cyclophosphamide and haemodialysis is required [89,90]. There are occasional reports of bronchiolitis obliterans, although this is sometimes hard to distinguish from the lung involvement of rheumatoid arthritis untreated by drugs [91].

F. Musculoskeletal

Striated muscle fiber damage may be induced by low-dose D-penicillamine producing elastosis, although this is unusual [92].

Myasthenia gravis is a rare but important complication, particularly prevalent when the drug is used to treat rheumatoid arthritis. The syndrome is clinically indistinguishable from the spontaneous disease. Electromyography shows typical changes and the condition, which responds well to anticholinesterase therapy, is reversed when D-penicillamine is discontinued [93–95]. Antibodies to acetyl choline receptors have been described in this condition [96,97]. Thymic aplasia, but not frank thymoma, has been described in a single case [97].

Polymyositis and dermatomyositis have also been described [98]. Exceptionally, this may be associated with complete heart block [99].

G. Immunological Abnormalities

D-penicillamine has been associated with several autoimmune-mediated disorders, including drug-induced systemic lupus erythematosus [100], pemphigus, hemolytic anemia [101], and thrombotic thrombocytopenic purpura [102] in addition to those already described. D-penicillamine is associated with the appearance of a number of autoantibodies, including antinuclear antibodies, antiacetylcholine receptor antibodies, antistriated muscle antibodies, and antiheart muscle antibodies. The fact that such complications have also been described in patients receiving D-penicillamine for Wilson's disease suggests that these effects may be drug rather than disease related.

H. Infrequent Adverse Events

Infrequent adverse effects associated with D-penicillamine include drug fever, occurring 7–10 days after the commencement of high-dose therapy, occasional breast enlargement, and acute colitis

1. Overdosage

D-penicillamine overdosage treatment should be prompt and symptomatic, emptying the stomach by emesis or gastric lavage. There is no specific antidote. Bone marrow suppression is the most serious risk, although renal impairment and failure may also occur. Patients should be monitored meticulously for these complications.

VI. SPECIAL CIRCUMSTANCES

There are no data on D-penicillamine administration to neonates, nor on the excretion of penicillamine in breast milk, although the extensive protein binding is unlikely to allow a high concentration. In children, the starting dose of D-penicillamine should be correspondingly lower than in adults. No special precautions are required in the elderly.

D-penicillamine can be continued through pregnancy in Wilson's disease and cystinuria. Normal pregnancies have resulted from patients taking D-penicillamine for rheumatoid arthritis throughout gestation, although slow withdrawal is normally attempted, and there have been isolated case reports of an Ehlers-Danlos type of defect in children of mothers treated with D-penicillamine [103,104].

A. Concurrent Disease

It is always prudent to reduce the dose of D-penicillamine in patients with renal failure or hepatic failure.

B. Drug Interactions

Interactions have not been described between D-penicillamine, a nonsteroidal anti-inflammatory agent, or other drugs. Food substantially reduces the availability of penicillamine [15]. Dosing should normally be on an empty stomach, although it is more important that it should be consistent. Absorption is reduced in patients with rheumatoid arthritis taking concomitant oral iron [63]. Iron tablets should be appropriately spaced away from penicillamine ingestion.

REFERENCES

1. Abraham EP, Chain E, Baker W, Robinson R. Penicillamine: A characteristic degradation product of penicillin. Nature 1943; 151:107.
2. Walshe JM. Wilson's disease; new oral therapy. Lancet 1956; 1:25–26.
3. Crawhall JC, Sowen EF, Watts RWE. Effects of penicillamine on cystinuria. Br Med J 1963; 1:588–590.
4. Deutsch HF, Morton JI. Dissociation of human serum macroglobulins. Science 1957; 125:600.
5. Ritzmann SE, Coleman SL, Levin WC. The modification of a macrocryogelglobulin by penicillin, penicillamine, and cysteamine. J Lab Clin Med 1959; 54:938.
6. Dresner E, Trombly P. Dissociation of the rheumatoid factor *in vitro* and *in vivo*. Clin Res 1960; 8:16.
7. Griffin SW, Ulloa A, Henry M, et al. Effect of penicillamine on circulating rheumatoid factor. Clin Res 1960; 8:87.
8. Jaffe IA. Intra-articular dissociation of the rheumatoid factor. J Lab Clin Med 1962; 60:409–442.
9. Jaffe IA. The effect of penicillamine on the laboratory parameters in rheumatoid arthritis. Arthritis Rheum 1965; 8:1064–1079.
10. Miehlke von K, Kohlhardt I. Uber die immuno-depressonische Wirkung von D-penicillamin in der behandlung der progredient-chronischen Polyarthritis. Rheumaforschung 1967; 26:56–68.
11. Golding JR, Wilson JV, Plunkett TG. Laboratory observations on the use of penicillamine in rheumatoid disease. Postgraduate Med J (Oct Suppl):40–41.
12. Leading Article. Penicillamine in the treatment of rheumatoid arthritis. Br Med J 1973; ii:464.
13. Miners JO, Fearnley I, Smith KJ, Birkett DJ, Brooks PM, Whitehouse MW. The analysis of D-penicillamine in plasma by fluorescence derivitisation with N-(p-(benzoxazolyl)-phenyl) maleimide and high performance liquid chromatography. J Chromatogr 1983; 275:89–96.
14. Lipsky PE. Remission-inducing therapy in rheumatoid arthritis. Am J Med 1983; 75:40–49.
15. Schuna A, Osman MA, Patel RB, Welling PG, Sundstrom WR. Influence of food on the bioavailability of penicillamine. J Rheumatol 1983; 10:95–97.
16. Wiesner RH, Dickson ER, Carlson GL, McPhaul LW, Go VLW. Pharmacokinetics of D-penicillamine in man. J Rheumatol 1981; 8(Suppl 7):51–55.
17. Bergstrom RF, Kay DR, Harcome TM, Wagner JG. Penicillamine kinetics in normal subjects. Clin Pharmacol Ther 1981; 30:404–413.
18. Joyce DA. Variability and response to D-Penicillamine: pharmacokinetic insight. In: Variability and Response to Anti-rheumatoid dysfunction. Basle: Birkhäuser Verlag, 1993:203–207.
19. Madhok R, Zoma A, Torley HI, Capell HA, Waring R, Hunter JA. The relationship of sulfoxidation status to efficacy and toxicity of penicillamine in the treatment of rheumatoid arthritis. Arthritis Rheum 1990; 33:574–577.
20. Huskisson EC, Jaffe IA, Scott J, Dieppe PA. F-Thiopyridoxine in rheumatoid arthritis: Clinical and experimental studies. Arthritis Rheum 1980; 23:106–110.

21. Jaffe IA. Penicillamine in rheumatoid arthritis: Clinical pharmacology and biochemical properties. Scand J Rheumatol 1979; 28(Suppl):58–64.
22. Jaffe IA, Merryman P, Ehrenfeld E. Further studies of the anti-viral effect of D-penicillamine. Postgrad Med J 1974; 50(Suppl 2):50–55.
23. Harvey W, Henderson DRF, Graham R. Observations on *in vivo* skin elasticity and skin thickness of patients with rheumatoid arthritis treated with D-penicillamine and gold salts. Postgrad Med J 1974; 40(Suppl 2):33–36.
24. Scheinberg IH. D-penicillamine with particular relation to Wilson's disease. J Chronic Dis 1964; 17:293.
25. Nimni ME, Gerth N, Bavetta LA. Reversibility of a penicillamine induced defect in collagen aggregation. Nature 1967; 213:921–922.
26. Harkness JA, Blake DR. Penicillamine nephropathy and iron. Lancet 1982; 2:1368–1369.
27. Mowat AG. Neutrophil chemotaxis in rheumatoid arthritis. Effect of D-penicillamine, gold salts and levamisole. Ann Rheum Dis 1978; 37:1–8.
28. Froland SS, Munthe E, Abrahamsen T, et al. In: Munthe E, ed. Penicillamine Research in Rheumatoid Dis. Fabritius and Sonner, 1976:185–192.
29. Zuckner J, Ramsey RH, Dorner RW, et al. D-penicillamine in rheumatoid arthritis. Arthritis Rheum 1970; 13:131.
30. Roath S, Wills R. The effects of penicillamine on lymphocytes in culture. Postgrad Med J 1974; 50(suppl 2):56–57.
31. Schumacher K, Maerker-Alzer G, Preuss R. Effect of D-penicillamine on lymphocyte function. Arzneimittelforsch 1975; 25:603–606.
32 Lipsky PE. Immunosuppression by D-penicillamine *in vitro*. Inhibition of human T lymphocyte proliferation by copper- or ceruloplasmin-dependent generation of hydrogen peroxide and protection by monocytes. J Clin Invest 1984; 73:53–65.
33. Lipsky PE. Modulation of human antibody production *in vitro* by D-penicillamine and $CuSO_4$: Inhibition of helper T cell function. J Rheumatol, 1981; 7(Suppl):69–73.
34. Munthe E, Jellum E, Aaseth J. Some aspects of the mechanism of action of penicillamine in rheumatoid arthritis. Scand J Rheumatol 1979; 28(Suppl):6–12.
35. Multi Centre Trial Group. Controlled trial of D-penicillamine in severe rheumatoid arthritis. Lancet, 1973; 1:275–280.
36. Dixon AStJ, Davis J, Dormandy TL, et al. Synthetic D-penicillamine in rheumatoid arthritis. Ann Rheum Dis 1975; 34:416–421.
37. Williams HJ, Ward JR, Reading JC, et al. Low dose D-penicillamine therapy in rheumatoid arthritis. Arthritis Rheum 1983; 26:581–592.
38. Hill HFH. Treatment of rheumatoid arthritis with penicillamine. Semin Arthritis Rheum 1977; 6:361–388.
39. Gibson T, Huskisson EL, Wojtulewski JA, et al. Evidence that D-penicillamine alters the course of rheumatoid arthritis. Rheumatol Rehab 1976; 18:211.
40. Sternlieb I, Bennett B, Scheinberg IH. D-penicillamine induced Goodpasture's syndrome in Wilson's disease. Ann Intern Med 1975; 82:673–676.
41. Jaffe IA. Rheumatoid arthritis and arteritis. Report of a case treated with penicillamine. Ann Intern Med 1964; 61:556.
42. Lake BJ, Andres G. Rheumatoid arthritis with secondary amyloidosis and malabsorption syndrome: Effect of d-penicillamine. Am J Med 1968; 44:105–115.
43. Lorber A. Penicillamine therapy for rheumatoid lung disease: Effects on protein sulphydryl groups. Nature 1966; 210:1235–1237.
44. Gibson T, Huskisson EC, Wojtulewski JA, et al. Evidence that D-penicillamine alters the course of rheumatoid arthritis. Rheumatol Rehab 1976; 15:211–215.
45. Berry H, Liyanage SP, Durance RA, et al. Azathioprine and penicillamine in treatment of rheumatoid arthritis: a controlled trial. Br Med J 1976; 1:1052–1054.
46. Bunch TW, O'Duffy JD, Tompkins RB, O'Fallon WM. Controlled trial of

hydroxychloroquine and D-penicillamine singly and in combination in the treatment of rheumatoid arthritis. Arthritis Rheum 1984; 27:267–276.
47. Situnayacke RD, Gurindulis KA, McConkey B. Long term treatment of rheumatoid arthritis with sulphasalazine, gold or penicillamine; A comparison using life table methods. Ann Rheum Dis 1987; 46:177–183.
48. Capell HA, Marabani M, Madhock R, Torley A, Hunter JA. Degree and extent of response to sulphasalazine or penic therapy for rheumatoid arthritis: Results from a routine clinical environment over a two year period. Q J Med 1990; 75:335–344.
49. Hakoda M, Taniguchi A, Kamatani N, Akahoshi T, Kashiwazaki S. Intermittent treatment with D-penicillamine is effective in lower doses with fewer adverse effects in patients with rheumatoid arthritis. J Rheumatol 1994; 21:1637–1641.
50. Yasuda M, Sakai K, Orbe M, et al. Efficacy of additive DMARD therapy in patients with rheumatoid arthritis. Double blind controlled trial using bucillamine and placebo with maintenance doses of gold sodium thiomalate. J Rheumatol 1994; 21:44–50.
51. Schairer H, Stoeber E. In: Munthe E, ed. Penicillamine Research in Rheumatoid Disease. Oslo: Fabritius and Sonner, 1976:279–281.
52. Ansell BM, Hall MA. Penicillamine in chronic arthritis of childhood. J Rheumatol 1981; 7(Suppl):112–115.
53. Ansell BM. International symposium on levamisole in rheumatoid arthritis. Introduction to the symposium. J Rheumatol 1978; 4(Suppl 5):1–2.
54. Bird HA, Dixon JS. Failure of d-penicillamine to affect peripheral joint involvement in ankylosing spondylitis of HLA B27-associated arthropathy. Ann Rheum Dis 1977; 36:289.
55. Golding DN. In: Munthe E, ed. Penicillamine Research in Rheumatoid Disease. Oslo: Fabritius and Sonner, 1976:282–283.
56. Leca AP, Camus JP. Spondylarthrite ankylosante echec due traitement par la D-penicillamine. Nouv Presse Med 1975; 04:12.
57. Baum J. The use of penicillamine in the treatment of rheumatoid arthritis and scleroderma. Scand J Rheumatol 1979; (Suppl 28):65–70.
58. Steen VD, Medsger TA Jr, Rodnan GP. D-penicillamine therapy in progressive systemic sclerosis (sclerodmera): a retrospective analysis. Ann Intern Med 1982; 97:652–659.
59. Falanga N, Medsger TA. D-penicillamine in the treatment of sclerodmera. Arch Dermatol 1980; 126:609–612.
60. Jimenez SA, Sigal SA. A 15 year prospective study of treatment of rapidly progressive systemic scleroderma with D-penicillamine. J Rheumatol 1991; 18:496–508.
61. Alarcon GS, Casas JA, Saway PA, et al. 5-fluorouracil in the treatment of scleroderma: a randomised double-blind placebo controlled international collaborative study. Ann Rheum Dis 1990; 49:926–928.
62. Furst DE, Clements PJ, Hillis S, et al. Immunosuppression with clorambucil versus placebo for scleroderma. The results of a three year parallel randomised double blind study. Arthritis Rheum 1989; 32:584–593.
63. Mowat AG, Huskisson EC. D-penicillamine in rheumatoid arthritis. Clin Rheum Dis 1975; 1:319–333.
64. Hewitt J, Benveniste M, Lessana-Leibowitch M. Pemphigus induced by D-penicillamine, an "experimental" pemphigus. Br J Dermatol 1975; 93(Suppl 11):12.
65. Hewitt J, Lessana-Leibowitch M, Beneveniste M, Saporta L. Un cas de pemphigus injuit par la D-penicillamine. Le pemphigus iatrogene existe t'il? Ann Med Interne (Paris) 1971; 122:1003.
66. Hill HFH. Penicillamine in rheumatoid arthritis: Adverse effects. Scand J Rheumatol, 1979; 28(Suppl):94–99.
67. Goldberg A, Smith JA, Lochhead AC. Treatment of lead-poisoning with oral penicillamine. Br Med J 1963; 1:1270.

68. Lyle WH. Penicillamine. In: Huskison EC, ed. Anti-rheumatic Drugs: Clinical Pharmacology and Therapeutics, Vol. 3. East Sussex, England: Prager Scientific, 1983:521–567.
69. Jaffe IA, Treser G, Suzuki Y, Ehrenreich T. Nephropathy induced by D-penicillamine. Ann Intern Med 1968; 69:549–556.
70. Stockman A, Richter D, Barraclough D, et al. Difficulties in the use of D-penicillamine in the treatment of rheumatoid arthritis. Aust NZ J Med 1979; 9:495–503.
71. Hill HFH, Hill AGS, Davison AM. Resumption of treatment with penicillamine after proteinuria. Ann Rheum Dis 1979; 38:229–231.
72. Neild GH, Gatner H-V, Bohle A. Penicillamine induced membranous glomerulonephritis. Scand J Rheumatol 1979; 28(Suppl):79–90.
73. Sternlieb I. Penicillamine and the nephrotic syndrome. JAMA 1966; 198:1311–1312.
74. Golding JR, Wilson JV, Day AT. Observations on the treatment of rheumatoid disease with penicillamine. Postgrad Med J 1970; 46:599–605.
75. Huskisson EC, Hart FD. Penicillamine in the treatment of rheumatoid arthritis. Ann Rheum Dis 1972; 31:402.
76. Multicentre Trial Group. Controlled trial of D(-)penicillamine in severe rheumatoid arthritis. Lancet 1973; 1:275–280.
77. Bacon PA, Tribe CR, Mackenzie JC, et al. Penicillamine nephropathy in rheumatoid arthritis. Q J Med 1976; 45:661–684.
78. Jaffe IA. Effects of penicillamine on the kidney and on taste. Symposium on penicillamine. Postgrad Med J 1968; 44:(Oct Suppl):15.
79. Dische FE, Swinson DR, Hamilton EBD, Parsons V. Immunopathology of penicillamine-induced glomerular disease. J Rheumatol 1976; 3:145–154.
80. Jaffe IA. D-penicillamine. Bull Rheum Dis 1978; 28:948.
81. Hill HFH. Treatment of rheumatoid arthritis with penicillamine. Semin Arthritis Rheum 1977; 6:361–388.
82. Willaims HJ, Ward JR, Reading JC, et al. Low dose D-penicillamine therapy in rheumatoid arthritis. A controlled, double-blind trial. Arthritis Rheum 1983; 26:581–592.
83. Corcos JM, Soler-Bechara J, Mayer K, et al. Neutrophilic agranulocytosis during administration of penicillamine. JAMA 1964; 189:265–268.
84. Halverson PB, Kozin F, Bernhard GC, Goldman AL. Toxicity of penicillamine. A serious limitation to therapy in rheumatoid arthritis. JAMA 1978; 240:1870–1871.
85. Kay AGL. Myelotoxicity of D-penicillamine. Ann Rheum Dis 1979; 32:232–236.
86. Jaffe IA. The treatment of rheumatoid arthritis and necrotizing vasculitis with penicillamine. Arthritis Rheum 1970; 13:436–443.
87. Jacobs JWG, van der Weide FR, Kruijsen MWM. Fatal cholestatic hepatitis caused by D-penicillamine. Br J Rheumatol 1994; 33:770–773.
88. Editorial. Penicillamine: More lessons from experience. Br Med J 1975; 3:120–121.
89. Gavaghan T, McNaught PJ, Ralston M, Hayes I. Penicillamine induced Goodpasture's syndrome: Successful treatment of a fulminant case. Aust NZ J Med 1981; 11:2610265.
90. Lockwood CM, Ree RJ, Pearson TA, et al. Immunosuppression and plasma-exchange in the treatment of Goodpasture's syndrome. Lancet 1976; 1:711–715.
91. Chakravarty K, Webley M. A longitudinal study of pulmonary function in patients with RA treated with gold and D-penicillamine. Br J Rheumatol 1992; 31:829–833.
92. Dakziel KL, Burge SM, Frith PA, Ryan TJ, Mowat A. Elastic fibre damage induced by low dose D-penicillamine. Br J Dermatol 1990; 123:305–312.
93. Balint G, Szobor A, Temesvari P, et al. Myasthenia gravis developed under D-penicillamine treatment. Scand J Rheumatol 1975; 4(Suppl 3):Workshop 21, Abs. 12.
94. Bucknall RC, Dixon ASJ, Glick EN, et al. Myasthenia gravis associated with penicillamine treatment for rheumatoid arthritis. Br Med J 1975; 1:600–602.
95. Gordon RA, Burnside JW. D-penicillamine-induced myasthenia gravis in rheumatoid arthritis. Ann Intern Med 1977; 87:578–579.

96. Russell AS, Lindstrom JM. Penicillamine-induced myasthenia gravis associated with antibodies to acetylcholine receptor. Neurology 1978; 28:847–849.
97. Vincent A, Newsom-Davis J, Martin V. Antiacetylcholine receptor antibodies in D-penicillamine-associated myasthenia gravis. Lancet 1978; 1:1254.
98. Doyle DR, McCurley TL, Sergent JS. Fatal polymyositis in D-penicillamine-treated rheumatoid arthritis. Ann Intern Med 1983; 98:327–330.
99. Wright GD, Wilson C, Bell AL. D-penicillamine induced polymyositis causing complete heart block. Clin Rheumatol 1994; 13:80–82.
100. Chalmus A, Thompson D, Stein HE, et al. Systemic lupus erythematosus during D-penicillamine therapy for rheumatoid arthritis. Ann Intern Med 1982; 97:659–663.
101. Harrison HE, Hickman JW. D-penicillamine and haemolytic anaemia. Lancet 1976; 1:38.
102. Ahmed F, Sumalnop V, Spain DM, Tobin MS. Thrombohemolytic thrombocytopenic purpura during penicillamine therapy. Arch Intern Med 1978; 1292–1293.
103. Mjolnerod OK, Dommerud SA, Rassmussen K, Gjeruldsen ST. Congenital connective tissue defect probably due to D-penicillamine treatment in pregnancy. Lancet 1971; 1:673–675.
104. Lyle WH. Penicillamine in pregnancy. Lancet 1978; 1:1064.

9
Gold Therapy

Anne McEntegart and Hilary A. Capell
Royal Infirmary, Glasgow, United Kingdom

I. INTRODUCTION

Despite increasing interest in the development of novel biological therapies, gold compounds, given either by intramuscular injection or as an oral preparation, retain an important position in the hierarchy of treatment of inflammatory joint disease. In use since the 1920s [1], the clinical efficacy of gold is well established as is its extensive toxicity profile. Intriguingly, the precise mechanisms of action remain elusive, although as our understanding of the complex inflammatory pathways which lead to joint destruction increases, several levels of gold-mediated inhibition emerge in the cascade.

Intramuscular administration of any anti-inflammatory therapy offers a potential advantage to the clinician. Specifically, the certainty of compliance, noting the potentially serious adverse effect profile, are attractive, as is the opportunity for ongoing patient education by health-care professionals administering therapy. The oral equivalent of intramuscular sodium aurothiomalate, auranofin, however is more acceptable to some patients, thereby offering those who decline parenteral drug administration the benefit of chrysotherapy, although, as will be discussed, the expected efficacy and toxicity profile may be altered. Intramuscular gold and auranofin therapy, therefore, will be considered separately in this chapter.

II. ORAL GOLD

A. Pharmacology

1. Chemistry

Auranofin (AUR) (triethylphosphic gold) is a lipid-soluble monomer of molecular weight 678.5 containing 29% gold by weight.

2. Pharmacokinetics

After a single 6-mg dose, auranofin is rapidly, although incompletely, absorbed. The peak concentration achieved is 60–90 $\mu g/L^{-1}$ after 1–2 h. In the region of 13–33% of dose is absorbed, and the remainder is excreted over 7 days. At a dose of 3 mg bid, steady state is reached over 8–12 weeks at about 700 μg/L^{-1} (these levels are lower than those achieved with intramuscular [IM] gold). It is noteworthy that 40% is RBC associated, a much higher proportion than with IM gold, whereas 60% is protein bound, lower than the 90%+ observed with IM gold. Excretion patterns also differ for those observed with injectable gold. During auranofin treatment, 85% of absorbed gold is excreted in feces and only 15% by the renal route. The plasma half-life if 17–25 days. Passage across the placenta and secretion in breast milk has not been established.

Serum gold levels do not correlate with efficacy or toxicity and are of no value in monitoring patients (except possibly when compliance is in doubt).

3. Mechanism of Action

Auranofin has been demonstrated in vitro to be a more potent inhibitor of monocyte and polymorph activity than IM gold. Inhibition of chemotaxis, phagocytosis, chemiluminescence, and superoxide production have been found. Recently, auranofin has been shown to inhibit the production of leucotriene B_4, a proinflammatory mediator which activates human polymorphs with respect to chemotaxis and aggregation [2].

Case reports of auranofin-induced diarrhea and enterocolitis have postulated a direct toxic effect on the mucosa of the bowel evidenced by high excretion of oral gold in feces [3] and gold deposits in the mucosal layer on electron microscopy [4]. Auranofin-induced stimulation of enteric nerves and neurotransmitter release has been demonstrated in vitro [5].

B. Clinical Efficacy

1. Placebo-controlled Studies

The benefits of auranofin therapy over placebo have been demonstrated in several trials [6–9]. These are summarized in Table 1. Improvement in both clinical and laboratory indices have been shown in patients who continue therapy to 6 months [7,9]. Despite this, a substantial number of patients are withdrawn from therapy owing to lack of effect [7,8]. Similarly, a 24-month double-blind Scandinavian study of 132 patients with early rheumatoid arthritis (RA) showed benefit in clinical, laboratory, and radiographic measures in the auranofin group over placebo. Thirty-five of 67 (52%) patients remained on auranofin for 2 years—The majority of withdrawals were due to cutaneous and gastrointestinal side effects [9]. Champion et al. found that by 45 months follow-up, 3.5% of the patients has stopped auranofin owing to lack of efficacy and 14.5% owing to toxicity (mainly rash and diarrhea) [10].

2. *Comparison with Other DMARDs* (see Table 2)

Available evidence suggests that although auranofin is undoubtedly efficacious as a disease-modifying antirheumatic drug (DMARD), the benefit observed is less than that of most other second-line agents.

Intramuscular Gold. As outlined in Section III on IM gold, auranofin appears slightly less efficacious than IM gold therapy. Attempts to switch patients from parenteral gold therapy to auranofin have on the whole been unsuccessful, resulting in a flare of RA or side effects leading to withdrawal of therapy [11]. In addition, in a group of patients unresponsive to auranofin 50% subsequently responded to IM gold.

Table 1 Comparison of Auranofin with Placebo

Treatment	Reference	No. enrolled	Duration (months)	Outcome
AUR vs placebo	Wenger et al. [6]	340	6	AUR superior to placebo. Subsequent follow-up for further year showed AUR reduced erosion rate.
AUR vs placebo	Katz et al. [7] Crofton et al. [8]	252	6 12	AUR superior to placebo in clinical parameters assessed and in a reduction in radiographic score.
AUR vs placebo	Johnson et al. [9]	132	24	Greater improvement in clinical and laboratory parameters in AUR group. Gastrointestinal and cutaneous adverse reactions most common reason for discontinuing AUR

Table 2 Auranofin Compared with Other DMARDs

Treatment	Reference	No. enrolled	Duration (months)	Outcome
AUR vs d-penicillamine	Manthorpe et al. [12]	40	12	No difference in efficacy or toxicity.
AUR vs d-penicillamine	Hoonberg et al. [13]	90	12	Greater efficacy with d-penicillamine but fewer side effects in AUR group.
AUR vs SASP	Porter et al. [14]	200	12	No difference in efficacy or toxicity.
	McEntegart et al. [15]	200	60	SASP more effective than AUR with significantly more patients still on SASP (31%) vs AUR (15%) at 60 months.
AUR vs MTX	Weinblatt et al. [16]	281	9	Significantly lower rate of radiographic progression on MTX compared with AUR.

D-Penicillamine. Comparing penicillamine 500 mg/day with auranofin 6 mg/day in 40 RA patients, no difference in efficacy was demonstrated [12]. In a 12-month trial of auranofin 6 mg/day versus penicillamine 750 mg/day fewer side effects occurred on auranofin but penicillamine was more effective [13].

Sulfasalazine. A prospective trial comparing auranofin with sulfasalazine in 200 RA patients showed little difference between the two therapies at 12 months [14]. These patients, however, have now been followed up for 5 years. Thirty-one percent on sulfasalazine for 5 years compared with 15% on auranofin ($P < .05$). Patients continuing on sulfasalazine showed a substantial response in clinical and laboratory parameters over the 5-year period. No significant improvement in those remaining on auranofin for 5 years was demonstrated [15].

Methotrexate. Weinblatt et al. conducted a 9-month randomised, multicenter trial comparing the effect of methotrexate versus auranofin on radiographic progression in RA patients. They found a significantly lower rate of progression in joint space narrowing and erosion score in the methotrexate-treated group [16].

Meta-analysis. A meta-analysis of 66 published clinical trials of second-line drugs found auranofin to be less efficacious but less toxic than other second-line agents (only hydroxychloroquine was less toxic) [17,18].

3. *Use of Auranofin in Combination Therapy* (Table 3)

Auranofin has been used in combination with methotrexate (MTX), sulfasalazine, and hydroxychloroquine. Williams et al. compared auranofin, methotrexate, and both combined in 335 RA patients over 48 weeks [20]. No significant difference in clinical or laboratory variables was demonstrated between the three groups. Side effects resulting in discontinuation of treatment were more common in the group on combination therapy. A multicenter trial comparing the effect of auranofin, methotrexate, or both drugs on radiographic progression in RA reported worsening scores for erosions and joint space narrowing in all three groups. Only in the auranofin group, however, did this differ significantly from the baseline leading the investigators to conclude that progression of disease radiographically may be slowed by methotrexate [21]. A more recent Japanese study looked at three treatment groups in RA patients who had not responded sufficiently to auranofin therapy. One group continued on auranofin only; sulphasalazine was added to auranofin in the second group and methotrexate to auranofin in the third. Clinical improvement appeared to be better in the groups on combination therapy compared with auranofin only. No unexpected adverse reactions were demonstrated in any of the treatment groups [22].

C. Clinical Use

1. *Indications*

Auranofin is of proven value in RA. As with injectable gold, patients with clinical synovitis, functional impairment, acute phase response, and progressive erosive disease should be considered for treatment. Auranofin may be of limited use in patients in whom IM gold has failed [14,23].

The onset of benefit is slower than injectable gold and often takes as much as 6 months to become apparent.

Table 3 Auranofin in Combination Therapy

Treatment	Reference	No. enrolled	Duration (months)	Outcome
AUR vs MTX vs AUR + MTX	Williams et al. [20]	355	12	No significant difference in clinical/laboratory parameters assessed between three groups.
AUR vs MTX vs AUR + MTX	Lopez-Mendez et al. [21]	211	12	Suggested MTX and MTX + AUR slowed radiographic progression but not AUR alone.

A practical guide to prescribing with a need for monitoring, education, and explanation of the delayed onset of action to patient is given in Table 4. Management of adverse reactions is given in Table 5.

2. Contraindications

Auranofin should not be used in the presence of IM gold-induced side effects such as necrotizing enterocolitis, pulmonary fibrosis, exfoliative dermatitis, bone marrow aplasia, or other blood dyscrasia. It is also not appropriate in patients with progressive renal disease, severe active hepatitis, or systemic lupus erythematosus (SLE).

3. Special Groups

Oral gold is contraindicated in pregnancy and should be avoided in lactating women.

Reduction of dose in the elderly to 3 mg/day is suggested, although several RA studies include patients older than 64 years and do not report increased toxicity in these groups.

4. Drug Interactions

Ataxia resulting from increased phenytoin levels during auranofin therapy has been reported [24].

III. INTRAMUSCULAR GOLD

A. Pharmacology

1. Chemistry

There are several water-soluble polymeric gold complexes that are administered intramuscularly, with the best known being sodium aurothiomalate and aurothioglucose. Most work on the chemistry and pharmacology of these complexes has been conducted on aurothiomalate, and this is discussed briefly below. Absorption of aurothiomalate is more rapid than aurothioglucose, but otherwise the properties of these two water-soluble complexes appear similar. In addition, both appear to be equally efficacious [25,26].

Table 4 Recomended Regimen for Use of Auranofin

Discuss need for DMARD/delay in onset of effects (3–6 months)/side effects with patient.
Baseline full blood count/urinalysis/chest X-ray. Urea and electrolytes, liver function tests.
Supply *Auranofin Information Sheet* to patient and family doctor who will share care.
Supply *Drug Monitoring Card* to patient.
Commence auranofin 3 mg bid.
Monthly FBC and urinalysis.
Dose of auranofin can be increase to 3 mg tid at 6 months if no response to therapy.
Suggest family doctor should withhold treatment and contact hospital if:
WBC $< 4 \times 10^9$/L
Platelets $< 150 \times 10^9$/L
Hb < 9g/dL
Urine 1 + protein or more
Severe diarrhea/rash/mouth ulcers

Table 5 Management of Adverse Effects of Auranofin

Mucocutaneous	
	Withhold auranofin and look for an alternative cause. (Not all mucocutaneous events during chrysotherapy are related to auranofin.) If side effect is mild and settles promptly, rechallenge cautiously if the patient agrees.
	Alopecia is rare.
Gastrointestinal	
	Diarrhea: Auranofin commonly causes mild diarrhea. Bran or other bulking agent could be tried, but if it does not resolve or is severe, auranofin should be discontinued.
	Abnormal liver function tests. Withhold therapy. Exclude other causes. Discontinue auranofin if none found.
Hematological	
	Fall in WBC to $<4000 \times 10^9/L$: Withhold auranofin and verify WBC. In general, further auranofin is inadvisable. Monitor WBC until normal. Give supportive care as necessary. Granulocyte colony-stimulating factor may be tried if WBC remains low.
	Fall in platelet count to $<150{,}000 \times 10^9/L$. *Mild, gradual, and no evidence of bleeding*: Withhold auranofin. Repeat count and request film; clumped platelets may give a falsely low result. If confirmed, discontinue auranofin and monitor until normal.
	Sudden precipitous fall to $<10{,}000 \times 10^9/L$ *with bruising, etc*. This is rare with auranofin.
	Rise in mean cell volume with or without fall in hemoglobin level. Look for alternative cause (e.g., check B_{12} folate). If none found, monitor closely. Does not usually pose a major problem.
Renal	
	Proteinuria trace: No action necessary but continue to monitor.
	One or more plus of proteinuria: Withhold auranofin. Look for and treat infection. Perform 24-h quantitative protein estimation. If > 0.5 g/24 hr, discontinue auranofin, and if no alternative cause is found, do not give further gold. If amyloidosis is diagnosed as a cause of proteinuria and a good joint response has been obtained, continue auranofin therapy cautiously.
	Hematuria: Look for infection or other cause. Continue auranofin therapy cautiously.
Rare	
	Pulmonary fibrosis: Seek expert respiratory help.

2. Pharmacokinetics

The peak plasma concentration of sodium aurothiomalate is reached 2 h after intramuscular injection (7 mg/L) and falling to 3 mg/L some 7 days later. Weekly gold administration therefore gives an effective serum concentration of about 3 mg/L, >90% of which is protein bound as opposed to that of 0.75–1.25 mg/L when treatment is offered monthly, as is common practice in clinically stable disease. Low levels of gold are found in RBC after 7 days and also in white cell series.

Between 30 and 50% of administered gold is excreted each week. Excretion is 70% renal, especially initially and up to 24 h; 30% of excretion is fecal. The half-life in serum is 5.5 days and somewhat longer in synovial fluid (6–7 days) [27]. There is widespread tissue distribution in involved (but not normal) joints—gold is found in synovial fibroblasts and macrophages (EM studies [28]). After prolonged therapy, the total body half-life is about 250 days, with consequences for toxicity, subsequent DMARD choice and interpretation of later toxicity. Serum gold varies but does not correlate with toxicity except perhaps a high free gold concentration [29]. Gold deposition is seen in the cornea in a concentration proportional to the cumulative dose. This deposition reverses when gold therapy is stopped and does not lead to ocular toxicity. Of the gold which accumulates in the skin, almost all is deposited in the dermis. Gold is, however, distributed throughout the body during chrysotherapy, with spleen, kidneys, and adrenals showing particularly high concentrations.

3. Mechanism of Action of Gold Compounds

The mechanism of action of auranofin and intramuscular gold has not been satisfactorily elucidated. Many in vitro and in vivo studies have explored avenues none of which entirely explain the mode of action of these drugs on disease activity in inflammatory arthropathies. Findings in vitro are difficult to extrapolate to in vivo activity—highlighted by the paradoxical observation that auranofin, which in some respects has greater effects in vitro than aurothiomalate, appears to be the less active drug in vivo. Improvement in disease activity clinically may be associated with better immunoregulation and control of inflammation. Whether this is a cause or a consequence of the control of disease activity is unclear and makes interpretation of changes in cellular and humoral responses difficult. Concentrations of serum immunoglobulins and rheumatoid factor fall during gold therapy [30]. This change is, however, usually observed after and not before demonstrable clinical benefit.

There have been several reports of a reduction in lymphocyte counts in patients on gold therapy [31,32] but no changes in T-cell subset ratios or killer T-cell function have been demonstrated. In vitro lymphocyte studies have in contrast shown auranofin and IM gold to inhibit cellular proliferation [33]. This effect may well be monocyte dependant.

More recently, interest has focused on the effect of chrysotherapy on cytokine activity. Interleukin-1 (IL-1) production is inhibited by auranofin but not IM gold in vitro [34]. Sfikakis et al. postulated suppression of IL-2 and IL-2 receptor production by auranofin and IM gold [35]. However, Crilly et al. found no correlation between concentrations of the soluble IL-2 receptor and clinical parameters of disease activity. In addition, no change in the concentration of serum IL-2 (sIL-2) receptor could be demonstrated by treatment with auranofin, IM gold, or sulfasalazine [34]. This result was confirmed in a 24-week study of 40 RA patients treated with IM gold with or without steroids—no change in sIL-2R levels was demonstrated despite the improvement in clinical measures assessed [35]. Yanni et al. examined synovial biopsies from 10 RA patients on IM gold (at 1, 2, and 12 weeks of therapy) after staining the tissue with a panel of monoclonal antibodies to various cytokines. They found a significant decrease in IL-1α, IL-1β, IL-6, and tumor necrosis factor-α (TNF-α) expression at 12 weeks. In addition, a reduction in the number of monocytes and macrophages in the synovium was noted with no significant reduction in T- or B-cell counts. They concluded that gold, by influencing monocytes and macrophages and thus cytokine production, could suppress disease activity in RA [38].

There has been recent interest in synoviocytes as the effector cells in cytokine secretion in the RA joint. Loetscher et al. have found IM gold inhibits chemotactic cytokines (IL-8 and monocyte chemoattractant protein-1 [MCP-1]) produced by RA synoviocytes. They postulate that subsequent recruitment of neutrophils and monocytes into the joint would therefore diminish with reduction in inflammatory effects [39].

B. Clinical Efficacy

1. *Placebo-controlled Trials* (Table 6)

In the Empire Rheumatism Council Study, 199 RA patients were randomized to receive either a 5-month course of 20 weekly injections of 50 mg sodium aurothiomalate (99 patients) or 0.5 μg weekly of the same substance (100 patients) as a control group. Considerable improvement was found in the treatment group in all variables assessed except radiological progression from 3 months onward and was maintained up to 18 months (1 year after completion of "the course") [40]. A smaller North American trial involved 68 patients involved up over 18 months and showed significant improvement in only the erythrocyte sedimentation rate (ESR) in the gold group when compared with placebo. However, the number of patients studied was small and only one patient withdrew from the gold group because of inefficacy compared with eight withdrawals from the placebo-treated group [41]. Sigler et al. found IM gold significantly better than placebo in 27 patients studied over 30 months; in particular a reduction in the number of erosions in the gold-treated group was found [42].

2. *IM Gold Versus Auranofin in RA* (Table 7)

Several trials have compared intramuscular gold and auranofin. Davis et al. studied 120 patients over a period of 1 year and found no statistically significant difference between the two therapies in any of the clinical variables measured. They noted, however, that withdrawal from the study through lack of effect was twice as frequent for auranofin as for IM gold. Toxicity in contrast was the commonest reason for stopping IM gold [43]. In a study of 193 patients followed up for 20 months, Ward et al. found IM gold more effective than auranofin [44]. Similarly, a 3-year follow-up of 90 patients receiving auranofin, IM gold, or placebo found benefit from both active compounds when compared with placebo [45]. Fourteen of the 30 patients treated with auranofin had therapy withdrawn because of lack of effect, and subsequently 50% of those patients responded to IM gold. More recently, a randomized trial switching RA patients in remission on injectable gold to auranofin found that only 29% remained on auranofin at 2 years compared with 64% still on IM gold therapy [46]. In addition, radiographic deterioration was significantly worse in the auranofin group than in those on IM gold. Van Riel et al. studied 40 RA patients treated with auranofin or aurothioglucose over a 12-month period. They found a significant increase in the mean number of new erosions and in the total radiographic score in the auranofin group at 6 and 12 months. In the aurothioglucose-treated patients, radiographic progression of joint destruction was also seen, but it did not reach statistical significance [47]. Thus, parenteral gold therapy appears more efficacious than auranofin in retarding radiographic progression.

3. *Comparison with Other DMARDs* (Table 8)

Intramuscular gold has been compared with other DMARDs in a number of different trials. When compared with D-penicillamine over a 6-month period, similar efficacy was found in 89 patients [48]. Similarly, Thomas et al. followed 50 patients in a double-blind study for 21 weeks initially and found no significant difference between either drug in terms of clinical outcome or toxicity: Those patients who remained on therapy at 21 weeks were followed up to 55 months. Six of 10 patients on IM gold and 6 of 13 on penicillamine who had completed the study remained on treatment at 55 months [49].

Table 6 Placebo-controlled Trials of Gold Sodium Aurothiomalate

Reference	No. enrolled	Duration (months)	Outcome
Empire Rheumatism Council [40]	199	30	Gold better than placebo when clinical and laboratory parameters assessed. No difference in radiographic progression.
Cooperating Clinics Committee of the ARA [41]	68	18	Gold-treated group showed significant improvement in ESR only compared with placebo (however, numbers small).
Sigler et al. [42]	27	30	Gold significantly better than placebo with reduction in number of erosions in gold-treated group.

Table 7 Gold Sodium Aurothiomalate Compared with Auranofin

Treatment	Reference	No. enrolled	Duration (months)	Outcome
GSTM vs AUR	Davis et al. [43]	120	12	No significant differences between GSTM or AUR but lack of effect twice as frequent with AUR.
GSTM vs AUR	Ward et al. [44]	193	20	GSTM better than AUR.
GSTM vs AUR	Capell et al. [45]	90	36	Suggested GSTM better than AUR (50% of patients discontinuing AUR through lack of effect subsequently responded to IM gold.
GSTM vs AUR	Prete et al. [46]	46	24	Patients in remission on GSTM continued IM gold or switched to AUR. Radiographic progression significantly worse in AUR group.

Table 8 Gold Sodium Aurothiomalate Compared with Other DMARDs

Treatment	Reference	No. enrolled	Duration	Outcome
GSTM vs penicillamine	Huskisson et al. [48]	89	6 months	No difference in efficacy.
GSTM vs penicillamine	Thomas et al. [49]	50	55 months	No significant difference in efficacy or incidence of side effects.
GSTM vs SASP	Pullar et al. [50]	90	6 months	No significant difference in improvement of clinical and laboratory parameters.
GSTM vs SASP	Williams et al. [51]	186	37 weeks	SASP similar efficacy to GSTM but better tolerability.
GSTM vs MTX	Suarez-Almazor et al. [53]	40	26 weeks	Equal efficacy but greater number adverse reactions in gold group.
GSTM vs MTX	Morassut et al. [54]	35	26 weeks	Equal efficacy but greater number adverse reactions in gold group.
GSTM vs MTX	Rau et al. [55]	57	6 months	Equal efficacy MTX tolerability better.

Two placebo-controlled trials comparing IM gold with sulfasalazine demonstrate equal efficacy in active RA patients. Pullar et al. studied 90 patients with active RA treated with sulfasalazine, IM gold, or placebo [50].

At 6 months, sulfasalazine and gold showed significant clinical and laboratory improvement, whereas placebo-treated patients showed no benefit. In a similar study of 186 patients followed for 37 weeks, IM gold and sulfasalazine again were found to be equally efficacious [51]. Forty-one percent of patients on IM gold were withdrawn from the study because of adverse reactions (rash, stomatitis, and proteinuria) compared with 16% on sulfasalazine. Thus, in this study, sulfasalazine appeared to be better tolerated than IM gold.

Porter et al. studied 675 RA patients treated with sulfasalazine, IM gold, or penicillamine in prospective trials in Glasgow. At 5 years, ESR and morning stiffness were significantly better in the gold-treated groups, and with penicillamine, there was a greater improvement in articular index. There was no significant difference in the number of patients remaining on gold (34%), SASP (26%), or penicillamine (22%) after 5 years follow-up [52].

More recently, comparison with methotrexate in several trials has demonstrated similar efficacy between the two therapies. These studies to date have been small and of short duration; however, 40 patients with active RA were randomized to receive either 10 mg IM methotrexate weekly or 50 mg gold weekly [53]. Equal efficacy was demonstrated in all but one of the parameters (proximal interphalangeal joint circumferance measured. The number of adverse reactions in the gold group, however, was significantly greater than in the methotrexate-treated group ($p < .01$). Similarly, Morassut et al. found no significant difference between 12.5 mg of oral methotrexate weekly and 50 mg of gold IM weekly in 35 patients at 26 weeks [54]. During this period, however, 6 of 17 gold-treated patients withdrew from the study owing to drug toxicity compared with only 2 of 18 patients in the methotrexate group. More recently Rau et al. compared 15 mg IM methotrexate weekly with 50 mg IM gold weekly in 57 RA patients over 6 months of follow-up [55]. Again, no difference in efficacy was demonstrated in either number of swollen joints involved or radiographic progression of disease, but tolerability of methotrexate seemed greater. No serious methotrexate-related side effects (pneumonitis, pancytopenia) were seen in these three studies. One patient developed abnormal liver function that was found to be secondary to chronic cholecystitis.

Intramuscular gold is as effective as azathioprine (2.5 mg/kg/day) and cyclophosphamide (1.5 mg/kg/day) with no significant difference in improvement in clinical parameters assessed [56].

Meta-analysis. A meta-analysis of 66 published clinical trials assessing efficacy and toxicity for several second-line drugs found auranofin to be less efficacious than other second-line agents. Intramuscular gold was in contrast among the most efficacious and was comparable with sulfasalazine, methotrexate, and penicillamine. It is noteworthy, however, that the toxicity index for IM gold was high, whereas auranofin was less toxic [17].

4. *Use of IM Gold in Combination Therapy* (Table 9)

Hydroxychloroquine. Intramuscular gold has been used in combination with hydroxychloroquine in several studies with differing outcomes. Scott et al. studied 101 RA patients who were randomized to receive gold and hydroxychloroquine or gold and

Table 9 IM Gold in Combination Therapy

Treatment	Reference	No. enrolled	Duration (months)	Outcome
IM gold + HCQ	Scott et al. [57]	101	12 months	Combination therapy slightly more efficacious than gold alone but more adverse reactions in gold + HCQ group.
IM gold + HCQ	Porter et al. [58]	142	6 months	No significant difference between gold + HCQ vs gold + placebo.
IM gold + d-PEN	Bitter et al. [59]	71	18 months	Combination therapy resulted in greater number of patients in remission than either drug alone but toxicity greater.
IM gold + d-PEN	McKenna et al. [60]	45	6 months	No difference in efficacy or toxicity in combination therapy group compared with either drug alone.
IM gold + cyclosporin A	Bensen et al. [61]	20	6 months	Significant improvement in clinical parameters. Nephrotoxicity in 3 of 20 patients leading to treatment withdrawal.

placebo from the outset and followed for 12 months [57]. Results suggested a possible slight advantage to combination therapy but a greater number of withdrawals owing to adverse reactions in this group [57]. Porter et al. randomized 142 patients with a suboptimal response to IM gold after 6 months to receive in addition either 400 mg hydroxychloroquine or placebo. After 6 months of the combination, no significant difference between the two groups was demonstrated for any variable analyzed (ESR, C-reactive protein [CRP], HAQ, articular index, grip strength). Thus, no benefit of combination therapy over treatment with IM gold alone was demonstrated [58].

D-Penicillamine. Two studies using D-penicillamine and IM gold in combination again found differing results. Bitter et al. used 71 RA patients who had not responded adequately to IM gold or D-penicillamine alone [59]. When both drugs were used in combination, 8 of 12 patients achieved remission compared with only 2 of 24 patients on either drug alone. However, subsequently, 40% of the patients on combination therapy withdrew because of toxicity. In contrast, no improved efficacy could be demonstrated on a combination of D-penicillamine (500 mg/day) and sodium aurothiomalate (50 mg/week) compared with either drug alone over a 6-month period in 45 patients with active RA [60].

Cyclosporin. Recently, Bensen et al. have reported on two uncontrolled pilot studies of cyclosporin A in combination with methotrexate or IM gold [61]. Twenty patients were assigned to either group. All patients had shown continual disease activity despite treatment with IM gold (50 mg every 2–4 weeks) for at least 22 weeks or oral methotrexate (mean dose 10 mg/week) for at least 6 months. After 6 months of cyclosporin A therapy, there was a significant improvement in joint count, joint score, swelling, and joint pain in both groups. Three of the 20 patients in the gold/cyclosporin A group discontinued therapy because of a 30–50% increase in serum creatinine above baseline, otherwise adverse reactions were mild and temporary.

C. Clinical Use

1. *Indications*

The preceding description of studies has provided ample evidence of the clinical efficacy of injectable gold in RA. Studies in psoriatic arthritis [62], seronegative spondyloarthropathies, palindromic rheumatism, and juvenile chronic arthritis have shown evidence of a beneficial effect from gold.

2. *Anticipated Benefit*

In all the above conditions, the expectation is that inflammatory synovitis and the acute phase response will be suppressed with an anticipated effect on progression of erosive disease and functional outcome. This effect takes 8–20 weeks to become apparent.

3. *Magnitude of Response*

A median 50% improvement in pain score and ESR and 75% in morning stiffness has been observed over the first 6–12 months and can be sustained in those who continue treatment over 5 years.

4. *Method of Administration* (see Table 10)

It is recommended that in the absence of toxicity, gold should not be discontinued for lack of effect until an attempt has been made to increase the dose to 100 mg for 6 weeks.

Table 10 Recommended Regimen for Use of IM Gold

Discuss need for DMARD/delay in onset of effects (3–6 months)/side effects with patients.
Baseline full blood count and urinalysis, urea and electrolytes, liver function tests, chest x-ray.
Supply *IM gold Information Sheet* to patient and family doctor.
Supply *Drug Monitoring Card* to patient.
Test dose 10 mg GSTM. If no adverse reaction, give 50 mg weekly until response. Injections can then be reduced to 2 weekly, 3 weekly, and then 4 weekly maintenance therapy.
If no response by 6 months: 100 mg IM gold weekly for 6 weeks.
FBC and urinalysis before each injection of gold.
Withhold treatment and contact hospital if:
- WBC $<4 \times 10^9$/L
- Platelets $<150 \times 10^9$/L
- Hb <9 g/dL
- Urine 1 + protein or more
- Severe rash or mouth ulcers

Table 11 Management of Adverse Effects of IM Gold

Mucocutaneous

Withhold gold and look for an alternative cause. (Not all mucocutaneous events during chrysotherapy are related to gold.) If side effect is mild and settles promptly, rechallenge cautiously if the patient agrees.

Nitritoid reaction: Reassure patient that the reaction will resolve after a few injections; if patient is reluctant to continue, try alternative second-line drug. Where available, an alternative oil-based gold preparation may be tried (reputed to be less likely to produce nitritoid reaction).

Gastrointestinal

Diarrhea: Intramuscular gold rarely causes diarrhea, but if it does, it should be discontinued.

Abnormal liver function tests. Withhold therapy. Exclude other causes. Discontinue gold if none found.

Hematological

Fall in WBC to $<4000 \times 10^9$/L: Withhold gold and verify WBC. In general, further gold is inadvisable. Monitor WBC until normal. Give supportive care as necessary. Granulocyte/macrophage colony-stimulating factor may be helpful if WBC remains low.

Fall in platelet count to $<150{,}000 \times 10^9$/L. Mild, gradual, and no evidence of bleeding: Withhold gold. Repeat count and request film; clumped platelets may give a falsely low result. If confirmed, discontinue gold and monitor until normal.

Sudden precipitous fall to $<10{,}000 \times 10^9$/L with bruising, etc. Hospitalize patient and monitor closely. Prednisolone 40–60 mg po is usually required for a few weeks with or without platelet transfusion. IV immunoglobulins may be tried. This side effect usually reverses in 1–2 weeks. Decrease dose of prednisolone as soon as possible.

Renal

Proteinuria trace: No action necessary but continue to monitor.

One or more plus of proteinuria: Withhold gold. Look for and treat infection. Perform 24-h quantitative protein estimation. If >0.5 g/24 hr, discontinue gold, and if no alternative cause is found, do not give further gold. If amyloidosis is diagnosed as a cause of proteinuria and a good joint response has been obtained, continue gold therapy cautiously.

Hematuria: Look for infection or other cause (e.g., renal calculi). Abdominal ultrasound should be obtained. Continue gold therapy cautiously.

Rare

Pulmonary fibrosis: Seek expert respiratory advice.

In some instances, simply increasing the frequency of gold injections at conventional doses (50 mg) is sufficient to regain response.

5. Contraindications to Injectable Gold

These include marrow toxicity (relative), previous severe reaction to gold, pregnancy (relative), and exfoliative dermatitis.

6. Special Groups

In juvenile chronic arthritis (Stills), there is evidence of an increased incidence of toxicity [63]. Breast-feeding is considered safe, since gold is absorbed in only small amounts by the neonate gut.

7. Concurrent Disease

Exercise caution in the face of severe renal or liver disease or marrow-based malignancy.

8. Drug Interactions

It has been noted that patients receiving angiotensin-converting enzyme (ACE) inhibitors are more likely to exhibit prominent and prolonged nitritoid reactions [64,65].

The management of adverse reactions is shown in Table 11.

REFERENCES

1. Forestier J. L'Aurothiopie dans les rhumatisme chronique. Bull Mem Soc Med Hop Paris 1929; 53:323.
2. Elmgreen J, Annfelt-Ronne I, Nielsen OH. Inhibition of human neutrophils by auranofin: chemotaxis and metabolism of arachidonate via the 5-lipoxygenase pathway. Ann Rheum Dis 1989; 48:134–138.
3. Jarner D, Mertz Nielsen A. Auranofin induced enterocolitis in rheumatoid arthritis. Scand J Rheumatol 1983; 12:254–256.
4. Langer HE, Hartmann G, Heinemann G, Richter K. Gold colitis induced by auranofin treatment of rheumatoid arthritis: case report and review of the literature. Ann Rheum Dis 1987; 46:787–792.
5. De Beaux A, Keenan CM, Tytgat K, Rangachan PK. Responses of the colonic epithelium to auranofin: evidence for involvement of enteric nerves. J Rheumatol 1990; 17:1137–1141.
6. Wenger ME, Alexander S, Bland JH, et al. Auranofin versus placebo in the treatment of RA. Am J Med 1983; 75(Suppl. 6A):123–127.
7. Katz WA, Alexander S, Bland JH, et al. The efficacy and safety of auranofin compared to placebo in RA. J Rheumatol 1982; 9(Suppl. 8):173–178.
8. Gofton JP, O'Brien WM, Hurley JN, Scheffler BJ. Radiographic evaluation of erosion in rheumatoid arthritis: double blind study of auranofin versus placebo. J Rheumatol 1984; 11:768–771.
9. Johnsen V, Borg G, Trang LE, et al. Auranofin in early rheumatoid arthritis: results from at 24 month double-blind, placebo controlled study. Effect on clinical and biochemical assessments. Scand J Rheumatol 1989; 18:251–260.
10. Champion GD, Cairns DR, Bieri D, et al. Dose response studies and longterm evaluation of auranofin in rheumatoid arthritis. J Rheumatol 1988; 15:28–34.
11. Blackburn WD. Auranofin: its use in rheumatoid arthritis patients maintained on parenteral chrysotherapy. J Rheumatol 1987; 14:863.

12. Manthorpe R, Horbor S, Sylrest J, Vinterberg H. Auranofin versus penicillamine in rheumatoid arthritis. One year results from a perspective clinical investigation. Scand J Rheumatol 1986; 15:13–22.
13. Hochberg MC. Auranofin or d-penicillamine in the treatment of rheumatoid arthritis. Ann Intern Med 1986; 195:528.
14. Porter D, Madhok R, Hunter JA, Capell HA. Prospective trial comparing the use of sulphasalazine and auranofin as second line drugs in patients with rheumatoid arthritis. Ann Rheum Dis 1992; 51:461–464.
15. McEntegart A, Porter D, Capell HA, et al. Five year prospective study of 200 RA patients on sulphasalazine or auranofin. Arthritis Rheum 1995; 38(Supppl 9):5369.
16. Weinblatt ME, Polisson R, Blother SD, et al. The effects of drug therapy on radiographic progression of rheumatoid arthritis. Results of a 36 week randomised trial comparing methotrexate and auranofin. Arthritis Rheum 1993; 36:613–619.
17. Felson DT, Anderson JJ, Meenan RF. The comparative efficacy and toxicity of second line drugs in rheumatoid arthritis. Results of two meta-analyses. Arthritis Rheum 1990; 33:1449–1461.
18. Felson DT, Anderson JJ, Meenan RF. Use of short-term efficacy/toxicity tradeoffs to select second line drugs in rheumatoid arthritis. A meta-analysis of published clinical trials. Arthritis Rheum 1992; 35:1117–1125.
19. Fries JF, Williams CA, Ramey D, Block DA. The relative toxicity of disease-modifying antirheumatic drugs. Arthritis Rheum 1993; 36:297–306.
20. Williams HJ, Ward JR, Reading JC, et al. Comparison of auranofin, methotrexate and the combination of both in the treatment of rheumatoid arthritis. A controlled clinical trial. Arthritis Rheum 1992; 35:1406–1407.
21. Lopez-Mendez A, Daniel WW, Reading JC, et al. Radiographic assessment of disease progression in rheumatoid arthritis patients from the Cooperative Systematic Studies of the Rheumatic Diseases clinical trial of auranofin versus methotrexate versus a combination of the two. Arthritis Rheum 1993; 36:1364–1369.
22. Fuju T, Suwa A, Yosida T, et al. Study on combinations of auranofin, salazosulfapyridine and methotrexate in rheumatoid arthritis. Rynmachi 1994; 34:571–82.
23. Davis P, Landon M. Treatment with auranofin in patients with rheumatoid arthritis previously experiencing drug related side-effects with sodium aurothiomalate. J Rheumatol 1985; 12:622.
24. Barraclough D, Boyden K, Brooks P, et al. A comparative study of auranofin, gold sodium thiomalate and D-penicillamine in rheumatoid arthritis: a progress report. In: Proceedings of a Smith, Kline & French International Symposium, November 15–16, Amsterdam, 1982. Amsterdam: Excerpta Medica, 1982:240–248.
25. Lawrence JS. Comparative toxicity of gold preparations in the treatment of rheumatoid arthritis. J Rheumatol 1976; 35:171–173.
26. Pothermich NO, Philips VK, Bergen W, Thomson MH. Chrysotherapy. a prospective study. Arthritis and Rheumatism 1976; 19:1321–1327.
27. Freedman PS. Myocrisin: review of pharmacology. In: Nuki G, Gumpell JM, eds. Proceedings of an International Symposium, MCI Symposium Series No. 11 1985:25–30.
28. Norton WL, Lewis DC, Ziff M. Electron-dense deposits following injection of gold sodium thiomalate and thiomalic acid. Arthritis Rheum 1968; 11:436–443.
29. Heath MJ. Measurement of "free" gold in patients receiving disodium aurothiomalate and the association of high free to total gold levels with toxicity. Ann Rheum Dis 1988; 47:18–21.
30. Hanly JG, Hassan J, Whelan A, et al. Effects of gold therapy on the synthesis and quantity of serum and synovial fluid IgM, IgG and IgA rheumatoid factors in rheumatoid arthritis

patients. Arthritis Rheum 1986; 29:480–487.
31. Hanly JG, Bresnihan B. Reduction in peripheral lymphocytes in patients receiving gold therapy for rheumatoid arthritis. Ann Rheum Dis 1985; 44:299–301.
32. Smith MD, Smith A, Fehr M, et al. Effects ofchrysotherapy on circulating lymphocyte numbers and subsets. Ann Rheum Dis 1988; 47:15–17.
33. Lipsky PE, Ziff M. Inhibition of antigen and mitogen-induced human lymphocyte proliferation by gold compounds. J Clin Invest 1977; 59:455–466.
34. Davis VA, Kulesz A, Nelson BS, Brooks PM. Bimodal effect of gold on IL-1 production by blood monocytes. J Rheumatol 1989; 16:1160–1161.
35. Sfikakis PP, Souliotis VL, Panayiotidis PP. Suppression of interleukin-2 and interleukin-2 receptor biosynthesis by gold compounds in in-vitro activated human peripheral blood mononuclear cells. Arthritis Rheum 1993; 36:308–312.
36. Crilly A, Madhok R, Watson J, Capell HA. Serum concentrations of soluble interleukin-2 receptor in patients with rheumatoid arthritis: effect of second line drugs. Ann Rheum Dis 1993; 52:58–60.
37. Kirkham BW, Davison SC, Corkhill MM, et al. Serial soluble interleukin-2 receptor levels in rheumatoid arthritis: differences in response to glucocorticoid treatment and chrysotherapy. J Rheumatol 1993; 20:935–939.
38. Yanniu G, Nabil M, Farahat MR, et al. Intramuscular gold decreases cytokine expression and macrophage numbers in the rheumatoid synovial membrane. Ann Rheum Dis 1994; 53:315–22.
39. Loetscher P, Dewald B, Baggiolini M, et al. Monocyte chemoattractant protein 1 and interleukin-8 production by rheumatoid synoviocytes. Effects of anti-rheumatic drugs. Cytokine 1994; 6:162–170.
40. Empire Rheumatism Council. Gold therapy in rheumatoid arthritis: final report of a multicentre controlled trials. Ann Rheum Dis 1961; 20:315.
41. The Cooperative Clinics Committee of the ARA. A controlled trial of gold salt therapy in rheumatoid arthritis. Arthritis Rheum 1973; 16:353.
42. Sigler JW, Bluhm GB, Duncan H, et al. Gold salts in the treatment of rheumatoid arthritis: a double-blind study. Ann Intern Med 1974; 80:21.
43. Davis P, Menard H, Thompson J, et al. One year comparative study of gold sodium thiomalate and auranofin in the treatment of rheumatoid arthritis. J Rheumatol 1985; 12:60.
44. Ward J, Williams H, Egger M, et al. Comparison of auranofin, gold sodium thiomalate and placebo in the treatment of rheumatoid arthritis: a controlled clinical trial. Arthritis Rheum 1983; 26:1303–1315.
45. Capell HA, Lewis D, Carey J. A three year follow-up of patients allocated to placebo or oral or injectable gold therapy for rheumatoid arthritis. Ann Rheum Dis 1986; 46:705–711.
46. Prete PE, Zane J, Krailo M, Bulanowski M. Randomised trial of switching rheumatoid arthritis patients in remission with injectable gold to auranofin. Clin Rheumatol 1994; 13:60–69.
47. Van Riel PLCM, Larsen A, Van de Putte LBA, Gribnau FWJ. Effects of aurothioglucose and auranofin on radiographic progression in rheumatoid arthritis. Clin Rheumatol 1986; 5:359–364.
48. Huskisson EC, Gibson TJ, Balme HW. Trial comparing D-penicillamine and gold in rheumatoid arthritis. Ann Rheum Dis 1974; 33:532.
49. Thomas MH, Rothermich NO, Philips VK, et al. Gold versus D-penicillamine double blind study and follow-up. J Rheumatol 1984; 11:764.
50. Pullar T, Hunter JA, Capell HA. Sulphasalazine in rheumatoid arthriis. A double-blind comparison of sulphasalazine with placebo and sodium aurothiomalate. Br Med J 1982; 287:1102.
51. Williams HJ, Ward DR, Dahl SL, et al. A controlled trial comparing sulphasalazine, gold sodium thiomalate and placebo in rheumatoid arthritis. Arthritis Rheum 1988; 31:702.
52. Porter DR, McInnes I, Hunter JA, Capell HA. Outcome of second line therapy in rheumatoid arthritis. Ann Rheum Dis 1994; 53:812–815.

53. Suarez-Almazor ME, Fitzgerald A, Grace M, Russell AS. A randomised controlled trial of parenteral methotrexate compared with sodium aurothiomalate in the treatment of rheumatoid arthritis. J Rheumatol 1988; 15:753.
54. Morassut P, Goldstein R, Cyr M, Karsh J, McKendry RJ. Gold sodium thiomalate compared to low dose methotrexate in the treatment of rheumatoid arthritis—a randomised, double-blind 26 week trial. J Rheumatol 1989; 16:302.
55. Rau R, Herborn G, Menninger H, et al. One year randomised double-blind study of methotrexate and gold sodium thiomalate in early erosive rheumatoid arthritis. Arthritis Rheum 1990; 33:539.
56. Currey HLF, Harris J, Mason RM. Comparison of azathioprine, cyclophosphamide and gold in treatment of rheumatoid arthritis. Br Med J 1974; 3:763.
57. Scott DL, Dawes PT, Tunn E, et al. Combination therapy with gold and hydroxychloroquine in rheumatoid arthritis: a prospective randomised, placebo-controlled study. Br J Rheumatolo 1989; 28:128–133.
58. Porter DR, Capell HA, Hunter J. Combination therapy in rehumatoid arthritis—no benefit of addition of hydroxychloroquine to patients with a suboptimal response to intramuscular gold therapy. J Rheumatol 1993; 20:645–649.
59. Bitter T. Combined disease-modifying chemotherapy for intractable rheumatoid arthritis. Clin Rheum Dis 1984; 10:413–428.
60. McKenna F, Hopkins R, Hinchcliffe KP, et al. Gold and penicillamine alone and in combination in active rheumatoid arthritis [abstr]. 16th International Congress of Rheumatology, Sydney, Australia, May 1985.
61. Bensen W, Tugwell P, Roberts RM, et al. Combination therapy of cyclosporin with methotrexate and gold in rheumatoid arthritis (2 pilot studies). J Rheumatol 1994; 21:2034–2038.
62. Palit J, Hill J, Capell HA, et al. A multicentre double blind comparison of auranofin, intramuscular gold thiomalate and placebo in patients with rheumatoid arthritis. Brit J Rheumatol 1990; 29:280–283.
63. Brewer EJ, Giannini EH, Barkley E. Gold Therapy in the management of juvenile rheumatoid arthritis. Arth Rheum 1980; 24:404–411.
64. Healey LA, Backes MB. Nitritoid reactions and angiotensin-converting-enzyme inhibitors [letter]. N Engl J Med 1989; 321:763.
65. Fort JG,. Abruzzo JL. Nitritoid reaction following initiation of ACE inhibitors in patients with rheumatoid arthritis treated with i.m. gold [abst]. Arth Rheum 1992; 35(Suppl.):R10.

10
Sulfasalazine

Maxime Dougados
Hôpital Cochin, Paris, France

I. INTRODUCTION

Sulfasalazine was developed and manufactured to cure rheumatoid arthritis by eliminating the then putative cause, a group B streptococcal intestinal infection. In fact, it has long been accepted as the drug of choice in the treatment of inflammatory bowel disease [1]. After temporary disfavor, sulfasalazine has regained a position as a second-line disease-modifying antirheumatic drug (DMARD). Before looking at the potential clinical use of sulfasalazine in rheumatoid arthritis, it appears of interest to review the pharmacokinetics of the compound, which might have consequences not only for the mechanism of action of the drug but also for the clinical monitoring of patients treated with sulfasalazine.

II. PHARMACOKINETICS

A. Human Pharmacokinetics and Bioavailability

The pharmacokinetics of sulfasalazine have been extensively investigated mainly in humans [2].

1. Absorption

Following a single oral dose of sulfasalazine in healthy volunteers, the individual variations in plasma concentrations are large [3]. The reasons for these variations are not fully understood, although the conditions of absorption, such as the intraluminal milieu of the gastrointestinal tract, are probably of great importance. Small differences were observed between old (>70 years) and young (<50 years) groups of rheumatoid arthritis patients [4,5]. The plasma half-life was about twice as long in the elderly as in the young patients.

2. Distribution

The apparent volume of distribution calculated after an intravenous dose of sulfasalazine in nine healthy volunteers indicates restricted distribution. Autoradiographic studies show that sulfasalazine has a very uniform distribution pattern in the body [6]. Sulfasalazine is shown to bind to serum protein [7], as well as to the warfarin site on albumin, which is also the primary binding site for bilirubin. Displacement of warfarin was seen at a concentration of sulfasalazine that was much higher than therapeutic levels. The distribution of sulfasalazine to synovial fluid has been studied in rheumatoid arthritis patients [8]. Sulfasalazine was found to be present in the synovial fluid at similar concentrations as in plasma. Human studies on pregnant women have shown that at full-term, both sulfasalazine and its metabolites equilibrate completely across the placenta [9,10]. Owing to the risk of bilirubin displacement by the high protein binding of sulfasalazine, caution should be taken during late pregnancy. Sulfasalazine passes into the milk, in which it can be found at concentrations of about 40% of the serum concentration [11].

3. Metabolism (Fig. 1)

About 10% of orally administered sulfasalazine is absorbed via the small intestine and is returned unchanged to the gut via the bile. As sulfasalazine reaches the colon, azoreductive cleavage occurs by the intestinal bacteria, resulting in the formation of sulfapyridine and 5-aminosalicylic acid (5-ASA) in equimolar amounts. This has been elucidated by studies in germ-free and conventional rats [12,13] and in patients with ileostomy [14]. In these patients, only about 7% of the administered dose was excreted as sulfapyridine compared with 60% in healthy subjects or patients with colitis but with preserved colon.

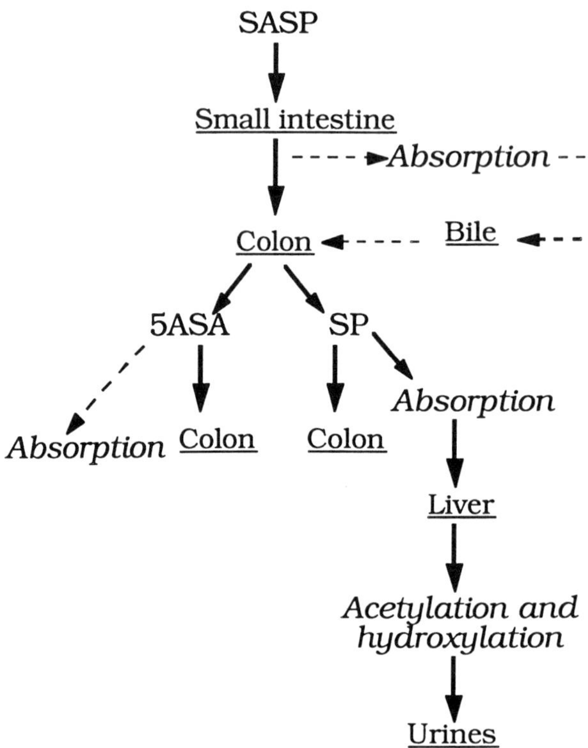

Figure 1 Pharmacokinetics of sulfasalazine. SASP, sulfasalazine; 5ASA, 5-aminosalicylic acid; SP, sulfapyridine.

Sulfapyridine liberated in the colon is to a large extent absorbed and subsequently metabolized [15]. Owing to the higher absorption of sulfapyridine compared with sulfasalazine, plasma concentrations of sulfapyridine have been used in bioequivalence studies. The metabolism of sulfapyridine (hydroxilation and acetylation) is to a large extent dependent on the rate of acetylation, which is determined by genetic factors [16]. Patients can be phenotyped as slow or fast acetylators on the basis of the ratio of sulfapyridine and acetylsulfapyridine concentration in serum or urine. Approximately 60% of the white population are slow acetylators [15]. The half-life and the protein binding of sulfapyridine are dependent on acetylation phenotype [5].

5-Aminosalicylic acid remains largely in the colon; only a small portion of this metabolite is absorbed and excreted in the urine [6]. Most 5-aminosalicylate is recovered unchanged in the feces, but some may be found in the acetylated form. Some data suggest that 5-aminosalicylate may be subject to gut as well as systemic acetylation [17].

When 5-amino salicylate and sulfapyridine are administered as single agents orally, both are absorbed in the proximal gastrointestinal tract and excreted in the urine [18].

4. Factors Influencing the Pharmacokinetics of Sulfasalazine

The absorption of sulfasalazine is subject to considerable interindividual variation. The bioavailability of the parent compound is low (<10%), and absorption is largely determined by factors such as intestinal mobility, transit time, and intraluminal milieu. Concerning these factors, patients with rheumatoid arthritis have fewer problems with increased mobility or other changes in the intestinal milieu than patients with inflammatory bowel disease. The pharmacokinetics of sulfasalazine do not vary with gender [15]. The small variation due to age seems thus to be of minor importance. The acetyl phenotype does not influence the pharmacokinetics of sulfasalazine but does influence the plasma levels of sulfapyridine.

B. Clinical Consequences

Knowledge of the human pharmacokinetics of sulfasalazine in the human and of the characteristics of rheumatoid arthritis raises two questions:

1. What is the active moiety of sulfasalazine in rheumatoid arthritis?
2. Is the acetylator status of the patients of clinical relevance in influencing the efficacy and/or the toxicity of sulfasalazine?

1. Active Moiety of Sulfasalazine

Studies in inflammatory bowel disease suggest that 5-ASA is the therapeutically active moiety of sulfasalazine, whereas sulfapyridine may be responsible for most of the toxicity of the drug [1]. In rheumatoid arthritis, 60 patients were enrolled in a prospective double-blind controlled study of 24 weeks' duration comparing sulfapyridine (2 g daily) and 5-aminosalicylic acid (1–2 g daily) [18]. This study showed an unequivocal effect (i.e., improvement in both laboratory and clinical indices of inflammation) in the rheumatoid patients receiving sulfapyridine, and therefore suggests that sulfapyridine is the active moiety of sulfasalazine, although previous work did not show any relation between serum concentrations of sulfapyridine or its metabolites and the therapeutic efficacy of sulfasalazine in rheumatoid arthritis [19]. This evidence raises the question whether we should use sulfapyridine in preference to sulfasalazine in the treatment of rheumatoid arthritis. In fact, in the study previously discussed, sulfapyridine appeared less well tolerated than 5-aminosalicylic acid and also less well tolerated than sulfasalazine in patients treated in the same unit [19]. Although sulfapyridine is the active moiety of sulfasalazine in rheumatoid arthritis, its ratio of efficacy to toxicity is no better than that of sulfasalazine.

2. Acetylator Status of the Patient

The percentage of slow acetylators is similar in rheumatoid arthritis patients and in the general white population [20–22]. Fast- and slow-acetylator rheumatoid arthritis patients do not differ in age or sex and/or in disease characteristics (seropositivity, disease activity, and disease severity). There are some differences concerning the percentage of patients who experienced minor laboratory abnormalities (e.g., increase in hepatic enzyme aspartate transaminases) according to acetylator status. However, in such studies, the level of efficacy and the level of toxicity of sulfasalazine with regard to acetylator status does not relate significantly to either a favorable response or an incidence of side effects in patients with rheumatoid arthritis treated with sulfasalazine. It is possible that hepatic metabolism is affected by sulfasalazine treatment, particularly in patients with slow-acetylator status, but this does not lead to clinically identifiable problems.

III. MODES OF ACTION

Despite decades of research efforts, the etiology of rheumatoid arthritis is largely unknown. This situation makes evaluation of the mode of action of disease-modifying drugs difficult and conclusions from experimental data concerning these types of drugs should be interpreted with caution. Sulfasalazine has been shown to have several biological activities, all of which could contribute to its beneficial clinical effects in rheumatoid arthritis.

Better knowledge of the pharmacokinetics of sulfasalazine permits considering two different modes of action: a local activity of the drug at the gut level and a systemic activity.

1. Local Gut Effects

Antibacterial Effects. Studies in vitro have shown that both sulfasalazine and its main metabolites inhibit bacterial growth [23]. A reduction in several bacterial species of the gut flora has also been observed after clinical treatment with sulfasalazine [24–27]. The relationship between this antibacterial effect and the clinical efficacy in rheumatoid arthritis is unknown, but it should be recalled that the abnormal mucosal permeability observed in rheumatoid arthritis could be important for the transport of bacterial antigens across the intestinal wall [28,29].

Anti-inflammatory Effects. Together with abnormally increased mucosal permeability, a higher than normal incidence of intestinal inflammation has also been observed in rheumatoid arthritis patients [30]. Sulfasalazine could have an effect on the disease via the anti-inflammatory effects of its 5-aminosalicylic acid component. To identify the source of intestinal blood loss in rheumatoid arthritis patients being treated with nonsteroidal anti-inflammatory drugs (NSAIDs) and assess the response to sulfasalazine, intestinal inflammation (evaluated using ^{111}indium leukocyte studies), blood loss (evaluated using ^{51}chromium red blood cell studies) and gastroduodenal damage (evaluated by performing endoscopy) were assessed in 46 patients taking NSAIDs [31]. The conclusions of this study were that the small intestine is the main site of mild chronic blood loss in patients receiving NSAIDs and that this blood loss could be reduced with sulfasalazine treatment.

Immunomodulatory Effects. To analyze whether the intestinal mucosa in rheumatoid arthritis is immunologically abnormal and whether sulfasalazine possesses any local intestinal immunoregulatory effect, lymphocyte subpopulations and HLA-DR expression were evaluated from the duodenal-jejunal mucosa and in peripheral blood samples obtained from 17 patients with rheumatoid arthritis both before and after 16 weeks of sulfasalazine treatment [32]. The conclusion of this study was that no signs of inflammation or immunological abnormalities were seen in the duodenal-jejunal mucosa of rheumatoid arthritis patients, but that sulfasalazine exerted immunoregulatory effects that were not encountered in the peripheral blood (reduction in mucosal CD_3^+ and γ/δ^+ lymphocyte numbers).

2. Systemic Effects

Effects on Immunological Functions. Both T-cell proliferation and natural killer cell activity are inhibited by sulfasalazine and in vitro systems [33–36]. In addition, both immunoglobulin and rheumatoid factor production is depressed by sulfasalazine in vitro, indicating an effect on B-cell function [35].

Effects on Inflammatory Cells. Sulfasalazine has been shown to inhibit several inflammatory cell functions, including superoxide production by granulocytes stimulated by immune complexes or formyl peptides. Granulocyte functions inhibited by sulfasalazine include degranulation, chemotaxis, and random migration [37–39].

Effects on Enzymes. Sulfasalazine is a relatively weak inhibitor of cyclooxygenase but a potent inhibitor of 15 prostaglandin dehydrogenase [40]. Sulfasalazine has also been shown to inhibit both 5- and 15-lipooxygenase and the glutathion transferase involved in the formation of leukotriene C_4 [41,42]. Sulfasalazine can also interfere with other enzymes such as xanthine oxidase and granulocyte protease [43,44].

Effects on Folate Metabolism. Sulfasalazine has been shown to inhibit both folate transport across the intestine and folate metabolizing enzymes. These antifolate properties of sulfasalazine could have relevance for the inhibition of rapidly proliferating immunological cells [45,46].

IV. CLINICAL USE

Sulfasalazine has been in wide use for over 40 years [1]. There is a wealth of clinical experience in the literature documenting both the efficacy and the various adverse events reported with the drug.

A. Efficacy

Numerous clinical trials have been conducted to evaluate the efficacy of sulfasalazine in rheumatoid arthritis. Most of them are open, uncontrolled studies. However, the seven double-blind placebo-controlled studies [47–53] and the double-blind comparative studies [50–54,55] permit us to formulate an idea of the place of sulfasalazine in the treatment of rheumatoid arthritis.

1. Characteristics of Sulfasalazine-treated Patients

Diagnosis. In all (except one) [50] published studies so far conducted using sulfasalazine, patients have had a definite diagnosis of the disease to enter the study. In the Australian multicenter study, patients with a probable diagnosis could also be recruited. It is therefore not surprising that in this study the radiographic findings were less severe than in other studies also evaluating radiographic damage.

Activity. All the recruited patients had a disease which was active at entry (activity usually defined by the number of swollen or tender joints).

Severity. Most patients had previously failed on at least two or three DMARDs and had long-term disease. Consequently, the subjects used have been relatively old. However, in three studies (two European and one Australian), only early rheumatoid arthritis patients were recruited. It is difficult to compare the treatment effect across the different studies. However, based on the data obtained in these studies, it is not clear whether the clinical and/or biological effects of sulfasalazine were related to the duration of the disease and, particularly, whether these effects were more impressive in patients with early disease.

2. Parameters Influenced by Sulfasalazine

Clinical Parameters. The following parameters assessing rheumatoid arthritis activity were used in the different trials; most were significantly improved after sulfasalazine therapy.

- Pain evaluated on either a visual analogue scale or using an articular index.
- Function evaluated using different indices. The most frequent was the Health Assessment Questionnaire, but others such as the Lee Functional Index or the Arthritis Impact Measurement Scale were also favorably influenced by sulfasalazine.
- Inflammation evaluated by the duration of early morning stiffness and the amount of synovitis.

Biological Parameters. Biological parameters evaluating inflammation (i.e., acute phase reactants such as C-reactive protein) also improved after sulfasalazine therapy.

The effects of sulfasalazine on cytokine levels were described in a subset of patients enrolled in the Australian Multicenter Clinical Trial [56]. In the subgroup of 17 patients who completed the 6 months of treatment with sulfasalazine, there was a progressive and significant decline in interleukins IL-1α and IL-1β and tumor necrosis factor-α (TNF-α) levels. These reductions were associated with an improvement in clinical and laboratory variables. In 22 patients completing 6 months on placebo, there was no reduction in cytokine levels or improvement in clinical and laboratory variables.

At variance, in the published studies, rheumatoid factor titers were not influenced by sulfasalazine therapy.

Radiological Parameters. Cartilage and bone damage due to rheumatoid arthritis was evaluated in three controlled trials conducted in early patients; one of them enrolled both definite and probable rheumatoid arthritis. In both the Dutch and Finnish trials, erosions and joint space narrowing in multiple joints on radiographs were interpreted using a modification of the method originally published by Sharp [57,58]. In the Dutch study comparing sulfasalazine with hydroxychloroquine, patients showed both an increase in total joint erosion and total joint narrowing score from baseline to weeks 24 and 48. However, intergroup differences were significantly in favor of sulfasalazine at weeks 24 and 48 for both the erosion and the narrowing scores. In the Finnish study comparing sulfasalazine to placebo, radiographs at week 48 did not show any significant differences between treatment groups, although deterioration in both joint erosion and joint narrowing score was less in the sulfasalazine than the placebo patients. The large number of dropouts during this study and the fact that by week 48, almost all of these patients had received oral or intramuscular gold may have confused the results of the radiographic images at week 48.

In the Australian multicenter study, radiographic studies were performed at weeks 0 and 26 and scored for the presence or absence of erosions, not for the number of erosions; there were no significant differences between the two treatment groups.

Apart from the question of whether sulfasalazine might have an effect on the directional progression of the disease, these studies are interesting from a methodological point of view. The demonstration of a treatment effect on this parameter is not easy and encounters at least three problems:

1. Since the progression of the disease is more rapid during the first years of evolution, it seems logical to focus the studies on early rheumatoid arthritis. However, at this stage, the diagnosis is not so easy to establish, since the criteria have been devised to classify rheumatoid arthritis patients and not with the aim of diagnosis. It must be recalled that the performance of a set of classification criteria is better at a later stage of the disease than at an early stage. The lack of effect of sulfasalazine in the Australian study might be explained in part by inclusion of "probable" rheumatoid arthritis patients; only a small percentage of patients worsened after 6 months in terms of radiographic damage.
2. The duration of these studies has to be long enough to show progression. However, with such duration, the number of dropouts might hamper the interpretation of the obtained results.
3. The scoring system is also important to consider. The modifications proposed to the Sharp method by van der Heidje lead to a more sensitive system. Two main modifications have to be stressed: the quantification system and the inclusion of small joints of the feet, which are frequently affected at an early stage of the disease.

3. Dose-related Effect

Two double-blind, controlled-dose ranging studies have been conducted [49,52]. The analysis of the results obtained in these studies together with those obtained in uncontrolled studies suggests that the most appropriate dose of sulfasalazine is 2 g daily. If tolerated, and in case of inefficacy after 4 weeks of therapy, the dose may be increased to 3 g per day to achieve clinical benefit.

4. Clinical Pharmacokinetics Effects

A detailed analysis of the changes caused by sulfasalazine in some selected clinical and laboratory variables shows that its onset of action occurs as soon as week 4 after initiation of therapy and reaches a plateau after about 16 weeks. Therefore, in practice, in case of clinical inefficacy, it seems logical to increase the dosage of sulfasalazine from 2 to 3 g daily after 4 weeks of therapy but also to wait for week 16 before considering this drug as inefficient.

Patients who respond to sulfasalazine therapy but have to discontinue it because of side effects usually experience a flare of their disease 4–8 weeks after discontinuation.

5. Degree of Efficacy

The degree of efficacy of a drug is very difficult to evaluate but can be estimated using three different approaches.

1. Analyze the parameters influenced by the treatment. From this point of view, data from the trials indicate that sulfasalazine is not only a symptomatic treatment but is also potentially a disease-modifying anti-rheumatic drug, since it is able to reduce the two parameters known to be important predisposing factors for long-term disability in rheumatoid arthritis (i.e., synovitis and acute phase reactants). Moreover, one of the three studies evaluating radiographic progression of the disease suggests that sulfasalazine could slow the progression of cartilage and bone damage due to rheumatoid arthritis.
2. Check if the level of results obtained in the trials reaches not only statistical significance but also clinical relevance. The first step of this methodological approach is to define clinical relevance. This was the objective of the OMERACT Conference during which a consensus was reached among both clinicians and statisticians dealing with rheumatoid arthritis. As an example, a difference in at least three joints between two drugs in terms of reduction in swollen joints was considered clinically relevant [59]. In the placebo-controlled trials conducted with sulfasalazine, the drug was superior to placebo by seven joints for joint count and to 6 joints for joint swelling, suggesting that the degree of efficacy of sulfasalazine is of clinical relevance.
3. Compare the results obtained to those with other disease-modifying anti-rheumatoid drugs. Several controlled comparative trials have been conducted with sulfasalazine in comparison with intramuscular gold, oral gold, Lobenzarit, D-penicillamine, and hydroxychloroquine. In all these studies, there were either no statistically significant differences between sulfasalazine and the comparator or a statistically significant difference in favor of sulfasalazine. Moreover, in 1990, Felson and colleagues published two landmark meta-analyses of placebo-controlled and comparative trials of second-line antirheumatic drugs [60,61]. The objective was to evaluate the comparative efficacy and toxicity of the different agents. These analyses were subsequently updated to include additional data from more recently published studies. Altogether a total of 79 trials were analyzed, including more than 6500 patients with rheumatoid arthritis. Agents evaluated included azathioprine, antimalarial drugs, injectable gold, oral gold, methotrexate, D-penicillamine, sulfasalazine, and placebo. Efficacy was defined by using a composite index comprising assess-

ments of joint count, grip strength, and erythrocyte sedimentation rate, as well as the proportion of patients who did not withdraw because of lack of drug efficacy. Methotrexate and sulfasalazine were found to be the most potent drugs. A British study evaluating the percentage of rheumatoid arthritis patients who had to discontinue their drug because of inefficacy with regard to duration of treatment (by using life-table analysis) by treatment group suggests that 61% of patients receiving sulfasalazine are still on treatment after 6 months, but only 32% are still on treatment after 2 years. These percentages are similar to those obtained with other drugs [62]. Using this methodology, recent studies suggest that methotrexate could be superior to sulfasalazine [63].

6. Combination Therapy

Chapter 14 is particularly focused on the reasons for the use of and the different reported experiences of various combination therapies.

To our knowledge, only three controlled studies have been reported evaluating the potential effect of a combination of sulfasalazine with another active so-called disease-modifying antirheumatic drug. In the study reported by Faarvang et al., all three treatment groups (sulfasalazine 2 g/day, hydroxychloroquine 250 mg/day, and a combination of the two) improved during the course of 6 months of treatment as determined by a reduction in swollen joints, a decrease in erythrocyte sedimentation rate, and improvement in the physician's and patient's overall assessment [64]. Although patients treated with the drug combination appeared to respond faster, there was no overall statistically significant differences between the treatment groups. The efficacy and the tolerability of sulfasalazine-methotrexate combination to sulfasalazine and to methotrexate given alone were compared in a prospective, randomized 1-year study including 105 patients. Although all efficacy variables favored the combination, no statistically significant differences existed between the treatment groups [65]. In the study reported by Taggart, only two groups of patients were evaluated [66]: one receiving sulfasalazine alone and the second sulfasalazine plus D-penicillamine. This open, prospective, randomized controlled study suggests that combination therapy might lead to a faster response to treatment without increasing the percentage and/or severity of side effects. Various uncontrolled open studies have been reported evaluating the efficacy and the toxicity of sulfasalazine when combined with other drugs such as D-penicillamine [66–68], azathioprine [69], gold [67], and sulfasalazine [70].

B. Tolerability

1. Description of Observed Side Effects

The adverse events associated with sulfasalazine can be divided into two categories [71–75] (Table 1). The first is dose related and the second comprises idiosyncratic or hypersensitivity reactions. Knowledge of this classification might be helpful for the clinician monitoring rheumatoid arthritis patients: the less severe dose-related effects may resolve with a reduction of sulfasalazine dose; for the idiosyncratic reactions, sulfasalazine treatment should be withdrawn immediately, and rechallenge should not be attempted. Aside from this clear classification, there are some other side effects for which the mechanism of action is not clear.

Table 1 Side Effects of Sulfasalazine

Dose-related side effects
1. Gastrointestinal disturbances
2. Central nervous system effects
3. Hematological disorders
⇒ leukopenia
⇒ hemolytic anemia
⇒ megaloblastic anemia
Hypersensitivity reaction
1. Skin reactions
2. Hepatitis
3. Pneumonitis
4. Agranulocytosis and aplastic anemia
Other side effects
1. Autoimminue effects
2. Male infertility

Dose-related Side Effects. This group includes the common effects such as nausea, vomiting, headache, and malaise, and perhaps the rare effects such as hemolytic anemia.

1. *Gastrointestinal disturbances*: Nausea, vomiting, anorexia, dyspepsia, and abdominal pain are the most common adverse effects reported by patients on sulfasalazine, and these side effects account for approximately two-thirds of treatment withdrawals due to adverse effects. Nausea generally disappears within a day or two after discontinuing sulfasalazine. It may also respond to a reduction in sulfasalazine dose and to antiemetics.
2. *Central nervous system effects*: Headache, irritability, depression, and/or dizziness may affect up to 10% of patients and generally occur early during sulfasalazine treatment. These symptoms can be sufficiently severe and persistent to require sulfasalazine withdrawal; however, they often respond adequately to dose reduction.
3. *Hematological problems*
   a. Leukopenia [76–79]: Both toxic and hypersensitivity hematological reactions can be observed with sulfasalazine. Leukopenia is observed in 1–10% of treated patients. Most episodes of leukopenia occur within the first 6 months of sulfasalazine treatment but may appear later. Continuation of treatment has occasionally been possible after temporary withdrawal of sulfasalazine and reintroduction at a lower dose.
   b. Hemolytic anemia [80]: Hemolytic anemia may occur both with and without Heinz body formation. There is some evidence that this effect may be associated with high serum concentrations of sulfapyridine. Some patients are genetically predisposed; for example, those with glucose-6-phosphate dehydrogenase deficiency.

c. Megaloblastic anemia: Megaloblastic anemia has been reported in a small number of rheumatoid arthritis patients, usually after several months of treatment. It is commonly associated with low folate levels. Patients respond to temporary withdrawal of sulfasalazine and folate supplementation.

Hypersensitivity Reaction. This category includes both frequent adverse events such as rash and uncommon events, including toxic hepatitis, pneumonitis, aplastic anemia, and agranulocytosis.

1. *Skin reactions* [57–60]: Rash and other cutaneous adverse effects account for about 15% of treatment withdrawals during long-term treatment with sulfasalazine. Most of them are nonspecific maculopapular lesions which occur soon after the beginning of treatment and improve quickly following cessations. However, sulfasalazine may induce more severe adverse effects, including toxic epidermal necrolysis, Steven-Johnson syndrome, and exfoliate dermatitis which might be life threatening.
2. *Hepatitis* [81–84]: Transient, mild liver enzyme elevations are noted occasionally in patients on sulfasalazine; in these cases, resolution usually occurs after sulfasalazine is discontinued. However, more toxic or allergic hepatitis in patients receiving sulfasalazine can occur. Patients develop clinical symptoms (fever, rash) and physical examination shows hepatomegaly and lymphadenopathy; laboratory abnormalities include elevation of liver enzymes, hyperbilirubinemia, and, in some cases, eosinophilia. Liver biopsy may show hepatocellular necrosis similar to that seen in viral hepatitis, cholestasis, or granulomatous hepatitis.
3. *Pneumonitis* [81,89–91]: Allergic interstitial pneumonitis with or without eosinophilia has been described in patients receiving sulfasalazine. The presenting symptoms include cough, dyspnea, and fever. Following discontinuation of sulfasalazine, recovery and radiographic resolution has occurred within a few weeks.
4. *Agranulocytosis and aplastic anemia* [92–96]: Less frequent than leukopenia, hematological adverse events suggesting a hypersensitivity reaction may occur in patients receiving sulfasalazine. These effects on white cells usually resolve rapidly after treatment is discontinued, although fatalities following agranulocytosis have occurred, usually as a result of gram-negative sepsis.

Other Side Effects.

1. *Autoimmune effects* [97–102]: Sulfonamides are among those drugs capable of inducing systemic lupus erythematosus. Several patients receiving sulfasalazine have developed clinical and/or serological evidence of systemic lupus erythematosus. The syndrome is usually reversible when sulfasalazine is discontinued but may recur on rechallenge.
2. *Male infertility* [103–105]: An effect of sulfasalazine on sperm count, motility, and morphology may develop within 2 months of starting treatment and may result in infertility. The changes are reversible within 2 or 3 months of sulfasalazine withdrawal. The mechanism is unclear, but antifolate and antiprostaglandin activity have both been suggested. There is no associated teratogenesis.

2. Factors Predisposing to Sulfasalazine Toxicity

Based on the knowledge of the pharmacokinetics of sulfasalazine, some potential predisposing factors to drug toxicity can be evoked: age, acetylator status, concomitant therapies, sulfasalazine dose, and disease. Age, acetylator status, and sulfasalazine dose are well known as factors predisposing to sulfasalazine toxicity. In rheumatoid arthritis, it is interesting to discuss the potential toxicity due to the disease itself and the concomitant therapies.

In a meta-analysis, Wijnands et al. described the adverse event profile and incidence rates each month for the various indications of sulfasalazine [106]. The side-effect profile of adverse drug reactions leading to withdrawal was similar for inflammatory bowel disease and rheumatoid arthritis. However, in this analysis, there was a trend toward greater hematological and hepatic toxicity in rheumatoid arthritis patients. Moreover, patients suffering from Still's disease represented a subgroup particularly predisposed to severe sulfasalazine toxicity; these adverse effects include high fever, generalized exanthema, and pneumonitis [107]. For pediatricians dealing with rheumatic disease, sulfasalazine has to be considered contraindicated in this particular subgroup of diseases (A.M. Prieur personal communication).

Concomitant therapies necessitated by persistent activity of the disease are frequently needed in rheumatoid arthritis patients receiving sulfasalazine. These concomitant therapies include anti-inflammatory drugs (nonsteroidal and steroidal agents) and other slow-acting drugs. Sulfasalazine, like nonsteroidal anti-inflammatory drugs has multiple effects on both the cyclooxygenase and the lipoxygenase pathways of arachidonic acid metabolism and can cause some gastric distress. However, it does not seem that there is a synergistic and/or additional effect with the concomitant use of these two compounds in terms of gastric toxicity. At variance, recent data suggest that sulfasalazine could reduce both intestinal inflammation and intestinal blood loss induced by nonsteroidal anti-inflammatory drugs [31].

Similarly, sulfasalazine toxicity is not increased when combined with corticosteroids. At variance, it has been suggested that corticosteroids might have a protective effect on sulfasalazine toxicity in rheumatoid arthritis [108].

The emerging problem is the potentially higher toxicity of combination therapy when using several second-line drugs, especially a combination of sulfasalazine with methotrexate [109]. Side effects occurring during methotrexate therapy are quite similar to those during sulfasalazine therapy; that is, gastrointestinal disturbances, hepatic toxicity, bone marrow suppression, and allergic pneumonitis. Sulfa-containing drugs, sulfasalazine included, increase the bone marrow suppression caused by methotrexate. Despite this potentially higher toxicity, the rare reported studies evaluating this combination do not indicate a higher incidence of side effects [110,111].

3. Sulfasalazine Monitoring in Practice

Several recommendations can be proposed for the use of sulfasalazine:

- Sulfasalazine should not be given to patients with ileostomy.
- Special monitoring has to be performed in patients concurrently taking other compounds such as methotrexate.
- Full information should be given to the patient before starting therapy, especially concerning the possibility of occurrence of skin reaction and nausea.
- To try to avoid gastrointestinal side effects, the following are recommended: (a) start at a low dose and increase it gradually up to 2–3 g daily. As an ex-

ample: 500 mg b.i.d. during the first 4 days, then 1000 mg b.i.d. during the next 4 days and then 1000 mg t.i.d.; if this 3000-mg daily dosage is well tolerated when taken three times per day, it is possible to propose taking the same dosage twice daily (i.e., 1500 mg b.i.d.); and (b) a complete blood count, including a differential white cell count and liver function tests, should be performed before starting and at least every 4 weeks during the first 6 months of therapy (some workers propose laboratory monitoring every second week during the first 3 months of therapy). After the sixth month of therapy, laboratory monitoring once every 3 months is sufficient but still necessary, since it is possible that, with time, new adverse events of sulfasalazine may emerge in rheumatoid arthritis. Moreover, the patient should be instructed to perform a blood evaluation in case of clinical symptoms such as rash or fever.

REFERENCES

1. Peppercorn MA. Sulfasalazine: pharmacology, clinical use, toxicity and related new drug development. Ann Intern Med 1984; 101:377–386.
2. Das KM, Dubin R. Clinical pharmacokinetics of sulfasalazine. Clin Pharmacokinet 1976; 1:406–425.
3. Schröder H, Campbell DES. Absorption, metabolism and excretion of salicylazosulfapyridine in man. Clin Pharmacol Ther 1972; 13:539–551.
4. Astbury C, Taggart AJ, Juby L, Zebouni L, Bird HA. Comparison of the single dose pharmacokinetics of sulfasalazine in rheumatoid arthritis and inflammatory bowel disease. Ann Rheum Dis 1990; 49:587–590.
5. Taggart AJ, McDermott BJ, Roberts SD. The effect of age and acetylator phenotype on the pharmacokinetics of sulfasalazine in patients with rheumatoid arthritis. Clin Pharmacokinet 1992; 23:311–320.
6. Peppercorn MA, Goldman P. Distribution studies of salicylazosulfapyridine and its metabolites. Gastroenterology 1973; 64:240–245.
7. Sjöholm I, Ekman B, Kober A, Ljungstedt-Pahlman I, Seiving B, Sjödin T. Binding of drugs to human serum albumin: XI. The specificity of three binding sites as studied with albumin immobilized in microparticles. Mol Pharmacol 1979; 16:767–777.
8. Farr M, Brodrick A, Bacon PA. Plasma and synovial fluid concentrations of sulphasalazine and two of its metabolites in rheumatoid arthritis. Rheumatol Int 1985; 5:247–251.
9. Hensleigh PA, Kauffman RE. Maternal absorption and placental transfer of sulfasalazine. Am J Obstet Gynecol 1977; 127:443–444.
10. Järnerot G, Into-Malmberg MB, Esbjörner E. Placental transfer of sulphasalazine and sulphapyridine and some of its metabolites. Scand J Gastroenterol 1981; 16:693–697.
11. Järnerot G, Into-Malmberg MB. Sulphasalazine treatment during breast feeding. Scand J Gastroenterol 1979; 14:869–871.
12. Peppercorn MA, Goldman P. The role of intestinal bacteria in the metabolism of salicylazosulfapyridine. J Pharmacol Exp Ther 1972; 181:555–562.
13. Schröder H, Gustafsson BE. Azo reduction of salicyl-azosulphapyridine in germ-free and conventional rats. Xenobiotica 1973; 3:225–231.
14. Schröder H, Lewkonia RM, Price Evans DA. Mettabolism of salicylazosulfapyridine in healthy subjects and in patients with ulcerative colitis. Effects of colectomy and of phenobarbital. Clin Pharmacol Ther 1973; 14:802–809.
15. Schröder H, Evans DAP. Acetylator phenotype and adverse effects of sulphasalazine in healthy subjects. Gut 1972; 13:278–284.

16. Schröder H. Simplified method for determining acetylator phenotype. Br Med J 1972; 3:506–507.
17. Pieniaszek HJ Jr, Bates TR. Capacity-limited gut wall metabolism of 5-aminosalicylic acid, a therapeutically active metabolite of sulfasalazine in rats. J Pharm Sci 1979; 68:1323–1325.
18. Pullar T, Hunter JA, Capell HA. Which component of sulphasalazine is active in rheumatoid arthritis? Br Med J 1985; 290:1535–1538.
19. Pullar T, Hunter JA, Capell HA. Sulphasalazine in the treatment of rheumatoid arthritis: relationship of dose and serum level to efficacy. Br J Rheumatol 1985; 24:269–276.
20. Kitas GD, Farr M, Waterhouse L, Bacon PA. Influence of acetylator status on sulphasalazine efficacy and toxicity in patients with rheumatoid arthritis. Scand J Pheumatol 1992; 21:220–225.
21. Pullar T, Hunter JA, Capell HA. Effect of acetylator phenotype on efficacy and toxicity of sulphasalazine in rheumatoid arthritis. Ann Rheum Dis 1985; 44:831–837.
22. Bax DE, Greaves MS, Amos RS. Sulphasalazine for rheumatoid arthritis: relationship between dose, acetylator phenotype and response to treatment. Br J Rheumatol 1986; 25:282–284.
23. Sandberg-Gertzen H, Kjellander J, Sundberg-Gilla B, Järnerot G. In vitro effects of sulphasalazine, azodisal sodium and their metabolites on clostridium difficile and some other fæcal bacteria. Scand J Gastroenterol 1985; 20:607–612.
24. West B, Lendrum R, Hill MJ, Walker G. Effects of sulphasalazine (Salazopyrin) on fæcal flora in patients with inflammatory bowel disease. Gut 1974; 15:960–965.
25. Danielsson D, Kjellander J, Järnerot G. The effect of metronidazole and sulfasalazine on the fecal flora in patients with Crohn's disease. Scand J Gastroenterol 1981; 16:183–192.
26. Neumann VC, Grindulis KA. Sulphasalazine in rheumatoid arthritis: an old drug revived. J R. Soc Med 1984; 77:169–172.
27. Neumann VC, Shinebaum, R, Cooke EM, Wright V. Effects of sulphasalazine on fæcal flora in patients with rheumatoid arthritis: a comparison with penicillamine. Br J Rheumatol 1987; 26:334–337.
28. Segal AW, Isenberg DA, Hajirousou V, Tolfree S, Clark J, Snaith ML. Preliminary evidence for gut involvement in the pathogenesis of rheumatoid arthritis? Br J Rheumatol 1986; 25:162–166.
29. Bjarnason I, Zanelli G, Smith T, Prouse P, Williams P, Smethurst P, Delacey G, Gumpel MJ, Levi AJ. Nonsteroidal antiinflammatory drug-induced intestinal inflammation in humans. Gastroenterology 1987; 93:480–489.
30. Marcolongo R, Bayeli PF, Montagnani M. Gastrointestinal involvement in rheumatoid arthritis: A biopsy study. J Rheumatol 1979; 6:163–173.
31. Hayllar J, Smith T, MacPherson A, Price AB, Gumpel M, Bjarnason I. Nonsteroidal antiinflammatory drug-induced small intestinal inflammation and blood loss: Effects of sulfasalazine and other disease-modifying antirheumatic drugs. Arthritis Rheum 1994; 37:1146–1150.
32. Kanerud L, Scheynius A, Hafström I. Evidence of a local intestinal immunomodulatory effect of sulfasalazine in rheumatoid arthritis. Arthritis Rheum 1994; 37:1138–1145.
33. Ali ATMM, Basran GS, Morley J. Mode of action of sulphasalazine: an alternative view. Lancet 1982; 1:506–507.
34. Gibson PR, Jewell DP. Sulphasalazine and derivatives, natural killer activity and ulcerative colitis. Clin Sci (Colch) 1985; 69:177–184.
35. Comer SS, Jasin HE. *In vitro* immunomodulatory effects of sulfasalazine and its metabolites. J Rheumatol 1988; 15:580–586.
36. Symmons DPM, Salmon M, Farr M, Bacon PA. Sulfasalazine treatment and lymphcyte function in patients with rheumatoid arthritis. J Rheumatol 1988; 15:575–579.
37. Harvath L, Yancey KB, Katz SI. Selective inhibition of human neutrophil chemotaxis to N-formyl-methionyl-leucyl-phenylalanine by sulfones. J Immunol 1986; 137:1305–1311.

38. Molin L, Stendahl O. The effect of sulfasalazine and its active components on human polymorphonuclear leukocyte function in relative to ulcerative colitis. Acta Med Scand 1979; 206:451–457.
39. Rhodes JM, Bartholomew TC, Jewell DP. Inhibition of leucocyte motility by drugs used in ulcerative colitis. Gut 1981; 22:642–647.
40. Hoult JRS, Moore PK. Sulphasalazine is a potent inhibitor of prostaglandin 15-hydroxydehydrogenase: possible basis for therapeutic action in ulcerative colitis. Br J Pharmacol 1978; 64:6–8.
41. Sircar JC, Schwender CF, Carethers ME. Inhibition of soybean lipoxygenase by sulfasalazine and 5-aminosalicylic acid: a possible mode of action in ulcerative colitis. Biochem Pharmacol 1983; 32:170–172.
42. Bach MK, Brashler JR, Johnson M. Inhibition of sulfasalazine of LTC synthetase and of rat liver glutathione S-transferases. Biochem Pharmacol 1985; 34:2695–2704.
43. Klessen C. Inhibition of neutral proteases from polymorphonuclear (PMN) neutrophils by salicylazosulfapyridine (SASP). Histochemistry 1980; 66:43–47.
44. Carlin G, Djursäter G, Smedegärd G. Inhibitory effects of sulfasalazine and related compounds on superoxide production by human polymorphonuclear leukocytes. Pharmacol Toxicol 1989; 65:121–127.
45. Franklin JL, Rosenberg HH. Impaired folic acid absorption in inflammatory bowel disease: effects of salicylazosulfapyridine (azulfidine). Gastroenterology 1973; 64:517–525.
46. Selhub J, Dhar GJ, Rosenberg IH. Inhibition of folate enzymes by sulfasalazine. J Clin Invest 1978; 61:221–224.
47. Pinals RS, Kaplan SB, Lawson JG, Hepburn B. Sulfasalazine in rheumatoid arthritis. A double-blind, placebo-controlled trial. Arthritis Rheum 1986; 29:1427–1434.
48. Williams HJ, Ward JR, Dahl SL, Clegg DO, Willkens RF, Oglesby T, Weisman MH, Schlegel S, Michaels RM, Luggen ME, Polisson RP, Singer JZ, Kantor SM, Shiroky JB, Small RE, Gomez MI, Reading JC, Egger MJ. A controlled trial comparing sulfasalazine, gold sodium thiomalate, and placebo in rheumatoid arthritis. Arthritis Rheum 1988; 31:702–713.
49. Skosey JL. Comparison of responses to and adverse effects of graded doses of sulfasalazine in the treatment of rheumatoid arthritis. J Rheumatol 1988; 16:(Suppl):5–8.
50. Nuver-Zwart IH, van Riel PLCM, van de Putte LBA, Gribnau FWJ. A double-blind comparative study of sulphasalazine and hydroxychloroquine in rheumatoid arthritis: Evidence of an earlier effect of sulphasalazine. Ann Rheum Dis 1989; 48:389–395.
51. Pullar T, Hunter JA, Capell HA. Sulphasalazine in rheumatoid arthritis: a double-blind comparison of sulfasalazine with placebo and sodium aurothiomalate. Br Med J (Clin Res Ed) 1983; 287:1102–1104.
52. Nishioka N, Nobunaga M, Sakuma A. [A double-blind comparative study of 1 g/day, 2 g/day salazosulfapyridine and placebo in rheumatoid artrittis.] Ryumachi 1991; 31:327–345.
53. Australian Multicentre Clinical Trial Group. Sulfasalazine in early rheumatoid arthritis. J Rheumatol 1992; 19:1672–1677.
54. Neumann VC, Grindulis KA, Hubball S, McConkey B, Wright V. Comparison between penicillamine and sulphasalazine in rheumatoid arthritis: Leeds-Birmingham trial. Br Med J (Clin Res Ed) 1983; 287:1099–1102.
55. Nishioka K, Azuma T, Iwasaki Y. [A double-blind comparative study between salazosulfapyridine enteric-coated tablets (PJ-306) and lobenzarit disodium (CCA) in rheumatoid arthritis.] Ryumachi 1991; 31:346–367.
56. Danis VA, Franic GM, Rathjen DA, Laurent RM, Brooks PM. Circulating cytokine levels in patients with rheumatoid arthritis: results of a double-blind trial with sulfasalazine. Ann Rheum Dis 1992; 51:946-950.
57. Sharp JT, Lidsky MD, Collins LC, Moreland J. Methods of scoring the progression of

radiologic changes in rheumatoid arthritis. Correlation of radiologic, clinical, and laboratory abnormalities. Arthritis Rheum 1971; 14:706–720.
58. van der Heijde DM, van Riel PL, Nurrer-Zwart IH, Gribnau FW, van de Putte LB. Effects of hydroxychloroquine and sulphasalazine on progression of joint damage in rheumatoid arthritis. Lancet 1989; 1:1036-1038.
59. Goldsmith CH, Boers M, Bombardier C, Tugwell P, for the OMERACT Committee. Criteria for clinically important changes in outcomes: Development, scoring and evaluation of rheumatoid arthritis patient and trial profiles. J Rheumatol 1993; 20:561–565.
60. Felson DT, Anderson JJ, Meenan RF. The comparative efficacy and toxicity of second-line drugs in rheumatoid arthritis: results of two metaanalyses. Arthritis Rheum 1990; 33:1449-1461.
61. Felson DT, Anderson JJ, Meenan RF. Use of short-term efficacy/toxicity tradeoffs to select second-line drugs in rheumatoid arthritis: a metaanalysis of published clinical trials. Arthritis Rheum 1992; 35:1117–1125.
62. Situnayake RD, McConkey B. Clinical and laboratory effects of prolonged therapy with sulfasalazine, gold or penicillamine: the effects of disease duration on treatment response. J Rheumatol 1990; 17:1268–1273.
63. Anaya JM, Jorgensen C, Daures JP, Combe B, Sany J. Taux de maintenance thérapeutique du méthotrexate au cours de la polyarthrite rhumatoïde. Etude propspective de 191 cas. Rev Rhum Mal Osteoartic 1992; 59:181–187.
64. Faarvang KL, Egsmose C, Kryger P, Podenphant J, Ingeman-Nielsen M, Hansen TM. Hydroxychloroquine and sulfasalazine alone and in combination in rheumatoid arthritis. A randomized double-blind trial. Ann Rheum Dis 1993; 52:711–715.
65. Haagsma C, van de Putte L, van Riel P. Sulfasalazine (SAS), Methotrexate (MTX) and the combination (COMBI) in early RA: a double blinb randomized study [abstr]. Arthritis Rheum 1995; 38(Suppl 9):1290.
66. Taggart AJ, Hill J, Astbury C, Dixon JS, Bird HA, Wright V. Sulphasalazine alone or in combination with D-penicillamine in rheumatoid arthritis. Br J Rheumatol 1987; 26:32–36.
67. Farr M, Kitas G, Bacon PA. Sulphasalazine in rheumatoid arthritis: combination therapy with D-penicillamine or sodium aurothiomalate. Clin Rheumatol 1988; 7:242–248.
68. Scott DL, Huskisson EC. Assessing combination therapy in rheumatoid arthritis: treatment with sulphasalazine and penicillamine. Br J Rheumatol 1990; 29:313–314.
69. Waterworth RF. The use of sulphasalazine and azathioprine in combination to treat rheumatoid arthritis. Br J Rheumatol 1989; 28:456.
70. Morand EF, Axtens RSK, Littlejohn GO. Combination methotrexate and sulfasalazine therapy in patients with rheumatoid arthritis. Arthritis Rheum 1993; 36(Suppl):S53.
71. Pullar T. Adverse effects of sulphasalazine. Advserse Drug React Toxicol Rev 1992; 11:93–109.
72. Amos RS, Pullar T, Bax DE, Situnayake D, Capell HA, McConkey B. Sulphasalazine for rheumatoid arthritis: toxicity in 774 patients monitored for one to 11 years. Br Med J (Clin Res Ed) 1986; 293:420–423.
73. Farr M, Scott DGI, Bacon PA. Side effect profile of 200 patients with inflammatory arthritides treated with sulfasalazine. Drugs 1986; 32(Suppl 1):49–53.
74. Donovan S, Hawley S, MacCarthy J, Scott DL. Tolerability of enteric-coated sulfasalazine in rheumatoid arthritis: Results of a co-operating clinics study. Br J Rheumatol 1990; 29:201-204.
75. Scott DL, Dacre RE. Adverse reactions to sulphasalazine: The British experience. J Rheumatol 1988; 16(Suppl):17–21.
76. Amos RS, Bax DE. Leucopenia in rheumatoid arthritis: relationship to gold or sulphasalazine therapy. Br J Rheumatol 1988; 27:465–468.
77. Farr M, Tunn EJ, Symmons DPM, Scott DGI, Bacon PA. Sulfasalazine in rheumatoid

arthritis: hæmatological problems and changes in hæmatological indices associated with therapy. Br J Rheumatol 1989; 28:134–138.
78. Hopkinson NK, Saiz Garcia F, Gumpel JM. Hæmatological side-effects of sulphasalazine in inflammatory arthritis. Br J Rheumatol 1989; 28:414–417.
79. Marabani M, Madhok R, Capell HA, Hunter JA. Leucopenia during sulphasalazine treatment for rheumatoid arthritis. Ann Rheum Dis 1989; 48:505–507.
80. Wijnands MJ, Nuver-Zwart IH, van Riel PL, van't Hof MA, Gribnau FW, van de Putte LB. Hemolysis during low-dose sulfasalazine treatment in rheumatoid arthritis patients. Scand J Rheumatol 1991; 20:52–57.
81. Timmer R, Duurkens VAn van Hees PA. Sulphasalazine-induced eosinophilic pneumonia. Neth J Med 1992; 41:153–157.
82. McKenna KE, Burrows D. Leucopenia, thrombocytopenia and lymphadenopathy associated with sulphasalazine. Clin Exp Dermatol 1994; 19:419–420.
83. Gabay C, de Bandt M, Palazzo E. Sulphasalazine-related life-threatening side effects: is N-acetylcysteine of therapeutic value? Clin Exp Rheumatol 1993; 11:417–420.
84. Marce S, Schaeverbeke T, Bannwarth B, Marty L, Dehais J. Pustulose exanthematique aiguë généralisée après prise de sulfasalazine. Presse Med 1993; 22:271.
85. Rubin R. Sulfasalazine-induced fulminant hepatic failure and necrotizing pancreatitis. Am J Gastroenterol 1994; 89:789–791.
86. Brooks H, Taylor HG, Nichol FE. The three week sulphasalazine syndrome. Clin Rheumatol 1992; 11:566–568.
87. Marinos G, Riley J, Painter DM, McCaughan GW. Sulfasalazine-induced fulminant hepatic failure. J Clin Gastroenterol 1992; 14:132–135.
88. Caspi D, Fuchs D, Yaron M. Sulphasalazine induced hepatitis in juvenile rheumatoid arthritis. Ann Rheum Dis 1992; 51:275–276.
89. Kolbe J, Caughey D, Rainer S. Sulphasalazine-induced sub-acute hyper-sensitivity pneumonitis. Respir Med 1994; 88:149–152.
90. Gabazza EC, Taguchi O, Yamakami T, Machishi M, Ibata H, Suzuki S, Matsumoto K, Kitagawa T, Yamamoto J. Pulmonary infiltrates and skin pigmentation associated with sulfasalazine. Am J Gastroenterol 1992; 87:1654–1657.
91. Hamadeh MA, Atkinson J, Smith LJ. Sulfasalazine-induced pulmonary disease. Chest 1992; 101:1033–1037.
92. Canvin JM, el-Gabalawy HS, Chalmers IM. Fatal agranulocytosis with sulfasalazine therapy in rheumatoid arthritis. J Rheumatol 1993; 20:909–910.
93. Keisu M, Ekman S. Sulfasalazine associated agranulocytosis in Sweden 1972–1989. Clinical features, and estimation of its incidence. Eur J Clin Pharmacol 1992; 43:215–218.
94. Keisu M, Ekman E, Wiholm BE. Comparing risk estimates of sulphonamide-induced agranulocytosis from the Swedish Drug Monitoring System and a case-control study. Eur J Clin Pharmacol 1992; 43:211–214.
95. Kuipers EJ, Vellenga E, de Wolf JT, Hazenberg BP. Sulfasalazine induced agranulocytosis treated with granulocyte-macrophage colony stimulating factor. J Rheumatol 1992; 19:621–622.
96. Chakravarty K, Scott DG, MacCann BG. Fatal neutropenic enterocolitis associated with sulphasalazine therapy for rheumatoid arthritis. Br J Rheumatol 1992; 31:351–353.
97. Mongey AB, Hess EV. Sulphasazine-induced systemic lupus erythematosus. Br J Rheumatol 1994; 33:789–790.
98. Caulier M, Dromer C, Andrieu V, Le Guennec P, Fournie B. Sulfasalazine induced lupus in rheumatoid arthritis. J Rheumatol 1994; 21:750–751.
99. Walker EM, Carty JE. Sulphasalazine-induced systemic lupus erythematosus in a patient with erosive arthritis. Br J Rheumatol 1994; 33:175–176.
100. Siam AR, Hammoudeh M. Sulfasalazine induced systemic lupus erythematosus in a patient with rheumatoid arthritis. J Rheumatol 1993; 20:207.

101. Vyse T, So AK. Sulphasalazine induced autoimmune syndrome. Br J Rheumatol 1992; 31:115–116.
102. Farr M, Kitas GD, Tunn EJ, Bacon PA. Immunodeficiencies associated with sulphasalazine therapy in inflammatory arthritis. Br J Rheumatol 1991; 30:413–417.
103. Wu FC, Aitken RJ, Ferguson A. Inflammatory bowel disease and male infertility: effects of sulfasalazine and 5-aminosalicylic acid on sperm-fertilizing capacity and reactive oxygen species generation. Fertil Steril 1989; 52:842–845.
104. Giwercman A, Skakkebaek NE. The effect of salicylazosulphapyridine (sulphasalazine) on male fertility. A review. Int J Androl 1986; 9:38–52.
105. Steeno OP. Side-effects of salazopyrin on male fertility. Eur J Obstet Gynecol Reprod Biol 1984; 18:361–364.
106. Wijnands MJA, van't Hof MA, van de Putte LBA, van Riel PLCM. Rheumatoid arthritis: A risk factor for sulphasalazine toxicity? A meta-analysis. Br J Rheumatol 1993; 32:313–318.
107. Hertzberger-ten Cate R, Cats A. Toxicity of sulfasalazine in systemic juvenile chronic arthritis. Clin Exp Rheumatol 1991; 9:85–88.
108. Gran JT, Myklebust G. Toxicity of sulphasalazine in rheumatoid arthritis. Possible protective effects of rheumatoid factors and corticosteroids. Scand J Rheumatol 1993; 22:229–232.
109. Schwarzer AC, Arnold MH, Kelly D, Jones M, Beller E, McNaught PJ, Schrieber L, Brooks PM. The cycling of combination antirheumatic drug therapy in rheumatoid arthritis. Br J Rheumatol 1990; 29:445–450.
110. Haagsma C, van Riel P, de Rooij DJ, Vree TB, Russel FJ, van't Hof MA, van de Putte LB. Combination of methotrexate and sulphasalazine vs. Methotrexate alone: a randomized open clinical trial in rheumatoid arthritis patients resistant to sulphasalazine therapy. Br J Rheumatol 1994; 33:1049–1055.
111. Shiroky JB, Neville C, Ballachey ML. Combination methotrexate and sulfasalazine in the treatment of rheumatic diseases. Arthritis Rheum 1993; 36(Suppl):S268.

11
Methotrexate

Michael Ahern
Flinders University of South Australia, Adelaide, South Australia, Australia

I. INTRODUCTION

Methotrexate (2-4-diamino-N^{10}-methylpteroyl glutamic acid) is an antimetabolite of folic acid with an amino substitution for the hydroxyl at position 4 and a methyl substitution for a hydrogen at position 10 (Fig. 1).

The drug's metabolic effects are illustrated in Figure 2.

Methotrexate enters cells using an active transport system shared by folate N^5 - methyl - FH_4 and N_5 - formyl - FH_4 (leucovorin). A second mechanism, probably involving diffusion, occurs at high concentrations of methotrexate (20 μM). After entering the cells, methotrexate binds to and inactivates dihydrofolate reductase (DHFR), leading to depletion of intracellular pools of reduced folate [1]. This in turn inhibits thymidylate synthesis which requires $N^{5\text{-}10}$-methylene-FH_4. N^{10}-formyl-FH_4 is also depleted, leading to cessation of purine synthesis. Hence, inhibition of thymidylate synthesis or purines suppresses DNA synthesis.

Similar to the physiological folates, methotrexate is metabolized intracellularly to polyglutamate derivatives. Methotrexate polyglutamate synthesis increases with higher drug concentration of methotrexate and duration of exposure, leading to progressive lengthening of the polyglutamate chain and increased amounts of methotrexate polyglutamate formation [1]. The formation of methotrexate polyglutamates allows accumulation of intracellular drug; the polyglutamates have a similar affinity for DHFR to the parent compound and probably dissociate from DHFR at a slower rate. The formation of polyglutamate allows the cells to retain these compounds, as retention is proportional to chain length. Polyglutamate derivatives have been demonstrated in red cells and hepatic cells in patients with rheumatoid arthritis on low-dose methotrexate [2,3].

II. ADSORPTION

Methotrexate can be administered orally, intravenously, or intramuscularly. When given orally, methotrexate is rapidly absorbed with peak serum concentrations between 1 and 3 h [4–6]. Bioavailability after oral administration is greater with smaller doses [5–7],

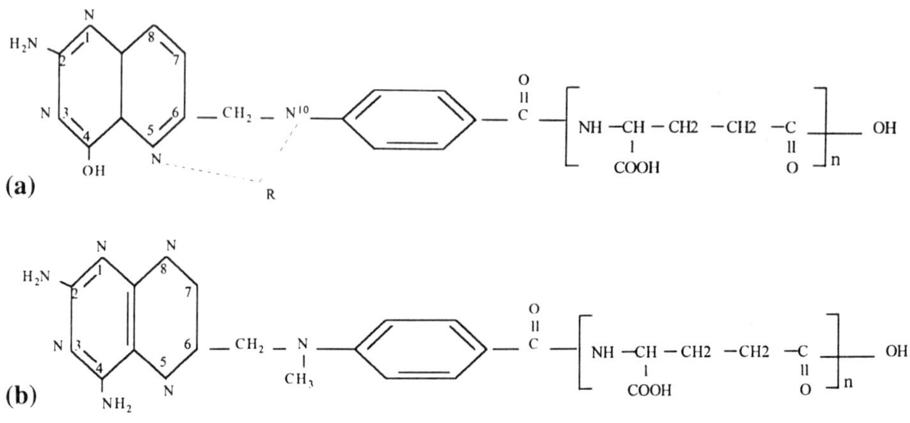

Figure 1 (a) Tetrahydrofolate; (b) methotrexate.

although significant interindividual variability has been described [4,5]. Bioavailability after a single low oral dose of methotrexate is usually 60–80% [4,5].

Factors reported to decrease the rate or extent of absorption include food [8], intestinal bacteria [9], and non absorbable antibiotics [10]. Time to peak concentration was increased from 1.3 to 2.0 h when methotrexate was taken with food [11]. However, Kremer et al. found no significant effect of food on methotrexate absorption or bioavailability [12].

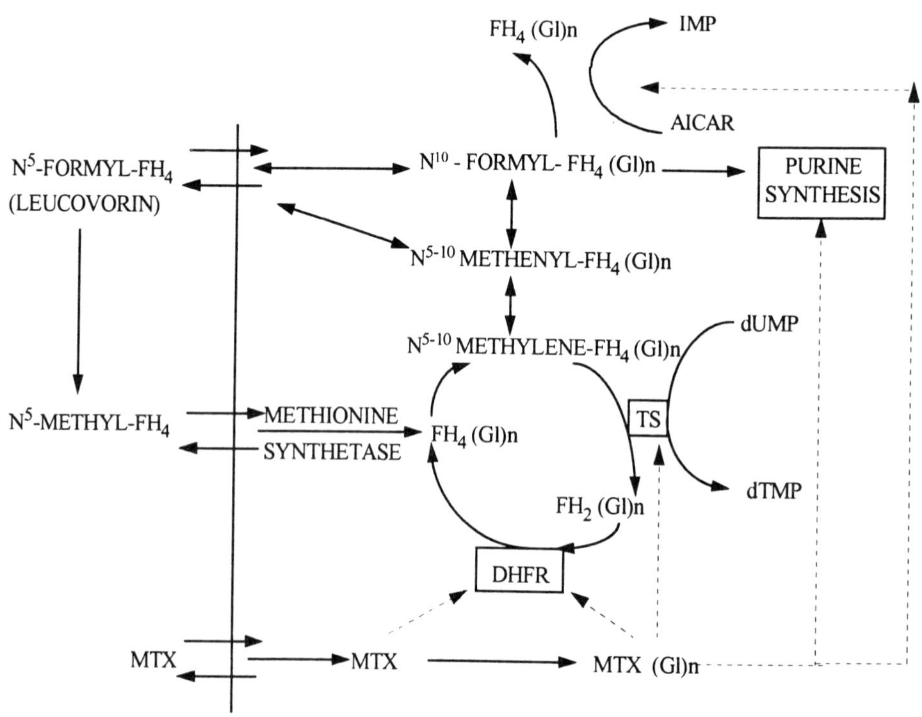

Figure 2 Mechanism of action of methotrexate.

III. ASSAY SYSTEMS

Methotrexate levels can be measured by spectrophotometry, high-performance liquid chromatography, and immunochemical techniques by either enzyme multiplied immunoassay or fluorescence polarization. Most recent studies measuring plasma levels of methotrexate use fluorescence polarization immunoassay (TDx), which has high sensitivity and specificity [13].

IV. PHARMACOKINETICS

Methotrexate pharmacokinetics in both adults and children given low weekly oral doses (7.5–15.0 mg/week) have ben studied by several groups [4,6,14,15]. After oral low-dose methotrexate, peak concentrations are usually within the range of 0.31–0.72 μM, and levels may be measurable 24 h after a single oral dose [6].

The disappearance of methotrexate from serum after low doses is generally biphasic; a third phase may be discerned in some patients [4,14]. The initial phase predominantly reflects renal elimination, whereas the terminal phase is the result of a combination of factors, including renal excretion, enterohepatic circulation, and release from tissues and third spaces [16]. The terminal half-life of low-dose oral methotrexate in patients with rheumatoid arthritis is 3–10 h [4,14,15]. No significant differences in mean elimination half-life have been found after intravenous, oral, or intramuscular administration [17].

Methotrexate excretion is primarily renal. At higher concentrations of methotrexate, active secretion by renal tubules occurs, but the mechanism is saturable [5,6,18]. A significant reduction in renal clearance of methotrexate and creatinine have been described in patients with rheumatoid arthritis (RA) after 6 months of methotrexate therapy [19]. Biliary excretion may contribute to a small but significant component of methotrexate clearance [20]. Measuring methotrexate excretion from a postoperative bile duct in a patient with normal renal function, Nuernberg et al. estimated that 9–26% of methotrexate elimination occurred through the biliary tree [21].

V. DRUG INTERACTIONS

Renal methotrexate clearance is consistently higher than creatinine clearance in keeping with the known tubular secretion of methotrexate which can be competitively inhibited by organic acids such as probenecid [22] and nonsteroidal anti-inflammatory drugs (NSAIDs) [23]. NSAIDs have been reported to enhance methotrexate toxicity both with high-dose therapy for cancer and with low-dose treatment of psoriasis and rheumatoid arthritis. Thus, salicylates [24], diclofenac [25], indomethacin [26,27], and ketoprofen [28], have been implicated in the former setting, whereas phenylbutazone [29], azapropazone [30], and naproxen [31] have been involved in the latter.

With low doses of methotrexate (i.e., 7.5 mg weekly), these interactions are probably not clinically significant [5,32]. However, with higher doses (> 15 mg weekly), decreases in renal function and renal clearance of methotrexate have been reported [33]. Caution must be used in coprescribing drugs which impair glomerular filtration, such as aminoglycosides, and cyclosporin A. NSAIDs may impair glomerular filtration,

Table 1 The Effects of Methotrexate Implicated in Its Mechanism of Action

Rheumatoid factor	Nature of study	References
No effect	Ex vivo	34, 62, 63
Decreased production	In vitro, in vivo	39, 64, 65
Acute phase response		
Reduced	In vivo	36
Lymphocyte, mononuclear cell populations		
No effect	Ex vivo	34
Increased T cells	Ex vivo	63
Increased TH cells	Ex vivo	38
Lower Ts cells	Ex vivo	66
Decreased monocytes	Ex vivo	41
Lymphocyte proliferative response		
No effect (^{3}H - UdR)	Ex vivo	42
Proliferation enhanced (^{3}H - TdR)	Ex vivo, in vitro	34, 39, 40
Proliferation enhanced (^{3}H - TdR)	Ex vivo	41
Proliferation enhanced (^{3}H - UdR)	Ex vivo	43
Proliferation enhanced (^{3}H - UdR)	Ex vivo	39, 67
Cytokine activity		
No effect on IL-1 production	In vitro, in vivo	40, 68
Inhibition IL-1 activity	In vitro	40, 65
Inhibition IL-1 production	Animal model	52
Increased IL-2 production	Ex vivo	53
Decreased soluble IL-2 receptors	Ex vivo	57, 69
Decreased IL-6	Ex vivo	53, 57
Decreased IL-8	Ex vivo	53
Decreased sTNF receptor	Ex vivo	57
Eicosanoid production		
No effect on leukotrienes	Animal model, ex vivo	48, 70
Inhibition of leukotrienes	Ex vivo	46, 47, 71
Neutrophil function		
Inhibition of chemotaxis	Ex vivo	45
Inhibition of adherence	In vitro	50
Miscellaneous		
Inhibition of proteases in rheumatoid arthritis cartilage and synovium	In vivo	60

particularly in the setting of prerenal volume contraction; hence methotrexate clearance may be reduced in these clinical settings when NSAIDs are used (e.g., congestive cardiac failure, ascites).

VI. MECHANISMS OF ACTION

Major research efforts have been undertaken to define the mechanisms of action of methotrexate. Because of the antifolate effect, methotrexate impairs DNA, RNA, and protein synthesis and inhibits transmethylation reactions and polyamine synthesis (see Fig. 2). The relatively rapid onset of clinical effect in rheumatoid arthritis [34,35] and changes in acute phase response have supported an anti-inflammatory effect of methotrexate [36]. The effects on inflammatory cells and cytokines are described below.

A. Mononuclear Cells

High-dose methotrexate in rheumatoid arthritis patients reduced activated circulating lymphocytes [37]. The effects of methotrexate on DNA synthesis in lymphocytes from patients with rheumatoid arthritis have been studied by several groups with variable results. Weinblatt reported an increase in peripheral blood lymphocyte proliferative responses using tritiated thymidine uptake [34,38]. Other groups have also reported enhanced lymphocyte proliferative responses [39,40], whereas yet others have demonstrated decreased responses with methotrexate [41]. Tritiated thymidine assays may give inaccurate results with methotrexate, because it inhibits thymidilate synthetase [42].

Using tritiated deoxyuridine uptake, mononuclear proliferative responses following methotrexate have been reported to be increased [43], suppressed [39], or not altered [42].

Methotrexate (MTX) at 10^{-6} M concentration was toxic to peripheral blood mononuclear cells in culture [39]. Using a colorimetric proliferation assay, 10^{-6} MTX inhibited peripheral blood mononuclear cell proliferation by 48% [39] and suppressed immunoglobulin production [44]. This effect on immunoglobulin production was reversed by folinic acid, S-adenosylmethionine (SAM) or spermidine. It was suggested that methotrexate inhibited SAM and polyamine release through inhibition of methionine regeneration resulting in decrease responsiveness of lymphocytes to mitogens [44].

B. Neutrophils

Methotrexate inhibits the chemotactic response of neutrophils of patients with rheumatoid arthritis [45]. Inhibition of neutrophil 5-lipooxygenase metabolism and leukotriene B^4 production after methotrexate have been reported [46,47], although not confirmed, by a recent study [48].

Methotrexate also inhibits purine biosynthesis by inhibition of aminoimidazole carboxamide ribonucleotide transformylase, leading to accumulation of adenosine, an inhibitor of neutrophil chemotaxis [49]. Using the murine air pouch model, Cronstein demonstrated a methotrexate - mediated reduction in leukocyte accumulation, which was reversed by a specific adenosine A receptor antagonist [50]. These results suggest that methotrexate in low doses has an anti-inflammatory effect inhibiting neutrophil chemotaxis as a result of increased adenosine accumulation at inflamed sites.

C. Cytokines

Interleukin-1 (IL-1) is an important mediator of inflammation and joint destruction in rheumatoid arthritis [51]. In vivo studies have reported reduced IL-1 synthesis by methotrexate [52]; decreases in serum and synovial fluid concentration of IL-1β have been described in rheumatoid arthritis patients on methotrexate [53,54]. The evidence from in vitro and in vivo studies of patients on methotrexate as well as animal models suggest that methotrexate may inhibit the proliferative effects of IL-1 and decrease monocyte IL-1 production in the short term in certain patients, but this effect is not sustained and is unlikely to explain the long-term efficacy of methotrexate [55].

In vitro, methotrexate inhibits IL-6 but not TNF bioactivity [56,57]. Treatment with methotrexate reduces circulating IL-6, IL-8, and p55 soluble tumor necrosis factor (TNF) receptor concentrations in rheumatoid arthritis patients but does not effect circulating levels or monocyte production of TNF-α [53,57].

Lymphocyte IL-2 synthesis increases with methotrexate, whereas circulating soluble IL-2 receptor levels were decreased [57,58]. Recent studies suggest that methotrexate may also downregulate Th2-derived cytokines [55]: treatment with methotrexate reduced IL-4 and IL-10 produced from mononuclear cells from rheumatoid arthritis patients [59] and others have reported decreases in serum IL-4 [53].

VII. OTHER MECHANISMS OF ACTION

Methotrexate decreases the level of neutral proteases in human rheumatoid arthritis cartilage and synovium [60]. Methotrexate has an antiangiogenic effect through the reduction of small blood vessels associated with mononuclear cell infiltration and proliferation of synovial tissue [61]. The same workers showed that rabbit corneal neovascularisation in vivo was also suppressed by low-dose weekly methotrexate.

VIII. LOW-DOSE METHOTREXATE IN RHEUMATOID ARTHRITIS

In 1951, aminopterin was first reported to be efficacious in reducing synovitis in six patients with rheumatoid arthritis [72]. However, on the one hand, these observations were overshadowed by the success of the folate antagonists in leukemia therapy leading to their identification with more toxic chemotherapeutic agents and, on the other hand, by the advent of corticosteroids with their dramatic anti-inflammatory effects in patients with rheumatoid arthritis. Thus the use of methotrexate in rheumatoid arthritis was delayed. However, following the widespread use of methotrexate for psoriasis and the observation that psoriasis-associated arthritis was also responsive to the drug, reports of its use in rheumatoid arthritis appeared [73,74].

Low-dose methotrexate was found to be effective in open studies of short duration. Short-term placebo-controlled studies demonstrated significant improvement in clinical parameters such as joint swelling, joint tenderness, and duration of early morning stiffness (Table 2). A dose-response relationship has been suggested by Furst et al., who compared 5 and 10 mg of MTX/m^2 weekly [76]. A rapid initial response to methotrexate was noted in two placebo-controlled studies [35,63] with significant differences from the placebo group evident at 6 weeks for painful/tender joint counts and scores [35].

Following the encouraging experience obtained with short-term studies, data on the long-term use of methotrexate emerged [78–81]. Long-term prospective observational studies have demonstrated that methotrexate remains efficacious as long as 8 years, and more patients can continue methotrexate in the long term than with other antirheumatic drugs. However, sustained remission rates vary from none [82] to 8% to a maximum of 14% [83]. A plateau effect in clinical response was reported with clinical im-

Table 2 Short-term Placebo-controlled Studies of Methotrexate (MTX) in Rheumatoid Arthritis

Study	Design	No. of subjects	Duration (weeks)	MTX dose (per week)	Outcome	Withdrawals due to side effects	References
1.	MTX: placebo double-blind randomized	189	18	7.5–15.0 mg/	MTX > placebo	30/95	35
2.	MTX: placebo crossover double-blind randomized	35	24	7.5–15.0 mg/	MTX > placebo	1/35	34
3.	MTX: placebo randomized	48	12	10 mg/ 25 mg/	MTX > placebo 10 mg = 25 mg	1/48	75
4.	MTX: placebo crossover double blind	15	27	10–25 mg/	MTX > placebo	1/17	63
5.	MTX: placebo double-blind randomized	46	18	$5mg/m^2$/ $10mg/m^2$/	MTX > placebo	2/30	76
6.	MTX: placebo crossover double-blind	19	24	7.5mg/	MTX > placebo	1/19	77

provement noted between 3 and 12 months in one study [84] and a plateau effect at 6 months in another study [79].

A steroid-sparing effect of methotrexate was observed in both placebo-controlled and long-term open studies [79,82,84]. Changes in laboratory variables with significant reduction in ESR have been demonstrated [82,84].

The effects of methotrexate on radiographic changes have been reported. Methotrexate was cited to retard the progression of erosive disease in patients with disease unresponsiveness to gold therapy [85] and was associated with significantly less radiographic progression in comparison with azathioprine [86]. Both improvement in erosive changes [78] and progressive erosive disease while on methotrexate therapy have been described [84]. A fair conclusion of long-term prospective studies of methotrexate in the treatment of rheumatoid arthritis is that generally patients show radiographic progress, but a small number of patients stabilize.

IX. COMPARATIVE STUDIES OF METHOTREXATE AND OTHER DISEASE-MODIFYING ANTIRHEUMATIC DRUGS

Methotrexate has been compared with oral gold [86], injectable gold [87–89], and azathioprine [90–92]. Methotrexate has a greater and earlier clinical response that oral gold and has similar efficacy to intramuscular gold. Radiographic progression was observed in both methotrexate- and intramuscular gold–treated groups [89].

Weekly oral methotrexate was found to be equally efficacious [92] or superior to azathioprine [90,91]. In a multicenter study comparing methotrexate with azathioprine, the rate of radiographic progression was less in the methotrexate group than in the azathioprine group [93].

A. Meta-analysis

Felson et al. [94,95] performed a meta-analysis of the major antirheumatic drugs. The main clinical endpoints were drug efficacy and drug toxicity. Data were analyzed from placebo-controlled trials of methotrexate, auranofin, parenteral gold, penicillamine, sulfasalazine, and the antimalarials. The cytotoxic drugs were not included in the first analysis.

The final outcome of the meta-analysis showed that with regard to efficacy, patients receiving placebo had the least improvement in the measured parameters. Methotrexate was the most efficacious when the number of tender joints was measured and sulfasalazine was best when decreases in ESR were considered. The antimalarials, auranofin, and methotrexate were the least toxic agents followed by penicillamine, sulfasalazine, and gold in that order of increasing toxicity.

A subsequent meta-analysis included azathioprine [95]. The same clinical indices and toxicity measurements were used, but a new concept of efficacy toxicity ratio (ETR), was introduced as a measurement of the efficacy of a drug compared with its toxicity. For example, a drug with a high ETR is one that is very efficacious and/or has low toxicity. Included in this measurement is whether the patient stops taking the drug because of its lack of benefit (low efficacy) or adverse effects (high toxicity).

Again, the antimalarial drugs and methotrexate had the best ETR. Methotrexate was consistently one of the most efficacious drugs and among the efficacious drugs had the most benign toxicity profile. Sulfasalazine also had relatively high efficacy and only modest toxicity. Although the antimalarials were not placed among the most efficacious, their relative safety made their ETR high.

From this information, it would appear that for moderate to severe rheumatoid arthritis, methotrexate should be the drug of choice. However, in mild rheumatoid arthritis, hydroxychloroquine with its low toxicity may be more appropriate.

B. Combination Studies of Methotrexate and Other Antirheumatic Drugs

Methotrexate in combination with azathioprine or alone was superior in efficacy to azathioprine alone [90], methotrexate and cyclosporin was superior to methotrexate alone [96], and combination methotrexate and sulfazalazine was superior to methotrexate alone [97]. Surprisingly, there was no increase in toxicity with these combinations, but these results must be regarded as preliminary in nature, as the latter two studies had small numbers of patients.

X. SIDE EFFECTS

The frequency of side effects due to methotrexate has been reported to be as high as 90% [78], although discontinuation rates are much lower. Approximately 20–30% of patients with rheumatoid arthritis discontinue methotrexate within the first year of treatment [98–100]. Most studies report side effects as the most frequent cause of cessation of methotrexate than lack of efficacy. One of the lowest rates of withdrawal due to side effects is Weinblatt's study [101] which reported a prospective 5-year experience of 123 patients with a withdrawal rate of only 7%. This may reflect more experience in modifying the dosage or implementing other changes (see below) with increased use of methotrexate.

No association between adverse reactions and HLA antigens in patients with rheumatoid arthritis has been found [79,102].

Although not statistically significant, side effects tend to occur more commonly at higher doses of methotrexate, particularly the gastrointestinal side effects. Clinical experience would indicate that the majority of side effects can be eliminated by brief cessation of methotrexate, generally up to 2 weeks, without inducing a flare of the activity of the arthritis.

A. Minor Adverse Reactions

Minor adverse reactions to methotrexate are common but usually do not result in treatment discontinuation [103]. These reactions include stomatitis, alopecia, nausea, mouth ulcers, rashes, and diarrhea. A postdose reaction consisting of arthralgia/myalgia and fatigue/malaise occurs in up to 10% of patients on methotrexate [103].

Side effects effecting the gastrointestinal tract occur in up to 50% of patients taking methotrexate for prolonged periods [80,81]. Nausea, vomiting, and diarrhea are the most frequent complaints and may be related to methotrexate effecting the gastrointestinal epithelium [104]. The side effects can be alleviated by dose adjustment, altering the route of administration, using divided weekly doses, or topical treatment.

B. Liver Toxicity

For many years, there has been debate concerning the frequency and severity of methotrexate hepatotoxicity in patients with rheumatoid arthritis. Hepatotoxicity has been identified as a problem in patients with psoriasis treated with methotrexate [105–107]. Guidelines for monitoring hepatotoxicity in psoriasis patients treated with methotrexate were established in 1982 and revised in 1988 by the Psoriatic Task Force [108,109] (Table 3).

Initially, rheumatologists adopted these guidelines, but as clinical experience increased with the use of methotrexate in rheumatoid arthritis, it became evident that clinically serious liver toxicity occurred less frequently in RA patients than in psoriasis patients [110–113]. The reasons for the differences in liver toxicity of methotrexate in patients with rheumatoid arthritis and in those with psoriasis are unknown, but heavy alcohol consumption, cumulative dose of methotrexate, and better selection of patients are possible explanations.

Hepatic involvement due to rheumatoid arthritis is described [114]. Findings on liver histology are nonspecific and include Kupffer cell hyperplasia, fatty infiltration, and mild inflammation of portal triads [114]. Liver biopsies in patients taking methotrexate have usually been graded using the Roenigk classification [109]. Serial liver biopsies in patients taking methotrexate using light microscopy have demonstrated worsening histological grade and the development of mild fibrosis (grade IIIA of Roenigk) in 52% [110]. The clinical significance of these changes is not known. Increasing hepatic collagen after 2 years of methotrexate therapy has been documented on serial liver biopsies using electron microscopy [115] and videoimage analysis [116].

Table 3 Methotrexate in Psoriasis: Revised Guidelines

A. Premethotrexate evaluation
   1. Urine analysis
   2. Blood urea nitrogen or serum creatinine determination
   3. Creatinine clearance determination.
   4. Serum AST, ALT, alkaline phosphatase, bilirubin, and albumin determinations
   5. Those at high risk for AIDS, an HIV antibody determination
   6. If long-term methotrexate treatment is anticipated, initial (premethotrexate) liver biopsy should be performed.

B. Continuing laboratory studies.
   1. Intervals of 1–4 weeks: complete blood cell count with differential and platelet count
   2. Intervals of 3–4 months:
      a. Urine analysis
      b. Blood urea nitrogen or serum creatinine determination
      c. ALT, AST, alkaline phosphatase, and serum albumin determinations

C. More frequent monitoring, which may be useful in the following circumstances:
   1. During initial treatment
   2. When changing dose
   3. During episodes of increased risk of increased blood concentrations of methotrexate (dehydration, impaired renal function)

D. A liver biopsy is recommended after a cumulative methotrexate dose of approximately 1.5 g and thereafter at 1.0–1.5 g intervals.

AST, aspartate aminotransferase; ALT, alanine aminotransferase; AIDS, acquired immunodeficiency syndrome; HIV, human immunodeficiency virus.

It has been suggested in a preliminary study that the progression of fibrosis was related to the accumulation of hepatic methotrexate polyglutamates [117].

The 5-year cumulative incidence of cirrhosis and liver failure has been calculated at 1/1000 [118]–9.4/1000 [119], with late age at first use of methotrexate and duration of therapy predictors of serious clinical liver disease [118]. Other identifiable risk factors were alcohol ingestion and frequent dosage interval. Other reported associations for liver disease include total methotrexate dose, renal insufficiency, and perhaps diabetes and obesity [110].

Elevation of transaminases has been noted in up to 88% of patients taking methotrexate over a 53-month period [79]. Histological abnormalities have not been predicted by isolated liver function tests apart from low serum albumin which characterizes grade IV changes (frank cirrhosis with loss of normal architecture, fibrosis, and nodular regeneration) [120]. Serial increases in transaminases, however, appear to be more predictably associated with liver biopsy abnormalities [110]. These findings have led to the publication of guidelines for monitoring and the need for liver biopsies in patients with rheumatoid arthritis taking methotrexate [121]. They have been found to be clinically useful and cost effective [122]. These guidelines are listed in Table 4.

C. Pulmonary Toxicity

Methotrexate pneumonitis is an infrequent, but potentially serious complication occurring in 2.0–5.5% of patients with rheumatoid arthritis [123–125]. Thought to be a

Table 4 Recommendation for Monitoring Hepatic Toxicity in Patients with Rheumatoid Arthritis (RA) Receiving Methotrexate

A. Baseline
   1. Tests for all patients
      a. Liver blood tests (AST, ALT, alkaline phosphatase, albumin, bilirubin), hepatitis B and C serological studies
      b. Other standard tests, including complete cell count and serum creatinine
   2. Pretreatment liver biopsy (Menghini suction-type needle) only for patients with:
      a. Prior excessive alcohol consumption
      b. Persistently abnormal baseline AST values
      c. Chronic hepatitis B or C infection

B. Monitor AST, ALT, albumin at 4- to 8-week intervals

C. Perform liver biopsy if:
   1. Five of nine determinations of AST within a given 12-month interval (6 of 12 if tests are performed monthly) are abnormal (defined as an increase above the upper limit of normal)
   2. There is a decrease in serum albumin below the normal range (in the setting of well controlled RA).

D. If results of liver biopsy are:
   3. Roenigk grades I, II, or IIA, resume methotrexate and monitor as in B, C1, and C2 above.
   4. Roenigk grade IIIB or IV, discontinue methotrexate.

E. Discontinue methotrexate in patients with persistent liver test abnormalities, as defined in C1 and C2 above, or who refuse liver biopsy.

AST, aspartate aminotransferase; ALT, alanine aminotransferase

hypersensitivity reaction, clinical features include dry cough, tachypnea, fever, bibasalar rales in association with hypoxia, and a restrictive ventilatory defect on lung function tests [126]. Diffuse interstitial or alveolar infiltrates are seen on chest radiography and biopsy findings include patchy and diffuse alveolar damage with interstitial infiltrates characterized by a predominance of T lymphocytes [124]. A set of diagnostic guidelines has been published which proposes distinctions between definite, probable, and possible methotrexate pneumonitis [126].

Preexisting pulmonary disease [126,127] and history of smoking are reported to be potential risk factors. Corticosteroids have been used in the majority of patients with methotrexate pneumonitis and are thought to be beneficial [126].

D. Hematological Toxicity

Leukocytopenia or thrombocytopenia may occur in up to 22% of patients with RA. [78,128–130] There is an increased risk of toxicity in patients with prior hematological disorder, Felty's syndrome, and red cell macrocytosis. Weinblatt et al. advise monitoring the mean corpuscular volume (MCV), as a rising MCV may indicate an increase risk of severe cytopenia [131]. Other identified risk factors for pancytopenia include increasing age, elevated creatinine, and concomittant trimethoprim-sulfamethoxazole therapy [132,133].

Management of severe cytopenias include supportive therapeutic measures, withdrawal of methotrexate, and high-dose folic or folinic acid.

E. Infections

Reports of opportunistic infections have been greater with methotrexate (17/1000) than with other disease-modifying antirheumatic drugs such as gold, hydroxychloroquine, D-penicillamine, and azathioprine (5/1000) [134]. There have been several case reports of *Pneumocystis carinii* infection in patients with rheumatoid arthritis taking methotrexate [135,136], and in some, RA patients, an associated CD_8 lymphopenia has been described [136]. An increased incidence of herpes zoster in a cohort of patients on methotrexate has been described [137].

An increased risk of postoperative infections in patients taking low-dose methotrexate has been reported [138]. No increased incidence of postoperative infection or significant impairment of wound healing were seen in a study of patients who continued low-dose methotrexate at the time of orthopedic surgery [139]. Longer prospective studies are required to answer these questions.

F. Accelerated Nodulosis

Accelerated nodule development and cutaneous vasculitis have been reported in patients with rheumatoid arthritis taking low-dose methotrexate [140]. Regression of nodules following cessation of methotrexate may indicate a causal relationship, which is supported by a recurrence of nodules on rechallenging with methotrexate [141]. The nodules that develop on methotrexate tend to be small and occur predominantly in the hands, and they are histologically identical to typical rheumatoid nodules [141].

G. Oncogenicity and Teratogenicity

There are several case reports describing tumors arising in patients treated with methotrexate, particularly non-Hodgkin's lymphoma in rheumatoid arthritis patients receiving methotrexate [142–144]. It has been suggested that methotrexate is a cocarcinogen for non-Hodgkin's lymphoma in patients with rheumatoid arthritis, increasing an already present malignancy risk [143]. There are no cohort studies to deny or support this suggestion.

Methotrexate is a potent abortifacient and teratogen [104]. Reported teratogenic effects include anencephaly, hydrocephaly, and palatal and skeletal abnormalities [145]. Methotrexate also causes a transient, but reversible, oligospermia in men [146].

H. Central Nervous System

Mild cognitive effects in patients taking methotrexate for rheumatoid arthritis have been reported and include dysphonia, depressed mood, unpleasant cranial sensation, and impaired concentration [130,147].

I. Supplementation with Folates

There is evidence to support the use of supplemental folic acid to diminish methotrexate-induced side effects without altering efficacy (Table 5). The dose of folate and its timing in relation to the methotrexate dose appear to be critical. The optimal dosing schedule of folate supplements in relation to methotrexate is not known. Safety and cost would suggest folic acid is the better supplement, but a controlled trial of folic acid and folinic acid has not been performed.

These studies suggest that folic acid or folinic acid can be prescribed in patients on methotrexate leading to a reduction in side effects without altering efficacy.

J. Use of Methotrexate in Other Rheumatic Diseases

Although there are many case reports of methotrexate being used successfully in a variety of rheumatic diseases (i.e., adult-onset Still's disease, diffuse and limited systemic sclerosis [scleroderma], systemic lupus erythematosus, Reiter's syndrome, ankylosing spondylitis, rheumatoid vasculitis, Felty's syndrome), very few controlled studies have been performed.

In observational studies, methotrexate has been shown to be effective in reducing the corticosteroid dose in polymyalgia rheumatica/giant cell arteritis and polymyositis/dermatomyositis. Controlled studies assessing the efficacy of methotrexate have been performed in patients with psoriatic arthritis and juvenile rheumatoid arthritis.

1. Psoriatic Arthritis

Two controlled trials of the use of methotrexate in psoriatic arthritis have been published (Table 6). [156,157]. Willkens performed a randomized placebo-controlled trial of 7.5–15 mg oral weekly methotrexate in patients with psoriatic arthritis [157]. Methotrexate was superior to placebo only in the physician assessment of arthritis activity and in the improvement of the amount of skin surface area effected by psoriasis. Black's

Table 5 Effects of Folates on Methotrexate (MTX) Efficacy and Side Effects in Rheumatoid Arthritis

Study no.	Study design	No. of subjects	Weekly folate to MTX ratio	Timing of folate relative to MTX dose	Effects on MTX efficacy	Side effects of MTX	References
Folic acid (FA)							
1.	Placebo-controlled DB. Randomized	79	0.53:1 and 2.85	FA given on 2 days when oral MTX not taken	No change	Reduced	148
2.	Placebo-controlled DB. Randomized	32	0.93:1	Not specified	No change	Reduced	149
Folinic acid (FNA)							
3.	Placebo-controlled DB. Randomized	16	0.05:1	Oral FNA given simultaneously with oral MTX	No change	Reduced	150
4.	Placebo-controlled DB. Randomized	97	0.09:1	Oral FNA 24 h after oral MTX	No change	Reduced	151
5.	Placebo-controlled Crossover DB. Randomized	20	0.5:1	Oral FNA 4 h after oral MTX	No change	Reduced	152
6.	Placebo-controlled Cross-over DB. Randomized	13	0.5:1	Oral FNA for 2 days, 4 days before IM MTX	No change	No change	153
7.	Open/case-controlled	7	0.95:1	Oral FNA for 3 days, 4–6 h after IV MTX	Diminished	Reduced	154
8.	Placebo-controlled Crossover DB. Randomized	27	2.3:1	Oral FNA 2 h after oral MTX	Diminished	No change	155

DB, double blind; IM, intramuscular IV, intravenous.

Table 6 Methotrexate in Psoriatic Arthritis

Study no.	Ref.	Nature of study	No. of subjects	Doses of MTX	Efficacy	Side effects
1	156	Double-blind crossover randomized	21	Up to 3mg/kg parenterally every 10 days	Improvement in skin and joint scores	33% leukopenia 60% nausea
2	157	Double-blind placebo-controlled	37	7.5–15.0 mg/weekly	Minimal	8% stomatitis
3	158	Prospective open study	40	5–25 mg/weekly	Effective	Cirrhosis in one patient

study used doses that are not comparable with current dosage practices and found a high occurrence of side effects. There is a need for controlled studies of methotrexate in psoriatic arthritis, particularly in the subgroup that has "rheumatoid-like" inflammatory joint disease, as this is the subgroup that intuitively should benefit from methotrexate.

2. *Juvenile Rheumatoid Arthritis*

Methotrexate has been studied in a placebo-controlled trial of juvenile rheumatoid arthritis [159]. In 127 patients treated with 5 or 10 mg/m^2/week over 6 months, methotrexate had a 63% response rate at 10 mg/m^2/week, whereas the lower-dose group had similar efficacy to placebo.

XI. CONCLUSIONS

Methotrexate has become the antirheumatic drug of choice with patients with active, moderate to severe rheumatoid arthritis because of its demonstrated efficacy and long-term tolerability. Studies have documented that the drug remains efficacious for at least 8 years, and more patients are able to remain on therapy with methotrexate than with other antirheumatic drugs.

Most clinicians begin therapy with 7.5 mg orally weekly and increase the dose at 6–8 weeks to achieve maximal efficacy. However, in some patients, doses up to 25 mg weekly may be necessary to achieve therapeutic efficacy. Side effects, particularly gastrointestinal side effects, can be reduced without altering efficacy by adding folate supplements.

Monitoring methotrexate treatment should consist of a full blood count, liver function tests, serum creatinine, and chest radiographs initially; a full blood count should be performed every 2 weeks and liver function tests every 4–6 weeks for the first few months. Thereafter, a full blood count and liver function tests should be performed every 4–8 weeks. Excessive dosing, such as with daily instead of weekly administration, has led to toxicity and several fatalities. It is recommended to nominate the day of methotrexate administration (e.g., Wednesday) to avoid the possibility of daily administration.

Methotrexate rarely induces clinical remission. When the drug is ceased, worsening of disease manifestation occurs 2–4 weeks after cessation.

Hepatic toxicity of methotrexate in rheumatoid arthritis appears to be less of a concern than earlier experiences with psoriasis, and recently published guidelines offer clinical utility for monitoring hepatotoxicity. Methotrexate-induced pulmonary disease may be a greater concern than hepatotoxicity.

REFERENCES

1. Jolivet J, Cowan KH, Chabner BA, et al. The pharmacology and clinical use of methotrexate. N Engl J Med 1983; 309:1094–1102.
2. Kremer JM, Galivan J, Kamen B, et al. Methotrexate metabolism analysis in blood and liver of rheumatoid arthritis patients. Arthritis Rheum 1986; 29:832–835.
3. Ahern MJ, Kevat S, Hall P, et al. Hepatic methotrexate content and progression of hepatic fibrosis: preliminary findings. Ann Rheum Dis 1991; 50:477–480.

4. Furst DE. Clinical pharmacology of very low dose methotrexate for use in rheumatoid arthritis. J Rheumatol 1985; 12:11–14.
5. Ahern MJ, Meffin P, Kevat S, et al. Methotrexate kinetics in rheumatoid arthritis: Is there an interaction with nonsteroidal anti-inflammatory drugs. J Rheumatol 1988; 15:1356–1360.
6. Sinnett MJ, Groff GD, Raddatz DA, et al. Methotrexate pharmacokinetics in patients with rheumatoid arthritis. J Rheumatol 1989; 16:745–748.
7. Kremer JM. The changing face of therapy for rheumatoid arthritis. Rheum Dis Clin North Am 1995; 21:845–852.
8. Pinkerton CR, Welshman SG, Dempsey SI, et al. Absorption of methotrexate under standardized conditions in children with acute lymphoblastic leukemia. Br J Cancer 1980; 42:613–615.
9. Wau SH, Huffman DH, Azarnoff DL. Effects of route of administration and effusions on methotrexate pharmacokinetics. Cancer Res 1974; 34:3487–3491.
10. Shen DD, Azaroff DL. Clinical pharmacokinetics of methotexate. Clin Pharmacokinet 1978; 3:1–13.
11. Ogucy K, Kölliker F, Gerber NJ, et al. Effect of food on the bioavailability of low-dose methotrexate in patients with rheumatoid arthritis. Arthritis Rheum 1992; 35:611–614.
12. Hamilton RA, Kremer JM. The effects of food on methotrexate absorption. J Rheumatol 1995; 22:630–632.
13. Slordal L, Prytz PS, Pettersen L, et al. Methotrexate measurements in plasma: comparison of enzyme multiplied immunoassay technique, TDx fluorescence polarization immunoassay and high pressure liquid chromatography. Ther Drug Monit 1986; 8:368–372.
14. Edelman J, Biggs DF, Jamali F, et al. Low-dose methotrexate kinetics in arthritis. Clin Pharmacol Ther 1984; 35:382–386.
15. Herman DA, Veng-Pedersen P, Furst DE, et al. Pharmacokinetics of low-dose methotrexate in rheumatoid arthritis patients. J Pharmaceut Sci 1989; 78:165–171.
16. Huffman DH, Wan SH, Azarnoff DL, et al. Pharmacokinetics of methotrexate. Clin Pharmacol Ther 1973; 14:572–579.
17. Campbell MA, Perrier DG, Dorr RT, et al. Methotrexate: bioavailability and pharmacokinetics. Curr Treat Rep 1985; 69:833–838.
18. Hendel J, Nyfors A. Nonlinear renal elimination kinetics of methotrexate estimated by the use of the D-isomer as a reference marker. Eur J Clin Pharmacol 1984; 26:121–124.
19. Kremer JM, Petrillo JF, Hamilton RA. Pharmacokinetics and renal function in patients with rheumatoid arthritis receiving a standard dose of oral weekly methotrexate. J Rheumatol 1995; 22:38–40.
20. Furst DE. Practical clinical pharmacology and drug interactions of low-dose methotrexate therapy in rheumatoid arthritis. Br J Rheumatol 1985; 34(Suppl 2):20–25.
21. Nuernberg B, Koehnke R, Solsky M, et al. Biliary elimination of low-dose methotrexate in humans. Arthritis Rheum 1990; 33:898–902.
22. Bourke RS, Cheda G, Bremer A, et al. Inhibition of renal tubular transport of methotrexate by probenecid. Cancer Res 1975; 35:110–116.
23. Leigler EG, Henderson ES, Hahn MA, et al. The effects of organic acids on renal clearance of methotrexate in man. Clin Pharmacol Ther 1969; 10:849–857.
24. Mandel MA. The synergistic effect of salicylates on methotrexate toxicity. Plastic Reconst Surg 1976; 57:733–737.
25. Rooney RW, Furst DE, Koehnke R, et al. Aspirin is not associated with more toxicity than other NSAID in patients with RA treated with methotrexate. J Rheumatol 1993; 20:1297–1302.
26. Ellison NM, Servi RJ. Acute renal failure and death following sequential intermediate-dose methotrexate and 5-FU: a possible adverse effect due to concomitant indomethacin administration. Cancer Treat Rep 1985; 69:342–343.

27. Maiche AG. Acute renal failure due to concomitant action of methotrexate and indomethacin. Lancet 1986; 1:1390.
28. Thyss A, Milano G, Kubar J, et al. Clinical and pharmacokinetic evidence of a life-threatening interaction between methotrexate and ketoprofen. Lancet 1986; 1:256–258.
29. Adams JD, Hunter GA. Drug interactions in psoriasis. Aust J Dermatol 1976; 17:39–40.
30. Daly H, Boyle J, Roberts C, et al. Interaction between methotrexate and non-steroidal anti-inflammatory drugs. Lancet 1986; 1:559.
31. Sing RR, Malaviya AN, Pandey JN, et al. Fatal interaction between methotrexate and naproxen. Lancet 1986; 1:1390.
32. Furst DE, Herman RA, Koehnke R, et al. Effect of aspirin and sulindac on methotrexate clearance. J Pharm Sci 1990; 79:782–786.
33. Kremer JM, Hamilton RA. The effects of non-steroidal anti-inflammatory drugs on methotrexate (MTX) pharmacokinetics. J Rheumatol 1995; 22:2072–2077.
34. Weinblatt ME, Coblyn JS, Fox DA, et al. Efficacy of low dose methotrexate in rheumatoid arthritis. N Engl J Med 1985; 312:818–822.
35. Williams HJ, Willkens RF, Samuelson CO, et al. Comparison of low-dose oral pulse methorexate and placebo in the treatment of rheumatoid arthritis: a controlled clinical trial. Arthritis Rheum 1985; 28:721–730.
36. Segal R, Caspi D, Tishler M. Short term effects of low dose methotrexate on the acute phase reaction in patients with RA. J Rheumatol 1989; 16:914–917.
37. Shiroky J, Allegra C, Inghirami G, et al. High dose intravenous methotrexate with leucovorin rescue in rheumatoid arthritis. J Rheumatol 1988; 15:251–255.
38. Weinblatt ME, Trentham DE, Fraser PA, et al. Long-term prospective trial of low-dose methotrexate in rheumatoid arthritis. Arthritis Rheum 1988; 31:167–175.
39. Olsen NJ, Murray LM. Antiproliferative effects of methotrexate on peripheral blood mononuclear cells. Arthritis Rheum 1989; 32:378–385.
40. Chang DM, Baptiste P, Schur PH. The effect of antirheumatic drugs on interleukin 1 activity and IL-1 and IL-1 inhibitor production of human monocytes. J Rheumatol 1990; 17:1148–1157.
41. Johnston CA, Russell AS, Kovithavongs T, et al. Meausures of immunologic and inflammatory responses in vitro in rheumatoid arthritis patients treated with methotrexate. J Rheumatol 1986; 13:294–296.
42. Martinez-Osuna P, Zwolinska JB, Sikes DH, et al. Lack of immunosuppressive effect of low-dose-oral methotrexate on lymphocytes in rheumatoid arthritis. Clin Exp Rheumatol 1993; 11:249–253.
43. Kremer JM, Lawrence DH. Correlation of immune parameters with clinical and laboratory effects in a prospective cohort of patients with rheumatoid arthritis receiving methotrexate [abstr]. Arthritis Rheum 1992; 35:S144.
44. Nesher G, Moore TL. The in vitro effects of methotrexate on peripheral blood mononuclear cells. Modulation by methyl donors and spermidine. Arthritis Rheum 1990; 33:954–959.
45. O'Callaghan JW, Forrest MJ, Brooks PM. Inhibition of neutrophil chemotaxis in methotrexate treated rheumatoid arthritis patients. Rheumatol Int 1988; 8:41–45.
46. Sperling RI, Benincaso AI, Anderson RJ, et al. Acute and chronic suppression of leukotriene B_4 synthesis ex vivo in neutrophils from patients with rheumatoid arthritis beginning treatment with methotrexate. Arthritis Rheum 1992; 35:376–384.
47. Sperling RI, Coblyn JS, Larkin JK, et al. Inhibition of leukotriene B_4 synthesis in neutrophils from patients with rheumatoid arthritis by a single oral dose of methotrexate. Arthritis Rheum 1990; 33:1149–1155.
48. Hawkes JS, Cleland LG, Proudman SM, et al. The effect of methotrexate on ex vivo lipoxygenase metabolism in neutrophils from patients with rheumatoid arthritis. J Rheumatol 1994; 21:55–58.
49. Cronstein BN, Eberle MA, Gruber HE, et al. Methotrexate inhibits neutrophil function by

stimulating adenosine release from connective tissue cells. Proc Natl Acad Sci 1991; 88:241–245.
50. Cronstein BN, Naime D, Ostad E. The anti-inflammatory mechanism in methotrexate—increased adenosine release at inflamed sites diminishes leukocyte accumulation in an in-vivo model of inflammation. J. Clin Invest 1993; 92:2675–2682.
51. Arend WP, Dayer JM. Cytokines and cytokine inhibitors or antagonists in rheumatoid arthritis. Arthritis Rheum 1990; 33:305–314.
52. Hu S-K, Mitcho YL, Oronsky AL, et al. Studies on the effect of methotrexate on macrophage function. J Rheumatol 1988; 15:206–209.
53. Kremer JM, Petrillo GF, Lawrence DH. Methotrexate induces significant changes in IL-1, IL-2, IL-6 and IL-8 but not lymphocyte markers in patients with rheumatoid arthritis [abstr]. Arthritis Rheum 1993; 36:S77.
54. Thomas R, Carroll GJ. Reduction of leukocyte and interleukin-1-β concentration in the synovial fluid of rheumatoid arthritis patients treated with methotrexate. Arthritis Rheum 1993; 36:1244–1252.
55. Barrera P, Boerbooms AM, van de Putte L, et al. Effects of anti-rheumatic agents on cytokines. Semin Arthritis Rheum 1996; 25:234–253.
56. Segal R, Yaron M, Tartakovsky B. Rescue of interleukin-1 activity by leucovorin following inhibition by methotrexate in a murine in vitro system. Arthritis Rheum 1990; 33:1745–1748.
57. Barrera P, Boerbooms AMT, Janssen EM, et al. Circulating soluble tumor necrosis factor receptors, interleukin-2 receptors, tumor necrosis factor α, and interleukin-6 levels in rheumatoid arthritis. Longitudinal evaluation during methotrexate and azathioprine therapy. Arthritis Rheum 1993; 36:1070–1079.
58. Aaron SL. Augmentation of IL-2 secretion by methotrexate therapy of rheumatoid arthritis. Arthritis Rheum 1989; 32:1070–1079.
59. Taylor R, Xie C, Beckenbaugh R, et al. Disease specific lymphokine pattern in rheumatoid arthritis: selective modulation by methotrexate. Arthritis Rheum 1994; 37:S277.
60. Pelletier JM, Cloutier J-M, Pelletier J-P. In vivo effects of anti-rheumatic drugs on neutral collagenolytic proteases in human rheumatoid arthritis cartilage and synovium. J Rheumatol 1988; 15:1198–1204.
61. Hirata S, Matsubara T, Tateishi H, et al. Inhibition of in vitro vascular endothelial cell proliferation and in vivo neovascularization by low dose Methotrexate. Arthritis Rheum 1989; 32:1065–1073.
62. Kremer JM, Phelps CT. Long-term prospective study of the use of methotrexate in the treatment of rheumatoid arthritis. Update after a mean of 90 months. Arthritis Rheum 1992; 35:138–145.
63. Andersen PA, West SG, O'Dell JR, et al. Weekly pulse methotrexate in rheumatoid arthritis. Clinical and immunologic effects in a randomized, double-blind study. Ann Intern Med 1985; 103:489–496.
64. Olsen NJ, Callahan LF, Pincus T. Immunologic studies of rheumatoid arthritis patients treated with methotrexate Arthritis Rheum 1987; 30:481–488.
65. Alarcon GS, Schrobenloher RE, Bartolucci AA, et al. Suppression of rheumatoid factor production by methotrexate in patients with rheumatoid arthritis. Evidence for differential influence of therapy and clinical status on IgM and IgA rheumatoid factor expression. Arthritis Rheum 1990; 33:1156–1161.
66. Kremer JM. Lymphocyte subset analysis after long-term methotrexate therapy for rheumatoid arthritis [abstr]. Arthritis Rheum 1986; 29:S75.
67. Kremer JM, Lawrence DH. Correlation of immune parameters with clinical response to methotrexate in patients with rheumatoid arthritis: A prospective study [abstr]. Arthritis Rheum 1991; 34:S159.

68. Segal R, Mozes E, Yaron M, et al. The effects of methotrexate on the production and activity of interleukin-1. Arthritis Rheum 1989; 32:370–377.
69. Kremer JM, Stocker RP, Rynes RI, et al. Methotrexate therapy causes a significant decrease in soluble interleukin-2 receptors in patients with rheumatoid arthritis [abstr]. Arthritis Rheum 1991; 35:R37.
70. Welles WL, Silkworth J, Oronsky AL, et al. Studies on the effect of low dose methotrexate on rat adjuvant arthritis. J Rheumatol 1985; 12:904–906.
71. Leroux JL, Damon M, Chavis C, et al. Effects of a single dose of Methotrexate on 5- and 12-lipoxygenase products in patients with rheumatoid arthritis. J Rheumatol 1992; 19:863–866.
72. Gubner R, August S, Ginsberg V. Therapeutic suppression of tissue reactivity. II. Effect of aminopterin in rheumatoid arthritis and psoriasis. Am J Med Sci 1951; 221:176–182.
73. Hoffmeister RT. Methotrexate therapy in rheumatoid arthritis [abstr.] Arthritis Rheum 1972; 15:S114.
74. Mackenzie AH, Scherbel AL. Management of rheumatoid arthritis in the surgical patients. Orthop Clin North Am 1971; 2:277–299.
75. Thomson RN, Watts C, Edelman J, et al. A controlled two centre trial of parenteral methotrexate therapy for refractory rheumatoid arthritis. J Rheumatol 1984; 11:760–763.
76. Furst DE, Koehnke R, Burmeister LE, et al. Increasing Methotrexate effect with increasing dose in the treatment of resistant rheumatoid arthritis. J Rheumatol 1989; 16:313–320.
77. Wilke WS, Segal AS, Calabrese LH, et al. 24 week double-blind study of methotrexate in rheumatoid arthritis. Clin Res 1995; 33:884A.
78. Kremer JM, Lee JK. The safety and efficacy of the use of methotrexate in long-term therapy for rheumatoid arthritis. Arthritis Rheum 1986; 29:822–831.
79. Kremer JM, Lee JK. A long-term prospective study of the use of methotrexate in rheumatoid arthritis. Arthritis Rheum 1988; 31:577–584.
80. Kremer JM, Phelps CT. Long-term prospective study of methotrexate in the treatment of rheumatoid arthritis. Arthritis Rheum 1992; 35:138–145.
81. Weinblatt ME, Weissman BN, Holdsworth DE, et al. Long-term prospective study of the use of methotrexate in the treatment of rheumatoid arthritis. Arthritis Rheum 1992; 35:129–137.
82. Tishler M, Caspi D, Rosenbach TO, et al. Methotrexate in rheumatoid arthritis: a prospective study in Israeli patients with immunogenetic correlation. Ann Rheum Dis 1988; 47:654–659.
83. Weinstein A, Marlowe S, Korn I, et al. Low-dose methotrexate treatment of rheumatoid arthritis. Am J Med 1985; 79:331–337.
84. Sany J, Anaya JM, Lussiez V. Treatment of rheumatoid arthritis with methotrexate: a prospective open long term study of 191 cases. J Rheumatol 1991; 78:1323–1327.
85. Rau R, Herborn G, Karger T, et al. Retardation of radiologic progression in rheumatoid arthritis with methotrexate therapy. Arthritis Rheum 1991; 34:1236–1244.
86. Weinblatt KE, Kaplan H, Germain BF, et al. Low-dose methotrexate compared with auranafin in adult rheumatoid arthritis. Arthritis Rheum 1990; 33:330–338.
87. Suarez-Alnazor ME, Fitzgerald A, Grace M, et al. A randomized controlled trial of parenteral methotrexate compared with sodium aurothiomalate in the treatment of rheumatoid arthritis. J Rheumatol 1988; 15:753–756.
88. Morassut P, Goldstein R, Cyr M, et al. Gold sodium thiomalate compared to low dose methotrexate in the treatment of rheumatoid arthritis—a randomized, double blind 26-week trial. J Rheumatol 1989; 16:302–306.
89. Rau R, Herborn G, Karger T, et al. A double-blind randomized parallel trial of intramuscular methotrexate and gold sodium thiomalate in early erosive rheumatoid arthritis. J Rheumatol 1991; 18:328–333.
90. Willkens RF, Urowitz MB, Stablein DM, et al. Comparison of azathioprine, methotrexate

and the combination of both in the treatment of rheumatoid arthritis. Arthritis Rheum 1992; 35:849–856.
91. Jeurissen MEC, Boerbooms ANT, van de Putte LBA, et al. methotrexate versus azathioprine in the treatment of rheumatoid arthritis. Arthritis Rheum 1991; 34:961–972.
92. Arnold MH, O'Callaghan J, McCredie M, et al. Comparative controlled trial of low-dose methotrexate versus azathioprine in rheumatoid arthritis: 3 year prospective study. Br J Rheumatol 1990; 29:120–125.
93. Jeurissen MEC, Boerbooms AMT, van de Putte LBA, et al. Influence of methotrexate and azathioprine on radiologic progression in rheumatoid arthritis. A randomized, double-blind study. Ann Intern Med 1991; 114:999–1004.
94. Felson DT, Anderson J, Meenan R. The comparative efficacy and toxicity of second-line drugs in rheumatoid arthritis: results of two meta-analyses. Arthritis Rheum 1990; 33:1449–1461.
95. Felson DT, Anderson J, Meenan RF. Use of short-term efficacy/toxicity trade offs to select second-lind drugs in rheumatoid arthritis. Arthritis Rheum 1992; 35:1117–1125.
96. Bensen W, Tugwell P, Roberts RM, et al. Combination therapy of cyclosporine with methotrexate and gold in rheumatoid arthritis. J Rheumatol 1994; 21:2034–2038.
97. Hagsma CJ, Van Riel PLCM, de Rooy DJRAM, et al. Combination of methotrexate and sulphasalazine vs methotrexate alone: a randomized open clinical trial in rheumatoid arthritis patients resistant to sulphasalazine therapy. Br J Rheumatol 1994; 33:1049–1055.
98. Fehlauer CS, Carson CW, Cannon GW, et al. Methotrexate therapy in rheumatoid arthritis: 2-year retrospective followup study. J Rheumatol 1989; 16:307–312.
99. McKendry RjR, Cyr M. Toxicity of methotrexate compared with azathioprine in the treatment of rheumatoid arthritis. Arch Intern Med 1989; 149:685–689.
100. Wolfe F, Hawley DJ, Cathey MA. Termination of slow acting antirheumatic therapy in rheumatoid arthritis: A 14-year prospective evaluation of 1017 consecutive starts. J Rheumatol 1990; 37:994–1002.
101. Weinblatt ME, Kaplan BN, Holdsworth DE, et al. Methotrexate in rheumatoid arthritis. Arthritis Rheum 1994; 10:1492–1498.
102. Gispen JG, Alarcon GS, Johnson JJ, et al. Toxicity to methotrexate in rheumatoid arthritis. J Rheumatol 1987; 14:74–79.
103. Halla JT, Hardin JC. Under recognised post dosing reactions to methotrexate in patients with rheumatoid arthritis. J Rheumatol 1994; 21:1224–1226.
104. Goodman TA, Polisson RP. Methotrexate: adverse reactions and major toxicities. Rheum Dis Clin North Am 1994; 20:518–528.
105. Coe R, Bull FE. Cirrhosis associated with methotrexate treatment of psoriasis. JAMA 1968; 206:1515–1520.
106. Epstein EH, Crafts JD. Cirrhosis following methotrexate administration for psoriasis. Arch Dermatol 1969; 100:531–534.
107. Zachariae H, Kragabule K, Sogaard H. Methotrexate induced liver cirrhosis: studies including serial liver biopsies during continued treatment. Br J Dermatol 1980; 102:407–412.
108. Roenigk HH, Auerbach R, Mailbach HI, et al. Methotrexate guidelines revised. J Am Acad Dermatol 1982; 6:145–155.
109. Roenigk HH, Auerbach R, Mailbach HI, et al. Metotrexate in psoriasis: revised guidelines J Am Acad Dermatol 1988; 19:145–156.
110. Kremer JM, Lee RG, Tolman KG. Liver histology in rheumatoid arthritis patients receiving long term methotrexate therapy: a prospective study with baseline and sequential biopsy samples. Arthritis Rheum 1989; 32:121–127.
111. Whiting - O'Keefe QE, Fye KH, Sack KD. Methotrexate and histologic hepatic abnormalities: a meta analysis Am J Med 1991; 90:711–716.
112. Hassan W. Methotrexate and liver toxicity: role of surveillance liver biopsy. Ann Rheum Dis 1996; 55:273–275.

113. Kevat S, Ahern MJ, Hall P. Hepatotoxicity of methotrexate in rheumatic diseases Med Toxicol 1988; 3:197–208.
114. Fernandes L, Sullivan S, McFarlane IG, et al. Studies on the frequency and pathogenesis of liver involvement in rheumatoid arthritis. Ann Rheum Dis 1979; 38:501–506.
115. Bjorkman DJ, Boschert M, Tolman KG, et al. The effect of long-term methotrexate therapy on hepatic fibrosis in rheumatoid arthritis. Arthritis Rheum 1993; 36:1697–1701.
116. Hall P, Ahern MJ, Jarvis LR, et al. Two methods of assessment of methotrexate hepatotoxicity in patients with rheumatoid arthritis. Ann Rheum Dis 1991; 50:471–476.
117. Ahern MJ, Kevat S, Hill W, et al. Hepatic methotrexate content and progression of hepatic fibrosis: preliminary findings Ann Rheum Dis 1991; 50:477–480.
118. Walker AM, Finch D, Dreyer NA, et al. Determinants of serious liver disease among patients receiving low-dose methotrexate for rheumatoid arthritis. Arthritis Rheum 1993, 36:329–335.
119. Chandran G, Ahern MJ, de la Hall P, et al. Cirrhosis in patients with rheumatoid arthritis receiving low-dose methotrexate. Br J Rheumatol 1994; 33:981–984.
120. Willkens AF, Leonard DA, Clegg DO, et al. Liver histology in patients receiving low-dose pulse methotrexate for the treatment of rheumatoid arthritis. Ann Rheum Dis 1990; 49:591–593.
121. Kremer JM, Alarcon GS, Lightfoot RW, et al. Methotrexate for rheumatoid arthritis: suggested guidelines for monitoring liver toxicity. Arthritis Rheum 1994; 37:316–328.
122. Erickson AL, Reddy V, Vogelgesang SA, et al. Usefulness of the American College of Rheumatology recommendations for liver biopsy in methotrexate-treated rheumatoid arthritis patients. Arthritis Rheum 1995; 38:1115–1119.
123. St Clair EW, Rice JR, Snyderman R. Pneumonitis complicating low-dose methotrexate therapy in rheumatoid arthritis. Ann Intern Med 1985; 145:2035–2038.
124. Carson CW, Cannon GW, Egger MJ, et al. Pulmonary disease during the treatment of rheumatoid arthritis with low-dose pulse methotrexate. Semin Arth Rheum 1987; 16:186–195.
125. Newman ED, Harrington TM. Fatal methotrexate pneumonitis in rheumatoid arthritis Arthritis Rheum 1988; 31:1585–1586.
126. Searles G, McKendry RJR. Methotrexate pneumonitis in rheumatoid arthritis J. Rheumatol 1987; 14:1164–1171.
127. Carroll GJ, Thomas R, Phatouros CG, et al. Incidence, prevalence and possible risk factors for pneumonitis in patients with rheumatoid arthritis receiving methotrexate. J Rheumatol 1994; 21:51–54.
128. Mielants H, Veys EM, van der Straten C, et al. The efficacy and toxicity of a constant low dose of methotrexate as a treatment for intractable rheumatoid arthritis: an open prospective study. J Rheumatol 1991; 18:978–983.
129. McKendry RJR, Dale P. Adverse effects of low dose methotrexate therapy in rheumatoid arthritis. J Rheumatol 1993; 20:1850–1856.
130. Schnabel A, Gross WL. Low dose methotrexate in rheumatic diseases—efficacy side effects and risk factors for side effects. Semin Arth Rheum 1994; 23:310–327.
131. Weinblatt ME, Fraser P. Elevated mean corpuscular volume as a predictor of haematologic toxicity due to methotrexate therapy. Arthritis Rheum 1989; 32:1592–1596.
132. Kevat S, Hill WR, Ahern MJ, et al. Pancytopenia induced by low-dose methotrexate for rheumatoid arthritis. Aust NZ J Med 1988; 18:697–700.
133. Al-Awadhi A, Dale P, McKendry RJR. Pancytopenia associated with low dose methotrexate therapy. A regional survey. J Rheumatol 1993; 20:1121–1125.
134. Singh G, Fries JF, Williams CA, et al. Toxicity profiles of disease modifying antirheumatic drugs in rheumatoid arthritis. J Rheumatol 1994; 18:188–194.
135. Leff RL, Case JP, McKenzie R. Rheumatoid arthritis, methotrexate therapy and pneumocystis pneumonia. Ann Intern Med 1990; 112:716.

136. Huntman PM, Stenger AA, Bruyn A, et al. Methotrexate may affect certain lymphocyte subsets in rheumatoid arthritis resulting in susceptibility to pneumocystis carinii infection [letter]. J Rheumatol 1994; 21:1168–1170.
137. Antonelli MAS, Moreland LW, Bruck JL. Herpes zoster in patients with rheumatoid arthritis treated with weekly, low-dose methotrexate. Am J Med 1991; 90:295–298.
138. Bridges LS, Lopez-Mendez A, Han KH. Should methotrexate be discontinued before elective orthopaedic surgery in patients with rheumatoid arthritis. J Rheumatol 1991; 18:984–988.
139. Sany J, Anaya J, Canovas F, et al. Influence of methotrexate on the frequency of postoperative infectious complications in patients with rheumatoid arthritis. J Rheumatol 1993; 20:1129–1132.
140. Segal R, Caspi D, Tishler M, et al. Accelerated nodulosis and vasculitis during methotrexate therapy for rheumatoid arthritis. Arthritis Rheum 1988; 31:1182–1185.
141. Kerstens PJSM, Boerbooks AMT, Jeurissen MLC, et al. Accelerated nodulosis during low dose methotrexate therapy for rheumatoid arthritis An analysis of ten cases. J Rheumatol 1992; 19:867–871.
142. Ellman MH, Hurwitz H, Thomas C. Lymphoma developing in a patient with rheumatoid arthritis taking weekly low dose methotrexate. J Rheumatol 1991; 18:1741–1743.
143. Kingsmore SF, Hall BD, Allen NB, et al. Association of methotrexate, rheumatoid arthritis and lymphoma: report of two cases and literature review. J Rheumatol 1992; 19:1462–1465.
144. Taillon B, Garnier G, Ferrari E, et al. Lymphoma developing in a patient with rheumatoid arthritis taking methotrexate. Clin Rheumatol 1993; 12:93–94.
145. Milunski MB, Graef JW, Gaynor MF. Methotrexate-induced congenital malformations: review of the literature. J Pediatr 1968; 72:790–795.
146. Sussman A, Leonard JM. Psoriasis, methotrexate and oligospermia. Arth Dermatol 1980; 116:215–217.
147. Wernick R, Smith DL. Central nervous system toxicity associated with weekly low-dose methotrexate treatment. Arthritis Rheum 1989; 32:770–775.
148. Morgan SL, Baggott JE, Vaughn WH, et al. Supplementation with folic acid during methotrexate therapy for rheumatoid arthritis. Ann Intern Med 1994; 121:833–841.
149. Morgan SL, Baggott JE, Vaughn WH, et al. The effect of folic acid supplementation on the toxicity of low-dose methotrexate in patients with rheumatoid arthritis. Arthritis Rheum 1990; 33:9–18.
150. Weinblatt ME, Maier AL, Coblyn JS. Low dose leucovorin does not interfere with the efficacy of methotrexate in rheumatoid arthritis: an 8 week randomized placebo controlled trial. J Rheumatol 1993; 20:950–952.
151. Shiroky JB, Neville C, Esdaile JM, et al. Low-dose methotrexate with leucovorin (folinic acid) in the management of rheumatoid arthritis. Results of a randomized, double-blind, placebo-controlled trial. Arthritis Rheum 1993; 36:795–803.
152. Buckley LM, Vacek PM, Cooper SM. Administration of folinic acid after low dose methotrexate in patients with rheumatoid arthritis. J Rheumatol 1990; 17:1158–1161.
153. Hanrahan PS, Russell AS Concurrent use of folinic acid and methotrexate in rheumatoid arthritis. J Rheumatol 1988; 15:1078–1080.
154. Tishler M, Caspi D, Fishel B, et al. The effects of leucovorin (folinic acid) on methotrexate therapy in rheumatoid arthritis patients. Arthritis Rheum 1988; 31:906–908.
155. Joyce DA, Will RK, Hoffman DM, et al. Exacerbation of rheumatoid arthritis in patients treated with methotrexate after administration of folinic acid. Ann Rheum Dis 1991; 59:913–914.
156. Black RL, O'Brien WM, Van Scott EI, et al. Methotrexate therapy in psoriatic arthritis. JAMA 1964; 189:743–747.
157. Willkens RF, Williams HJ, Ward JR, et al. Randomized, double blind, placebo controlled

trial of low-dose pulse methotrexate in psoriatic arthritis. Arthritis Rheum 1984; 27:376–381.

158. Epinoza LR, Zakraoki L, Espinoza CG, et al. Psoriatic arthritis: Clinical response and side effects to methotrexate therapy. J. Rheumatol 1992; 19:872–877.
159. Giannini EH, Brewer EJ, Kuzmina N, et al. Methotrexate in resistant juvenile rheumatoid arthritis. Results of the USA - USSR double-blind, placebo-controlled trial. N Engl J Med 1992; 326:1043–1049.

12

Newer Second-line Agents: Cyclosporin

Theresa Podrebarac and Peter Tugwell
University of Ottawa, and Ottawa General Hospital, Ottawa, Ontario, Canada

I. INTRODUCTION

Cyclosporin is a lipophilic, cyclic polypeptide isolated from the fungi *Tolypocladium inflatum* and Cyclindrocarpon lucidium [1]. Discovered in 1972, it has been used extensively in human subjects since 1978 and has been shown to have impressive immunosuppressive activity without causing myelotoxicity. Cyclosporin quickly proved to be an effective therapy in organ transplantation.

Knowledge of the effects of the drug spawned several research efforts to evaluate its therapeutic potential in various conditions suspected to be due to enhanced immune reactivity. It has been studied in animal models of uveitis, myasthenia gravis, systemic lupus erythematosus, diabetes mellitus, and adjuvant arthritis. In humans, it has been shown to be effective therapy in acute ocular Behçet's syndrome, psoriasis, atopic dermatitis, acute ulcerative colitis, and rheumatoid arthritis [2]. In this chapter, the pharmacology of cyclosporin will be reviewed along with recommendations for its clinical use with special emphasis on rheumatoid arthritis.

II. PHARMACODYNAMICS

Nine cyclosporins have been isolated but only cyclosporins A, C, and G have immunological properties [1]. Cyclosporin A is a lipophilic, cyclic polypeptide of 11 amino acids. It acts reversibly and specifically on lymphocytes, especially CD4-positive T cells [2] (Figure 1).

Cyclosporin has several effects on the immune system. The primary action of cyclosporin is the inhibition of interleukin-2 (IL-2) synthesis and expression [1]. Cyclosporin diffuses across the cell membrane then binds with the protein cyclophilin in the cytoplasm of the cell where it forms a complex with calcineurin in a calcium-

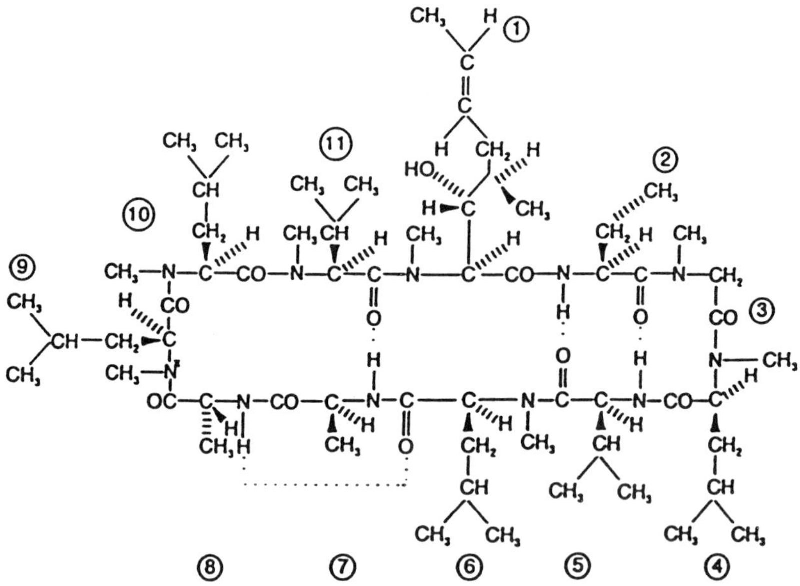

Figure 1 Structural formula of cyclosporin. Numbers indicate the standard numeration of the amino acid residues: 1, (4R)-4-[(E)-2-butenyl]-4,N-dimethyl-L-threonine; 2, l-α-aminobutyric acid; 3, sarcosine; 4, methyl-leucine; 5, valine; 6, methyl-leucine; 7, alanine; 8, d-alanine; 9, methyl-leucine; 10, methyl-leucine; 11, methylvaline.

dependent manner [2]. Inhibition of calcineurin phosphatase activity by the cyclosporin-cyclophilin complex prevents the binding of nuclear factors responsible for the regulation of transcription of the gene for IL-2 and other cytokines [2]. Thus IL-2 production and the expression of IL-2 receptors are blocked.

IL-2 production is critical in the early immune response. The clonal activation and expansion of T cells as well as stimulation of B cells and monocytes are mediated by IL-2. Most of the effects of cyclosporin on other cells are indirect and are mediated by the inhibition of T cell–dependent processes [2].

III. IMMUNOPATHOGENESIS OF RHEUMATOID ARTHRITIS

What is the rationale of using cyclosporin as a treatment in rheumatoid arthritis? Rheumatoid arthritis is a chronic, inflammatory, erosive arthropathy marked by intense synovitis, systemic manifestations, and significant disability and early mortality [3].

Among the earliest events in the inflammatory process is thickening of the synovial layer due to infiltration of macrophages and monocytes and hypertrophy and hyperplasia of type A and B synovial cells [4]. There are considerable microvascular changes and fibroblast proliferation. Neutrophils are in abundance in the synovial fluid but are sparse in the membrane. Endothelial cells are critical in the early stages of inflammation and play an instrumental role in leukocyte recruitment and adhesion [1]. As part of the immune response, macrophages are activated as is indicated by the intense expression of major histocompatibility complex (MHC) class II molecules, including HLA-DR molecules [1]. Somewhat later in the process, the synovium is filled with T cells primarily of the $CD4^+CD45RO^+$ phenotype but B cells and $CD8^+$ T cells are also present. In the later stages of the disease, cartilage and bone destruction predominate owing to the increased proteinase activity of the milieu.

In the T-cell–centric paradigm of the pathogenesis of rheumatoid arthritis, T cells are implicated in the initiation and perpetuation of the disease by activating resident inflammatory cells and their mediators. The role of the $CD4^+$ T cell is supported by the observation that patients with rheumatoid arthritis who then develop acquired immunodeficiency syndrome (AIDS) have an improvement in their clinical symptoms [1]. There is a strong association of HLA DR4/DR1 with rheumatoid arthritis offering the most striking support for the T-cell hypothesis, since the only known function of the MHC is to present antigen to T cells via T-cell receptors [4]. Several possible "rheumatoid antigens" have been proposed.

In contrast, there is substantial evidence suggesting alternative models of joint destruction in the pathogenesis of rheumatoid arthritis. For example, T-cell products such as interferon-γ, IL-2, and IL-4 have not been found in synovial fluids or tissue extracts [5,6]. MRL/*lpr* mice spontaneously develop an arthritis in the absence of T lymphocytes, whereas T-cell–deficient SCID mice develop a destructive arthritis on exposure to *Borrelia*. These animal models further argue against the T-cell–centric hypothesis.

In summary, there is suggestive evidence for a role of the T cell in the pathogenesis of rheumatoid arthritis, supporting the rationale for the use of cyclosporin. However, our knowledge of the etiology of the disease remains incomplete. This may in part account for the lack of a universal benefit to rheumatoid arthritis patients taking cyclosporin.

IV. PHARMACOKINETICS

The pharmacokinetic properties of cyclosporin vary considerably between patients. The drug is poorly absorbed orally with a bioavailability of about 30% (2–89% in healthy volunteers). The capsular and the liquid formulations are felt to have equal bioavailabilities. The primary site of absorption is the small intestine, and peak blood concentrations occur at 1–8 hr. A second blood peak is noted in some patients [2].

Cyclosporin is rapidly and widely distributed between the blood cells and plasma within 10 min. The apparent volume of distribution is 4–8 L/kg. Approximately 60–70% of the drug is taken up by the blood cells, mainly erythrocytes, and the remainder is bound to lipoproteins [2]. Cyclosporin does not cross the blood-brain barrier. However, it does cross the blood-retinal barrier, and it crosses into the placenta and has been located in both the fetal blood circulation as well as in amniotic fluid. Cyclosporin is also excreted into breast milk [2].

The primary route of elimination is via the biliary system, which removes 90% of the drug. Only 6% is eliminated through the urine. Cyclosporin is metabolized by the cytochrome P450 IIIA enzymes primarily in the liver and to a lesser extent in the gastric mucosa [2]. More than 30 metabolites have been observed. The active metabolites do have 10–20% of the immunosuppressive activity but do not appear to act synergistically with the parent drug. Metabolism is age dependent, with children requiring higher doses and older individuals a dosage reduction. Hepatic failure and biliary obstruction significantly decrease its metabolism [2]. Assays for cyclosporin levels should be made by a cyclosporin-specific method on whole blood for the most accurate results.

V. DRUG INTERACTIONS

Since the drug is metabolized through the cytochrome P450 enzymes, it is subject to several drug interactions. Metabolism is decreased by the following drugs: macrolide antibiotics such as erythromycin, azole antifungals, calcium channel antagonists, H_2 antagonists, oral contraceptives, and high-dose corticosteroids. Anticonvulsants and antitubercular medications tend to increase metabolism, hence lowering cyclosporin concentrations [2]. Nephrotoxicity may be increased if other potentially nephrotoxic agents are coadministered such as aminoglycosides or nonsteroidal anti-inflammatories (NSAIDs).

VI. PREGNANCY AND LACTATION

Cyclosporin does cross into the amniotic fluid through the placenta and is also excreted into breast milk. Experience with cyclosporin in pregnancy is limited. Over 100 babies have been born to mothers on cyclosporin. Organ transplant data indicates that compared with other immunosuppressive therapy, there is no increased risk of adverse outcomes with cyclosporin. Males on cyclosporin have fathered normal children [7]. As there are no controlled trials in pregnancy, its use is to be discouraged unless the potential benefit for the mother outweighs the potential harm to the fetus. Mothers should not breast feed [2].

VII. SIDE EFFECTS

Patients with autoimmune disorders have a similar tolerability profile as compared with transplant recipients. The most common adverse events have been gastrointestinal effects, including nausea, vomiting, cramps, and diarrhea followed by renal effects. Hypertrichosis, gingival hyperplasia, and neurological effects are also relatively common, including paraesthesias, headache, and tremor (Table 1). These are usually of mild to moderate severity and respond to dosage reduction [2]. Hyperuricemia is a common problem owing to underexcretion of uric acid caused by cyclosporin. The exact mechanism remains unknown.

VIII. RENAL TOXICITY

The major obstacle to the use of cyclosporin is its nephrotoxicity. Several mechanisms to explain the renal effects have been explored. Vasoconstriction leading to ischemia, disruption of the mitochondrial membranes, increased procollagen synthesis, and a

Table 1 Frequency of Adverse Effects Associated with Cyclosporin Rheumatoid Arthritis Patients

System	Frequency (%)	Features
Gastrointestinal	30–40	Nausea/vomiting
	20	Abdominal discomfort
	10–15	Gum disorders
	6	Diarrhea
	<1	Hepatotoxicity
Genitourinary	100	Increased creatinine
	20	Hypertension
	<5	Interstitial fibrosis
CNS	15–20	Paresthesias
	15	Headache
	10–15	Tremor
	5	Cramps
	5	Dizziness
Autonomic	5	Flushing
Skin	30–35	Hypertrichosis
	3	Rash
Other	5	Fatigue
	5	Flu-like symptoms

Source: Data summarized from five rheumatoid arthritis trials of 264 patients on cyclosporin [18–22,25].

possible coagulopathy have all been described [8]. The histological morphology of cyclosporin nephrotoxicity can be nonspecific. This can lead to confusion attributing changes on renal biopsies to the drug rather than the underlying disease. Interstitial fibrosis, either focal or diffuse with a striped pattern, is well described. Vasculopathy in addition to tubular toxicity and atrophy with features such as giant mitochondria and microcalcifications are felt to be more characteristic of cyclosporin toxicity [8].

Although rheumatoid arthritis (RA) is not associated with any specific renal lesion, approximately 14% of RA patients will have renal pathology [9,10]. Hematuria, proteinuria, and tubular dysfunction are common, but significant nephropathy can occur in the absence of clinical or laboratory abnormalities. The most common abnormality is a mesangial proliferative glomerulonephritis. Interstitial fibrosis is frequently seen in patients with long-standing disease. Upward of 40% of patients, with one autopsy series of 76 patients reporting an incidence of 46%, will have interstitial fibrosis. Some arteriosclerosis is common on biopsy, whereas renal vasculitis is rare. Amyloid has a reported incidence of ≤5% [8]. Rheumatoid arthritis patients have three characteristics which increase their risk of cyclosporin-related renal dysfunction. They include advanced age when initiating treatment, concomitant use of NSAIDs, their underlying disease, and previous second-line treatments that can adversely affect the kidneys.

A recent retrospective analysis to evaluate the long-term risk of irreversible kidney damage and cyclosporin in autoimmune diseases, excluding rheumatoid arthritis, showed 41 of 192 patients to have cyclosporin nephropathy [11]. The mean dosage of cyclosporin was 8.2 ± 2.8 mg/kg/day and the duration of treatment was a median of

13 months. The patients who developed nephropathy on average received higher initial dosages of 9.3 ± 2.8 mg/kg/day, had larger increases in serum creatinine, and were older. The study suggested that toxicity could be avoided by limiting the dose of cyclosporin to no higher than 5 mg/kg/day and avoiding large increases in serum creatinine to no higher than 30% above the patient's baseline [11].

This prompted a study to evaluate rheumatoid arthritis patients and cyclosporin. The International Kidney Biopsy Registry of Cyclosporin in autoimmune diseases obtained kidney biopsies in 41 RA patients treated with cyclosporin (average maximum dose 4.6 ± 1.2 mg/kg/day) for a median of 17 months and compared them with 11 RA patients not treated with cyclosporin, 3 of whom later took cyclosporin and had a repeat biopsies. Forty-one subjects who were kidney donors were used as sex- and age-matched controls [12]. The biopsies in all but one of the cyclosporin-treated patients were done as part of the research protocol and not because of suspected renal toxicity. Thirteen patients had stopped cyclosporin from 1 to 10 months before the biopsy and the remaining 28 patients were still taking the drug.

Four patients in the cyclosporin group but none of the controls had morphological features of cyclosporin nephrotoxicity. The dosage of cyclosporin and the initial serum creatinine level, but *not* treatment duration, were higher in the patients with cyclosporin changes. Of the patients whose dose did not exceed 5 mg/kg/day, none developed renal dysfunction, which reconfirmed the validity of the dosage recommendations [12].

A more recent study by the Canadian Multicentre Rheumatology Group examined 14 renal biopsies from patients with severe rheumatoid arthritis with no evidence of compromised renal function following completion of a course of cyclosporin [9]. Interstitial fibrosis was noted in nine specimens. It was considered to be mild in five, mild-moderate in three, and striped fibrosis was seen in one patient. Mild tubular atrophy was also seen in nine patients, amyloid in one, and obsolescent glomeruli were observed in five specimens. Although it was felt that there were minimal changes in 13 patients and characteristic changes of cyclosporin nephropathy in 1 patient, a greater frequency of adverse events due to the cyclosporin could not be excluded. In the absence of more long-term data, cyclosporin must be used cautiously in rheumatoid arthritis patients, who often have some underlying renal pathology.

IX. EFFICACY

Rheumatoid arthritis is a progressive, disabling disease which has been recognized as being associated with early mortality [3]. Despite current treatments, there are high levels of work disability and comorbidity. There is increasing interest in the concept that earlier, more aggressive treatment may be more successful at controlling the early stages of inflammation and perhaps halt disease destruction and progression.

During the 1980s, several studies were conducted to evaluate the efficacy and toxicity of cyclosporin in the treatment of rheumatoid arthritis. The early work was in rheumatoid arthritis patients with intractable disease using starting dosages of 10 mg/kg/day [13–16]. However, with accumulating evidence on renal dysfunction, lower dosage regimens were later employed. Between 1988 and 1994, seven controlled double-blinded studies were conducted employing lower initial dosages of cyclosporin in the range of 2.5–5.0 mg/kg/day. Six of these trials were randomized. An eighth randomized double-blinded trial compared high-dose to low-dose cyclosporin [17]. In well-established disease, cyclosporin was compared with either placebo (two trials) [18,19], azathioprine (two trials) [20,21], or D-penicillamine (one trial) [22]. Cyclosporin was compared with chloroquine in the only early disease intervention Dutch trial [23]. Most recently, a methotrexate and cyclosporin combination was compared with methotrexate and placebo in a randomized double-blind multicenter trial (Table 2) [24].

X. PLACEBO TRIALS

The first low-dose cyclosporin double-blind randomized placebo-controlled trial by Dougados et al. evaluated 52 rheumatoid arthritis patients with long-standing disease. Of the 26 patients randomized to cyclosporin, 14, or 54%, had a good to very good response compared with only 2 of 26, or 8% in the placebo group ($P < .0001$) [18]. Four patients discontinued cyclosporin because of side effects, whereas two placebo patients discontinued the treatment owing to inefficacy. Improvement was observed in five of the seven clinical variables measured in the active treatment group, but there was no change in the sedimentation rate. Thirteen patients on cyclosporin had renal dysfunction defined as a ≥50% increase in serum creatinine. Within 1 week, 12 of 13 patients had a return of their creatinine to basal levels with a dosage reduction. At the end of the trial, the mean plasma creatinine rose from 81 to 105 μmol/L. A second larger randomized placebo-controlled multicenter trial of 144 rheumatoid arthritis patients starting cyclosporin at a dosage of 2.5 mg/kg/day confirmed the superiority of cyclosporin to placebo [19]. Major clinical outcome measures such as active joint count, pain, and global improvement improved >20%. Thirty percent of patients had a >50% reduction in joint count. Biological parameters such as the sedimentation rate did not change. Serum creatinine increased on average by 15.6 μmol/L, but resulted in only one patient withdrawing from the study. The philosophy of "go low, go slow" was born. Of note, patients first showed signs of benefit at 3 months which continued, nevertheless, until the medication was discontinued when the benefits gained were slowly lost.

XI. COMPARATIVE STUDIES

Two studies have compared azathioprine at dosages of 1.5–2.0 mg/kg/day to cyclosporin at dosages of 4.2–5.0 mg/kg/day following patients over 6 months [20,21]. Both drugs were comparable in terms of overall efficacy. The withdrawal rate due to either inefficacy or adverse events was slightly higher in the azathioprine group in the Ahern study. No patient was withdrawn because of nephrotoxicity from the cyclosporin group, but predictably hypertension and elevated serum creatinine did occur and were manageable without withdrawing patients from the study for these reasons [16].

A multicenter randomized, double-blind trial compared cyclosporin at 5 mg/kg/day as a starting dosage with D-penicillamine at a starting dosage of 250 mg/day over a 6-month period [22]. Ninety-two patients were enrolled with an average disease duration of 7 years. The clinical benefits were not impressive, and there was no signifi-

Table 2 Summary of Controlled Cyclosporin Studies in Rheumatoid Arthritis

References	Study design (length)	Initial dose (mg/kg)	No. of patients (no. at finish)	Mean age (years)	Mean disease duration (years)	Overall efficacy
19	mc,r,db (6 months)	CyA 2.5 Placebo	72 (62) 72 (50)	55	11	CyA > placebo
18	r,db (4 months)	CyA 5.0 Placebo	26 (22) 26 (24)	58	14	CyA > placebo
20	mc,r,db (6 months)	CyA 4.2 Aza 1.7	25 (18) 27 (15)	60	9	CyA = Aza
21	mc,db (6 months)	CyA 5.0 Aza 1.5–2	115 (92) ?	?	?	CyA = Aza
22	mc,r,db (24 weeks)	CyA 5.0 Pen 250 mg/day	46 (36) 46 (37)	55	13	CyA = Pen
23	r,db (24 weeks)	CyA 2.5 Chl 300 mg/day	22 (20) 22 (19)	?	0.54	CyA = Chl
17	r,db (6 months)	CyA 1.0 CyA 10.0	16 (13) 15 (12)	50	12	$CyA_{10} > CyA_1$

Abbreviations: CyA, cyclosporin; Aza, azathioprine; Chl, chloroquine; Pen, penicillamine; mc, multicenter, db, double-blind; r, randomized.
Source: Adapted from Drugs 45(6) 1993:953–1040.

cant difference between the two regimens. Renal dysfunction accounted for 5 of the 10 withdrawals in the cyclosporin group.

The only trial thus far completed in patients with early rheumatoid disease (duration <2 years) is a randomized double-blind controlled trial by Landewé et al. This study followed 44 patients for 24 weeks and compared cyclosporin (starting at 2.5 mg/kg/day) to chloroquine (initial dosage 300 mg base/day) [23]. The patients were initially followed for the 24 weeks, at which point both agents were found to be equally efficacious. However, when these patients were followed to 1 year, the patients in the cyclosporin group were significantly better when compared with the chloroquine group, and there was no significant difference in the creatinine clearance between the two groups. Despite the superior improvement clinically in the cyclosporin group, there was radiographic progression in both groups. It appears that the cyclosporin group had more erosions at the outset of the trial. This finding is in contrast to work by Førre, who followed 122 patients over 48 weeks on cyclosporin and found that there was only radiographic progression in the placebo group and not in the cyclosporin group [25].

XII. CYCLOSPORIN COMBINATION STUDIES

A recent multicenter trial conducted in Canada and the United States by Tugwell et al. confirmed the experimental rat data that cyclosporin in combination with methotrexate is superior to methotrexate alone [24]. This trial randomized 148 rheumatoid arthritis patients who were taking methotrexate but had had an incomplete response to either low dose cyclosporin (2.5–5.0 mg/kg/day) in combination with the methotrexate or to placebo for 6 months [24]. The data showed a significant relative reduction in both tender joint count of 25%, or 4.8 joints, and in swollen joint count of 25%, or 3.8 joints, in the cyclosporin-methotrexate group. The physician and patient global assessments, pain, and functional status were also clinically and statistically improved when compared with the methotrexate-placebo group. This is the first trial in which 36 patients, or 48%, of the treatment group met the 1993 American College of Rheumatology criteria for improvement (more than a 20% improvement in five of seven defined variables). Adverse events caused eight patients to withdraw from the combination therapy group, whereas five withdrew from the methotrexate-placebo group because of adverse effects. Serum creatinine concentrations increased by a mean of 12 $\pm$ 24 mmol/L in the cyclosporin group and by 4 $\pm$ 17 mmol/L in the placebo group (P = .02). Other combination studies are currently being evaluated in early rheumatoid arthritis.

In summary, cyclosporin has a beneficial effect on synovitis in both long-standing and early rheumatoid arthritis. On average, 10% of patients discontinue cyclosporin because of inefficacy [27]. This was more common at lower dosages, where it is felt that it takes longer for patients to appreciate a noticeable effect. A trial by Yocum et al. compared cyclosporin at 10 mg/kg/day with 1 mg/kg/day in patients with long-standing rheumatoid arthritis and found the higher dosage to be superior [17]. Of the patients who discontinue treatment prematurely, the majority do so because of adverse reactions (17%, range of 6–41%) [27]. The most common adverse effect is gastrointestinal intolerance especially at the higher dosages (30–50%). The other major reason for discontinuation is unacceptably high creatinine levels.

XIII. CURRENT RECOMMENDATIONS

A. Whom Should We Treat with Cyclosporin?

Recommendations on the appropriate pateints were established at the international consensus conference on cyclosporin [28]. Patients who are considered eligible for second-line agents and have failed other therapies are the best candidates to receive cyclosporin. Because of the lack of data on long-term follow-up, especially regarding renal dysfunction and the limited data that exist on the use of cyclosporin in early disease, it is recommended that it should be used with caution in new-onset rheumatoid arthritis until more data ensuring safety become available.

B. Whom Should We *Not* Treat with Cyclosporin?

Patients with known renal dysfunction, uncontrolled hypertension, current or past malignancy except for basal cell carcinoma, leukopenia or thrombocytopenia, abnormal liver enzymes defined as twice baseline values, or those with an immunodeficiency disorder should not be treated. Caution should be exercised when considering cyclosporin treatment in the following patients:

Age over 65 years
Controlled hypertension
Concomitant use of drugs with known cyclosporin interactions
Concomitant use of NSAIDs
Previous or concurrent use of alkylating agents
Premalignant conditions
Active infections
Pregnant or are breastfeeding

XIV. CURRENT TREATMENT GUIDELINES

These guidelines are adapted from the latest EULAR International consensus conference on cyclosporin [28].

1. Patients should have a complete history and physical examination prior to therapy which should include at least two blood pressure measurements on separate occasions. Baseline creatinine should be done on at least two occasions, and if abnormal, a creatinine clearance should be obtained along with possible consultation with a nephrologist.
2. Baseline laboratory work should also include a full liver profile, bilirubin, magnesium, uric acid, potassium, fasting lipids, urinary protein, and complete blood count.
3. The starting dosage should be 2.5 mg/kg/day to 3.5 mg/kg/day as a twice daily regimen, and the dosage should not exceed 5 mg/kg/day.
4. Expect a response by 8–12 weeks. After 4–8 weeks, the dose can be increased up to a maximum of 5 mg/kg/day by increments of 0.5 to 1.0 mg/kg/day at 1- to 2-month intervals.
5. Once the largest required dosage has been reached and no further response

is expected, after being stable for 3 months, begin to decrease the dosage by 0.5 mg/kg/day to the lowest effective dosage. If only partially effective at 3 months at maximal dosing of cyclosporin, the drug should be replaced or possibly another agent added.

6. If after 6 months there is no response, then discontinue the medication.

XV. ADVERSE EVENT MONITORING

If the creatinine increases to 30% above the patient's baseline, decrease the dosage by 0.5 to 1.0 mg/kg/day over a period of 1 month or discontinue the drug depending on the severity of the increase. Creatinine should be measured every 2 weeks initially for at least 3 months and then monthly if stable. If the dosage is still increasing or the creatinine is increasing, the monitoring should be done more frequently. The blood pressure should also be measured every 2 weeks. If hypertension develops, it should be treated by lowering the dosage of medication, or calcium channel blockers can be used with the exception of diltiazem and verapamil because of potential drug interactions.

NSAIDs should be discontinued when possible.

Drug levels are not essential but can be useful to assess certain drug interactions, erratic absorption of the drug, and compliance, and they may have some link with the drug's toxicity.

XVI. MALIGNANCY

The issue of potential malignancies and cyclosporin is a contentious one. In a review of 1000 rheumatoid arthritis patients who had been treated with cyclosporin, 17 developed tumors after treatment with the drug [29]. These results indicate that there is an increased relative risk for the development of malignancy, especially skin cancers and lymphoproliferative disorders, but the relative risk is about the same for cyclosporin and as with other disease-modifying anti-inflammatory drugs (DMARDs). Rheumatoid arthritis itself is felt to have an increased risk of lymphoproliferative disorders and hematological malignancies [30]. There was no difference in the pattern of the malignancies between cyclosporin and other DMARDs. Patients need to be carefully monitored while our experience grows in the use of this medication in rheumatoid arthritis.

XVII. CONCLUSIONS

Cyclosporin is a powerful drug which has been shown to have a place in the treatment of several autoimmune disorders. It has been shown to be of benefit in rheumatoid arthritis and its most appropriate role in therapy is still being investigated. As our knowledge in the immunopathogenesis of rheumatoid arthritis increases, future avenues of therapy will be explored. Along with its potent role as an immunomodulator, it can cause significant renal dysfunction, and therefore regular monitoring is essential along with close adherence to proper dosing regimens. If the recommended dosing schedule is not exceeded, cyclosporin is a safe addition to our current ammunition of second-line agents.

REFERENCES

1. Yocum D. Immunological actions of Cyclosporin A in rheumatoid arthritis. Br J Rheumatol 1993; 32(Suppl 1):38–41.
2. Faulds D, Goa KL, Benfield P. Cyclosporin. A review of its pharmacodynamic and pharmacokinetic properties, and therapeutic use in immunoregulatory disorders. Drugs 1993; 45:953–1040.
3. Pincus T, Callahan LF, Sale WG, Brooks AL, et al. Severe functional declines, work disability, and increased mortality in seventy-five rheumatoid arthritis patients studied over nine years. Arthritis Rheum 1984; 27:864–872.
4. Panayi GS. The immunopathogenesis of rheumatoid arthritis. Br J Rheumatol 1993; 32(Suppl 1):4–14.
5. Zvaifler NJ, Firestein GS. Pannus and pannocytes. Alternative models of joint destruction in rheumatoid arthritis. Arthritis Rheum 1994; 37:783–789.
6. Firestein GS, Alvaro-Garcia JM, Maki R. Quantitative analysis of cytokine gene expression in rheumatoid arthritis. J Immunol 1990; 144:3374–3383.
7. Sandimmune Product Information. CPS 1995.
8. Ludwin D, Alexopoulou I. Cyclosporin A nephropathy in patients with rheumatoid arthritis. Br J Rheumatol 1993; 32(Suppl 1):60–64.
9. Ludwin D, Alexopoulou I, Esdaile JM, Tugwell P. Renal biopsy specimens from patients with rheumatoid arthritis and apparently normal renal function after therapy with cyclosporin. Am J Kidney Dis 1994; 23:260–265.
10. Boers M. Renal disorders in rheumatoid arthritis. Semin Arthritis Rheum 1990; 20:57–68.
11. Feutren G, Mihatsch MJ. Risk factors for cyclosporin-induced nephropathy in patients with autoimmune diseases. N Engl J Med 1992; 326:1654–1660.
12. Sandimmun International Kidney Biopsy Registry in Autoimmune Diseases. Renal morphology after cyclosporin A therapy in rheumatoid arthritis patients. Br J Rheumatol 1993; 32(Suppl 1):65–71.
13. van Rijthoven AWAM, Dijkmans BAC, Goei The HS et al. Cyclosporin treatment for rheumatoid arthritis: a placebo controlled, double blind, multicentre study. Ann Rheum Dis 1986;45:726–731.
14. Weinblatt Me, Coblyn JS, Fraser PA, et al. Cyclosporin A treatment of refractory rheumatoid arthritis. Arthritis Rheum 1987; 30:11–17.
15. Forre O, Bjerkhoel F, Salvesen CF, et al. An open, controlled, randomized comparison of cyclosporin and azathioprine in the treatment of rheumatoid arthritis: a preliminary report. Arthritis Rheum 1987; 30:88–92.
16. Tugwell P, Bombardier C, Gent M, et al. Low dose cyclosporin in rheumatoid arthritis: a pilot study. J Rheumatol 1987; 14:1108–1114.
17. Yocum D, Klippel JH, Wilder RL, et al. Cyclosporin A in severe, treatment-refractory rheumatoid arthritis. A randomized study. Ann Intern Med 1988; 109:863–869.
18. Dougados M, Awada H, Amor B. Cyclosporin in rheumatoid arthritis: a double blind, placebo controlled study in 52 patients. Ann Rheum Dis 1988; 47:127–133.
19. Tugwell P, Bombardier C, Gent M, et al. Low-dose cyclosporin versus placebo in patients with rheumatoid arthritis. Lancet 1990; 335:1051–1055.
20. Ahern MJ, Harrison W, Hollingsworth P, et al. Randomised double-blind trial of cyclosporin and azathioprine in refractory rheumatoid arthritis. Aust NZ J Med 1991; 21:844–849.
21. Kruger K, Schattenkirchner M, Petersen AK, Shand N. Long-term treatment of rheumatoid arthritis with cyclosporin A [abstr]. Br J Rheumatol 1992; 31(Suppl 2):39.
22. van Rijthoven AWAM, Dijkmans BAC, Goeithé HS, et al. Comparison of cyclosporin and D-penicillamine for rheumatoid arthritis: a randomized, double blind, multicenter study. J Rheumatol 1991; 18:815–820.

23. Landewé RBM, Goei The HS, van Rijthoven AAM, et al. A randomized, double-blind, 24-week controlled study of low-dose cyclosporine versus chloroquine for early rheumatoid arthritis. Arthritis Rheum 1994; 37:637–643.
24. Tugwell P, Pincus T, Yocum D, Stein M, et al. Combination therapy with cyclosporine and methotrexate in severe rheumatoid arthritis. N Engl J Med 1995; 333:137–141.
25. Forre O. Cyclosporin A (Sandimmun) in rheumatoid arthritis a double-blind placebo-controlled study [abstr]. Scand J Rheumatol 1990; 19(Suppl 85):57.
26. Brahn E, Peacock DJ, Banquerigo ML. Suppression of collagen-induced arthritis by combination cyclosporin A and methotrexate therapy. Arthritis Rheum 1991; 34:1282–1288.
27. Dijkmans BAC, van Rijthoven AWAM, Goei The HS, et al. Cyclosporine in rheumatoid arthritis. Semin Arthritis Rheum 1992; 22:30–36.
28. Panayi GS, Tugwell P. The use of cyclosporin A in rheumatoid arthritis: conclusions of an international review. Br J Rheumatol 1994; 33:967–969.
29. Arellano F, Krupp P. Malignancies in rheumatoid arthritis patients treated with cyclosporin A. Br J Rheumatol 1993; 32(Suppl 1):72–75.
30. Symmons DPM. Neoplasias in rheumatoid arthritis. J Rheumatol 1988; 15:9.
31. Wells G, Tugwell P. Cyclosporin A in rheumatoid arthritis: overview of efficacy. Br J Rheumatol 1993; 32(Suppl 1):51–56.
32. Dougados M, Luchesne L, Awada H, et al. Assessment of efficacy and acceptability of low dose cyclosporin in patients with rheumatoid arthritis. Ann Rheum Dis 1989; 48:550–556.
33. Dougados M, Torley H. Efficacy of cyclosporin A in rheumatoid arthritis: worldwide experience. Br J Rheumatol 1993; 32(Suppl 1):57–59.

13

Cytotoxics (Azathioprine, Chlorambucil, and Cyclophosphamide)

Philip J. Clements
University of California, Los Angeles, Los Angeles, California

I. INTRODUCTION

The management of rheumatoid arthritis (RA) was revolutionized by Hench's discovery that adrenal cortical extracts could miraculously, at least temporarily, "cure" the disease [1]. Since adrenal extracts were not readily available at the time of Hench's discovery, other investigators eagerly sought different medications that could mimic the actions of the adrenal extracts. The path to these "different" antirheumatic drugs then took a detour through the development of anticancer compounds.

Chemists working to develop anticancer compounds which themselves were inactive (prodrugs) but which could be activated once in the body (preferably in neoplastic cells) first identified mechlorethamine (nitrogen mustard). Because nitrogen mustard was highly reactive and toxic to both neoplastic and normal cells, it found limited use in the clinic. Although the ideal drug was never developed, two alkylating agents, chlorambucil (CHLOR), introduced in 1955, and cyclophosphamide (CTX), introduced in 1958, did enjoy some popularity in the 1960s and 1970s in managing rheumatic disease as well as oncological disease. Fosdick [2] was the first to describe the beneficial effects of CTX in RA (75% of 38 RA patients). Over the next decade, numerous controlled trials of CTX clearly demonstrated that CTX was a potent antirheumatic drug; these same reports also clearly demonstrated that CTX was enormously toxic. As a result of this toxicity, the indications for the use of the alkylating agents in the management of RA have become increasingly restricted.

Azathioprine (AZA) was introduced in 1961, as a prodrug for the antileukemic agent 6-mercaptopurine (6-MP), with the hope that the molecule would be protected from rapid inactivation and would be better tolerated. Since the early 1970s multiple studies (against placebo and against other disease-modifying antirheumatic drugs [DMARDs]) have clearly demonstrated that AZA is a potent antirheumatic drug equal or nearly equal in clinical efficacy to gold sodium thiomalate (GSTM), D-penicillamine (DPA), methotrexate (MTX), cyclophosphamide (CTX), and cyclosporin A (CyA).

This chapter first reviews the clinically applicable pharmacology, putative mechanism of actions, and adverse effects of the two alkylating agents (CHLOR and CTX) and the one purine antagonist (AZA) which have most commonly been employed in the management of RA. The next section reviews the published studies which describe and define the clinical use of each agent in the management of RA. Finally, some guidelines will be presented regarding the most applicable present-day use of each agent in the management of RA.

II. CLINICAL PHARMACOLOGY/PHARMACOKINETICS (TABLE 1)

A. Azathioprine

The bioavailability of the AZA metabolite, 6-MP, following orally administered AZA is 60% [3]. After AZA is absorbed, 50–90% is metabolized to 6-MP plus other metabolites. Less than 10% of AZA is excreted in the urine as AZA or 6-MP [4]. 6-MP is then metabolized by three competing mechanisms: thiol methylation, oxidation, and phosphorylation (Fig. 1). Thiol methylation (catalyzed by the enzyme thiopurine methyltansferase [TPMT]) metabolizes 6-MP and metabolites to inactive thiopurines. Xanthine oxidase catabolizes 6-MP to the inactive metabolite 6-thiouric acid, the major renally excreted metabolic product. Hypoxanthine-guanine-phosphoribosyl transferase (HGPRTase) catalyzes 6-MP to the active metabolites, 6-thioinosinic acid and 6-thioguanine, which are then further metabolized to inactive metabolites. The major urinary metabolites are inactive [4].

After oral AZA administration, blood AZA and 6-MP levels both peak within 2 hr. AZA and 6-MP levels thereafter fall with an elimination half-life of 1.7 and 1.2 h, respectively [5]. Since active metabolites are formed within cells and are not themselves able to traverse the cell membrane and circulate in plasma, measuring plasma levels of AZA or metabolites have little therapeutic value. In addition, very large intra-individual variability (variability of area under the curve [AUC] [day 1 vs day 2] as large as 257%) makes it hard to use kinetics productively [5].

A major pathway of 6-MP metabolism is via TPMT. This enzyme exhibits genetic polymorphism and is found in very low concentrations in 1 of 300 individuals. Patients with low TPMT may be at increased risk of myelosuppression [5–7].

AZA (and its metabolite 6-MP) are eventually metabolized in part by xanthine oxidase, an enzyme inhibited by allopurinol [3]. Therefore, when allopurinol is administered concomitantly with AZA or 6-MP, the AZA dose should be reduced to one-third or one-fourth the usual dose.

The major excretory route for AZA and its metabolites is the urine; however, the conversion of AZA to active metabolites and then to inactive metabolites occurs in nonrenal tissue (RBC, liver, intestine), and theoretically renal failure should not influence toxicity. When renal failure supervenes, AZA and these metabolites accumulate, but the kinetics of AZA and 6-MP do not change appreciably [3]. Although some investigators claim that AZA-induced leukopenia occurs more frequently in the presence of renal failure, others have found no increase in marrow toxicity in these circumstances [3–5]. Data about how to use AZA in the presence of liver failure are scant. Reduced

Table 1 Pharmacokinetics of Slow-acting Antirheumatic Drugs

Drug	Bioavailability	Clearance (mL/min/kg)	Serum elimination $t_{1/2}$ (hours)	Bound fraction	Routes of elimination (%)	Site of metabolism	References
Azathioprine	0.6–0.8 (AZA) (6-MP)	21–200 (AZA) 114 (6MP)	1.7 (AZA) 1.2–1.5 (6-MP)	0.30 (AZA) 0.20 (6-MP)	Renal (20–45)	Liver, RBC, intestine	5, 6, 71
Chlorambucil	0.7	20	1.5–1.7 (CHLOR) 2.3–2.6 (mustard)	1.0 CHLOR	Renal (20–71)	Unkown	3, 72
Cyclophosphamide	0.97	1.2	3–12 (CTX) 8.7 (mustard)	0.13 (CTX) 0.60 (mustard)	Renal (CTX 50, metabolites 8–35)	Liver	3, 9, 12

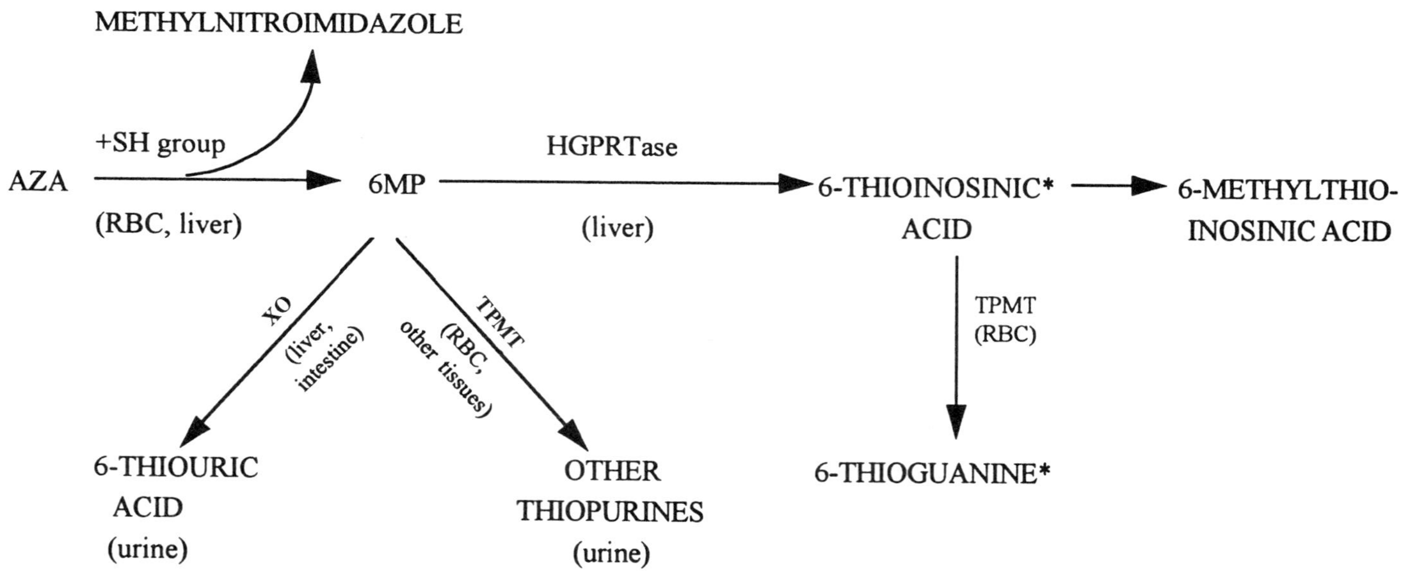

Figure 1 Metabolism of azathioprine. +SH group, sulfhydryl group; 6-MP, 6-mercaptopurine; HGPRTase, hypoxanthine-quanine-phosphoribosyltransferase; TPMT, thiopurine methyltransferase; XO, xanthine oxidase; RBC, red blood cell. *Cytotoxically active principle.

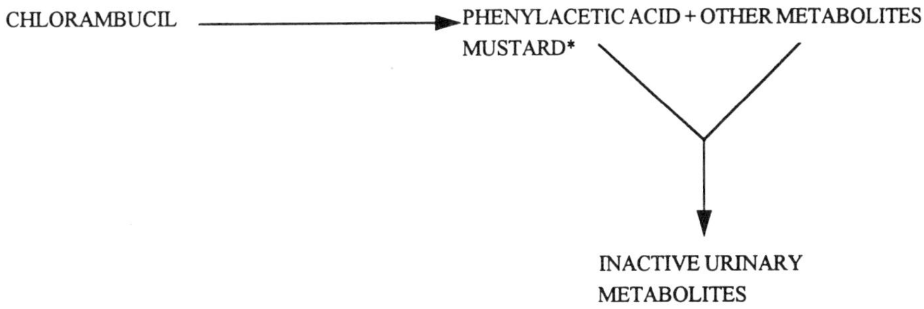

Figure 2 Metabolism of chlorambucil. *Cytotoxically active principle.

amounts of AZA should be given to subjects with severe liver impairment, since customary doses may lead to increased leukopenia and possibly coma [3].

About 30% of AZA and 20% of 6-MP are protein bound in the blood [3]. Little AZA or metabolites enter the cerebrospinal fluid (CSF) or breast milk [3,4]. However, when AZA was administered to pregnant females at term, reduction in white blood cell count was noted in the fetus, suggesting that active metabolites did in fact cross the placenta [3]. As expected, AZA and its metabolites were rapidly cleared by hemodialysis [3].

B. Chlorambucil

CHLOR is more than 70% absorbed by the oral route [8] and absorption occurs rapidly, being detectable in plasma within 15 min and peaking within 120 min. The plasma levels decay with a half-life of 1.5–1.7 h. The absorption rate does not vary over 3 successive days of 10 mg/day administration [8].

CHLOR, itself not cytoxic, is rapidly and almost completely metabolized in unknown sites to phenylacetic acid mustard (its major and most active metabolite) and several other poorly characterized metabolites (Fig. 2). Phenylacetic acid mustard appears in plasma within 15 min of oral CHLOR administration, its plasma level peaks within 2–4 h, and its elimination half-life is 2.3–2.6 h [8]. The elimination of intravenously and orally administered CHLOR occurs in two phases and the elimination half-lives are similar. Both CHLOR and phenylacetic acid mustard are bound extensively to plasma proteins. Other metabolites have not been well characterized or studied.

Although 20–70% of CHLOR metabolites are excreted in the urine within 24 h (and little more appears thereafter), less than 1% of the CHLOR appears in the urine as the parent drug or as phenylacetic acid mustard. Urinary metabolites have not been well characterized further nor has fecal CHLOR excretion been well studied [8]. ^{14}C label does not appear in the expired air following administration of radioactively labeled CHLOR. The effect of renal or liver failure on the metabolism or the efficacy of CHLOR has not been studied [8].

C. Cyclophosphamide

CTX (itself a racemic mixture of two enantomers) is not cytotoxic but must be enzymatically converted by hepatic microsomal enzymes (cytochrome oxidase P450 system) to multiple metabolites (Fig. 3) [9,10]. Phosphoramide mustard is the metabolite of CTX which is felt to be the active cytotoxic agent [9].

CTX is well absorbed from the gastrointestinal tract, and the systemic availability of orally administered drug is virtually 100% [8]. The kinetics of intravenous and oral CTX are very similar in doses up to 1 g/m^2 [8,9]. The disposition of CTX and phosphoramide mustard occurs in two phases. Following intravenous administration of CTX, phosphoramide mustard rapidly appears in the blood with peak levels occurring at 1 h. The elimination half-life of CTX is between 3 and 12 h and that of phosphoramide mustard is very similar, with a mean of 8.7 h [9,10]. There is a great deal of variation among individual subjects.

CTX and its metabolites are excreted largely by the kidney [9]. CTX is extensively metabolized before excretion, with less than 25% of the administered dose appearing in the urine unchanged [9]. Of the urinary metabolites, about half consist of carboxyphosphamide and about 15% of 4-ketocyclophosphamide [8,9,11]. In one study, about 60% of injected radioactivity (injected as ^{14}C-labeled CTX) appeared in the urine within 48 h and little additional radioactivity appeared in the urine thereafter. The fraction of CTX and its metabolites which appeared in the urine was independent of drug dosage [9].

About 12–14% of CTX and 60% of its metabolites are protein bound. Unmetabolized CTX was readily removed by hemodialysis: Grochow found a clearance of 78 mL/min during dialysis [9], whereas Wang reported that 72% of the CTX dose was found in the dialysate of patients undergoing a 6-h hemodialysis [9]. Less than 4% of the radioactive label appeared in the stool or in the expired air following ingestion of ^{14}C-labeled CTX [8]. Since biliary concentrations of CTX and metabolites parallel those in plasma and only a small fraction of drug appears in the stool, enterohepatic recirculation is extensive [12]. Conversely, alkylating metabolites passively diffuse into the interstitial fluid of effusions in concentrations up to 80% of the plasma levels [9]. Minute amounts of CTX itself have been detected in sweat, breast milk, saliva, and synovial fluid [8]. Cytotoxic material appears in the breast milk in quantities large enough to result in leukopenia in breast-fed infants [8]. Normally, only a small fraction of cytotoxic metabolites crosses the blood brain barrier in the CSF [9]. Patients with brain tumors receiving intravenous CTX, however, exhibited CSF concentrations which were 50% those in plasma. Elimination from the CSF occurred at a slower rate than that seen in plasma [12].

Hemorrhagic cystitis probably results from contact of the bladder with the metabolite acrolein. Ingestion of copious amounts of fluids and administration of CTX in a single morning dose reduces the incidence and degree of cystitis. The concurrent administration of 2-mercaptoethanesulfonate (Mesna), a sulfhydryl donor approved by the U.S. Food and Drug Administration (FDA) in 1989 to detoxify acrolein, may obviate or reduce the incidence and degree of cystitis [13]. Mesna is given intravenously and, usually in conjunction with intravenous CTX.

Since CTX and its metabolites are excreted primarily in the urine, the plasma levels of CTX and its metabolites increase in the presence of reduced renal function. Although contradictory observations have not yet resolved whether reduced renal function leads to increased clinical toxicity [9], the half-lives of CTX and metabolites are prolonged. Convention decrees that the initial CTX dose be reduced by one-quarter to one-half in the presence of significant azotemia. Conversely CTX dosage adjustment is not required in the presence of liver dysfunction.

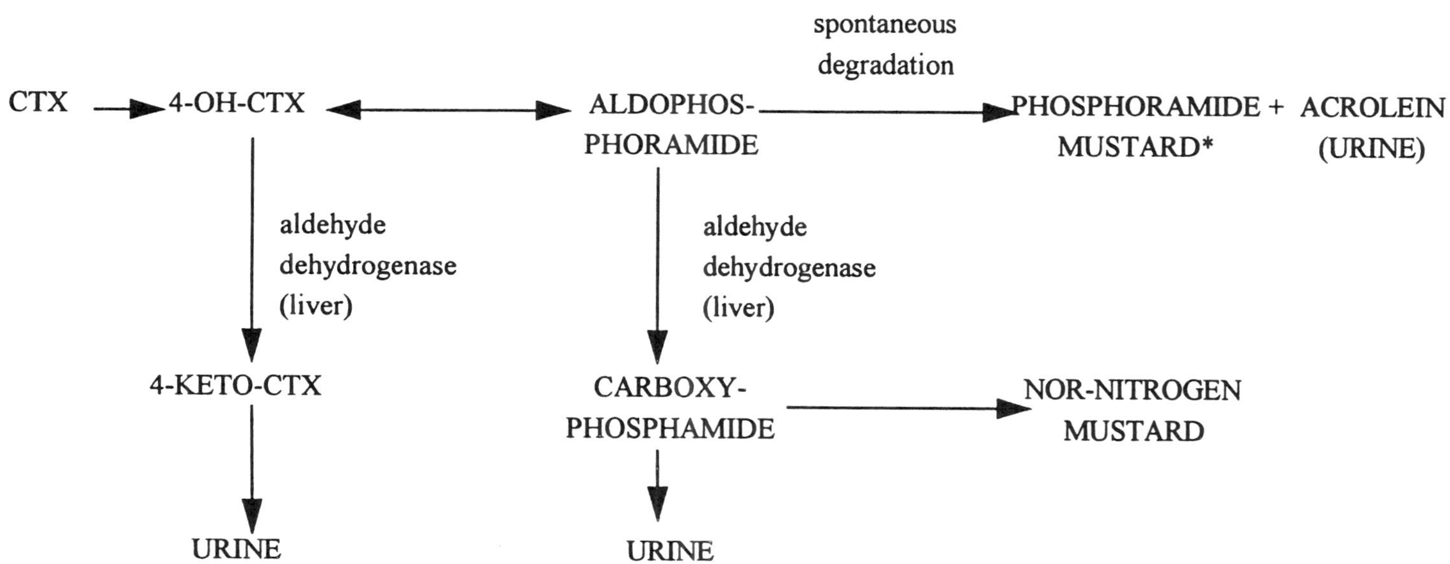

Figure 3 Metabolism of cyclophosphamide. 4-OH-CTX, 4-hydroxy-cyclophosphamide; 4-keto-CTX - 4-keto-cyclophosphamide. *Considered to be a cytotoxically active principle.

An increased incidence of leukopenia has been noted when allopurinol was administered concomitantly with CTX [14]. This presumably resulted from a prolongation of CTX half-life by allopurinol-mediated inhibition of hepatic microsomal enzymes [8]. During phenobarbital administration, the rate of CTX biotransformation is increased in two- to threefold (presumably by enzyme induction), but the quantity of metabolites measured in the urine is only minimally increased [9]. Shortening the CTX half-life is also noted when CTX has been administered for more than 6 months [8]. The alterations in kinetics associated with phenobarbital and prolonged CTX administration did not affect the toxic or chemotherapeutic properties of CTX, possibly because distribution of its cytotoxic metabolites is not influenced by hepatic enzyme induction [9]. CTX taken concomitantly with succinylcholine can prolong the action of succinylcholine; probably because CTX decreases plasma pseudocholinesterae activity [12].

III. MECHANISM OF ACTION

A. Azathioprine

AZA is converted to ribonucleotides of 6-MP (Fig. 1), which competitively inhibit enzymes needed in deoxyribonucleic acid (DNA) synthesis. The 6-MP ribonucleotides also produce feedback inhibition of 5-phosphoribosylamine, thus reducing purine biosynthesis. In RA, azathioprine reduces the numbers of circulating B and T lymphocytes (particularly suppressor, or CD8, cells) (15), mixed lymphocyte reactivity (16), immunoglobulin (Ig) M and G synthesis [15,16], and (interleukin-2) IL-2 secretion [17].

B. Alkylating Agents

The major effect of the alkylating agents is to crosslink DNA and proteins, which thereby prevents cell replication. The tissues most susceptible to the cytotoxic effects of these drugs are those undergoing the most rapid cellular turnover; namely, bone marrow cells, fetal cells, dermal epithelium, buccal and intestinal mucosa, mucosal cells of the urinary bladder, and hair follicles. These sites of action therefore are basic to an understanding not only of the efficacy of the alkylating agents but also their adverse effects.

1. Chlorambucil

Little is known about CHLOR's mechanism of action in RA. Chiappelli reported that monthly oral doses of 0.4–1.5 mg/kg in multiple sclerosis caused a dose- and time-dependent decrease in peripheral blood lymphocytes; T cells, B cells, and natural killer (NK)–effector cells, with B cells being preferentially decreased. Within the T-cell population, the number of T suppressor cells (CD8) was more profoundly reduced than the number of T helper cells (CD4) [18].

2. Cyclophosphamide

CTX is cytotoxic to both resting and dividing lymphocytes [16,19,20]. In RA patients, it suppresses helper cell function, decreases the number of activated T cells by 30–40% (which correlates with clinical improvement), and dramatically decreases B cells for months [21]. CTX suppresses primary cellular and humoral immune responses, especially if administered immediately after the antigen challenge, but it can also inhibit an established humoral or immune response. It effectively suppresses many cell-mediated immune responses, such as delayed hypersensitivity skin test, graft-versus-host reactivity of lymphoid cells, cell-mediated cytotoxicity, mitogen- and antigen-induced blastogenesis, and the production of soluble mediators. CTX also has anti-inflammatory properties [19,20].

IV. ADVERSE DRUG EXPERIENCES

The prevalence of adverse drug experiences is largely dose related. The prevalences for each agent are presented in Table 2 and are based largely on the reported experience in the rheumatic diseases, particularly where controlled studies are available.

A. Bone Marrow Suppression

Dose-related marrow suppression is the most frequent toxicity with all three cytotoxic drugs, and leukopenia is its most frequent expression [3,8,22–24]. With CHLOR lymphocyte suppression predominates, whereas with the other agents there is predominant granulocyte suppression. Nevertheless, with all three drugs it is usually granulocytopenia which is the dose-limiting bone marrow toxicity. Thrombocytopenia can occur with all three agents and is usually seen in association with leukopenia. Isolated thrombocytopenia is unusual except with CHLOR where it can be the initial evidence of marrow suppression. Anemia, like thrombocytopenia, is usually seen in association with leukopenia for all three agents. Isolated anemia or thrombocytopenia is unusual enough with

Table 2 Adverse Effects: Toxicity of DMARD

Adverse Effect	AZA	CHLOR	CTX
Dose-related marrow suppression			
Leukopenia	4–27	14–50	6–32
Thrombocytopenia	0–5	8–37	0–4
Susceptibility to infection			
Overall	0–9	18–27	0–22
Herpes zoster	0–6	4–27	5–30
GI Intolerance			
Nausea, vomiting	9–23	4	19–45
Diarrhea	≤1	—	3–18
Rash	1–6	0–18	0–2
Hair			
Alopecia	—	2	2
Hypertrichosis	—	—	2
Stomatitis	0–5	—	—
Abnormal liver function	0–5	—	—
Azoospermia/oligospermia	—	≤100	60–100
Amenorrhea	—	2–8	0–53
Cystitis	—	—	4–45
Teratogenesis	±	↑	↑
Neoplasia	↑	↑	↑
Pneumonitis	±	±	±

this group of drugs that when either occurs it should suggest other causes for the anemia or thrombocytopenia.

Although bone marrow suppression is evidence of cytotoxic action, it is not a prerequisite for efficacy, and the doses of these drugs do not have to be increased to the point of bone marrow toxicity to obtain clinical benefit. Although fatal outcomes from marrow suppression have been reported with all three agents (particularly CHLOR), suppression is usually temporary and the blood elements generally return to baseline levels when the drugs are withheld. With all three agents there is a time lag between the time the drug is administered and the time its full leukopenic effect is evidenced. The nadir of leukopenia following a single dose of any one of the three cytokines usually occurs between 7 and 14 days and, in the absence of further doses, leukopenia usually clears within 21 and 25 days. Evidence of cumulative marrow toxicity has been found with CHLOR and CTX even when examined after marrow "recovery" (usually 21–25 days). Experience suggests that daily CHLOR or CTX treatment over months can be accompanied by progressive marrow depression, so that the dosage tolerated after 2 years is lower than in the first 6 months (personal observation) [25,26]. Cumulative bone marrow suppression occurs regularly with chlorambucil and often requires discontinuation of the drug. In Cannon's study, only one of the initial 28 patients was able to continue the drug for no longer than 21 months [24]. This type of depression is usually reversible, and marrow function almost always returns to normal. It has been the observation of some investigators that after prolonged use of any of the three cytotoxics, marrow suppression can be more easily induced during administration of a second or third cytotoxic drug (personal observation) [27]. Marrow suppression can be adequately assessed by periodic complete blood counts, and the dosage of medication can be adjusted on the basis of changes in peripheral blood counts.

Bone marrow toxicity with AZA (both in renal transplant and RA patients) has been associated with genetic predisposition [5] and with low levels of purine methyltransference (which occurs in 0.3% of the population) [6,7].

B. Infections

The susceptibility to infection attributed to cytotoxic therapy probably relates to disease and/or drug-related alterations in humoral and cell-mediated immunity, to interference in the inflammatory response, to the degree of granulocytopenia, to abnormal host responses associated with the basic disease process, and to concomitant corticosteroid administration. There is an increased incidence of infectious diseases caused by ordinary as well as unusual microbes, and there is an increased morbidity and mortality as well [3,8,24,22,23,27,28]. There clearly is an increase in the prevalence of herpes zoster in all populations studied with CHLOR and CTX and probably with AZA. There is not, however, an increase in the frequency of herpes zoster dissemination beyond one or several dermatomes or in the mortality rate, which normally is 1–2% [3,8].

C. Gastrointestinal

Gastrointestinal upsets are unusual with CHLOR but are seen frequently with AZA and CTX (see Table 2). Nausea and vomiting are the principal adverse events leading to discontinuation of AZA. Vomiting with CTX may be severe, especially with high-dose intravenous CTX. In patients who are to receive intravenous CTX, this complication can usually be prevented or minimized by premedicating with antiemetics (i.e., phenothiazines, granisetron, ondansetron), corticosteroids (dexamethasone, methyl prednisolone), motility promotors (i.e., metaclopramide, cisapride), and/or hypnotics (i.e., benzodiazepines).

D. Rash

Cutaneous rashes occur with cytotoxics but only occasionally necessitate withdrawal of CHLOR, AZA, or CTX [3,8,23,24].

E. Pulmonary

The use of AZA, CHLOR, and CTX has rarely been associated with noninfectious pneumonitis and/or pulmonary fibrosis. This is characterized by chronic interstitial changes on chest radiograph and a pattern of restrictive lung disease on pulmonary function testing [3,8,24]. The onset is usually insidious, but it may be abrupt, and it usually occurs after prolonged cytotoxic therapy or after the high intravenous doses of CTX used in oncology. In some instances, the lung involvement may stabilize or improve once the cytotoxic is discontinued. Since RA itself can be associated with chronic interstitial pulmonary disease, it is often difficult to know whether the pulmonary disease is secondary to RA itself and/or to the cytotoxic therapy. The concurrent or sequential use of more than one cytotoxic drug or the use of a cytotoxic drug with radiation particularly predisposes the patients to this complication.

F. Alopecia

With AZA and CHLOR, hair loss usually consists of hair thinning rather than complete balding [3,8,22,23]. With CTX, thinning of hair may occur, but there is also a significant incidence of complete balding, particularly with intravenous administration or with higher oral doses [11]. Since the hair follicle remains intact, hair will usually regrow when the cytotoxic is discontinued, and in some subjects, hair may begin to regrow even though the cytotoxic is continued.

G. Fertility

Therapy with the alkylating agents (CHLOR and CTX) can result in male and female infertility [8,29–35]. One experience in systemic lupus erythematosus (SLE) nephritis reported that AZA plus prednisone was associated with an 18% rate of amenorrhea compared with 8% for prednisone alone [36]. The risk of infertility, azoospermia, and amenorrhea with CHLOR and CTX increases with increasing duration of therapy as well as with increasing doses [11,29]. Both agents produce the same constellation of findings. In postpubertal males, azoospermia and oligospermia are coupled with histological depletion of germinal epithelium and with elevations in plasma levels of follicle-stimulating hormone. This suggests that the alkylating agents cause a primary failure of spermatogenesis: as noted in Chapman's review [32], irreversible azoospermia was regularly produced in adult males who had received >18 g total dose of CTX or >400 mg of CHLOR. Conversely, plasma testosterone levels remained normal, as did the histological appearances of Leydig's and Sertoli's cells, suggesting sparing of hormonal function. Theoretically, therefore, libido and sexual function in males should not deteriorate solely because of cytotoxic therapy.

In postpubertal females, both gametogenesis and hormonal function are altered adversely, and menopause occurs. This drug-induced menopause occurs with increasing frequency as women age [29,32–35]: As noted in Damewood's review [33], the total mean dose of CTX needed to produce amenorrhea was 5.2 g in women >40 years of age, 9.3 g in 30- to 39-year-old women, and 20.4 g in 20- to 29-year-old women. Wang's recent report on 92 CTX-treated women with SLE [35] showed that rates of amenorrhea increased with increasing age and increasing cumulative oral CTX dose (Table 3), which supports Damewood's observations. This medication-induced menopause is characterized by decreased serum and urinary estrogen levels, increased levels of urinary gonadotropins, loss of follicular maturation, absence of ova, and increased amounts of ovarian fibrosis. These findings are consistent with total primary ovarian failure.

Reports of the reappearance of fertility following drug discontinuation have appeared, but azoospermia and amenorrhea are usually permanent once they have appeared. Less than 10% of CTX-treated women had a return of menses if the gonadotropin levels were elevated or ovarian histology was abnormal [33]. Younger women who were treated less than 9 months with CTX were more likely to have reversible amenorrhea [33]. Few men had a return of spermatogenesis once CTX was discontinued, and few reports have appeared of paternity in males who had stopped therapy with CTX even before they had become sterile [33]. The chances that fertility will return are inversely proportional to the length of time the drug was administered as well as to the drug doses employed.

In general, prepubertal males and females seem to be protected from the sterilizing effects of the alkylating agents as long as these agents are discontinued prior to the onset of puberty [30,32,33]. Several reports have appeared, however, describing sterility in subjects who had received high cumulative doses in their prepubertal years. In general, prepubertal and pubertal males developed normal spermatogenesis when the total CTX doses were <200 mg/kg, temporary oligospermia and azoospermia with doses between 200 and 365 mg/kg, and irreversible azoospermia with doses >365 mg/kg [33]. Ovulation and menses regularly developed in females who had been treated previously in prepuberty and puberty with CTX in total doses <525 mg/kg [37]. Permanent azoospermia virtually always developed in males who had been treated in prepuberty or puberty with doses of CHLOR > 25 mg/kg [37]. No data are available regarding the appearance of menses in females who had been treated in puberty and prepuberty with CHLOR.

Table 3 Rates (as %) of Permanent Amenorrhea Related to Different Age Groups and Cumulative Dose of Oral CTX

Age group	Cumulative dose of CTX (g)		
(years)	0–20	20–40	>40
14–20	0	0	30
21–30	0	38	25
31–40	33	58	100

Although recent studies employing oral contraceptives (OCPs) or progestins in humans [37] and inhibitors of gonadotropin-releasing hormone (GnRH) in mice, rats, and dogs [8] suggest promising strategies for protecting gonadal function from cytotoxic damage, their clinical efficacy is still unproven [38].

H. Cystitis

Urological problems are limited to CTX [8,29]. These urological adverse effects are thought to be related to the urinary metabolite, acrolein, rather than to CTX itself [11,29,39]. Hemorrhagic cystitis has been reported in about one-third of subjects receiving oral CTX daily. In a few instances, it has necessitated surgical removal of the bladder. There is, in addition, a significant but lesser incidence of bladder fibrosis and bladder carcinoma, with and without antecedent cystitis [38,39]. In many, but not all, subjects with cystitis, the urinary abnormalities (pyuria, hematuria) will be accompanied by symptoms of bladder irritability such as urinary frequency and dysuria.

Urological toxicity can probably be reduced if subjects take the drug as one dose daily in the morning coupled with copious fluid intake. The high fluid intake dilutes the toxic metabolites and flushes the bladder, reducing the metabolite concentration making contact with the bladder and reducing the time it is present. 2-Mercaptoethane sulfonate (Mesna) has recently been approved by the FDA to treat or prevent CTX-induced urological toxicity and is preferred over bladder irrigation [13]. Since Mesna is intravenously administered, its use is usually limited to those subjects receiving intermittent bolus intravenous CTX. Urological toxicity also decreases when CTX is administered intravenously on an intermittent schedule of once monthly or once every 3 months (even at 1000 mg/m^2) [40].

I. Teratogenesis

The available evidence (skimpy as it is) suggests that alkylating agents have teratogenic potential [29,41–43]. The issue is clouded by the fact that very few pregnancies occur in women taking alkylating agents, because the women quickly become infertile. The experience with teratogenesis is known for first-generation progeny; the risk to second-generation progeny is largely unknown.

Roubenoff's review [41] reported only nine living pregnancies were reported in women receiving CTX and six living pregnancies in those taking CHLOR. The malformation rate was 22% in CTX-treated and 33% in CHLOR-treated women compared with the expected congenital malformation rate of 2.0–3.5% in the general population, but the confidence intervals were very wide (10.2–44.0% for CTX; 6.8–96.4% for CHLOR). By its very design, Roubenoff's review was admittedly prone to report excessively high malformation rates with drugs, because the selection and publication biases in case reports is weighted toward poor outcomes.

The largest experiences of the use of AZA in pregnancy overall is in renal transplant patients, whereas in rheumatic diseases, it is in women with systemic lupus erythematosus (usually with glomerulonephritis). Although some data suggest that the risk of teratogenesis with AZA use is low [42–44], other data suggest that its use may be associated with intrauterine growth retardation, prematurity, transient immunosuppression of the neonate, and possible effects on the germline of the offspring [45].

J. Carcinogenesis

The uncertainty regarding the carcinogenic potential of the cytotoxics remains a major concern of patients and practitioners alike even though the cytotoxics have been available for almost four decades. Analysis of drug-related neoplasia in the rheumatoid diseases has been complicated by the unresolved issue of whether there is or is not an increased risk of malignancy (particularly of the hematopoietic and lymphatic systems) in RA patients untreated by cytotoxic drugs. Although some studies have suggested that RA patients have an increased relative risk as high as 8.7 times expected of developing cancers of the lymphatic and hematopoietic system (i.e., Hodgkin's and non-Hodgkin's lymphoma multiple myeloma, and leukemia), others have failed to substantiate such an increase [3,8].

A 50-fold increase in relative risk of malignant disease has been documented in azathioprine-treated renal transplant patients (particularly non-Hodgkin's lymphoma) [46]. In RA, the azathioprine -related risk of lymphoma (and non-Hodgkin's lymphoma) is confounded by the possibly increased relative risk secondary to RA per se [15]. Overall, there is probably a small added relative risk (about 1.3) of developing *some* type of malignancy when using azathioprine in RA [3] and a relative risk of between 2.2 and 8.7 for developing a lymphoproliferative disorder [3,15]. Reversible lymphoma has been documented during AZA use [47].

Kinlen reported a large clinical experience with cytotoxic therapy in the United Kingdom and Australia [48,49] involving 3823 renal transplant recipients and 1634 patients without transplants, of whom 643 were RA patients. The risk of cytotoxic-related neoplasia was clearly increased in transplant patients who had received CTX, but the risk of drug-related neoplasia in 1634 nontransplant patients (68% of whom received AZA and 28% CTX) was much less [49]. In the CTX treated RA group, the overall relative risk for all cancers combined was 12.8, for non-Hodgkin's lymphoma it was 10.9, and for bladder cancer it was 10.0.

Other evidence suggests that CTX and CHLOR may be associated with an increased risk of neoplasia, particularly of the skin and hematological systems [8,24,50–52]. In a case-control study of 119 RA patients treated with CTX, Radis [51] reported that the relative risk for the development of any type of malignancy in patients was 1.5. The risk was statistically significant for bladder ($P < .001$) and skin neoplasia ($P < .04$) with a trend toward hematological neoplasia ($P = .06$). Baltus [52] reported a relative risk of developing malignancy (particularly hematological and lymphoreticular) of 4.1 (95% confidence interval of 1.5–19.0) in 81 RA patients treated with CTX when compared with 81 RA patients who had not received CTX. Hazelman, in a small study of 34 patients with RA, presented data which conflicts with Kinlen's. Hazelman's data suggests that RA is itself associated with an increased risk of neoplasia and that patients treated with AZA and/or CTX had their risk of cancer reduced by almost 50% [53].

Some studies suggest that CHLOR and CTX may also be associated with an increased risk of acute leukemia [8]. In Kahn's study, an incidence of acute leukemia of 0.93% was reported in a group of 1711 RA patients (only two-thirds of whom were followed up) treated with chlorambucil. This incidence is considered by some investigators to be a severalfold increase in relative risk [8,50].

In summary, the overall risk of cytotoxic-related carcinogenesis appears to be severalfold (reports range from 1.0 to 12.8) for the alkylating agents. In particular, there is a significant increase in bladder cancer following oral CTX. The increase in the risk for neoplasia overall occurs both during and for some time following cytotoxic treatment. It probably increases in proportion to cumulative dose and increasing duration of cytotoxic therapy. Recent analysis of a small number of SLE-nephritis patients suggests that there may not be an increased malignancy risk associated with bolus, intermittent intravenous CTX [54].

V. CLINICAL EXPERIENCE

The alkylating agents are probably the most effective (and arguably among the most toxic) DMARDS presently available for the treatment of RA. Their efficacy in RA has been supported by multiple open trials of CHLOR and CTX. CTX is the only alkylating agent adequately evaluated in multiple controlled studies. Only one placebo-controlled trial of CHLOR has been reported.

Multiple studies (both open and controlled) support AZA's efficacy in RA. AZA is clearly superior to placebo. Multiple studies suggest that its efficacy is equal to CTX, GSTM, DPA, CyA, and chloroquine but marginally not as good as methotrexate.

A. Azathioprine

1. *Placebo-controlled Studies*

Azathioprine 1.25–3.0 mg/kg/day is clearly more effective than placebo in RA [3,15]. There appears to be a dose-response relationship in RA; comparing placebo, 1.25 mg/kg/day, and azathioprine and 2.50 mg/kg/day (although the data are not completely consistent) [15]. Cseuz reported that 300 mg of AZA given as a single oral dose on Monday, Wednesday, and Friday in 13 RA patients had a therapeutic advantage (without increased toxicity) over daily dosing (100–150 mg/day) in 15 comparison RA patients over the 12 weeks of study [55].

2. *Positively Controlled Comparative Studies*

There have been at least 12 double-blind controlled trials comparing AZA with other DMARDs [15,56–58] (see Table 4): AZA has been compared with CTX in two trials (one of which also compared AZA with chloroquine in the same trial), to DPA in three trials, to Cya in two trials, to MTX in four trials, and to GSTM in two trials. With the exception of MTX (for which two of the four trials showed a statistical superiority for MTX, whereas two 2 showed a trend in favor of MTX), there was not an overall difference in efficacy of AZA compared with CTX, DPA, CyA, GSTM, or chloroquine.

With the exception of four trials, which had 117, 121, 206, and 212 patients each, the remainder entered fewer than 100 patients. Most of the trials were, therefore, too small to be definitive. Furthermore, the trials were only of 6–24 months in duration.

In general, AZA takes 4–6 months to reach maximum effectiveness. No placebo-controlled trial showed AZA to retard bone destruction, although several experiences have suggested that AZA was as effective in retarding bone destruction as CTX and GSTM; agents for which there are data to suggest that they themselves may retard bone destruction [15,59]. Approximately 40–60% of RA patients stop taking AZA by 2 years; mostly for adverse effects rather than lack of efficacy [15]. In addition, crossover studies reveal that synovitis recurs within 3–6 weeks of switching from AZA to placebo [15].

Table 4 Trials in Which AZA was Compared with Other DMARDs (GSTM, DPA, CyA, MTX, CTX, Chloroquine)[a]

Trial		No. patients	Trial duration (months)	Outcome
GSTM				
Currey	1974[b]	121	18	GSTM = AZA
Dwosh	1977[c]	33	6	GSTM = AZA
DPA				
Berry	1976	65	12	DPA = AZA
Paulus	1984	206	6	DPA = AZA
Halberg	1984	74	24	DPA = AZA
CyA				
Førre	1987	24	6	CyA = AZA
Druger	1994	117	6	CyA = AZA
MTX				
Hamdy	1987	42	6	MTX = AZA
Bell	1988	34	5	MTX = AZA
Jeurrison	1991	64	11	MTX > AZA
Willkens	1992	212	6	MTX > AZA MTX + AZA > AZA
CTX				
Currey	1974[b]	121	18	CTX = AZA
Levy	1975	42	6	CTX = AZA
Miscellaneous				
Dwosh	1977[c]	33	6	Chloroquine = AZA

[a]These trials were cited or reviewed in references 15, 56–58.
[b]Currey 1974 compared GSTM, AZA, and CTX (cited twice).
[c]Dwosh 1977 compared AZA, chloroquine, and GSTM (cited twice).

3. Summary

The studies cited above allow us to make the following statements about AZA use in RA:

1. AZA is clinically effective in doses ≥1.25 mg/kg/day, with the usual dose being between 1.25–3.0 mg/kD/day. One small study suggested that 300 mg of AZA on Monday, Wednesday, and Friday may be more effective than smaller daily doses (100–150 mg/day).
2. There are not major differences between the clinical efficacies of AZA compared with CyA (1.0–3.0 mg/kg/day), CTX, GSTM, DPA, and chloroquine.
3. There are data which suggest that MTX is marginally superior to AZA in clinical efficacy, but the addition of AZA to methotrexate is not more efficacious than MTX alone.

B. Chlorambucil

1. Placebo-controlled Studies

One double-blind placebo-controlled study of CHLOR has been reported in RA and reviewed by Amor [3] (25 patients received CHLOR and 23 received placebo over 3 months). The mean dose of CHLOR in that study was 10 mg/day (the initial dose of 0.2 mg/kg/day was reduced as dictated by adverse effects). Multiple clinical and serological parameters improved significantly in the CHLOR-treated group as compared with the placebo-treated group. No long-term outcome (beyond 3 months of study) of this experience has been reported. When 13 of the patients initially allocated to placebo were later treated in an open fashion with CHLOR 0.2 mg/kg/day, 9 were declared "responders."

2. *Positively Controlled Comparative Studies*

One controlled, randomized study has addressed the addition of CHLOR to ongoing, well-tolerated but incompletely effective DMARD treatment over a 1-year period [60]. In that study, CHLOR was added to ongoing intramuscular GSTM, 60 mg weekly, or to ongoing DPA, 1.0–1.5 g daily. When the GSTM + CHLOR group of 6 patients was compared with the GSTM alone of 12 patients, and the DPA + CHLOR group of 5 patients was compared with the DPA alone group of 12 patients, it was evident that the addition of CHLOR resulted in significant improvements in inflammatory joint scores over the 2-year period study. A group of patients randomized to the combination of GSTM + DPA had better clinical outcomes than either of the CHLOR groups. "Cure-like remissions" or ARA-type remissions were seen in one-third of the GSTM + DPA group but less often in the GSTM + CHLOR or the DPA + CHLOR groups. Two of the 11 patients taking CHLOR with GSTM or DPA withdrew before the 2-year period (mainly for toxicity), whereas 6 of the 24 GSTM alone or DPA alone control groups withdrew (mainly for lack of efficacy).

3. *Uncontrolled Studies*

The reported uncontrolled experience in which CHLOR has been used to treat RA has been reviewed thoroughly previously and the reader is referred to these sources for details [8,24]. Suffice it to say that the reported experience has been largely from France (where it has been a favorite cytotoxic for the treatment of rheumatoid disease) and to a lesser extent from Australia, Russia, and the United States. The overall rate of response has been about 70% when the series are viewed as a whole, realizing that the definition of "response" varied widely from series to series. Although most series have employed doses of 0.1–0.3 mg/kg/day, at least initially, Cannon [24] used a mean dose of 0.06 mg/kg/day. Although Cannon's "response" rate was similar to the collective series using the higher doses, he noted a very high drop-out rate, with only 1 of the initial 28 subjects continuing drug for longer than 21 months. The drop-outs were from lack of efficacy in 9 patients and toxicity, mainly hematological, in 18 patients. Conversely, Thorpe was able to continue the majority of his patients on drug for longer than 5 years, albeit on much lower doses than his initial starting doses of 0.1–0.3 mg/kg/day [28].

No studies have addressed the issue of whether CHLOR retards bone destruction. The time lag before a therapeutic effect is obtained is somewhat dose dependent, but it is reported to be between 2 and 9 months. In patients who have responded, the time to flare after the drug has been discontinued is usually prolonged, with only 45–55% having flared at 6–12 months.

4. *Summary*

The studies cited above allow us to make the following statements about the use of CHLOR in RA:

1. CHLOR is probably effective clinically when given orally in doses ≥0.1 mg/kg/day and definitely effective in doses ≥0.2 mg/kg/day (good responses in about 70% of treated subjects).
2. If CHLOR has to be discontinued after patients have shown a favorable response, the ameliorative effect of CHLOR often remains for prolonged periods (i.e., only about 50% in one series flared at 6–12 months).
3. Many patients will be unable to take CHLOR for prolonged periods of time, because toxicity (primarily hematological) is often prolonged: In one study of 28 subjects, 27 discontinued CHLOR within 21 months even though CHLOR was used in a low mean dose of 0.06 mg/kg/day.
4. The addition of CHLOR to GSTM or DPA may improve the ameliorative effect of GSTM or DPA.

C. Cyclophosphamide

1. Placebo-controlled (Oral) Studies

In placebo-controlled trials, oral CTX has consistently been clinically better than placebo when used in doses ≥1.5 mg/kg/day [8]. It has not, however, been consistently effective in doses <1.0 mg/kg/day [8]. The measures that have consistently improved in these trials have included morning stiffness, joint counts (including joint tenderness and joint swelling), patient and physician overall assessments, grip strength, sedimentation rate, and rheumatoid factor assessments. CTX also has been shown to have steroid-sparing characteristics. CTX reaches its peak of effectiveness after approximately 16 weeks. Two small studies have shown that CTX can retard bone destruction: one study of CTX at 1.5 mg/kg/day for 18 months and a second study of CTX at 2.0 mg/kg/day for 8 months [8].

2. Positively Controlled Comparative Studies

When CTX has been compared with other DMARDs, it has been deemed equal or superior in clinical efficacy to GSTM, and it has been equal to AZA in clinical efficacy [8]. In the Currey study, CTX was found to be equal to AZA but superior to GSTM in retarding bone destruction [59].

All DMARDS are associated with frequent adverse effects, some of which are dose dependent. CTX is clearly more toxic than GSTM, DPA, hydroxychloroquine (HCQ), or AZA with particular concern for neoplasia, infertility, and hemorrhagic cystitis from CTX.

3. Uncontrolled (Oral) Studies

In addition to supporting the efficacy of CTX in the treatment of RA, uncontrolled studies have suggested several additional characteristics:

1. Long-term studies, some of which were extensions of controlled studies, have suggested that the peak level of effectiveness occurred after approximately 16 weeks and that the level of efficacy remained constant for at least 25 months [8,61].
2. Stajanovic [62] withdrew CTX from 32 patients who had improved during 19 months of CTX. Sixteen maintained remission for 41 months following withdrawal of CTX.
3. Several reports have suggested that some nonarticular complications of RA, such as necrotizing scleritis/keratitis, interstitial lung disease, cutaneous ul-

cers, and peripheral neuropathy, may respond to oral or intravenous CTX as well as to other DMARDS [8,63,64].

4. Alternative Methods of Administration

Intravenous Pulse Regimens. In Hall's study [65], intravenous CTX given as a 5–10 mg/kg dose every 7 days produced such severe nausea and vomiting that it was discontinued after only 1 month. On the other hand, when Hall gave intravenous CTX (5–10 mg/kg) coupled with bolus intravenous methyl prednisone (MP) (750 mg bolus) every 1–2 weeks for 5 doses in a 6-week period (followed by oral CTX 2 mg/kg/day on alternate weeks), it was relatively well tolerated. This latter regimen failed to alter the clinical assessments of arthritis, although it did significantly improve the "thermographic index" at 2 and 3 months. In Walter's study [66], one dose of intravenous CTX (1 g/m^2) given with intravenous MP alone or with intravenous MP + GSTM did not alter the outcome of intravenous MP alone or of intravenous MP + GSTM. In Arnold's study [67], 500–1000 mg of intravenous CTX given every 4–6 weeks for six doses did not provide any significant improvement over background treatment.

Conversely, Scott [63] reported that intravenous CTX (500–100 mg) plus intravenous MP (500–1000 mg) given at baseline to a group of patients with systemic rheumatoid vasculitis and again on days 8, 29, and 50 produced dramatic improvement in vasculitic lesions and reductions in relapse rates, serious complications, and mortality (usually within 4 months); in some instances, improvement was noted within 24 hs. After day 50, most of the patients were continued on oral maintenance therapy, including 2 mg/kg/day of AZA (15 patients) or 1.5 mg/kg/day of CTX (5 patients). Relapses were seen in 24% of the patients at 4–48 months after the initial intravenous CTX + intravenous MP treatment. Five of these patients developed sepsis during the 48 months of follow-up.

Intermittent Oral Regimens. In Hall's study [65], 1 mg/kg/day oral CTX was ineffective. In the same study, a second group of patients, who received alternating oral CTX at 2 mg/kg/day and no CTX on alternate weeks, failed to show significant clinical improvement over the 12-month study period. The "thermographic index" did, however, show significant improvement at 9 and 12 months in the alternate-week group.

Horslev-Peterson [68] reported the use of oral CTX given once every 4 days in three patients who had had leukopenia when receiving oral daily CTX for 5–22 months. Even though the three patients had incompletely responded to daily oral CTX in the face of leukopenia, they did respond over the next several months to doses of oral CTX every 4 days. It should be noted that two of these patients also received intermittent intravenous MP during the follow-up.

Combination Studies. In two open uncontrolled studies, low-dose oral CTX was given in combination with two other DMARDs: In Tiliako's study [69], 25 mg/day of oral CTX was given to 12 subjects, in combination with 400 mg/day of HCQ and 5 mg/week of oral MTX, with "good" improvement (50–90%) in clinical parameters. In the Csuka study [70], oral CTX at an average dose of 30 mg/day was given to 31 subjects in combination with 74 mg/day of AZA and 210 mg/day of HCQ, again with good clinical response (i.e., complete or partial "remission" in 30 of 31 patients). Recortication of erosions was noted in about 50% of patients in both studies; however, some of the same patients were also noted to have new erosions in other areas. Since most of the subjects in these two practice-based studies had been resistant to previous therapies, it was suggested that low-dose CTX in combination with two other DMARDs was more effective than previous, often single, DMARD therapy. Although it was hoped that CTX would have less toxicity when given in low-doses, four patients developed malignancies in the Csuka study [70]. Other subjects developed macular changes, herpes zoster, pneumonia, cystitis, and infections. It was the malignancies, however, which prompted the investigators to change the DMARD regimen to include MTX instead of CTX.

4. Summary

The studies cited above allow us to make the following statements about the use of CTX in the treatment of RA:

1. CTX is clearly effective clinically in oral doses ≥1.5 mg/kg/day and inconsistently effective or ineffective at doses <1 mg/kg/day, at least when given as a single DMARD.
2. CTX probably retards bone destruction in RA.
3. CTX is equivalent in clinical efficacy to AZA or GSTM and may be superior to GSTM in retardation of bone destruction.
4. At a dose of 2 mg/kg/day given on alternate weeks, CTX was not clinically effective.
5. CTX was not effective when given as a single bolus of 1 g intravenously or six intravenous doses (500–1000 mg each) administered intermittently every 4–6 weeks. This contrasts with the single experience where intravenous CTX combined with intravenous MP at the same setting (on days 1, 8, 29, 50) showed a favorable response of rheumatoid vasculitis. At that, 24% of the patients had a relapse of vasculitis during the 48-month follow-up period which usually included oral AZA or CTX.
6. The addition of intravenous MP to the intravenous CTX regimen seems to ameliorate the acute toxicity of intravenous CTX (i.e., nausea, vomiting, and leukopenia).
7. Even though oral CTX in combination with HCQ and MTX or with HCQ and AZA may provide good clinical efficacy with healing of erosions, toxicity is unacceptable.

VI. FINAL RECOMMENDATIONS

The alkylating agents (particularly CTX) are arguably the most effective DMARDs presently available. However, they cause too much toxicity (carcinogenicity, infertility, bone marrow suppression and, for CTX, hemorrhagic cystitis and bladder cancer) for routine use. They should be used primarily to treat patients with the most severe and recalcitrant type of rheumatoid arthritis. There are two situations where the potential benefits are likely to outweigh the nearly certain adverse effects.

1. The clearest indication for the use of alkylating agents is rheumatoid vasculitis (inflammatory arteritis) manifested by necrotizing scleritis/keratitis, cutaneous ulcerations, neuropathy (particularly mononeuritis multiplex), and/or other vascular complications which characterize periarteritis nodosa. These patients also usually have nodular, severely, deforming RA, their prognosis is poor, their life span is shortened, and there is high morbidity. This group of patients warrants oral CTX at doses of 2 mg/kg/day or the intravenous regimen of intravenous CTX with intravenous MP out-

lined by Scott above [63]. Even so, once the vasculitic component has come under control, an attempt to switch to a different, less risky DMARD is suggested.

2. A less clear indication might be the class II–III latex-positive patient with deforming RA who has failed all on other DMARDs (either for lack of effect or because of intolerance) and who still has active, severe RA. In this instance, oral CTX at 2 mg/kg/day or CHLOR at 0.1–0.2 mg/kg/day might be considered. Here too once the disease has come under control, switching to one or more less toxic DMARDs should be considered.

There is minimal evidence to suggest that RA patients can effectively be treated by intermittent pulses of oral or intravenous CTX alone. Therefore, oral CTX daily is the preferred route for most eligible patients. After 50 mg/day is started orally (start low to check for sensitivity), the dose should be increased gradually to 1.5–2.0 mg/kg/day. Toxicity should be screened in accord with recent guidelines [45]. A CBC should be obtained at baseline and every 2 weeks while the CTX dose is being changed. Once the CTX dose has been stable for 1–2 months, a CBC should be obtained every 1–3 months. For CTX, a routine urinalysis (RUA) should also be obtained at baseline and repeated every 1–3 months, screening for pyuria and/or hematuria. Urine should be evaluated for cytology every 6 months after CTX is discontinued. CTX doses should be reduced in the presence of renal failure and when given with concomitant succinyl choline or allopurinol. If intravenous CTX is administered, the patient can be given Mesna, antiemetics, steroids, and sedatives to prevent or reduce adverse effects.

Alternatively, CHLOR can be employed at a starting dose of 0.1–0.2 mg/kg/day. A CBC with platelet count should be obtained at baseline every 2 weeks while the CHLOR is being adjusted and every 1–2 months thereafter.

AZA is an easy agent to administer. If there were not concerns about its possible neoplastic potential, it would undoubtedly be more widely employed. As noted above, its efficacy is as good as, or better than, most of the other DMARDs, with the possible exception of MTX, which may be more efficacious; but because AZA may have neoplastic potential, it is often employed after HCQ, MTX, azulfidine, GSTM, and even DPA have failed.

Because some patients can be very sensitive to its leukopenic potential, AZA should be started at 50 mg/day. If leukopenia has not occurred in 1–2 weeks, the dose can be raised gradually to 1.5–3.0 mg/kg/day. A CBC should be obtained at baseline and every 2 weeks while the dose is being adjusted. Once the AZA dose is stable, a CBC should be obtained every 1–3 months. Liver and kidney function (i.e., ALT/AST, serum creatinine) should be screened at baseline and periodically thereafter. Dosage reductions are suggested with concomitant use of allopurinol or in the presence of liver or renal failure.

REFERENCES

1. Hench PS, Kendall EL, Slocumb CH, Polley HF. The effect of a hormone of the adrenal cortex (17-hydroxy-11-dehydroxycorticosterone; compound E) and of pituitary adrenocorticotropic hormone on rheumatoid arthritis: A preliminary report. Mayo Clin Proc 1949; 24:181–197.
2. Fosdick WM, Parsons JL, Hill DF. Long term cyclophosphamide therapy in rheumatoid arthritis. Arthritis Rheum 1968; 11:151–161.

3. Clements PJ. Cytotoxic immunosuppressive drugs. In: Paulus HE, Furst DE, Dromgoole SH, eds., Drugs for Rheumatic Diseases. New York: Churchill Livingstone, 1987:135–156.
4. Elion GB, Hitchings GH. Azathioprine. Handbook Exp Pharmacol 1975; 38:404–425.
5. Ohlman S, Albertioni F, Peterson C. Day-to-day variability in azathiprine pharmacokinetics in renal transplant recipients. Clin Trans 1994; 8(Suppl 3, Pt 1):217–223.
6. Lennard L, Van Loon JA, Weinshilboum RM. Pharmacogenetics of acute azathioprine toxicity: relationship to thiopurine methyltransferase genetic polymorphism. Clin Pharmacol Ther 1989; 46:146–154.
7. Weinshilboum RM. Methylation pharmcogenetics: thiopurine methyltranferase as a model system. Xenobiotica 1992; 22:1055–1071.
8. Clements PJ. Alkylating agents. In: Dixon J, Furst D, eds. Second Line Agents in the Treatment of Rheumatic Diseases. New York: Marcel Dekker, 1992:335–361.
9. Grochow LB, Colvin M. Clinical pharmacokinetics of cyclophosphamide. Clin Pharmacol 1979; 4:380–394.
10. Juma FD, Rogers HJ, Trounce JR. The pharmacokinetics of cyclophosphamide, phosphoramide mustard and nor-nitrogen mustard studied by gas chromatography in patients receiving cyclophosphamide therapy. Br J Clin Pharmacol 1980; 10:327–335.
11. Kovarsky J. Clinical pharmacology and toxicity of cyclophosphamide. Emphasis on use in rheumatic diseases. Semin Arthritis Rheum 1983; 12:359–372.
12. Moore JM. Clinical pharmacokinetics of cyclophosphamide. Clin Pharmacokinet 1991; 20:194–208.
13. Vose JM, Reed EC, Pippert GC, et al. Mesna compared with continuous bladder irrigation as uroprotection during high-dose chemotherapy and transplantation: a randomized trial. J Clin Oncol 1993; 11:1306–1310.
14. Boston Collaborative Drug Surveillance Program. Allopurinol and cytotoxic drugs. Interaction in relation to bone marrow depression. JAMA 1974; 227:1036.
15. McKendry RJR. Purine analogs. In: Dixon J, Furst DE, eds. Second Line Agents in the Treatment of Rheumatic Diseases. New York: Marcel Dekker, 1991:223–243.
16. Cannon GW, Ward JR. Cytotoxic drugs and combination drug therapy. In: McCarty DJ, Koopman WJ, eds. Arthritis and Allied Conditions, 12th ed. Philadelphia: Lea & Febiger, 1989:645–664.
17. Bacon PA, Salmon M. Modes of action of second line agents. Scand J Rheum 1987; 64(Suppl):17–24.
18. Chiappelli F, Myers LW, Ellison GW, et al. Preferential reductions in lymphocyte sub-populations induced by monthly pulses of chlorambucil: studies in patients with chronic multiple sclerosis. Int J Immunopharmacol 1991; 13:455–461.
19. Klinenberg JR, Reichman R, Clements PJ. Investigational therapy for rheumatoid arthritis. In: Cohen AS, ed. Progress in Clinical Immunology, Vol. 1. Orlando, FL: Grune & Stratton, 1984:111–144.
20. Tsokos GC. Immunomodulatory treatments in patients with rheumatic diseases: mechanism of action. Semin Arthritis Rheum 1987; 17:24–38.
21. Lacki JK, Schochat T, Sobieska M. Immunological studies in patients with rheumatoid arthritis treated with methotrexate or cyclophosphamide. Z Rheumatol 1994; 53:76–82.
22. Whisnant JK, Pelkey J. Rheumatoid arthritis: treatment with azathioprine: clinical side-effects and laboratory abnormalities. Ann Rheum Dis 1982; 41(Suppl):44–47.
23. Singh G, Fries JF, Spitz P, Williams CA. Toxic effects of azathioprine in rheumatoid arthritis. A national post-marketing perspective. Arthritis Rheum 1989; 32:837–843.
24. Cannon GW, Jackson CG, Samuelson CO Jr, et al. Chlorambucil therapy in rheumatoid arthritis: clinical experience in 28 patients and literature review. Semin Arthritis Rheum 1985; 15:106–118.
25. Lohrmann H-P. The problem of permanent bone marrow damage after cytotoxic drug treatment. Oncology 1984; 41:180–184.

26. Fauci AS, Young KR Jr. In: Kelly WN, Harris ED JR, Ruddy S, Sledge CB eds. Immunoregulatory Agents in Textbook of Rheumatology, 4th ed. Philadelphia: Saunders, 1993:797–821.
27. Fauci AS, Haynes BF, Katz P, Wolff SM. Wegener's granulomatosis: prospective clinical and therapeutic experience with 85 patients for 21 years. Ann Intern Med 1983; 98:76–85.
28. Thorpe P, Hassall JE, York JR. Rheumatoid arthritis treated with chlorambucil: a five-year follow-up. Med J Aust 1976; 2:197–199.
29. Schein PS, Winokur SH. Immunosuppressive and cytotoxic chemotherapy. Long-term complications. Ann Intern Med 1975; 82:84–95.
30. Schilsky RL, Lewis BJ, Sherins RJ, Young RC. Gonadal dysfunction in patients receiving chemotherapy for cancer. Ann Intern Med 1980; 93(Pt 1):109–114.
31. Tabbara KF. Chlorambucil in Behçet's disease. Ophthalmology 1983; 90:906–908.
32. Chapman RM. Gonadal injury resulting from chemotherapy. Am J Indust Med 1983; 4:149–161.
33. Damewood MD, Grochow LB. Prospects for fertility after chemotherapy or radiation for neoplastic disease. Fertil Steril 1986; 45:443–458.
34. Boumpas DT, Austin HA, Vaughn EM, et al. Risk for sustained amenorrhea in patients with systemic lupus erythematosus receiving intermittent pulse cyclophosphamide therapy. Ann Intern Med 1993; 119:366–369.
35. Wang, CL Want F, Bosco JJ. Ovarian failure in oral cyclophosphamide treatment for systemic lupus erythematosus. Lupus 1995; 4:11–14.
36. Austin HA III, Klippel JH, Balow JE, et al. Therapy of lupus nephritis. Controlled trial of prednisone and cytotoxic drugs. N Engl J Med 1986; 314:614–619.
37. Chapman RM, Sutcliffe SB. Protection of ovarian function by oral contraceptives in women receiving chemotherapy for Hodgkin's disease. Blood 1981; 58:849–851.
38. Klippel JH. Cyclophosphamide: ovarian and other toxicities [editorial]. Lupus 1995; 4:1–2.
39. Plotz PH, Klippel JH, Decker JL, et al. Bladder complications in patients receiving cyclophosphamide for systemic lupus erythematosus or rheumatoid arthritis. Ann Intern Med 1979; 91: 221–223.
40. Balow JE, Boumpas DT, Fessler BJ, Austin HA III. Management of lupus nephritis. Kidney Int 1996; 49:S88–S92.
41. Roubenoff R, Hoyt J, Petri M, et al. Effects of anti-inflammatory and immunosuppressive drugs on pregnancy and fertility. Semin Arthritis Rheum 1988; 18:88–110.
42. Ostensen M. Treatment with immunosuppressive and disease modifying drugs during pregnancy and lactation. Am J Reprod Immunol 1992; 28:148–152.
43. Bermas BL, Hill JA. Effects of immunosuppressive drugs during pregnancy. Arthritis Rheum 1995; 38:1722–1732.
44. Ramsey-Goldman R, Mientus JM, Kutzer JE, et al. Pregnancy outcome in women with systemic lupus treated with immunosuppressive drugs. J Rheumatol 1993; 20:1152–1157.
45. American College of Rheumatology Ad Hoc Committee on Clinical Guidelines. Guidelines for monitoring drug therapy in rheumatoid arthritis. Arthritis Rheum 1996; 39:723–731.
46. Kloppenberg M, Dijkmons BA, Breedveld FC, et al. Antimicrobial therapy for rheumatoid arthritis. Clin Rheumatol 1995; 9:759–769.
47. Larvol L, Soule JC, Le Tourneau A. Reversible lymphoma in the setting of azathioprine therapy for Crohn's disease. N Engl J Med 1994; 331:883–884.
48. Kinlen LJ, Scheil AGR, Peto J, Doll R. Collaborative United Kingdom-Australian study of cancer in patients treated with immunosuppressive drugs. Br Med J 1979; 2:1461–1466.
49. Kinlen LJ. Incidence of cancer in rheumatoid arthritis and other disorders with immunosuppressive treatment. Am J Med 1985; 78(Suppl A):44–49.
50. Kahn MF, Arlet J, Bloch-Michel H, et al. Leucemies aîgues après traîtement par agents cytotoxiques en rheumatologies: 19 obsérvations chez 2006 patients. Nouv Presse Med 1979; 8:1393–1397.

51. Radis CD, Kahl LE, Baker GL, et al. Effects of cyclophosphamide on the development of malignancy and on long-term survival of patients with rheumatoid arthritis. Arthritis Rheum 1995; 38:1120–1127.
52. Baltus JAM, Boersma JW, Hartman AP, Vandenbroucke JP. The occurrence of malignancies in patients with rheumatoid arthritis treated with cyclophosphamide: a controlled retrospective follow-up. Ann Rheum Dis 1983; 43:368–373.
53. Hazelman BL. Incidence of neoplasms in patients with rheumatoid arthritis exposed to different treatment regimens. Am J Med 1985; 78(Suppl A):39–43.
54. Pando JA, Gourley MF, Boumpas DT, et al. Risks of malignancy in patients with lupus nephritis treated with bolus cyclophosphamide (CY). Arthritis Rheum 1994; 37:S179.
55. Cseuz R, Zimmerman J, Panayi GS. Daily and alternate-day azathioprine treatment in rheumatoid arthritis: a twelve-week controlled clinical trial. Br J Rheumatol 1992; 31:501–504.
56. Jeurissen MEC, Boerbooms AMTH, van de Putte LBA, et al. Influence of methotrexate and azathioprine on radiologic progression in rheumatoid arthritis. A randomized double-blind study. Ann Intern Med 1991; 114:999–1004.
57. Willkens RF, Urowitz MB, Stablein DM, et al. Comparison of azathioprine, methotrexate, and the combination of both in the treatment of rheumatoid arthritis: a controlled trial. Arthritis Rheum 1992; 35:849–856.
58. Kruger K, Schattenkirchener M. Comparison of cyclosporin A and azathioprine in the treatment of rheumatoid arthritis—results of a double-blind multicentre study. Clin Rheumatol 1994; 13:248–255.
59. Currey HL, Harris J, Mason RM, et al. Comparison of azathioprine, cyclophosphamide, and gold in treatment of rheumatoid arthritis. Br Med J 1974; 3:763–766.
60. Bitter T. Combined disease-modifying chemotherapy for intractable rheumatoid arthritis. Clin Rheum Dis 1984; 10:417–428.
61. Fosdick WM, Parsons IL, Hill DF. Long term cyclophosphamide therapy in rheumatoid arthritis: A progress report, six years' experience. Arthritis Rheum 1969; 12:663.
62. Stojanovic I, Budincia M, Nikdic J. Duration of improvement of rheumatoid arthritis after good response to cyclophosphamide treatment. Scand J Rheumatol 1978; 7:1–2.
63. Scott DGI, Bacon PA. Intravenous cyclophosphamide plus methylprednisolone in treatment of systemic rheumatoid vasculitis. Am J Med 1984; 76:377–384.
64. Messmer EM, Foster CS. Destructive corneal and scleral disease associated with rheumatoid arthritis. Medical and surgical management. Cornea 1995; 14:408–417.
65. Hall ND, Bird HA, Ring EFJ, Bacon PA. A combined clinical and immunological assessment of four cyclophosphamide regimes in rheumatoid arthritis. Agents Action 1979; 9:97–102.
66. Walters MT, Cawley MID. Combined suppressive drug treatment in severe refractory rheumatoid disease: an analysis of the relative effects of parenteral methylprednisolone, cyclophosphamide, and sodium aurothiomalate. Ann Rheum Dis 1988; 47:924–929.
67. Arnold MH, Janssen B, Schrieber L, Brooks PM. Prospective pilot study of intravenous pulse cyclophosphamide therapy for refractory rheumatoid arthritis. Arthritis Rheum 1989; 32:933–934.
68. Horslev-Peterson K, Beyer JM, Helin P. Intermittent cyclophosphamide in refractory rheumatoid arthritis. Br Med J 1983; 287:711–712.
69. Tiliakos NA. Low-dose cytotoxic drug combination therapy in intractable rheumatoid arthritis. Two years later [abstr]. Arthritis Rheum 1986; 29(Suppl 4):S79.
70. Csuka ME, Carrera GF, McCarty DJ. Treatment of intractable rheumatoid arthritis with combined cyclophosphamide, azathioprine, and hydroxychloroquine. A follow-up study. JAMA 1986; 255:2315–2319.

14

Combination Disease-modifying Antirheumatic Drug Therapy In Rheumatoid Arthritis

H. James Williams
University of Utah,
Salt Lake City, Utah

I. INTRODUCTION

As our understanding of the pathogenesis and destructive nature of rheumatoid arthritis (RA) has increased, the treatment of the disease has become more aggressive. The recognition that the progression of RA may be most rapid in the first 2 years of the disease [1] and the desire to modify the disease process before erosive changes occur has resulted in the recommendation to use the so-called disease-modifying antirheumatic drugs (DMARDs) earlier in the course of the disease [2]. However, the means of identification of patients that may benefit from early aggressive therapy has not been clarified [3]. These individual DMARDs used singly with a background of nonsteroidal anti-inflammatory drugs (NSAIDs) and/or low doses of prednisone have shown efficacy in numerous short-term studies comparing these agents with placebo. These agents, the proposed mechanisms of action, and the efficacy and safety data are contained in other chapters in this book. The efficacy of the different agents appears to be similar in most comparative trials comparing two DMARDs.

Despite these apparent successes and the development of several drugs with "disease-modifying" potential, patients continue to have progressive deformity and disability. True remissions, as defined by the American College of Rheumatology [4], are exceptional. The implication that these medications are truly disease modifying is not well documented and the relentless progression of joint destruction continues in those patients most severely affected with RA [5,6]. Severe RA continues to result in both long-term morbidity and increase mortality [7,8]. It has been suggested that the mortality risk in patients with RA is similar to that seen in stage IV Hodgkin's disease or three-vessel coronary artery disease [9].

Many patients who initially respond to DMARDs eventually lose that response, and these patients experience persistent clinical and radiographic disease progression [10,11]. Fewer then half of the patients receiving a given DMARD continue to take that specific medication longer than 2 years [12,13], and less than 25% of the patients take a given drug for 5 years [13]. Methotrexate is an exception, with more than 50% of the patients continuing this medication for 5 years [13].

II. RATIONALE FOR USE OF COMBINATIONS OF DRUGS

Because of the paucity of long-term effective and remittive therapy, rheumatologists have looked at the success of oncologists and infectious disease specialists in using combinations of drugs to achieve improved treatment outcomes. Multiple-drug chemotherapy of lymphoproliferative malignancies has resulted in better patient survival and even eradication of some disease. Some observers have labeled RA as a "nonmalignant B-lymphoproliferative disease" [14], and others have suggested that the pannus leads to bony erosions by behaving like a locally invasive tumor [15]. This suggests that a similar approach to that of the oncologist may be beneficial.

There is a rationale for the use of combinations of DMARDs [3,16]. The inflammatory process is incredibly complex, and it is possible that two drugs with mechanisms of action at different sites in the process may have some synergy that results in greater efficacy than can be achieved with either drug alone. Alternatively, medications in combination could perhaps be used at lower individual doses than usually recommended with similar or greater efficacy but with less toxicity. Also, multiple simultaneous approaches to drug therapy may result in eradication of the disease process similar to the cure of certain cancers with multiple drugs or broad-spectrum coverage of infectious diseases. Out of a sense of desperation from lack of other approaches to treatment of patients with resistant disease, one investigator [16] has suggested that combinations might be used without strong scientific support.

III. EARLY UNCONTROLLED EXPERIENCE WITH COMBINATION DMARD THERAPY

A. Use by Practicing Rheumatologists

Many practicing rheumatologists have utilized combination DMARD therapy over the years either out of the desperation mentioned above or as an overlap of treatments to prevent a regression of the disease which might occur when one medication is discontinued before a replacement drug has time to become effective. Paul Young in North Carolina and Arthur Scherbel in Ohio used combinations of these drugs in their respective practices for several decades with apparent acceptable outcomes, but the results were never published or reported [17].

A mail survey to investigate the use of antimalarials by 92 Canadian and 77 Australian rheumatologists revealed that the combination of an antimalarial and parenteral gold was used by 45% of the Canadians and 31% of the Australians. The combination of penicillamine and an antimalarials was used by 31% of the rheumatologists in Canada and 18% of the rheumatologists in Australia [18].

McCarty described his personal experience with combination drug therapy in an editorial published in 1990 [19]. Over a 16-year period, McCarty had personally seen 196 new patients, of which he estimated that nearly 50% were referred by other rheumatologists for RA intractable to usual therapy. He had followed 97 of these patients for at least 1 year and some as long as 16 years. Of these 97 patients, only 11 had remained on single DMARD therapy and the other 86 had taken a combination of two or more DMARDs. All patients followed for more than 1 year were reported to have satisfactory disease control. Three patients required four DMARDs, whereas 31 were on two DMARD combinations, but the majority (52 patients) needed a combination of three DMARDs to obtain this control.

B. Response of RA to Cancer Chemotherapy

The experience of combination chemotherapy in RA patients who are treated for concurrent cancer also is enlightening. Two women with active erosive seropositive RA developed acute myelogenous leukemia. The RA and the leukemia went into remission after treatment with cytosine arabinoside, daunorubicin hydrochloride, and m-AMSA [20]. One patient remained in remission for both diseases after 8 months. The other woman had a recurrence of the RA after 13 months, although the leukemia remained in remission. However, the RA is reportedly much less aggressive than it had been prior to the chemotherapy. Her rheumatoid factor had fallen with the initial chemotherapy and had become elevated again at the time of consolidation therapy. The rheumatoid factor fell with consolidation therapy and has remained low even though the synovitis has returned.

Another woman with seropositive RA as well as immunoglobulin A deficiency subsequently evolved features suggestive of an overlap connective tissue disease. A few years later, she developed symptoms of fever and weight loss and was diagnosed with Hodgkin's disease. The woman was treated with nitrogen mustard (later changed to cyclophosphamide because of myelosuppression), vincristine, procarbazine, and prednisone, and her RA and overlap connective tissue disease remitted [21]. Severe RA, but not the other connective tissue disease symptoms, recurred after 3 years.

C. Early Combination DMARD Use in RA

The use of combination DMARD therapy to treat resistant RA patients was first reported in an open study of Sievers and Hurri in 1963 [22]. These investigators used the combination of an antimalarial (usually chloroquine) and parenteral gold in 248 patients and described increased improvement or remission in more patients on the combination therapy than in comparison groups of patients treated with either drug used alone.

However, it was not until the report of McCarty et al. [23], in 1982, that enthusiasm for combination therapy emerged. These investigators reported 17 patients with progressive erosive RA that was refractory to conventional therapy. The patients were on stable doses of hydroxychloroquine and were then treated with relatively small doses of either cyclophosphamide or azathioprine. The other cytotoxic drug was then added. The mean daily doses of these drugs were 221 mg for hydroxychloroquine, 38.5 mg for cyclophosphamide, and 55 mg for azathioprine. Disease suppression was reported within 16 months in 14 of the 17 patients with remissions described in 5 patients. Side effects of the treatment regimen were considered minor by the McCarthy et al. except for four patients in whom treatment was discontinued.

A follow-up study by the same group [24] reported that all but 1 of 31 RA patients responded to the regimen after a mean of 9 months. The three patients termed failures in the first report responded to longer therapy. Sixteen patients were considered to have gone into disease remission. The mean daily maintenance doses of the three drugs were 210 mg for hydroxychloroquine, 30 mg for cyclophosphamide, and 74 mg for azathioprine. However, three patients developed malignancies and one developed erythroleukemia. Three of these patients died. Seven other patients had one or more drugs stopped for adverse effects.

These dramatic efficacy results led to other trials and reports of combinations of DMARDs in the treatment of RA.

IV. TWO DMARD COMBINATIONS

Many studies employing combinations of two DMARDs have been reported, although the majority have been nonrandomized open trials. Several reviews of combination DMARD therapy have been written which summarize many of these trials [16,25–28]. Drugs that are considered DMARDs for this discussion include auranofin, injectable gold salts, hydroxychloroquine (or chloroquine), methotrexate, azathioprine, penicillamine, sulfasalazine, cyclosporin, cyclophosphamide, and chlorambucil. The latter two drug are used less frequently because of their oncogenicity [29,30]. Other agents are also being studied as potential DMARDs.

It was expected that combination DMARD therapy would be more efficacious than single-agent DMARD treatment, and this assumption is supported by the published case reports and uncontrolled or unblinded studies. These reports were even more remarkable, since many of them involved patients with severe RA that was considered intractable or refractory to conventional therapy.

However, randomized controlled trials have been less impressive. In the majority of these blinded studies, combination therapy has not been significantly better than a single agent. In a few studies, there is a suggestion that combination therapy may even be worse [31]. Although many of these studies suffered from small numbers of patients with the possibility of type II error, the actual measured differences among groups were generally small and probably not clinically meaningful. Also, a meta-analysis of controlled trials comparing combination therapy to single-drug therapy failed to demonstrate any meaningful advantage for a combination of drugs [32]. There was a small difference in the improvement of the tender joint count but at the cost of increased toxicity. Although randomized studies preclude bias by the observer or the patient, the study populations are also highly selected and may not represent the response of an individual patient or the population of patients seen in clinical practice [33].

The question of the benefit of combination DMARD therapy is still open, and well-designed randomized controlled trials with adequate numbers of patients are necessary to determine whether two drug combinations are effective and which drugs used in concert are most advantageous and which are the safest [16]. The sequence of administration of these agents also requires investigation. The combinations can be given with sequential or additive administration of different drugs, simultaneous institution of several drugs, or delivery of the drugs in some rotational manner or with intermittent pulses of one or more medications [3].

V. MULTIPLE DRUG COMBINATIONS

Part of the rationale for using combination DMARD therapy came from the success of the oncologists in treating hematological malignancies with multiple drugs. The use of multiple DMARDs in patients with RA has not been studied in randomized controlled trials but anecdotal reports have been encouraging. McCarty [19] continues to recommend small doses of several drugs with proven efficacy in controlled trials of single DMARD therapy; perhaps to prevent or delay the clonal expansion of resistant inflammatory cells. He recommends the use of whatever medication needed to suppress the inflammation.

Wilske and Healey [34] have proposed a "step-down bridge" concept of therapy. Patients with RA are initially treated with prednisone 10 mg per day for 1 month. Patients who do not adequately respond to the prednisone are then started on a combination of multiple DMARDs. Any combination is acceptable, but the investigators recommend methotrexate, injectable gold, auranofin, and hydroxychloroquine. As the arthritis responds to the therapy, drugs are discontinued, one at a time until a maintenance level of only one medication is achieved. In their example, they discontinue the methotrexate, then the injectable gold, followed by the auranofin, which leaves the patient on hydroxychloroquine. Methotrexate and prednisone can be used intermittently as needed for flares of the disease activity.

Wilke and Clough [27] have suggested a similar approach which they call "graduated-step therapy." New patients with RA are categorized by a disease activity index and then a treatment paradigm is used that is based on the severity of disease. The more severe the RA, the greater number of DMARDs used in treatment. Patients with mild disease receive hydroxychloroquine and NSAIDs. For those patients with moderate diseases, a second DMARD is added to the regimen. This additional DMARD may be auranofin, sulfasalazine, or methotrexate. Severe disease is treated with three DMARDs, adding parenteral gold, penicillamine, and azathioprine to the list of possible medications. Patients are evaluated regularly and a change in disease severity category may result in a change in therapy.

The use of multiple DMARDs in combination is intriguing but needs vigorous scientific evaluation before it can be considered anything more than experimental.

VI. SELECTION OF COMBINATIONS OF DMARDS

The challenge in the selection of reasonable combinations of DMARDs persists. Ideally, the combinations of DMARDs selected should be based on differing mechanisms of action, drug efficacy, and/or lack of overlapping toxicities.

A. Efficacy and Mechanism of Action

Unfortunately, a detailed understanding of the mechanism of action of these agents in RA is lacking or incomplete and selection is more often by differing drug class, such as an alkylating agent and a folic acid antagonist. This latter method is less logical than desired and may have no relevance. For example, it has been suggested that the use of two antifolate drugs may increase toxicity [35]. However, it has been shown that two drugs with antifolate activity, methotrexate and sulfasalazine, have been well-tolerated when used together without any increase in toxicity over methotrexate alone [36,37].

Direct comparisons of two DMARDs used as single-drug therapy often fails to identify significant differences in efficacy. Many of these trials have limited numbers of patients so that small differences will not be identified. Felson et al. [38] performed a large meta-analysis of controlled and comparative trials of DMARDs and concluded that there was little difference in efficacy among methotrexate, parenteral gold, penicillamine, or sulfasalazine but that auranofin and hydroxychloroquine were somewhat weaker agents. Furst [39] also reviewed multiple trials and determined that methotrexate and parenteral gold were the most effective DMARDs followed by azathioprine and penicillamine. Auranofin, hydroxychloroquine, and sulfasalazine were identified as the least effective DMARDs. Pincus et al. [13] evaluated the probability of continuation of DMARD therapy and demonstrated that methotrexate was the most likely to be continued, with 50% of courses continuing for more than 60 months. Auranofin was the agent most likely to be discontinued, with 50% of courses continuing for only 10 months. Hydroxychloroquine, penicillamine, parenteral gold, and azathioprine were comparable, with 50% of courses continuing for 20–27 months. With the variability of estimates of efficacy, it is difficult to select combination therapy based on this measure.

B. Toxicity

Toxicity is another variable in selecting combination therapy. It has been assumed that some DMARDs were less toxic than others, including auranofin, hydroxychloroquine, and sulfasalazine [40]. This assumption was based on the severity of the adverse reactions as well as their frequency. However, this assumption has not been directly investigated [38]. Felson et al. [38], in the meta-analysis mentioned above, evaluated withdrawals for toxicity and concluded that auranofin and hydroxychloroquine were the least toxic followed by penicillamine, azathioprine, and sulfasalazine, with injectable gold being the most toxic DMARD. The ARAMIS data identified relative toxicities among DMARDs by use of a toxicity index score [41]. Using the assistance of patients, rheumatologists, and other health professionals, they assigned weighting scales to certain untoward drug effects [42], although not all rheumatologists may agree with the weightings. For instance, diarrhea is weighed at 7.8, whereas rash is only 4.7, and heartburn is 3.8. The conclusion was reached that hydroxychloroquine was the least toxic DMARD followed by parenteral gold, which was followed by penicillamine, methotrexate, and azathioprine. Auranofin was the most toxic, and sulfasalazine was not evaluated.

C. Specific Adverse Reactions

Certain adverse effects of selected DMARDs may make them less desirable for use in combination therapy. Because of the oncogenic potential of cyclophosphamide, Csuka et al. [24] recommended that it should be replaced in the regimen that they reported. Also, a DMARD with nephrotoxicity, such as cyclosporin A, should only be used with great caution if combined with a DMARD that is dependent on the kidney for excretion. Many of the combinations will be determined safe only by the method of trial and error. The combination of gold and penicillamine seems to have several disadvantages. Toxicity is similar between the two drugs, and penicillamine is a chelator of heavy metals. However, the combination of the two has been tried successfully and without unreasonable toxicity [14]. In the published studies at this time, no unanticipated catastrophic events have been described [16].

Selecting an effective combination of drugs by mechanism of action, efficacy, or toxicity does not appear to be realistic at this time. Much of the future of combination therapy will still be intuitive or theoretical.

VII. SPECIFIC COMBINATION DMARD TRIALS

Two drugs frequently used in combination DMARD studies are hydroxychloroquine and methotrexate. Sulfasalazine is also becoming a frequent choice.

A. Two DMARD Combinations Including Antimalarials

1. Gold

Sievers and Hurri [22] compared 248 RA patients treated with antimalarial and gold injections with 240 patients treated with antimalarials alone in an unblinded, nonrandomized trial. Chloroquine was the antimalarial used in a dose of 200–400 mg/day, although a few patients received hydroxychloroquine 400 mg/day. Gold sodium thiomalate or aurothioglucose was given intramuscularly in a dose of 50 mg/week for at least 12 weeks. Patients were hospitalized for an average of 3.4 months. The investigators reported that 36% of the patients treated with antimalarials alone demonstrated major improvement or remission compared with 43% of the patients on the combination therapy. Patients with less severe disease did even better.

In a similar 12-month randomized, placebo-controlled trial, Scott et al. [43] treated 101 RA patients with sodium aurothiomalate 50 mg/week for 20 weeks and then 50 mg every 2 weeks. These patients were randomized to receive either hydroxychloroquine 400 mg per day for 6 months and then 200 mg/day or placebo. Fifty-two patients received the combination therapy. Although the patients who completed 12 months on combination therapy improved more than the patients on gold alone in all variables measured, this improvement was only statistically significant for the change in C-reactive protein and a disease activity index. However, 18 patients on hydroxychloroquine withdrew for adverse drug effects, whereas only 10 patients on placebo withdrew for this cause. It was concluded that the two-drug combination was more effective but also more toxic.

A different conclusion was reached by Porter et al. [44], who studied 142 patients with RA who had a suboptimal response to parenteral gold therapy after 6 months of treatment. These patients were randomized to hydroxychloroquine 400 mg/day or placebo and followed for another 6 months. There was no difference found in efficacy or toxicity between the two treatment groups.

2. Penicillamine

In a small 2-year randomized double-blind controlled trial, Bunch et al. [31] treated 56 patients with hydroxychloroquine (2.2 mg/kg/day), penicillamine (7 mg/kg/day), or the combination of both. The 17 patients on both drugs manifested less improvement than patients on either single-drug treatment. Interestingly, the combination therapy was associated with less toxicity than penicillamine alone and similar toxicity to hydroxychloroquine.

In a 1-year single-blind randomized study by Gibson et al. [45], 72 patients were assigned to chloroquine 250 mg/day, penicillamine 750 mg/day, or the combination of both. All groups showed improvement, but there were no differences in clinical response among the groups. Laboratory and radiological measures favored the two groups receiving penicillamine. Untoward drug effects were higher in patients on penicillamine and were slightly increased in the patients receiving both drugs. Withdrawals for adverse effects were higher on combination therapy.

Martin et al. [46] briefly reported a 6-month trial of penicillamine and hydroxychloroquine given singly and in combination to 45 patients in an open trial. The doses used are not given and there are no outcome results or statistics. They conclude that the results suggest an advantage for the combination therapy.

3. Methotrexate and Sulfasalazine

The HCQ/MTX Study Group reported an unusual trial in an abstract in 1993 [47]. One hundred and forty-one patients were treated for 24 weeks with hydroxychloroquine 400 mg/day and methotrexate with a mean dose of 9 mg/week. At the end of this open phase, 121 patients were randomized to a double-blind trial to continue hydroxychloroquine while using pulse methotrexate for any disease flares, a similar group with placebo for flares, and a group on placebo with pulse methotrexate for flares. All three groups showed significant improvement during both phases of the study, and the investigators concluded that patients improve on the combination therapy, that maintenance therapy with hydroxychloroquine delays onset and duration of flares, and that methotrexate-treated flares are shortened in duration in patients on maintenance hydroxychloroquine.

In a controlled trial, Ferraz et al. [48] randomized 82 patients to receive either methotrexate 7.5 mg/week and chloroquine 250 mg/day or methotrexate and placebo. Sixty-eight patients completed 6 months of treatment, and the combination group had a significantly lower joint count, greater grip strength, and better functional ability than the group on methotrexate alone. Fifteen patients on the combination therapy had mild adverse drug reactions compared with eight patients on methotrexate alone. Elevation of liver transaminases was more common in the group receiving the combination of drugs.

A group of investigators in Denmark compared hydroxychloroquine and sulfasalazine to hydroxychloroquine or sulfasalazine given alone in a randomized controlled trial of 91 patients [49]. After 6 months of therapy, there was no difference between the combination therapy and patients receiving sulfasalazine alone, but the combination therapy was statistically superior to hydroxychloroquine alone in the improvement in the number of swollen joints and in the patient assessment of disease activity. The two single-drug treatment groups were comparable in efficacy. Toxicity was similar among all three treatment groups.

Schwarzer et al. [50] performed an open pilot study of 16 patients who had failed three or more DMARDs given as single-drug therapy. The patients were treated with hydroxychloroquine 400 mg/day for 4 weeks and then 200 mg/day. Sulfasalazine 2 g/day and pulse oral methotrexate 10 mg/week were given in alternating months. The patients improved at 3 months, but after 12 months, the only improvement was in the pain score and in the erythrocyte sedimentation rate. Eight of the patients did not complete the study; four were withdrawn for lack of efficacy and four had adverse drug effects. Although open studies with a sample size this small cannot give definitive conclusions, the results of this study do not encourage the alternate use of combinations of second-line agents.

B. Two DMARD Combinations Including Methotrexate

1. Antimalarials

See Section VII.A.3.

2. Gold

Injectable gold has not been adequately evaluated in combination with methotrexate. Brawer [51] anecdotally reported seven patients who relapsed after a mean of 4 years on injectable gold therapy. Methotrexate, in a mean dose of 11.5 mg/week, was added to the gold with a recapture of the good response with an average follow-up of 19 months.

Auranofin was evaluated with methotrexate in a randomized controlled trial comparing the combination to each drug given alone [52]. Three hundred and thirty-five patients were followed for 48 weeks in the three-arm trial; auranofin 6 mg/day, methotrexate 7.5 mg/week, or the combination of both. No remissions were seen, and there were no statistically significant differences among the three groups in the clinical and laboratory variables measured. Patients taking auranofin alone had a slower onset of response than either group taking methotrexate. Withdrawals for adverse drug effect was slightly more common on the combination therapy, but withdrawals for lack of efficacy were slightly less common in this group. Except for this lesser withdrawal rate for lack of response, no advantage was seen for combination therapy.

In 267 patients who were previously untreated with DMARDs, Kantor et al. [53] started auranofin and methotrexate. After a 6-month open study phase, 89% of the patients had responded with at least a 50% reduction in total joint count and a physician's global assessment of good or very good. One hundred and seventy-four patients were randomized to another 6-month double-blind phase to either auranofin alone or to continue the combination. Benefits obtained during the 6-month open study were maintained in 74% of the combination patients and in 51% of the auranofin patients. Toxicity did not appear to be greatly increased on combination therapy.

3. Sulfasalazine

Nisar et al. [36] reported their experience with 32 patients treated with methotrexate and sulfasalazine and compared the tolerability and toxicity to 63 patients treated with methotrexate alone. Doses of the two medications were standard but variable. Mean duration of combination therapy was 23 months. Five patients on the combination discontinued methotrexate; one for lack of response and four for toxicity. Seventeen patients on methotrexate alone discontinued the drug; seven for toxicity. The conclusion was made that there was no increase in toxicity for combination therapy compared with methotrexate used alone.

Shiroky et al. [37] described four patients treated for a mean of 24 months with methotrexate and sulfasalazine. In three of these patients, adequate disease control was not accomplished with high-dose pulse methotrexate, but the patient responded to the addition of sulfasalazine. Attempts to discontinue either DMARD were unsuccessful. The other patient, who also had Crohn's disease, had RA that did not respond to sulfasalazine but improved after methotrexate was added to the regimen.

In a report of community experience with the combination of methotrexate and sulfasalazine, Morand et al. [54] described 31 courses of treatment in 29 patients. Fifteen of the courses were in patients who originally received methotrexate with the addition of sulfasalazine, whereas the other 16 were in the reverse order. Only one patient had the combination discontinued for adverse drug reaction and five patients stopped the treatment for lack of response. The investigators state that the cumulative probability of continuation of the combination at 24 months was 74%, which is at least equal to single-drug therapy.

A Dutch study [55] describes 40 patients without adequate response to 3 g of sulfasalazine who were then randomly assigned to methotrexate (7.5–15.0 mg per week) or to methotrexate and sulfasalazine. After 24 weeks in this unblinded study, the group on the combination therapy was significantly more improved than the group on methotrexate alone. Only one patient on the combination was withdrawn for a possible drug reaction.

4. *Penicillamine*

In a retrospective study [56] of 16 patients who had a partial response to penicillamine in a mean dose of 750 mg/day, methotrexate (mean dose of 10 mg/week) was added to the treatment program. There were no dropouts for drug intolerance. Eight patients achieved a complete remission which was sustained in seven of the patients for 3–72 months.

5. *Cytotoxics*

In 1971, Fosdick [57] reported his experience with 16 patients who had failed to respond to 12 months of cyclophosphamide therapy. Methotrexate was added in an unknown dose, and only one patient failed to respond and six were in complete remission after at least 8 weeks of treatment. Toxicity was tolerable but not well described.

Willkens et al. [58] described a 48-week prospective, randomized, double-blind trial of methotrexate and azathioprine. Two hundred and nine patients were assigned to three treatment groups: methotrexate (15 mg/week), azathioprine (150 mg/day), or methotrexate (7.5 mg/week) and azathioprine (100 mg/day). A crossover was allowed at 24 weeks. After 24 weeks of therapy, the groups receiving methotrexate alone and the combination had a similar response which was greater than azathioprine alone but not statistically significant. At 48 weeks, the methotrexate group had a higher response rate than the combination which was greater than sulfasalazine, but again there was no statistical significance.

6. *Cyclosporine*

In a study recently reported, Tugwell et al. [59] described 148 patients in a randomized, double-blind trial of 6 months' duration. All patients were receiving maximum tolerated doses of methotrexate (≤15 mg/week) with substantial, but only partial, response to disease activity. One group was given cyclosporin 2.5–5.0 mg/kg/day and the other received placebo. Patients on the cyclosporin had a net improvement of 25% in both tender and swollen joint count as compared with placebo. Significant differences were seen in patient and physician assessment of disease activity, joint pain, and degree of disability. Thirty-six patients on active drug met the criteria for remission, whereas only 12 patients on methotrexate and placebo met that definition. Withdrawals for adverse drug effect were slightly higher on the cyclosporin (nine patients versus five). Only one patient was withdrawn from the study for an unacceptable elevation of serum creatinine.

C. Two DMARD Combinations Including Sulfasalazine

1. *Antimalarials*

See Section VII.A.3.

2. *Methotrexate*

See Section VII.B.3.

3. *Gold and Penicillamine*

Dawes et al. [60] added sulfasalazine to 25 patients who had shown a partial response to gold or penicillamine. The combination therapy was given for 6 months, and 22 of the patients showed meaningful improvement in seven of eight clinical and laboratory measures.

The converse of the above study was done by Farr et al. [61], who selected 38 patients on established sulfasalazine therapy in a dose of 1.5–3.0 g per day and added either penicillamine, beginning at 125 mg/day and increasing to 1 g/day, or sodium aurothiomalate 50 mg/week until 1-g cumulative dose and then monthly injections. In this open study, 9 patients received the gold, whereas 29 were given penicillamine. Three patients on gold and nine on penicillamine were subsequently withdrawn for drug toxicity. A favorable response was seen in 70% of the patients, with two patients obtaining a remission. Farr et al. felt that the sequential approach to combination therapy helped to minimize the toxicity of combinations of DMARDs.

In another open study, Taggart et al. [62] divided 30 patients into two treatment groups. The first received 2 g of sulfasalazine daily and the second group received the same dose of sulfasalazine plus penicillamine 500 mg daily. After 6 months, the only remission was seen in a patient on combination therapy, and the combination group showed greater improvement with nine responders compared to only six responders in the sulfasalazine group. However, withdrawals for adverse drug effects were seen in six patients on combination therapy and in three patients on single-drug treatment.

4. *Azathioprine*

Waterman [63] treated 14 patients resistant to sulfasalazine or azathioprine alone with the combination of both drugs in an unblinded trial. Sulfasalazine was given in a dose of 1 g/day to 11 patients and in a dose of 2 g/day in three. The azathioprine was given in a dose of 50 mg/day in one patient and a dose of 100 mg/day in the remainder. After a mean of 14 months of treatment, the number of swollen joints had fallen in 9 patients and 11 patients were deemed by the physician to have had a good or excellent response.

D. Two DMARD Combinations Including Gold

1. *Antimalarials*

See Section VII.A.1.

2. *Methotrexate*

See Section VII.B.2.

3. *Sulfasalazine*

See Section VII.C.3.

4. *Penicillamine*

Paulus reported an abstract by McKenna et al. [16] in which they described 45 RA patients who were randomized to gold sodium thiomolate (50 mg/wk), penicillamine (500 mg/day), or the combination of both in a 6-month double-blind trial. Efficacy occurred earlier in the combination group, but efficacy and toxicity were otherwise similar among the three groups.

However, Bitter [14] took 42 patients who had failed approximately 1 year of high-dose injectable gold therapy (sodium thiopropanol 150 mg/week) and sequentially assigned them to one of four treatment groups. The first group continued gold therapy alone. The second group continued the gold with the addition of penicillamine 1 g/day. The third group continued the gold but added levamisole 150 mg/day for three consecutive days each week. The final group continued gold but added chlorambucil 5 mg/day. Patient dropouts were replaced so that all patients completed at least 18 months of treatment. Two of the 12 patients on gold alone achieved remission, whereas 8 of the twelve on gold and penicillamine achieved the same level of response. Six of 12 patients on gold and levamisole and 3 of 6 patients on gold and chlorambucil also achieved remission. Bitter concluded that high-dose gold and penicillamine were not antagonistic but induced remissions in some intractable patients without increased levels of toxicity.

5. Other

In the study mentioned above [14], Bitter was "disappointed" with the improvement seen in most of the combinations tested, including the combination of gold and chlorambucil. Only six patients received this regimen for 1 year. Nevertheless, one patient was considered to be in remission.

Walters and Cawley [64] selected 17 patients with severe RA and gave them a single intravenous bolus of methylprednisolone (15 mg/kg). Thirteen of the patients had improvement. A concomitant single intravenous pulse of cyclophosphamide (1 g/m^2) did not give any additional benefit, but the addition of 24 weekly injections of gold prolonged the improvement from the pulse methylprednisolone. The prolongation of response seen with gold was seen whether or not the patient also received cyclophosphamide.

E. Two DMARD Combinations Including Penicillamine

1. Antimalarials

See Section VII.A.2.

2. Methotrexate

See Section VII.B.4.

3. Sulfasalazine

See Section VII.C.3.

4. Gold

See Section VII.D.4.

5. Other

In the study by Bitter [14] that has been cited previously, an additional 29 patients were treated with penicillamine in a dose of 1 g/day with a inadequate response. These patients were sequentially assigned to remain on penicillamine alone, add levamisole to the penicillamine, or add chlorambucil (5 mg/day) to the penicillamine. Only five patients entered into the latter group. Bitter was "disappointed" in the combination of penicillamine and chlorambucil, although one patient achieved remission and the improvement appeared to be better than that seen with penicillamine alone. Three patients were considered failures on the combination treatment.

F. Multiple DMARD Combinations

The experience of McCarty and this coworkers [23,24] with multiple DMARD treatment in open studies has previously been discussed. The recommendation of Wilske and Healey [34] for the step-down bridge approach to therapy and the Wilke graduated-step therapy [27] utilizing several DMARDs simultaneously have also been discussed above.

In a report of an open study of the Wilke approach, Biro et al. [65] treated 20 patients on hydroxychloroquine, methotrexate, and azathioprine. All patients had failed previous therapy with either of the latter two drugs used in combination with hydroxychloroquine. The alternative drug was added to the regimen and improvement after 12 months was impressive. For example, the mean joint count decreased from 11.4 to 3.3. Toxicity was minimal, and only one patient was removed from the treatment for stomatitis.

Butler and Tiliakos [66] randomly assigned 18 patients with RA intractable to gold or penicillamine to one of three treatments: hydroxychloroquine (400 mg/day), methotrexate (5 mg/week), and cyclophosphamide (25 mg/day); methotrexate (10 mg/week); or previous therapy without immunosuppressive agents. After 6 months, the first two groups had similar clinical improvement, but four of five patients in the combination group demonstrated recortication of erosions, whereas patients in the other two groups developed new erosions.

In a follow-up report [67] after 16–25 months, 12 patients on the three-drug combination had improved 50–90%, whereas patients on methotrexate alone had improved 30–40% and the third group was unchanged. Recortication of erosions occurred in seven patients on the combination treatment. Only one patient discontinued the combination for stomatitis, although two others discontinued the hydroxychloroquine and one patient left the study as a personal preference.

Twelve other patients who were failures to single-DMARD therapy were treated by an Israeli group [68] with hydroxychloroquine (400 mg/day for 1 month and then 200 mg/day), methotrexate (5.0–12.5 mg/week), and azathioprine (25–50 mg/day). Four patients left the study after 3–4 months; three for lack of response and one for nausea. After 14–18 months of therapy, seven of the eight remaining patients had responded with one of the patients going into remission. The investigators considered the combination promising.

O'Dell et al. [69] have reported partial results of a randomized double-blind trial in 79 RA patients who have failed at least one DMARD. There were three treatment groups: methotrexate (7.5–17.5 mg/wk), hydroxychloroquine (200 mg twice daily), and sulfasalazine (500 mg twice daily); hydroxychloroquine and sulfasalazine; and methotrexate alone. The dose of methotrexate was adjusted for maximal results. The patients had to achieve and maintain at least 50% improvement in undefined improvement criteria to be considered responders. The three-drug combination was highly significantly better than the other two treatment groups. O'Dell et al. state that the triple combination therapy was well tolerated.

VIII. CONCLUSIONS AND RECOMMENDATIONS

Combination DMARD therapy is theoretically beneficial. More aggressive therapy should result in better disease control. It would appear that there may be some individual patients who will obtain a good response to two-DMARD combination therapy when other single-DMARD therapies have failed. This would be suggested by the number of anecdotal reports of such improvement. Open studies and anecdotal experience are encouraging, but randomized controlled trials are either lacking or have been disappointing. The possibility that more aggressive therapy with more than two DMARDs may alter the course of intractable RA is suggested by several open studies. New approaches using three or more DMARDs have been suggested but not tested.

Although it is recognized that randomized controlled trials look at a specialized patient population and may not be totally germane to the general population of patients, such trials are necessary to demonstrate efficacy of one treatment over another and to eliminate unintentional bias.

There has been no specific combination of DMARDs that has been shown to be superior to any other. The use of any combination must be considered experimental until further conclusive data are obtained. This is not to suggest that combinations should never be used. The desperation referred to by Paulus [16] will continue to exist and the intractable patient may respond to another approach. However, the physician should recognize the experimental nature of the therapy. This approach to RA therapy deserves more scrutiny, but well-designed controlled trials with adequate numbers of patients are required to authenticate the efficacy and safety of this approach.

REFERENCES

1. Wilke WS. Combination therapy for rheumatoid arthritis: new paradigms of treatment. Cleveland Clin J Med 1993; 60:101–102.
2. Ward JR. Earlier intervention with second line therapies. J Rheumatol 1990; 17(Suppl 25):18–23.
3. Klippel JH. Winning the battle, losing the war? Another editorial about rheumatoid arthritis. J Rheumatol 1990; 17:1118–1122.
4. Pinals RS, Masi AT, Larsen RA and the Subcommittee for Criteria of Remission in Rheumatoid Arthritis of the American Rheumatism Association Diagnostic and Therapeutic Criteria Committee. Preliminary criteria for clinical remission in rheumatoid arthritis. Arthritis Rheum 1981; 24:1308–1315.
5. Scott DL, Coulton BL, Symmons DPM, Popert AJ. Long-term outcome of treating rheumatoid arthritis: results after 20 years. Lancet 1987; 1:1108–1111.
6. Pincus T. Rheumatoid arthritis: disappointing long-term outcomes despite successful short-term clinical trials. J Clin Epidemiol 1988; 41:1037–1041.
7. Reilly PA, Cosh JA, Maddison PJ, Rasker JJ, Silman AJ. Mortality and survival in rheumatoid arthritis: a 25-year prospective study of 100 patients. Ann Rheum Dis 1990; 49:363–369.
8. Pincus TS. Is mortality increased in rheumatoid arthritis? J Musculoskeletal Med 1988; 5(6):27–46.
9. Pincus T, Callahan LF. Taking mortality in rheumatoid arthritis seriously—predictive markers, socioeconomic status and comorbidity. J Rheumatol 1986; 13:841–845.
10. Iannuzzi L, Dawson N, Zein N, Kushner I. Does drug therapy slow radiographic deterioration in rheumatoid arthritis? N Engl J Med 1983; 309:1023–1028.

11. Kushner I. Does aggressive therapy of rheumatoid arthritis affect outcome? J Rheumatol 1989; 16:1–4.
12. Wolfe F, Hawley DJ, Cathey MA. Termination of slow acting antirheumatic therapy in rheumatoid arthritis: a 14-year prospective evaluation of 1017 consecutive starts. J Rheumatol 1990; 17:994–1002.
13. Pincus T, Marcum SB, Callahan LF. Longterm drug therapy for rheumatoid arthritis in seven rheumatology private practices: II. second line drugs and prednisone. J Rheumatol 1992; 19:1885–1894.
14. Bitter T. Combined disease-modifying chemotherapy for intractable rheumatoid arthritis. Clin Rheum Dis 1984; 10:417–428.
15. Hamilton JA. Hypothesis—*in vitro* evidence for the invasive and tumor-like properties of the rheumatoid pannus. J Rheumatol 1983; 10:845–851.
16. Paulus HE. The use of combinations of disease-modifying antirheumatic agents in rheumatoid arthritis. Arthritis Rheum 1990; 33:113–120.
17. Ehrlich GE. Heroic treatment for nonmalignant disease. JAMA 1982; 248:1743–1744.
18. Bellamy N, Brooks PM. Current practice in antimalarial drug prescribing in rheumatoid arthritis. J Rheumatol 1986; 13:551–555.
19. McCarty DJ. Suppress rheumatoid inflammation early and leave the pyramid to the Egyptians. J Rheumatol 1990; 17:1115–1118.
20. Roubenoff R, Jones RJ, Karp JE, Stevens MB. Remission of rheumatoid arthritis with the successful treatment of acute myelogenous leukemia with cytosine arabinoside, daunorubicin, and m-AMSA. Arthritis Rheum 1987; 30:1187–1190.
21. Cohen MG, Janssen B, Webb J. Response of rheumatoid arthritis to chemotherapy for Hodgkin's disease in a patient with IgA deficiency and overlap connective tissue disease. Ann Rheum Dis 1988; 47:603–605.
22. Sievers K, Hurri L. Combined therapy of rheumatoid arthritis with gold and chloroquine. I. Evaluation of the therapeutic effect. Acta Rheum Scand 1963; 9:48–55.
23. McCarty DJ, Carrera GF. Intractable rheumatoid arthritis. Treatment with combined cyclophosphamide, azathioprine, and hydroxychloroquine. JAMA 1982; 248:1718–1723.
24. Csuka M, Carrera GF, McCarty DJ. Treatment of intractable rheumatoid arthritis with combined cyclophosphamide, azathioprine, and hydroxychloroquine. A follow-up study. JAMA 1986; 255:2315–2319.
25. Jaffe IA. Combination therapy of rheumatoid arthritis--rationale and overview. J Rheumatol 1990; 17(Suppl 25):24–27.
26. Boers M, Ramsden M. Longacting drug combinations in rheumatoid arthritis: a formal overview. J Rheumatol 1991; 18:316–324.
27. Wilke WS, Clough JD. Therapy for rheumatoid arthritis: combinations of disease-modifying drugs and new paradigms of treatment. Semin Arthritis Rheum 1991; 21(Suppl 1):21–34.
28. Brooks PM. Combination therapy in rheumatoid arthritis. Agents Actions 1993; 44(Suppl):95–103.
29. Baker GL, Kahl LE, Zee BC, Stolzer BL, Agarwal AK, Medsger TA. Malignancy following treatment of rheumatoid arthritis with cyclophosphamide. Long-term case-control follow-up study. Am J Med 1987; 83:1–9.
30. Cannon GW, Jackson CG, Samuelson CO, Ward JR, Williams HJ, Clegg DO. Chlorambucil therapy in rheumatoid arthritis: clinical experience in 28 patients and literature review. Semin Arthritis Rheum 1985; 15:106–118.
31. Bunch TW, O'Duffy JD, Tompkins RB, O'Fallon WM. Controlled trial of hydroxychloroquine and d-penicillamine singly and in combination in the treatment of rheumatoid arthritis. Arthritis Rheum 1984; 27:267–276.
32. Felson DT, Anderson JJ, Meenan RF. The efficacy and toxicity of combination in rheumatoid arthritis. A meta-analysis. Arthritis Rheum 1994; 37:1487–1491.

33. Pincus T. Limitations to standard randomized controlled clinical trials to evaluate combination therapies in rheumatic diseases. Agents Actions 1993; 44:(Suppl):83–91.
34. Wilske KR, Healey LA. Remodelling the pyramid--a concept whose time has come. J Rheumatol 1989; 16:565–567.
35. Morgan SL, Baggott JE, Alarcon GS. Methotrexate and sulfasalazine combination therapy: is it worth the risk? Arthritis Rheum 1993; 36:281–282.
36. Nisar M, Carlisle L, Amos RS. Methotrexate and sulphasalazine as combination therapy in rheumatoid arthritis. Br J Rheumatol 1994; 33:651–654.
37. Shiroky JB, Watts CS, Neville C. Combination methotrexate and sulfasalazine in the management of rheumatoid arthritis: case observations. Arthritis Rheum 1989; 32:1160–1164.
38. Felson DT, Anderson JJ, Meenan RF. The comparative efficacy and toxicity of second-line drugs in rheumatoid arthritis. Results of two metaanalyses. Arthritis Rheum 1990; 33:1449–1461.
39. Furst DE. Rational use of disease-modifying antirheumatic drugs. Drugs 1990; 39:19–37.
40. Williams HJ. Rheumatoid arthritis. Treatment. In: Schumacher HR Jr, Klippel JH, Koopman WJ, eds. Primer of the Rheumatic Diseases, 10th ed. Atlanta: Arthritis Foundation, 1993:96–99.
41. Fries JF, Williams CA, Ramey D, Bloch DA. The relative toxicity of disease-modifying antirheumatic drugs. Arthritis Rheum 1993; 36:297–306.
42. Fries JF, Spitz PW, Williams CA, Bloch DA, Singh G, Hubert HB. A toxicity index for comparisons of side effects among different drugs. Arthritis Rheum 1990; 33:121–130.
43. Scott DL, Dawes PT, Tunn E, Fowler PD, Shadforth MF, Fisher J, Clarke S, Collins M, Jones P, Popert AJ, Bacon PA. Combination therapy with gold and hydroxychloroquine in rheumatoid arthritis: a prospective, randomized, placebo-controlled study. Br J Rheumatol 1989; 28:128–133.
44. Porter DR, Capell HA, Hunter J. Combination therapy in rheumatoid arthritis—no benefit of addition of hydroxychloroquine to patients with a suboptimal response to intramuscular gold therapy. J Rheumatol 1993; 20:645–649.
45. Gibson T, Emery P, Armstrong RD, Crisp AJ, Panayi GS. Combined d-penicillamine and chloroquine treatment of rheumatoid arthritis—a comparative study. Br J Rheumatol 1987; 26:279–284.
46. Martin M, Dixon J, Hickling P, Bird H, Golding J, Wright V. A combination of D-penicillamine and hydroxychloroquine for the treatment of rheumatoid arthritis. Ann Rheum Dis 1982; 41:208.
47. Clegg DO for the HCQ/MTX Study Group. Combination hydroxychloroquine and methotrexate in the treatment of rheumatoid arthritis [abstr]. Arthritis Rheum 1993; 36(Suppl):S53.
48. Ferraz MB, Pinheiro GRC, Helfenstein M, Albuquerque E, Rezende C, Roimicher L, Brandao L, Silva SC, Pinheiro GC, Atra E. Combination therapy with methotrexate and chloroquine in rheumatoid arthritis. A multicenter randomized placebo-controlled trial. Scand J Rheumatol 1994; 23:231–236.
49. Faarvang KL, Egsmose C, Kryger P, Podenphant J, Ingeman-Nielsen M, Hansen TM. Hydroxychloroquine and sulphasalazine alone and in combination in rheumatoid arthritis: a randomised double-blind trial. Ann Rheum Dis 1993; 52:711–715.
50. Schwarzer AC, Arnold MH, Kelly D, Jones M, Beller E, McNaught PJ, Schrieber L, Brooks PM. The cycling of combination antirheumatic drug therapy in rheumatoid arthritis. Br J Rheumatol 1990; 29:445–450.
51. Brawer AE. The combined use of oral methotrexate and intramuscular gold in rheumatoid arthritis [abstr]. Arthritis Rheum 1988; 31(Suppl 1):R10.
52. Williams AJ, Ward JR, Reading JC, Brooks RH, Clegg DO, Skosey JL, Weisman MH, Willkens RF, Singer JZ, Alarcon GS, Field EH, Clements PJ, Russell IJ, Hochman RF, Boumpas DT, Marble DA. Comparison of auranofin, methotrexate, and the combination of both in the treatment of rheumatoid arthritis. A controlled clinical trial. Arthritis Rheum 1992; 35:259–269.

53. Kantor SM, Wallin BA, Grier CG, McCafferty JP, Wetherington JD, Fox MJ and the Auranofin Cooperating Group. Combination of auranofin and methotrexate as initial DMARD therapy in RA [abstr]. Arthritis Rheum 1990; 33(Suppl):S60.
54. Morand EF, Axtens RSK, Littlejohn GO. Combination methotrexate and sulfasalazine therapy in patients with rheumatoid arthritis [abstr]. Arthritis Rheum 1993; 36(Suppl):S53.
55. Haagsma C, van Riel P, de Rooij DJ, van de Putte L. Combination therapy in RA: sulphasalazine and methotrexate [abstr]. Arthritis Rheum 1993; 36(Suppl):S53.
56. Lee S, Solomon G. Treatment of rheumatoid arthritis (RA) with combination of d-penicillamine (DPCN) and methotrexate (MTX) [abstr]. Arthritis Rheum 1990; 33(Suppl):R39.
57. Fosdick WM. Combined cytotoxic therapy in rheumatoid arthritis (RA) [abstr]. Arthritis Rheum 1971; 14(Suppl):161–162.
58. Willkens RF, Urowitz ME, Sharp JE, Stablein DM. Combination therapy of RA with methotrexate and azathioprine; 48 week results [abstr]. Arthritis Rheum 1993; 36(Suppl):S53.
59. Tugwell P, Pincus T, Yocum D, Stein M, Gluck O, Kraag G, McKendry R, Tesser K, Baker P, Wells G, for the Methotrexate-Cyclosporine Combination Study Group. Combination therapy with cyclosporine and methotrexate in severe rheumatoid arthritis. New Engl J Med 1995; 333:137–141.
60. Dawes PT, Sheeran TP, Fowler PD, Shadforth MF. Improving the response to gold or D-penicillamine by addition of sulphasalazine—a pilot study of 25 patients with rheumatoid arthritis. Clin Exp Rheum 1987; 5:151–153.
61. Farr M, Kitas G, Bacon PA. Sulphasalazine in rheumatoid arthritis: combination therapy with D-penicillamine or sodium aurothiomalate. Clinical Rheumatol 1988; 7:242–248.
62. Taggart AJ, Hill J, Astbury C, Dixon JS, Bird HA, Wright V. Sulphasalazine alone or in combination with d-penicillamine in rheumatoid arthritis. Br J Rheumatol 1987; 26:32–36.
63. Waterworth RF. The use of sulphasalazine and azathioprine in combination to treat rheumatoid arthritis. Br J Rheumatol 1989; 28:456.
64. Walters MT, Cawley MID. Combined suppressive drug treatment in severe refractory rheumatoid disease: an analysis of the relative effects of parenteral methylprednisolone, cyclophosphamide, and sodium aurothiomalate. Ann Rheum Dis 1988; 47:924–929.
65. Biro JA, Segal AM, Mackenzie AH, Mazanec DJ, Wilkes WS. The combination of methotrexate (MTX) and azathioprine (AZA) for resistant rheumatoid arthritis (RA) [abstr]. Arthritis Rheum 1987; 30(Suppl):S18.
66. Butler D, Tiliakos N. Low-dose cytotoxic drug combination therapy in intractable rheumatoid arthritis [abstract]. Arthritis Rheum 1985; 28(Suppl):S15.
67. Tiliakos N. Low-dose cytotoxic drug combination therapy in intractable rheumatoid arthritis: two years later [abstr]. Arthritis Rheum 1986; 29(Suppl):S79.
68. Langevitz P, Kaplinsky N, Ehrenfeld M, Pras M. Intractable RA--treatment with combined methotrexate, azathioprine and hydroxychloroquine. Br J Rheumatol 1989; 28:271–272.
69. O'Dell J, Haire C, Erikson N, Drymalski W, Palmer W, Eckhoff J, Garwood V, Maloley P, Illera V, Klassen L, Wees S, Klein H, Moore G. Triple DMARD therapy for rheumatoid arthritis [abstr]. Arthritis Rheum 1994; 37(Suppl):S295.

15

When to Stop Second-line Drugs: Risk/Benefit Ratio of Continuation Versus Cessation in Patients with Rheumatoid Arthritis in Remission

S. ten Wolde
Leiden University Hospital, Leiden, The Netherlands

B. A. C. Dijkmans
Free University Hospital, Amsterdam, The Netherlands

I. INTRODUCTION

Drug therapy for patients with rheumatoid arthritis (RA) is divided in first- and second-line drugs. The first-line drugs include nonsteroidal anti-inflammatory drugs (NSAIDs); for example, indomethacin, diclofenac, and naproxen. These drugs are given to achieve both pain relief and reduction of the inflammatory component of the synovitis. There is, however, no evidence that NSAIDs influence the natural history of the disease.

Second-line drugs, such as antimalarials, gold salts, sulfasalazine, D-penicillamine, azathioprine, and methotrexate are thought to influence the disease process more fundamentally [1]. These drugs are also called slow-acting antirheumatic drugs (SAARDs) because of their delayed onset of action, remittive agents because of their ability to induce remission, or disease-modifying antirheumatic drugs (DMARDs) because of their alleged capacity to modify the course of the disease. Short-term significant clinical improvement has been documented for each of the second-line drugs as compared with placebo [2–8]. However, it is not clear how well short-term improvement correlates with long-term outcome of the disease [9,10]. Moreover, results of studies to the effect of second-line drugs on the rate of radiographic progression, a generally accepted parameter for long-term outcome of RA, are disappointing [11–16]. Besides this uncertainty about the long-term efficacy of second-line drugs, these drugs are potentially toxic [17,18]. Therefore, their use must depend on the careful assessment of the course of the disease in the individual patient and on the making of a balanced judgment between the likely effect on the disease and the possible toxicity of the treatment.

There are few established guidelines for treatment with second-line drugs, and their use is almost entirely based on empiricism [19–22]. They are usually started 3–6 months after treatment with NSAIDs have been judged unsatisfactory. This policy is now changing with the increasing evidence that most joint damage occurs early in the disease [23] and that RA is associated with shortened life expectancy [24,25]. Therefore, the early use of second-line drugs has been advocated to reverse the process before the onset of destruction [26,27]. However, spontaneous remissions occur quite frequently in the first months of the disease [28], whereas such remissions are infrequent after 1 year of sustained progressive disease. Thus, with the use of second-line drugs very early in the disease course, the patient's remission might be falsely attributed to the action of the drug rather than to the natural history of the illness [29]. To enable the selection of patients with a poor prognosis for early treatment, research has been done to establish factors early in the disease course which predict progressive disease. These studies have revealed that the presence of rheumatoid factor or HLA-DR4 is a predictor for sustained progression of RA [28,30–32].

Guidelines for discontinuation of second-line drugs are even more complex. First of all, it is obvious that a drug should be stopped when serious adverse events occur. Second, it seems reasonable to stop a second-line drug when it has failed to show any effect on the disease within 4–6 months of adequate treatment. And third, it feels safe to never change the winning team and continue second-line drugs even once a remission is achieved. The simplicity of these guidelines gives them a semblance of truth, whereas there are actually many uncertainties, such as the causality of adverse events, the duration of the delayed onset of action, and the risk/benefit ratio of continuous therapy in patients with a remission.

A review of studies on the termination of second-line treatment revealed that 1–7% of the stopped courses were because of remission [5,33–37]. However, the main reasons for treatment discontinuation were toxicity and lack or loss of efficacy. Overall 50% of the treatment courses were terminated within the first 2 years [36–38]. In the case of adverse events or lack of efficacy, the second-line drug will be replaced by another. During remission, the only situation where the cessation of second-line drug therapy could be definitive, it is advised to continue the drugs [19–21]. This leads to the suggestion that second-line drugs can never be stopped safely.

In this chapter, the risk/benefit ratio of continuation versus cessation of second-line drugs in RA patients who achieved a remission is discussed in order to answer the question if and when these drugs can be stopped.

II. REMISSION IN RA

Despite the general agreement that spontaneous or drug-induced remission may occur in RA, there is no clear definition of this state. The term *remission* implies the total absence of disease activity. But since this ideal state is rarely achieved in RA, consensus criteria were developed to describe a state of reduced disease activity (Table 1) [39]. According to these American Rheumatism Association (ARA) criteria for remission 18% of RA patients have one or more periods of remission during their disease course [40]. This in line with the results of studies on the course of disease activity in which overall 20–40% of RA patients had both remissions and flares, and 40–70% of RA patients had sustained progressive disease [25,41,42].

Table 1 Proposed ARA Criteria for Clinical Remission in Rheumatoid Arthritis

Five or more of the following requirements must be fulfilled for at least 2 consecutive months:	
1.	Duration of morning stiffness not exceeding 15 min
2.	No fatigue
3.	No joint pain (by history)
4.	No joint tenderness or pain on motion
5.	No soft tissue swelling in joints or tendon sheaths
6.	Erythrocyte sedimentation rate (Westergren method) less than 30 mm/h for a female or 20 mm/h for a male

Exclusions: Clinical manifestations of active vasculitis, pericarditis, pleuritis or myositis, and unexplained recent weight loss or fever attributable to RA will prohibit a designation of remission.
Source: From ref. 39.

The reported percentages of RA patients achieving remission during treatment with second-line drugs varies between 7% and 33%, with an average of about 20% [40,43–48]. Comparison of 1–7% treatment terminations because of remission with the occurrence of remission in about 20% of treated patients suggests that second-line drugs are stopped only in a minority of patients in remission.

III. RISK/BENEFIT RATIO OF CONTINUOUS THERAPY

In the decision to continue second-line drugs in patients with a remission, the risk for adverse events should be weighted by the prolonged benefit of the drugs during remission. In addition to this risk/benefit ratio, the costs and discomfort for the patient of continuous therapy should be taken into account.

A. Risk for Adverse Events

Adverse events during treatment with second-line drugs are common and occur in approximately 50% of treated patients [18,21]. Most adverse effects occur within the first year of therapy, but even after many years of treatment, serious adverse effects have been reported [18,49]. There are, however, no clear data on the risk for adverse effects during long-term maintenance therapy with second-line drugs. Fortunately, many adverse effects are transient and mild. And the incidences of adverse effects which shorten the life span or produce permanent damage are low for most second-line drugs. For instance, the estimated incidence of death related to intramuscular gold therapy, the drug with the highest toxicity rate [17], was 1.6 death per 10,000 prescriptions [50]. Therefore, it could be concluded that the risk for serious adverse effects is probably low in patients who are able to tolerate the drug for many years [51]. Recently, we confirmed this low risk for side effects in a placebo-controlled treatment-discontinuation study [52].

B. Benefit of Continuous Therapy

Once a remission is achieved with second-line drugs, their benefit can only be analyzed by comparing the flare rate during continuous therapy with the flare rate after the withdrawal of therapy. However, there is only scanty literature on this. Furthermore, there are no absolute criteria for a rheumatoid flare [53], which makes comparison of studies difficult. In most studies, a flare could be described as an increase in disease activity after a period of remission which requires resumption or a dosage increase of treatment.

Since the mean duration of remission is only 10 months [40] and the discontinuation rate of second-line drugs due to loss of efficacy is high [37], there is no doubt that flares occur also during continuous therapy. This is supported by Grindulus et al. [54], who reported flare rates between 4 and 16% within 2 years of treatment with intramuscular gold, sulfasalazine, or D-penicillamine, and by Bax et al. [55], who reported that about 10% of patients flared who were treated with sulfasalazine for more than 1 year and initially had responded well. Therefore, it can be concluded that continuous therapy is no guarantee for maintained remission.

The number of flares observed in placebo-controlled studies [46,56–59] on second-line drug discontinuation are shown in Table 2. The risk for a flare during continuous therapy varies between 0 and 20%. However, the number of patients randomized to continuous therapy is very small and not all patients were in remission at the start of the study. Nevertheless, these studies suggest a prolonged benefit of second-line drugs during remission, whereas in most studies, there was a higher flare risk in the patients switched to placebo than in the patients with continuous therapy. We recently confirmed this suggestion in a 1-year placebo-controlled treatment discontinuation study in patients with inactive disease [52].

C. Costs and Discomfort

The potential toxicity of second-line drugs has become an important factor in their clinical use. The main purpose of visits to the physician during the course of second-line drug therapy is to screen for early evidence of toxicity, and such screening accounts for much of the expense of second-line drug therapy [60]. discomfort associated with second-line drug therapy is difficult to measure. Minor adverse events not causing drug withdrawal, like mild rash or nausea, may cause discomfort. In our treatment-discontinuation study, the disappearance of side effects was indeed reported by some patients in the placebo group [52]. Moreover, frequent visits to the physician for toxicity screening might place a load on patients. From this point of view, one would prefer to stop the therapy.

D. Conclusion: Risk/Benefit of Continuous Therapy

The risk for serious adverse effects of second-line drugs is small, especially after many years of treatment, and there seems to be a prolonged benefit of second-line drugs during remission. Therefore, it can be concluded that the benefit is greater than the risk. But since continuous therapy is expensive and can cause discomfort in patients, it will depend on the actual risk for flare after cessation of second-line drugs to which side the balance will tip.

Table 2 Double-blind Placebo-controlled Studies to the Effect of Second-line Drug Discontinuation After Achievement of Remission in Patients with Rheumatoid Arthritis

				Patients with continuous therapy		Patients switched to placebo		
Ref.	Year	Second-line drug	Follow-up (months)	No. of patients	No (%) with flare	No. of patients	No. (%) with flare	Inclusion criteria
59	1986	Intramuscular gold	24	11	1 (9)	13	1 (8)	More than 6 g gold
46	1984	D-penicillamine	12	19	2 (11)	19	15 (79)	ARA criteria for remission
56	1986	Methotrexate	1–3	5	0 (0)	7	7 (100)	"Good or excellent improvement"
58	1987	Methotrexate	1	5	1 (20)	5	5 (100)	36 months' treatment
57	1981	Azathioprine[a]	8	14	1 (7)	18	12 (67)	"Long-term treatment"
71	1976	Azathioprine[b]	2			16	15 (94)	24 months' treatment

[a]Patients in both randomization groups continued with intramuscular gold and/or corticosteroids.
[b]Double-blind crossover study in which all patients received placebo.

IV. RISK FOR FLARE AFTER CESSATION OF THERAPY

The empirical guideline that second-line drugs must never be stopped during remission because a flare of the disease will usually occur [19–21] has to be based on the experiences of clinicians who have tried to withdraw RA patients from these drugs. Unfortunately, there is scanty literature published on the flare risk after the cessation of treatment. And despite their importance, placebo-controlled trials are especially scare. Therefore, we have conducted a large placebo-controlled treatment-discontinuation study of which the results have been recently published [52].

Only by comparing the flare rate in patients with continuous therapy with the flare rate in patients who stopped their second-line treatment will allow us to make a conscious choice between the two treatment options. Moreover, the severity of the flares and the effect of treatment resumption should also be taken into account.

The placebo-controlled studies on the cessation of second-line drugs are summarized in Table 2. Flare rates between 8 and 100% were observed in patients who switched to placebo. However, groups were very small and not all of these patients were in remission at study entry.

Observational studies with information on flare risk after treatment discontinuation are summarized in Table 3. Although there might be differences in flare risk between the different kinds of second-line drugs, they will be discussed separately.

A. Intramuscular Gold

From the study of van der Leeden et al. [59], the suggestion arose that discontinuation of intramuscular injections with aurothioglucose (ATG) might be possible. This is in line with an earlier observation that the beneficial effects of the aurothiomalate (ATM) may persist for at least 12 months after administration of gold 1 g [61,62]. These persisting effects may be ascribed to the tissue gold stores, which can led to measurable serum concentrations of gold 24 months after its discontinuation in patients who had received a cumulative dose of at least 6 g [59].

The crucial factor for gold discontinuation therfore might be the total cumulative dose received. This was already mentioned by Kean et al. in 1979 [63] in reference to 10 patients who discontinued intramuscular ATM during sustained remission. The six patients who stayed in remission had received an higher average cumulative dose than the four patients who flared. And a high flare rate of 74% was observed in 31 patients in remission who only received a mean cumulative dose of 400 mg, whereas ATG was stopped owing to side effects [64].

A high cumulative dose, however, does not always protect patients for a flare. In a recent randomized study [65] in patient with a mean cumulative dose of 5 g of gold (range 1–23 g), significant more deterioration was observed in RA patients in remission who switched from intramuscular ATG to oral gold (auranofin) than in patients who were continued on intramuscular ATG.

In our 1-year study, more patients flared in the placebo group than in the group of patients who continued parenteral gold, but this difference was not significant [52].

In conclusion, reported flare rates after the cessation of intramuscular gold salts (ATM or ATG) varies between 8 and 74% and seems to be only partly dependent on the total cumulative dose received.

Table 3 Observational and Open Randomized Studies with Information on the Effect of Cessation or Dose Reduction of Second-line Drugs in Patients with Rheumatoid Arthritis in Remission

Ref.	Year	Kind of study	Second-line drug	No. of patients who stopped drug during remission	No of patients with a flare after cessation	No. of patients with dose reduction during remission	No. of patients with a flare after dose reduction
64	1989	Retrospective	Intramuscular gold	31	23		
63	1979	Prospective	Intramuscular gold	10	4		
65	1994	Randomized[a]	Intramuscular gold			24	10 (?)
66	1981	Retrospective	D-penicillamine	4	4		
67	1993	Randomized[b]	D-penicillamine			14	2
69	1957	Prospective	Chloroquine	12	12		
33	1991	Prospective	Sulfasalazine	9 (?)	3		
72	1983	Prospective	Methotrexate	28	15		
73	1992	Prospective	Methotrexate			15	2

[a]Patients were randomized to either switching to oral gold (auranofin) or continuous ATG; no patients flared during continuous therapy.
[b]Patients were randomized to either dose reduction or continuous therapy; no flares were observed during continuous therapy.

B. D-Penicillamine

Discontinuation of D-penicillamine seems to induce flares in the majority of patients. A double-blind placebo-controlled study in 38 RA patients with a remission reported a flare rate of 79% in the patients receiving placebo compared with 11% in patients with continuous therapy [46]. This is in line with the results of a retrospective study in which all four patients who achieved remission for more than 6 months flared after stopping D-penicillamine [66]. However, in our study, there was no difference in flare risk between the two treatment groups, each consisting of only 10 patients [52].

Dose reduction of D-penicillamine on the other hand seems to be safer than discontinuation. In a recent study, poor treatment compliance in 39% of the studied patients, as assessed by urinary tests, was not associated with higher disease activity [67]. In the same article, the results of a randomized study on the effect of 75% dose reduction of D-penicillamine were reported. Two of the 14 patients randomized to intermittent treatment flared, whereas none of the 14 patients with continuous therapy did. Moreover, in an open prospective trial, no differences in efficacy were observed between intermittent and daily administration of D-penicillamine [68].

In conclusion, these studies suggest that a relatively low dose of D-penicillamine is able to maintain patients in remission, whereas complete withdrawal of the drug will lead to flares in the majority of the patients. However, the results of our own study in 20 patients treated with D-penicillamine did not support this suggestion [52].

C. (Hydroxy)chloroquine (Antimalarials)

The only information found on the flare risk after discontinuation of chloroquine in RA patients is from a study publiced in 1957 [69]. In this 4-year study of chloroquine therapy, all 12 RA patients whose chloroquine was stopped because of a remission flared within 1 year.

In patients with quiescent systemic lupus erythematosus (SLE), an other rheumatic disorder, withdrawal of hydroxychloroquine in a double-blind placebo-controlled study led to significantly more flares in the placebo group compared with the group with continuous therapy [70]. If RA patients can be compared with SLE patients, these studies suggest a continuous need for antimalarials once a remission is achieved.

In our placebo-controlled study, which included a large group of patients treated with (hydroxy)chloroquine, the flare risk was significantly higher for patients receiving placebo than for those continuing with antimalarials [52].

D. Sulfasalazine

Sulfasalazine has been rediscovered in the treatment of RA during the last 15 years. However, there are only scanty data on the cessation of sulfasalazine in RA patients with a remission. Jones et al. [33] prospectively followed a group of 86 RA patients treated with sulfasalazine for 5 years. Six of these patients stopped sulfasalazine because of a remission according to the ARA criteria [39] and none of these patients flared within 1–2 years. However, in the same article, another three patients with a remission were mentioned who all flared after discontinuation of sulfasalazine. On basis of this information, no conclusions could be drawn for the cessation of sulfasalazine during remission.

Our placebo-controlled study, which included 34 patients treated with sulfasalazine, showed a significant difference in flare rate between the two treatment groups [52].

E. Azathioprine and Methotrexate

Fear of the potential side effects of the prolonged use of cytostatic drugs has led to several studies on withdrawal of these drugs once remission had been achieved.

In a double-blind crossover study, using a placebo tablet in all patients, azathioprine was stopped in 16 patients once the disease was "stable" [71]. Fifteen of these 16 patients flared 3–8 weeks after switching to placebo. And in a double-blind placebo-controlled study, the substitution of placebo for the active drug resulted in clinical deterioration of 67% of the patients [57]. The results of these studies have discouraged further attempts to study withdrawal of azathioprine during remission. Therefore, we included only a very small group of patients treated with azathioprine in our study of which no conclusions can be drawn [52].

Hoffmeister reported in 1983 the results of 15 years of experience with methotrexate therapy in 78 patients [72]. From the 28 patients who stopped methotrexate because of a complete remission, 15 patients flared and resumed therapy. Two double-blind placebo-controlled trials were interrupted because of rapid deterioration in the placebo groups. In one of these studies, significant worsening was observed within 1 month in five patients and within 2 months in all seven patients assigned to placebo [49]. In the other terminated study, all five patients who received placebo had a flare within 1 month [58]. These dramatic results also halted further research on the effect of methotrexate withdrawal. We only included five patients with methotrexate in our study [52].

Dose reduction of methotrexate seems to be associated with a lower flare rate. Switching from a weekly to a fortnightly scale in 15 patients with a "stable disease" led to a flare in two patients within 12 months [73].

The impression from these studies is that discontinuation of azathioprine or methotrexate leads to rapid flares in nearly all patients. However, numbers of patients were small, patients were not necessarily in remission at study entry, and studies were prematurely terminated. The results of our study did support this impression, but it also included only a small number of patients.

F. Effect of Treatment Resumption

The resumption of second-line drugs does not always mean that there had been an obvious flare. Patients who feel some subjective deterioration after treatment discontinuation are eager to start their therapy again. Only placebo-controlled studies overcome this bias. In Table 4, the results of the resumption of second-line drugs after flares are summarized. In most studies, the majority of patients responded again to their prior second-line drug [33,46,47,58,63,71,73–75]; except in the retrospective study of Evers et al. [76], in which only 4 of 11 patients with complete remission during the first gold course regained a complete remission with the second gold course.

Although numbers of patients are small, the suggestion is that most patients who achieved remission during the first treatment course will regain remission on treatment resumption within several months.

Table 4 Double-blind Placebo-controlled and Observational Studies with Information on Response to Resumption of Second-line Treatment After a Rheumatoid Flare

Ref.	Year	Kind of study	Second-line drug	No. of flared patients who resumed therapy	No. of patients who responded to drug resumption	Maximum time to response (months)
63	1979	Prospective	Intramuscular gold	2	2	4
74	1980	Retrospective	Intramuscular gold	24	24	?
76	1983	Retrospective	Intramuscular gold	11	4	< 12
47	1981	Retrospective	Intramuscular gold	3	2	?
46	1984	Placebo-controlled	D-penicillamine	15	15	> 4
47	1981	Retrospective	D-penicillamine	2	2	?
69	1957	Prospective	Chloroquine	7	7	?
33	1991	Prospective	Sulfasalazine	3	3	?
71	1976	Blind crossover	Azathioprine	15	15	7
58	1987	Placebo-controlled	Methotrexate	5	5	> 1

V. CONCLUSIONS

From the above discussed studies, it can be concluded that cessation of second-line drugs leads to a considerable increase of the flare rate within several months, whereas the risk for adverse effects of continuous therapy is low. This confirmed the guideline that second-line drugs should be continued in RA patients after achievement of remission [19].

These studies also supported the opinion that RA is a life-long disease in which spontaneous remissions almost never occur [19–22]. However, with the new policy of earlier treatment with second-line drugs, there will be more patients in whom a remission is erroneously attributed to the drug action, whereas the remission is actually spontaneous. Hopefully, we will find ways to distinguish spontaneous remission from drug-induced remission in the future. In the meantime, it seems best to advise only a trial of discontinuation of the drug in case spontaneous remission is suspected [29]. If the disease flares, resumption of the drug will usually again produce remission within several months.

The results of our recent study showed a two times increased risk for flare after treatment discontinuation, but the majority of patients in the placebo group did not experience a flare within the study year [52]. An important risk factor for flare after treatment discontinuation was an ever-positive rheumatoid factor [52]. On the basis of these results, we advise continuance of second-line treatment, especially in rheumatoid factor–positive patients.

REFERENCES

1. Cash JM, Klippel JH. Second-line therapy for rheumatoid arthritis. N Engl J Med 1994; 330:1368–1375.
2. Cooperating Clinics Committee of the American Rheumatism Association. A controlled trial of gold salt therapy in rheumatoid arthritis. Arthritis Rheum 1973; 16:353–358.
3. Clark P, Casas E, Tugwell P, et al. Hydroxychloroquine compared with placebo in rheumatoid arthritis. A randomized controlled trial. Ann Intern Med 1993; 119:1067–1071.
4. Scull E. Chloroquine and hydroxychloroquine therapy in rheumatoid arthritis. Arthritis Rheum 1962; 5:30–36.
5. Hannonen P, Mottonen T, Hakola M, Oka M. Sulfasalazine in early rheumatoid arthritis. A 48-week double-blind, prospective, placebo-controlled study. Arthritis Rheum 1993; 36:1501–1509.
6. Urowitz MD, Gordon DA, Smythe HA, et al. Azathioprine in rheumatoid arthritis: a double-blind, cross over study. Arthritis Rheum 1973; 16:411–418.
7. Weinblatt ME, Coblyn JS, Fox DA, et al. Efficacy of low-dose methotrexate in rheumatoid arthritis. N Engl J Med 1985; 312:818–822.
8. Multicenter Trial Group. Controlled trial of d-penicillamine in severe rheumatoid arthritis. Lancet 1973; 1:275.
9. Pincus T. Rheumatoid arthritis: disappointing long-term outcomes despite successful short-term clinical trials. J Clin Epidemiol 1988; 41:1037–1041.
10. Hawley DJ, Wolfe F. Are the results of controlled clinical trials and observational studies of second line therapy in rheumatoid arthritis valid and generalizable as measures of rheumatoid arthritis outcome: analysis of 122 studies. J Rheumatol 1991; 18:1008–1014.

11. Sharp JT. Radiologic assessment as an outcome measure in rheumatoid arthritis. Arthritis Rheum 1989; 32:221–229.
12. Gabriel SE, Luthra HS. Rheumatoid arthritis: can the long-term outcome be altered? Mayo Clin Proc 1988; 63:58–68.
13. van der Heijde DM, van Riel PL, Nuver-Zwart IH, et al. Effects of hydroxychloroquine and sulphasalazine on progression of joints damage in rheumatoid arthritis. Lancet 1989; 1:1036–1038.
14. Lopez-Mendez A, Daniel WW, Reading JC, et al. Radiographic assessment of disease progression in rheumatoid arthritis patients enrolled in the cooperative systematic studies of the rheumatic diseases program randomized clinical trial of methotrexate, auranofin, or a combination of the two. Arthritis Rheum 1993; 36:1364–1369.
15. Weinblatt ME, Polisson R, Blotner SD, et al. The effects of drug therapy on radiographic progression of rheumatoid arthritis. Results of a 36-week randomized trial comparing methotrexate and auranofin. Arthritis Rheum 1993; 36:613–619.
16. Jeurissen ME, Boerbooms AM, van de Putte LB, et al. Influence of methotrexate and azathioprine on radiologic progression in rheumatoid arthritis. A randomized, double-blind study. Ann Intern Med 1991; 114:999–1004.
17. Felson DT, Anderson JJ, Meenan RF. The comparative efficacy and toxicity of second-line drugs in rheumatoid arthritis. Results of two metaanalyses. Arthritis Rheum 1990; 33:1449–1461.
18. Singh G, Fries JF, Williams CA, et al. Toxicity profiles of disease modifying antirheumatic drugs in rheumatoid arthritis. J Rheumatol 1991; 18:188–194.
19. McCarthy DJ. Personal experience in the treatment of seropositive rheumatoid arthritis with drugs used in combination. Semin Arthritis Rheum 1993; 23(Suppl):42–49.
20. McCarty DJ. Treatment of rheumatoid arthritis. In: McCarty DJ, Koopman WJ, eds. Arthritis and Allied Conditions, 12th ed. Philadelphia: Lea & Febiger, 1993:877–886.
21. Day RO. SAARDs-I. In: Klippel JH, Dieppe PA, eds. Rheumatology. London: Mosby, 1994:12.1–12.10.
22. Harris ED Jr. Treatment of rheumatoid arthritis. In: Kelly WN, Ruddy F, eds. Textbook of Rheumatology, 4th ed. Philadelphia: Saunders, 1993:912–923.
23. van der Heijde DM, van Leeuwen MA, van Riel PL, et al. Biannual radiographic assessments of hands and feet in a three-year prospective followup of patients with early rheumatoid arthritis. Arthritis Rheum 1992; 35:26–34.
24. Abruzzo JL. Rheumatoid arthritis and mortality. Arthritis Rheum 1982; 25:1020–1023.
25. Reilly PA, Cosh JA, Maddison PJ, et al. Mortality and survival in rheumatoid arthritis: a 25 year prospective study of 100 patients. Ann Rheum Dis 1990; 49:363–369.
26. Wilske KR. Inverting the therapeutic pyramid: observations and recommendations on new directions in rheumatoid arthritis therapy based on the author's experience. Semin Arthritis Rheum 1993; 23(Suppl 1):11–18.
27. Ward JR. Challenging the pyramid. A new look at therapeutic approaches for rheumatoid arthritis. Earlier intervention with second line therapies. J Rheumatol 1990; 25(Suppl):18–23.
28. Wolfe F, Ross K, Hawley DJ, et al. The prognosis of rheumatoid arthritis and undifferentiated polyarthritis syndrome in the clinic—a study of 1141 patients. J Rheumatol 1993; 20:2005–2009.
29. Fries JF, Williams CA, Ramey D, Bloch DA. The relative toxicity of disease-modifying antirheumatic drugs. Arthritis Rheum 1993; 36:297–306.
30. van der Heijde DM, van Riel PL, van Rijswijk MH, van de Putte LB. Influence of prognostic features on the final outcome in rheumatoid arthritis: a review of the literature. Semin Arthritis Rheum 1988; 17:284–292.
31. van Zeben D, Hazes JM, Zwinderman AH, et al. Clinical significance of rheumatoid factors in early rheumatoid arthritis: results of a follow up study. Ann Rheum Dis 1992; 51:1029–1035.

32. van Zeben D, Hazes JM, Zwinderman AH, et al. Association of HLA-DR4 with a more progressive disease course in patients with rheumatoid arthritis. Results of a followup study. Arthritis Rheum 1991; 34:822–830.
33. Jones E, Jones JV, Woodbury JF. Response to sulfasalazine in rheumatoid arthritis: life table analysis of a 5-year followup. J Rheumatol 1991; 18:195–198.
34. Bendix G, Bjelle A. Outcome of parenteral gold therapy in RA patients: a comparison between two periods using life-table analysis. Br J Rheumatol 1991; 30:407–412.
35. Rothermich NO, Phillips VK, Bergen W, Thomas MH. Followup study of chrysotherapy. Arthritis Rheum 1979; 22:423.
36. Wolfe F, Hawley DJ, Cathey MA. Termination of slow acting antirheumatic therapy in rheumatoid arthritis: a 14-year prospective evaluation of 1017 consecutive starts. J Rheumatol 1990; 17:994–1002.
37. Wijnands MJ, van't Hof MA, van Leeuwen MA, et al. Long-term second-line treatment: a prospective drug survival study. Br J Rheumatol 1992; 31:253–258.
38. Pincus T, Marcum SB, Callahan LF. Longterm drug therapy for rheumatoid arthritis in seven rheumatology private practices: II. Second line drugs and prednisone. J Rheumatol 1992; 19:1885–1894.
39. Pinals RS, Masi AT, Larsen RA. Preliminary criteria for clinical remission in rheumatoid arthritis. Arthritis Rheum 1981; 24:1308–1315.
40. Wolfe F, Hawley DJ. Remission in rheumatoid arthritis. J Rheumatol 1985; 12:245–252.
41. Short CL. Rheumatoid arthritis: types of course and prognosis. Med Clin North Am 1968; 52:549–557.
42. Masi AT. Articular patterns in the early course of rheumatoid arthritis. Am J Med 1983; 75:16–26.
43. Veys EM, Mielants H, Verbruggen G. Goldsalts, levamisole and D-penicillamine as first choice slow-acting antirheumatic drugs in rheumatoid arthritis—a long-term follow-up study. Clin Exp Rheumatol 1987; 5:111–116.
44. Sambrook PN, Browne CD, Champion GD, et al. Terminations of treatment with gold sodium thiomalate in rheumatoid arthritis. J Rheumatol 1982; 9:932–934.
45. Marcus RE, Sebba A. Remission and toxicity using single and combination DMARD therapy in 196 patients with rheumatoid arthritis. Arthritis Rheum 1993; 54(Suppl):127.
46. Ahern MJ, Hall ND, Case K, Maddison PJ. D-penicillamine withdrawal in rheumatoid arthritis. Ann Rheum Dis 1984; 43:213–217.
47. Hoh KF, Dwosh IL, Ford PM, et al. Drug-related disease remissions in rheumatoid arthritis. Arthritis Rheum 1981; 24(Suppl 72):86.
48. Kutsuna T, Maeda K, Okamoto T, Kawaguchi M. Frequency and prognostic features of rheumatoid patients with remission-inducing agents—a comparison of different kinds of medication. Ryumachi 1990; 30:336–342.
49. Szanto E. Low-dose methotrexate treatment of rheumatoid arthritis; long-term observation of efficacy and safety. Clin Rheumatol 1989; 8:323–320.
50. Davis P. Undesirable effects of gold salts. J Rheumatol 1979; 5(Suppl):18–24.
51. Paulus HE. An overview of benefit/risk of disease modifying treatment of rheumatoid arthritis as of today. Ann Rheum Dis 1982; 41(Suppl):26–29.
52. ten Wolde S, Breedveld FC, Hermans J, et al. Randomised placebo-controlled study of stopping second-line drugs in rheumatoid arthritis. Lancet 1996; 347:347–352.
53. Scott DL. Rheumatoid flare. In: Klippel JH, Dieppe PA, eds. Rheumatology. London: Mosby, 1994:15.2.
54. Grindulis KA, McConkey B. Outcome of attempts to treat rheumatoid arthritis with gold, penicillamine, sulphasalazine, or dapsone. Ann Rheum Dis 1984; 43:398–401.
55. Bax DE, Amos RS. Sulphasalazine in the long term management of rheumatoid arthritis. Drugs 1986; 32(Suppl 1):73–76.
56. Szanto E. Low-dose methotrexate in rheumatoid arthritis: effect and tolerance. Scand J Rheumatol 1986; 15:97–102.

57. De Silva M, Hazleman BL. Long-term azathioprine in rheumatoid arthritis: a double-blind study. Ann Rheum Dis 1981; 40:560–563.
58. Kremer JM, Rynes RI, Bartholomew LE. Severe flare of rheumatoid arthritis after discontinuation of long-term methotrexate therapy. Am J Med 1987; 82:781–786.
59. van der Leeden H, Dijkmans BAC, Hermans J, Cats A. A double-blind study on the effect of discontinuation of gold therapy in patients with rheumatoid arthritis. Clin Rheumatol 1986; 5:56–61.
60. Borg G, Allander E, Goobar JE. Disease-modifying anti-rheumatic drug therapy. An expensive therapy despite inexpensive drugs. Scand J Rheumatol 1990; 19:115–121.
61. Empire Rheumatism Counsil. Gold therapy in rheumatoid arthritis. Ann Rheum Dis 1960; 19:95–119.
62. Empire Rheumatism Counsil. Gold therapy in rheumatoid arthritis. Ann Rheum Dis 1961; 20:315–334.
63. Kean WF, Anastassiades TP. Long term chrysotherapy: incidence of toxicity and efficacy during sequential time periods. Arthritis Rheum 1979; 22:495–501.
64. Caspi D, Tischler M, Yaron M. Association between gold induced skin rash and remission in patients with rheumatoid arthritis. Ann Rheum Dis 1989; 48:730–732.
65. Prete PE, Zane J, Karilo M, Bulanowski M. Randomized trial of switching rheumatoid arthritis patients in remission with injectable gold to auranofin. Clin Rheumatol 1994; 13:60–69.
66. Camp AV. Penicillamine in the treatment of rheumatoid arthritis. J Rheumatol 1981; 7(Suppl):103–106.
67. Doyle DV, Perrett D, Foster OJF, et al. The long-term use of d-penicillamine for treating rheumatoid arthritis: is continuous therapy necessary? Br J Rheumatol 1993; 32:614–617.
68. Hakoda M, Taniguchi A, Kamantani N, et al. Intermittent treatment with d-penicillamine is effective in lower doses and with fewer adverse effects in patients with rheumatoid arthritis. J Rheumatol 1994; 21:1637–1641.
69. Bagnall AW. The value of chloroquine in rheumatoid disease: a four-year study of continuous therapy. Can Med Assoc J 1957; 77:182–194.
70. The Canadian Hydroxychloroquine Study Group. A randomized study of the effect of withdrawing hydroxychloroquine sulfate in systemic lupus erythematosus. N Engl J Med 1991; 324:150–154.
71. Cade R, Stein G, Pickering M, et al. Low dose, long-term treatment of rheumatoid arthritis with azathioprine. South Med J 1976; 69:388–392.
72. Hoffmeister RT. Methotrexate therapy in rheumatoid arthritis: 15 years experience. Am J Med 1983; 75:69–73.
73. Tischler M, Caspi D, Yaron M. Methotrexate treatment of rheumatoid arthritis: is a fortnightly maintenance schedule enough? Ann Rheum Dis 1992; 51:1330–1331.
74. Sagransky DM, Greenwals RA. Efficacy and toxicity in retreatment with gold salts: a retrospective review of 25 cases. J Rheumatol 1980; 7:474–478.
75. Klinkhoff AV, Teufel A. The second course of gold. J Rheumatol 1995; 22:1655–1666.
76. Evers AE, Sundstrom WR. Second course gold therapy in the treatment of rheumatoid arthritis. Arthritis Rheum 1983; 26:1071–1075.

16
Do Corticosteroids Have a Disease-modifying Role in Rheumatoid Arthritis?

Keith Lim* and John R. Kirwan
University of Bristol,
Bristol, United Kingdom

I. INTRODUCTION

Rheumatoid arthritis (RA) is a systemic disease that affects primarily the synovial joints. It is chronic, results in considerable morbidity, is associated with an increase in mortality, and is currently incurable. The prevalence of RA in Europe ranges from 1–3% [1]. In southwest England, patients with RA make up 25% of all new hospital referrals to the rheumatology clinics and 75% of follow-up work [2]. The management of RA requires a multidisciplinary approach with an important medical input. The roles of the clinician are to support the patients in the management of symptoms, to help maintain normal joint function and activity, and to try to prevent complications from the disease and its treatment. Much debate has focused on whether or not it is possible to modify sufficiently the natural history of RA to make a difference to patient outcome [3,4]. This is a difficult question to answer because of the chronic nature of the disease and the limitations of present instruments to measure its impact, but the clinical impression is that medical intervention does have a positive effect on RA and improves outcome as measured by clinical, functional, and structural change.

Corticosteroids offer one avenue of treatment of RA. The history of their use is linked with some of the most important advances in medical science in this century. Philip Hench and his colleagues were rewarded the Nobel Prize for discovering the anti-inflammatory properties of corticosteroids and were the first to use them in RA with dramatic results [5]. On September 21, 1948, Hench treated a 29-year-old woman bedridden with RA by giving three daily intramuscular injections of hydrocortisone. The effect was miraculous. The subsequent widespread use of corticosteroids as anti-inflam-

**Current affiliation*: Subang Jaya Medical Centre, and University Hospital, Kuala Lumpur, Malaysia.

matory agents made its mark in many conditions. Initial euphoria gave way to disillusionment as clinicians and the public became aware of the serious adverse effects that can occur with prolonged use of high dosages corticosteroids (Table 1). In many countries, corticosteroids became relegated to the bottom of the league table of "second-line" therapy and were often used only as a last resort for symptom control. However, recent recognition of their potential disease-modifying ability in improving function and possibly structural damage has led to a renewed interest and resurgence in their use [6–9]. This chapter considers the evidence for disease modification and addresses the question of how this evidence might affect clinical practice.

II. SCIENTIFIC BASIS

Glucocorticoid hormones have a core structure of four interlinked carbon rings with principal hydroxyl groups determining their activity on tissue receptors [10]. The various synthetic compounds currently in wide use have different levels of efficacy, durations of action, and adverse effects related to their pharmacokinetics, but they have the same

Table 1 Adverse Effects Associated with Long-term of High-dose Corticosteroids

System	Features
Gastrointestinal	Dyspepsia
	Peptic ulceration (often gastric)
	Bleeding
	Intestinal perforation
Metabolic and endocrine	Weight gain
	Centripetal obesity (cushingnoid habitus)
	Hirsuitism
	Hyperlipidaemia
	Percipitating or worsening of diabetes
	Suppression of hypothalamic-pituitary adrenal system
	Growth failure in children
	Secondary amenorrhea
Musculoskeletal	Muscle weakness, atrophy
	Osteoporosis: vertebral compression, fractures
	Avascular necrosis of bone
	Impaired wound healing
	Subsutaneous skin atrophy, skin breakdown, easy bruising
Cardiovascular and renal	Hypertension
	Sodium and water retention—edema
	Hypokalaemic alkalosis
Suppression of immune response	Opportunistic infections:
	skin
	systemic
	reactivation of TB
Central nervous system and eye	Mood changes (euphoria)
	Glaucoma
	Cataracts

mode of action (Table 2). Compounds such as deflazacort may demonstrate tissue specificity due to selective tissue access and so increase the potential for reducing adverse effects [11].

About 80% of serum glucocorticoid is bound to transcortin (glucocorticoid-binding globulin). Free cortisol, the active moiety, diffuses into individual cells and combines with specific receptors in the cytoplasm [12]. Having undergone conformational change, the steroid-receptor complex enters the nucleus and binds reversibly with specific chromatin sites. Increased messenger ribonucleic acid (mRNA) production follows, resulting in coding for enzymes and other proteins. The main protein thus produced is lipocortin, which has an anti-inflammatory effect by inhibiting phospholipase A_2, the first enzymatic step in prostaglandin and ecosanoid synthesis (Fig. 1). Corticosteroids can affect the action of cytokines, especially those with proinflammatory activity [13–15]. They are antipyretic and anti-inflammatory. They also have wide-ranging effects on the immune response, causing downregulation of immune function, inhibition of cell-mediated immunity, reduced cellular accumulation at inflammatory sites, and reduced vascular responses during inflammation [16]. Recent evidence suggests that patients with RA may have a defect in the regulation of corticosteroid-releasing factor (CRF) by the hypothalamus [17,18]. In active inflammatory RA, serum cortisol levels are reduced and the cortisol response during surgical stress is dampened compared with patients who have osteomyelitis, another chronic inflammatory condition [18]. This raises the possibility that alterations in corticosteroid action or control may play a more fundamental role in the development and progress of RA than previously thought.

The immune dysfunction in RA is multilevel, and corticosteroids have the potential to influence the immune and inflammatory response at various stages (Fig. 2). It seems logical that an agent such as glucocorticoid, which has actions further "upstream" in the pathological pathways than do nonsteroidal anti-inflammatory drugs, is more likely to prevent structural damage.

III. CLINICAL TRIALS OF CORTICOSTEROIDS IN RA

Although they have been in use since 1948, there have been relatively few randomized, controlled trials of corticosteroids in RA, particularly in relation to long-term use. In the early 1950s, several attempts were made to define their role. The first of these was conducted by the Medical Research Council (MRC) in conjunction with the Nuffield

Table 2 Comparison of Commonly Used Glucocorticoids

Duration of action	Compound	Equivalent dose (mg)	Mineralocorticoid activity
Short acting:	Cortisol	20	1.0
$t_{1/2}$ 6–12 h	Cortisone	25	0.8
Intermediate:	Prednisone	5	0.8
$t_{1/2}$ 2–26 h	Methylprednisolone	4	0.5
	Triamcinolone	0.4	0
Long acting:	Dexamethasone	0.75	0
$t_{1/2}$ 36–72 h	Paramethasone	2	0
	Betamethasone	0.60	0

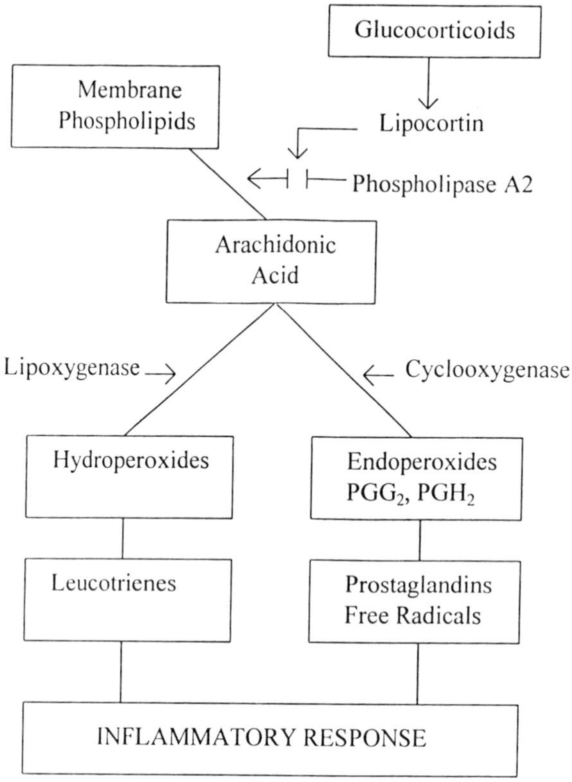

Figure 1 Mechanism of action of corticosteroids.

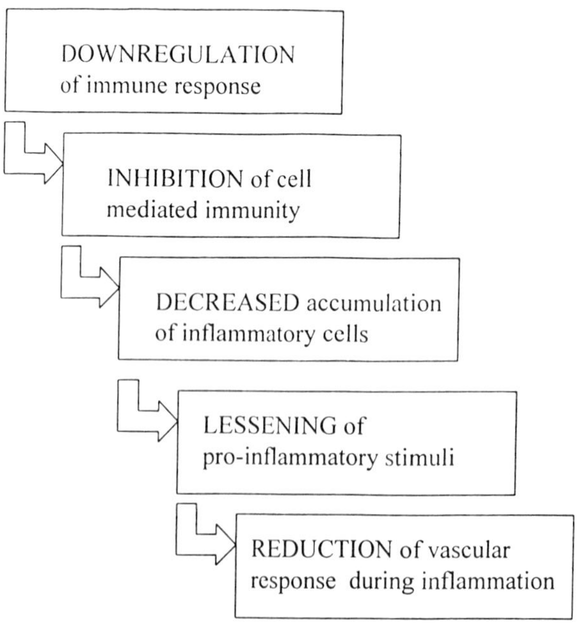

Figure 2 Influence of corticosteroids on the immune response.

Table 3 Proportion (%) of Radiographs with Definite Erosions After 2 Years of Treatment

Hands		Feet	
Cortisone (n = 30)	Aspirin (n = 27)	Cortisone (n = 26)	Aspirin (n = 24)
57	73	41	68

Source: From ref. 20.

Foundation in Great Britain [19]. In this study, 61 adult and pediatric patients were randomized to receive cortisone (mean dose 80 mg, equivalent to 16 mg prednisolone) or aspirin (mean dose 4.5 g daily) for 1 year. The study endpoints included clinical and laboratory parameters but radiographic progression was not followed. Patients had their treatment reduced in stages at the end of each 3-month period and final assessments were made 1 week after the drug had been discontinued. The results showed that the acute phase response (measured as the ESR) and hemoglobin levels responded better to cortisone. A series of clinical measures, including joint tenderness, range of joint movement, grip strength, disease activity, and functional capacity, showed improvement in both treatment groups. The investigators concluded that, although the patients on corticosteroids had some early advantage, by the end of the study, there was no difference between the treatments. They noted that patients on corticosteroids experienced significant withdrawal flares.

A study conducted by the Empire Rheumatism Council [20] randomized 100 adult patients to receive cortisone (mean dose 75 mg daily, equivalent to 14 mg prednisolone) or aspirin (mean dose 4 g daily) for 2 years. On this occasion radiographs of the hands and feet were taken during the second half of the second year and showed a higher erosion score in the aspirin-treated patients, although this did not reach statistical significance (Table 3). There were no radiographs at entry, so that progression during treatment could not be estimated.

A third trial [21] compared prednisolone (a synthetic analogue of cortisone with greater potency) with aspirin in 84 patients of whom 7 did not complete the study. The 41 patients receiving prednisolone had a daily mean dose of 12 mg at the end of the first year and 10 mg at the end of the second year. Thirty-six patients received aspirin. Radiographs were obtained of the hands and feet initially, and after 1 and 2 years of treatment. Radiographic progression was analyzed by assessing a variety of rheumatoid changes, including erosions. There were lower rates of progression in erosion scores in the prednisolone group (Table 4). At the end of the second year, eight patients on analgesics had fared badly and were given prednisolone. During the third year,

Table 4 Proportion (%) of Patients Showing Radiographic Progression After Different Periods of Treatment

Time	Prednisolone		Aspirin	
(years)	Hands	Feet	Hands	Feet
1	17	12	49	44
2	41	10	72	71

Source: From ref. 21.

5 of 26 (19%) of patients in the analgesic group progressed but only 4 of 49 (8%) of the prednisolone-treated patients did so [8,22]. Four years later, West [23] was able to follow up 74 of the original 77 patients in this study and reported that over 7 years only 9 of 39 (23%) patients who had continued on prednisolone developed new erosions compared with 32 of 34 (94%) patients who had continued on aspirin alone. Although this longer-term follow-up was uncontrolled, most patients had, in fact, continued with their initial therapy, and so this evidence appears persuasive. Published in 1967, in a journal not readily accessible and with a title which did not indicate the nature of the findings, this paper went unnoticed until referenced by Masi in 1983 [24].

Meanwhile, a variety of short-term inconclusive studies were published which did not satisfactorily address the question of alteration in radiological progression (Table 5). Berntsen [25] compared 183 RA patients on either hydrocortisone, cortisone, prednisolone, prednisone, dexamethasone, or triamcinolone against patients already on gold (n = 155) or analgesics alone (n = 50). The period of follow-up was at least 5 years. Radiographic progression was present in both groups, leading the investigators to conclude that corticosteroids were no better than gold or analgesics even though functional capacity was well maintained in the glucocorticoid-treated group. There are several important weaknesses in this study: The formulations and doses of glucocorticoids varied widely; the control group(s) had not been randomized; and (in keeping with thinking at that time) corticosteroids would have been used generally in more aggressive disease, certainly in comparison with an analgesic group. Indeed, 75% of patients in the steroid group had previously failed to respond to gold.

Three other randomized trials were published in 1981, 1983, and 1984 [26–28]. The first showed no advantage for monthly intravenous methylprednisolone compared with placebo over a 6-month period. The second was a small study involving only 18 patients. The investigators concluded that erosive progression was less in the prednisolone-treated group compared with placebo over a 10-month period. The third study compared patients treated with prednisolone (mean dosage 10.3 mg/day) with those without prednisolone. This study included 103 patients followed up over a period of 120 months. The suggestion from this study was that the hand radiographs showed significantly less erosions in the prednisolone-treated group. In a later study comparing pulse intravenous methylprednisolone with saline infusion, no long-term benefit was found in terms of clinical outcome or radiological progression [29].

In 1986, Byron and Kirwan [30] reviewed and reanalyzed the results of both the 1959 MRC trial [21] and the follow-up report by West [23] and concluded that there was a good cause for the disease-modifying potential of corticosteroid therapy. They proposed the conduct of a new randomized, double-blind, placebo-controlled trial of corticosteroids designed specifically to test the hypothesis that corticosteroids can suppress erosive progression. The results of that study, sponsored by the Arthritis and Rheumatism Council (ARC), have recently been published [9]. This multicenter trial recruited 128 patients with RA of less than 2 years since diagnosis and compared placebo treatment with prednisolone 7.5 mg/day. Patients were allowed to continue on routine medication, including second-line agents. The development of erosions and radiographic progression shown by changes in the Larsen score [31] were the primary outcome measures. After 2 years in the 106 patients available for full assessment, the Larsen scores increased by a mean of 0.72 units in the prednisolone group, indicating very little change, and by 5.37 units in the placebo group, indicating substantial joint destruction ($P = .004$). Of the 212 hands in these patients, 147 (69.3%) had no erosions at the start of the study. At 2 years, 15 of the 68 such hands in the prednisolone group (22.1%) and 36 of the 79 such hands in the placebo group (45.6%) had acquired

Table 5 Some Randomized Controlled Trials of Corticosteroids in Rheumatoid Arthritis

Ref.	Year	No. of patients	Treatment (mg/day)	Comparator	Duration (months)	Radiographic result	Comments
19	1954	61	Cortisone	Aspirin (80) 4.5 g/day	12	Not assessed	Withdrawal flares
20	1955	100	Cortisone (69)	Aspirin 4 g/day	12	Nonsignificant but higher porosis and erosion scores in aspirin group	Erosion score could have been refined. If cut-off taken at moderate to severe scores, cortisone did far better.
21 22	1959	77	Prednisolone (12 for year 1; 10 for years 2)	Aspirin	36	Less after 1 and 2 years	Followed up for 3 years. Prednisolone probably held advantage into third year.
25	1961	183	Hydrocortisone (25–100)	Analgesics, 50 IM gold	>60	No difference (steroid group had better functional outcome)	Poorly matched, different doses and formulations, steroid group worse at start.
23	1967	74	Prednisolone (<15)	Aspirin	84	Less progression	10 mg better than 7.5 mg. Publication not readily accessible.
26	1981	10	Methylprednisolone (a g/month)	Placebo	6	No difference	Very few patients
27	1983	18	Prednisolone (5)	Placebo crossover at 24/52	10	Less progression in steroid group (and better functional outcome)	Very few patients
28	1984	103	Prednisolone (10.3)	No steroids	120	Less erosions	Broad treatment comparison with contamination between groups
29	1990	97	Methyl-prednisolone (1 g/IV monthly)	IV saline	12	No difference in erosion scores	
9	1995	128	Prednisolone (7.5)	Placebo	24	Reduced erosive change	

erosions (difference, 23.5%, 95% confidence interval 5.9–40.7; $P = .007$). The patients in the prednisolone group had greater reductions than the patients in the placebo group in scores on an articular index and for pain and disability at 3 months; for pain at 6 months; and for disability at 6, 12, and 15 months (all $P < .05$). There was no difference between the groups for standardized scores for the acute phase response. One can conclude from this study that a fixed daily low dose of prednisolone (7.5 mg) can reduce the rate of radiographic progression over 2 years in patients with early RA who are taking concomitant treatment with other second-line agents. An important observation made in this study was that there was a dissociation between the response of three different aspects of RA in the prednisolone treatment. Compared with the placebo group, any increased suppression of the acute phase response had been lost by 3 months. Beneficial reduction in the symptoms of synovitis was evident in the prednisolone group, but only for 6–9 months. In contrast, control of radiographic progression was evident for the whole 2 years of treatment.

IV. ARE CORTICOSTEROIDS DISEASE-MODIFYING AGENTS?

The term *disease-modifying agent* was coined to describe compounds which not only relieved the symptoms of inflammation in RA (which can also be achieved by nonsteroidal anti-inflammatory drugs) but also reduced the acute phase response. The early compounds (gold, D-penicillamine, hydroxychloroquine, sulfasalazine) also shared the property of a delay of several months before the onset of their therapeutic benefit (hence their other name, "slow-acting" agents). Although there was no convincing evidence that these agents altered radiographic progression [32,33], they were seen to act in terms of the model of RA shown in Figure 3, in which erosive change is a direct consequence of synovitis. Evidence is now accumulating that the process of synovitis is T-cell driven, whereas that of cartilage and bone destruction may be more macrophage mediated [34]. In this regard, an important finding of the low-dose prednisolone study was the obser-

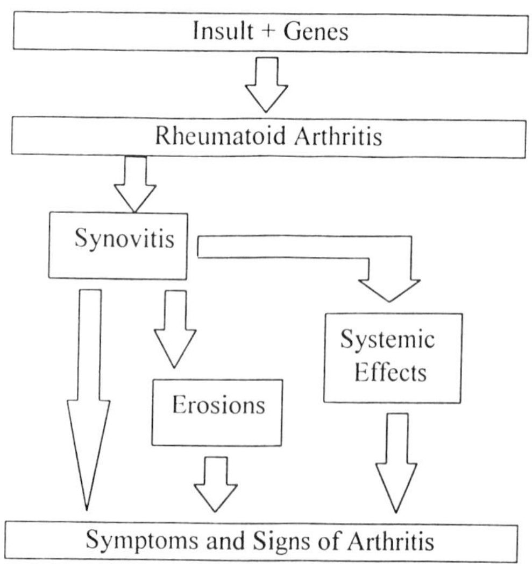

Figure 3 Traditional model of rheumatoid arthritis.

vation that the symptomatic benefits of corticosteroids (i.e., the reduction of synovitis) lasted only 6–9 months, whereas the suppressive effect on erosions persisted throughout the 2 years of study. Thus the causative link between synovitis and erosions is less convincing. Furthermore, in the ARC study, corticosteroids did not alter the acute phase response (except possibly in the very early weeks), suggesting that it too is not necessarily related to synovitis or erosions in a causal way. A more appropriate model of RA, which can accommodate these observations and is similar to that advocated by Kirwan and Currey [32], is shown in Figure 4. Thus the term *disease modifying* is an inappropriate one to describe drug actions, as all drugs used in RA modify the disease to some extent.

V. RECOMMENDATIONS FOR THE USE OF CORTICOSTEROIDS IN RA

Although corticosteroids cannot be recommended universally for all patients with RA, there are certain situations in which they may be the preferred treatment for symptom control. Owing to their relatively good safely profile, corticosteroids may be used for arthritic flares in pregnancy. Low-dose prednisolone may be a preferable alternative to nonsteroidal anti-inflammatory drugs in the elderly in order to avoid aggravation of renal or cardiac failure. The use of high-dose corticosteroids in systemic and vasculitic crises is widely practiced [16]. From the evidence of the MRC and ARC trials reviewed above, there is a case for using 7.5 mg prednisolone to treat some patients with RA in the early years of their disease (Table 6). Treating nonerosive patients more than 3 years after diagnosis will result in no benefit, as such patients are extremely unlikely to develop radiographic change [35]. The published findings for radiographic protection could

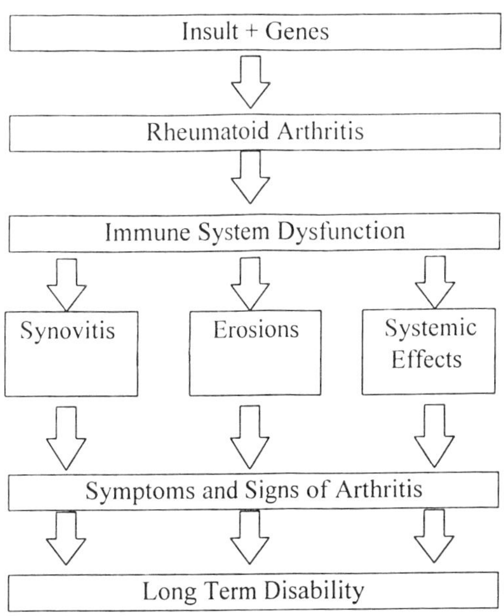

Figure 4 New model of rheumatoid arthritis showing possible sites of action of various drugs.

Table 6 Suggested Patients Suitable for Treatment with Low-dose Prednisolone Therapy

	Time since diagnosis (years)		
	0–2	3–5	>5
Erosions present	Treat	Probably treat	Probably do not treat
Erosions absent	Treat	Do not treat	Do not treat

reasonably be extrapolated into the fourth and fifth years of disease, but further extension of these findings would be difficult to justify without additional evidence of efficacy.

In the treatment of any disease which is not immediately fatal, the benefits must be weighed against the adverse effects that can be produced by the treatment. In studies of the frequency of adverse effects of corticosteroids at low doses, it has been shown that weight gain, skin changes, hypertension, peptic ulceration, and adrenal suppression are not increased [36,37]. Although some studies have shown an adverse effect of corticosteroids on bone loss even at small doses, the subject of osteoporosis is controversial. The evidence for glucocorticoid-induced osteoporosis cautions against routine use in postmenopausal women [38]. There is, however, an independent risk of osteoporosis in RA. Patients on corticosteroids tend to have more severe disease and as such are at greater risk of osteoporosis owing to the disease itself and the associated functional disability [4]. Corticosteroids used at higher doses in systemic lupus erythematosus (SLE) and in polymyalgia rheumatica do not seem to cause the same frequency of problems seen in RA. The improved function resulting from glucocorticoid treatment would reduce the rate of bone loss because of increased functional activity, which has a positive effect on bone density. Finally, even if low-dose glucocorticoid treatment does cause increased bone loss in RA, it is not entirely clear how this translates into clinically important fractures even though there is evidence that fracture risk is partially related to the total cumulative steroid dose [38]. There is some evidence that supplementation with biphosphanates and/or hormone-replacement therapy may retard bone loss with the potential to reduce the frequency of fractures [38,39]. One reasonable approach may be to avoid prescribing corticosteroids in patients at high risk of serious adverse effects. These include thin, frail, elderly women; patients with a history of serious cardiovascular disease (ischemic heart disease, hypercholesterolemia, and hypertension) and those with poorly controlled diabetes.

VI. SUMMARY

Corticosteroids have been shown to influence several aspects of RA, but to do so differentially. Following the addition of prednisolone to standard management regimens, the beneficial effects on symptoms of are relatively short lived, but reduction in radiographic progression in relatively early disease persists for 2 or 3 years. These findings open up new therapeutic avenues and also promote a new view of the pathogenesis of RA. The balance of evidence suggests that fixed, low-dose prednisolone does indeed modify some of the underlying process of RA. Given for 2 years in early disease, it produces clear benefit, but the benefit to risk ratio in the longer term awaits further clarification.

REFERENCES

1. Kirwan JR Silman AJ. Epidemiological, social and environmental aspects of rheumatoid arthritis and osteoarthritis. Bailliere's Clin Rheumatol 1987; 1:467–489.
2. Kirwan JR, et al. The effect of National Health Service reforms on outpatient rheumatology workload. Br J Rheumatol 1994; 33:1181–1183.
3. Pincus T. Rheumatoid arthritis: disappointing long-term outcomes despite successful short term-clinical trials. J Clin Epidemiol 1988; 41:1037–1041.
4. Scott DL, Spector TD, Pullar T, McConkey B. What should we hope to achieve when treating rheumatoid arthritis? Ann Rheum Dis 1989; 48:256–261.
5. Hench PS, Kendall EC, Slocumb CH, et al. Effects of a hormone of the adrenal cortex (17-hydroxy-11 dehydrocorticosterone compound E) and of pituitary adrenocorticotrophic hormone on rheumatoid arthritis. Preliminary report. Proc Staff Meetings of Mayo Clin 1949; 24:181–197.
6. Weisman MH. Should steroids be used in the management of rheumatoid arthritis? Rheum Dis Clin North Am 1993; 19:189–199.
7. Harris ED Jr, Emkey RD, Nicholas JE, et al. Low dose prednisolone therapy in rheumatoid arthritis. A double blind study. J Rheumatol 1983; 10:713–721.
8. Weiss MM. Corticosteroids in rheumatoid arthritis. Semin Arthritis Rheum 1989: 19:1:9–21.
9. Kirwan JR, Byron M, Dieppe P, et al. The effect of glucocorticoids on joint destruction in rheumatoid arthritis. N Engl J Med 1995; 333:142–146.
10. Mills LC. Adrenal cortex and adrenocortical hormone. In: DiPalma JD, ed. Drill's Pharmacology in Medicine, 4th ed. New York: McGraw-Hill, 1971:1526–1583.
11. Loftus J, Allen R, Hesp R, et al. Randomised, double-blind trial of deflazacort versus prednisolone in juvenile chronic (or rheumatoid) arthritis. A relatively bone-sparing effect of Deflazacort. Pediatrics 1991; 88:428–436.
12. Lim KKT, Kirwan JR. The place of glucocorticoid therapy in the treatment of rheumatoid arthritis. Rheum Rev 1994; 3:193–197.
13. Dinarello CA. Interleukin 1. Rev Infec Dis 1984; 6:51–95.
14. Grabstein K, Dower S, Gillis S, et al. Expression of interleukin 2, interferon-gamma and the IL-2 receptor by human peripheral blood lymphocytes. J Immunol 1986; 15; 136 (12):4503–4503.
15. Beutler B, Krochen N, Milsark IW, et al. Control of cachectin (TNF) synthesis mechanisms of endotoxin resistance. Science 1986; 232:977–980.
16. George E & Kirwan JR. Glucocorticoid therapy in rheumatoid arthritis. Bailliere's Clin Rheumatol 1990; 4:621–647.
17. Panayi GS. Heberden Oration, 1992. The pathogenesis of rheumatoid arthritis: From molecules to the whole patient. Br J Rheum 1993; 32:533–536.
18. Chikanza IC, Petrou P, Kingsley G, et al. Defective hypothalamic response to immune and inflammatory stimuli in patients with rheumatoid arthritis. Arthritis Rheumat 1992; 35:1281–88.
19. Joint Committee of the Medical Research Council and Nuffield Foundation. A comparison of cortisone and aspirin in the treatment of early cases of rheumatoid arthritis. Br Med J 1954; 29:1223–1227.
20. Empire Rheumatism Council. Multi-centre controlled trial comparing cortisone acetate and acetyl salicylic acid in the long-term treatment of rheumatoid arthritis. Ann Rheum Dis 1955; 14:353–367.
21. Joint Committee of the Medical Research Council and Nuffield Foundation. A comparison of prednisolone with aspirin or other analgesics in the treatment of rheumatoid arthritis. Ann Rheum Dis 1959; 18:173–187.
22. Joint Committee of the Medical Research Council and Nuffield Foundation. A comparison

of prednisolone with aspirin or other analgesics in the treatment of rheumatoid arthritis. Ann Rheum Dis 1960; 19:331–337.
23. West HF. Rheumatoid arthritis. The relevance of clinical knowledge to research activities. Abstr World Med 1967; 41:401–417.
24. Masi AT. Low dose glucocorticoid therapy in rheumatoid arthritis. J Rheumatol 1983; 10:675–678.
25. Berntsen CA, Freyberg RH. Rheumatoid patients after five or more years of glucocorticoid treatment: a comparative analysis of 183 cases. Ann Intern Med 1961; 54:938–953.
26. Leibling MR, Leib E, McLaughlin K. Pulse methyl-prednisolone in rheumatoid arthritis. Ann Intern Med 1981; 4:21–26.
27. Harris ED Jr, Emkey RD, Nichols JE, et al. Low dose prednisolone therapy in rheumatoid arthritis: A double blind study. J Rheumatol 1983; 10:713–721.
28. Million R, Poole P, Kellgren JH, et al. Long-term study of management of rheumatoid arthritis. Lancet 1984; 1:812–816.
29. Hansen TM, Kryger P, Elling H, et al. Double blind placebo controlled trial of pulse treatment with methylprednisolone combined with disease modifying drugs in rheumatoid arthritis. Br Med J 1990; 301:268–270.
30. Byron MA, Kirwan JR. Corticosteroids in rheumatoid arthritis: Is a trial of their 'disease modifying' potential feasible? Ann Rheum Dis 1986; 46:171–173.
31. Larsen A, Dale K, Eek M. Radiographic evaluation of rheumatoid arthritis and related conditions by standard reference films. Acta Radiol 1977; 18:481–491.
32. Kirwan JR, Currey HLF. Rheumatoid arthritis: disease modifying anti-rheumatoid drugs. Clin Rheum Dis 1983; 9:581–599.
33. Iannuzzi L, Dawson N, Zein N, Kushnev I. Does drug therapy slow radiographic deterioration in rheumatoid arthritis? N Engl J Med 1983; 309:1023–1028.
34. Bresnihan B, Mulherin D, FitzGerald O. Synovial pathology and articular erosions in rheumatoid arthritis. Rheumatol Eur 1995; 24(Suppl 2):158–160.
35. Brook A, Corbett M. Radiographic change in early rheumatoid disease. Ann Rheumat Dis 1977; 36:71–73.
36. Caldwell JR, Furst DE. The efficacy and safety of low-dose corticosteroids for rheumatoid arthritis. Semin Arthritis Rheum 1991; 21;1:1–11.
37. Sambrook PN, Eisman JA, Yeates MG, et al. Osteoporosis in rheumatoid arthritis: Safety of low dose corticosteroids. Annals of the Rheumatic Diseases 1986; 45:950–953.
38. Hall GM, Spector TD, Griffin AJ, et al. The effect of rheumatoid arthritis and steroid therapy on bone density in postmenopausal women. Arthritis Rheum 1993; 36:11:1510–1516.
39. Adachi JD, Cranney A, Goldsmith CH, et al. Intermittent cycle therapy with etidronate in the prevention of glucocorticoid induced bone loss. J Rheumatol 1994; 21:1922–1926.

17

Biological Agents Directed Against Cell Surface Antigens in the Treatment of Rheumatoid Arthritis

Ferdinand C. Breedveld
Leiden University Hospital, Leiden, The Netherlands

I. INTRODUCTION

Patients with rheumatoid arthritis (RA) have symmetrical synovitis of their peripheral joints and various degrees of joint destruction. In short-term studies, slow-acting antirheumatic drugs relieve symptoms and retard joint destruction, but many patients continue to have pain, stiffness, fatigue, and progressive disability [1]. Furthermore, there is a high frequency of potentially severe side effects which makes monitoring mandatory. Better treatments are needed. Our steadily increasing knowledge of mechanisms leading to tissue destruction in RA allows the utilization of the latest biotechnology techniques to develop more effective and less toxic therapies. Such therapies can be targeted at components of the immune response that are critical in the generation of rheumatoid inflammation. This chapter focuses on the experience with the use of biological agents directed against cell surface antigens in the treatment of RA.

II. INTERVENTION STRATEGIES

The results of several lines of research suggest that T-cell activation has a central role in the initiation and perpetuation of RA. These include morphological studies of the rheumatoid synovial membrane that show the dominant presence of T cells—in particular the $CD4^+$ helper subsets [2]; genetic studies that have established the association of RA with the expression of particular major histocompatibility complex (MHC) molecules [3], and clinical observations of an association between decreasing disease activity and decreased T-cell function [4,5]. Therefore, RA is thought to be driven by the presentation of an arthritogenic peptide complexed to MHC class II molecule on an antigen-presenting cell to a $CD4^+$ T-cell carrying the appropriate T-cell receptor (TCR). This results in T-cell activation which leads to activation of many other cells via the production of cytokines. The T-cell cytokine-activated cells considered to play a contributory role in immunologically driven inflammation of RA include B cells, macrophages, fibroblasts, and endothelial cells [5]. Not surprisingly, T-cell–targeted interventions were primary candidates to be selected for drug development.

Two types of intervention strategies have been developed using T-cell–targeted biological agents. A specific strategy would include interventions that influence the formation of the trimolecular complex of MHC molecules, antigens, and TCR and thereby abrogate the response of autoantigens in RA without compromising normal immune function. A second one has been selectively to target elements of the immune response irrespective of their antigen specificity. These interventions used agents that bind to the cell surface molecules of T cells, adhesion molecules, or cytokines.

III. AGENTS BINDING TO T-CELL SURFACE MOLECULES

The most frequently employed agents have been antibodies. Although earlier investigators had used polyclonal antibodies, more recently most groups have taken advantage of monoclonal antibody (mAb) technology. The mAbs have several advantages as therapeutic agents, with the most important being the possibility to produce unlimited quantities of uniform antibodies with a single specificity. The efficacy of mAbs with a particular specificity will depend on the characteristics of the targeted antigen such as its cell surface density and tissue distribution as well as the mAb characteristics, including fine specificity, affinity, and heavy chain isotype. mAbs directed against human targets are usually produced in animals and the commonest source is mice. By varying the immunoglobulin subclass mAbs can be designed to deplete cells or to bind to the cell surface and thereby inhibit their functions. In addition, killing of a target may be enhanced by the conjugation of mAbs with a cellular toxin, a so-called immunotoxin. This enhances cytotoxicity and may allow the usage of lower dosages. Some mAbs stimulate the target cells in vivo, which results in side effects through the release of cytokines and other inflammatory mediators.

A. CD4 Monoclonal Antibodies

Most information has been obtained with mAbs against the CD4 surface molecule. More than 150 RA patients with refractory disease have been enrolled in phase I and II studies. In general, daily dosages of 10–100 mg were administered, resulting in total dosages of 70–700 mg per treatment. It should be noted that the doses used in RA were much lower than those used in the treatment of animal models of autoimmune disease. Comparisons between the results of studies in RA are difficult, because they used different treatment regimens and different CD4 mAbs. In general, the side effects were mild but included flu-like symptoms, probably due to a cytokine-release syndrome. The injection of CD4 mAbs is followed by an immediate depression of the number of circulating $CD4^+$ cells lasting a few days in the case of murine antibodies but persisting for up to many months in the case of chimerized antibodies of the immunoglobulin G1 (IgG1) class. To date, the mechanism responsible for the prolonged depletion of circulating $CD4^+$ T cells has not been elucidated. Clinical results following administration of two murine IgG1 and three IgG2a mAbs were remarkably similar [6–10]. Clinical responses as judged by a significant reduction in the Ritchie index were observed in approximately 60–75% of the patients, but all evaluations were unblinded. Generally, 3 months of benefit was reported with a range of 1–12 months. Despite the strong effect on the number of circulating $CD4^+$ cells, there has been no consistent improvement in the traditional laboratory measures of disease activity such as acute phase proteins. To date, only the 16H5 [6] and BF-5 [7] produced a significant decrease in the serum C-reactive protein levels.

Three studies involved the cM-T412 CD4 mAb, which is a chimeric antibody with an IgG1 Fc region. One study reported a significant clinical response in patients treated with 50 mg in contrast to those treated with 10 mg CM-T412 daily for 7 days [11]. The other studies reported beneficial clinical effects of various dosages of mAbs given once or repeatedly to patients who were [12] or were not [13] concomitantly treated with a stable dose of methotrexate. These antibodies did not induce decreased levels of acute phase proteins.

Three placebo-controlled studies were performed on CD4 mAbs, all with cM-T412 [14–16]. In one study, single-dose infusions with placebo or 5, 10, or 50 mg Cd4 mAbs were given in 3 consecutive months in 64 methotrexate-treated RA patients [14]. In the other controlled study, two patients were randomized to placebo and seven to single-dose infusions with 50 mg cM-T412 [15]. A third controlled study has investigated the efficacy of multiple-dosage regimens of CD4 mAb treatment of RA patients in an early phase of the disease [16]. The main conclusion of these studies is that treatment with cM-T412 CD4 mAbs induces no improvement of arthritis activity. The results of these studies are in clear contrast with the therapeutic effect of multiple-dosage regimens of CD4 mAb treatment observed in previous open studies on RA patients. Several factors may account for the discrepancies, with the most obvious being the usage of a placebo-controlled design. Placebo effects in the treatment of rheumatoid arthritis have long been recognized. The discrepancy between the improvement in clinical parameters of disease and not in the objective laboratory parameters such as erythrocyte sedimentation rate (ESR) and serum C-reactive protein (CRP) levels are compatible with a placebo effect in the open studies. Another explanation may be that the type of CD4 mAb employed accounts for the difference in results between some studies. The CD4 mAbs investigated so far in the treatment of RA differ with respect to epitope specificity, affinity and Fc isotype, in vitro effects on T-cell functions, modulatory effect on the CD4 surface molecule, and in the capacity to induce a decrease in the number of circulating $CD4^+$ cells in vivo. Since the relation between these antibody characteristics and clinical efficacy is not known, further insight in possible differences in clinical efficacy between different CD4 mAbs has to come from direct clinical comparison. Synovial biopsies of patients treated with chimeric CD4 mAb cM-T412 showed a reduction in the number of inflammatory cells and decreased expression of adhesion molecules after treatment [17]. However, a significant number of lymphocytes remained in the synovia of CD4 mAb–treated RA patients. Furthermore, the synovial CD4/CD8 lymphocyte ratio remained unchanged, so that there was no preferential depletion of $CD4^+$ lymphocytes. It is conceivable that even the low numbers of $CD4^+$ cells found in the synovium of the patients treated with cM-T412 may have maintained enough inflammation to explain the lack of clinical effect in these patients.

The experience with IgG1 CD4 mAbs suggests that almost complete elimination of synovial lymphocytes is necessary to achieve therapeutic efficacy. This will also lead to blood lymphopenia and an immune compromised state. As an alternative strategy, tolerance induction by means of prolonged blockage of CD4 molecules with nondepleting CD4 mAbs has been suggested. It has been reported that mice develop antihuman antibodies on a transfusion with human IgG. However, if CD4 mAbs that did not induce T-cell depletion were coadministered, this response is suppressed [18]. A relatively nondepleting CD4 mAb has recently been used in refractory RA patients. Clinical improvement was variable but was found to be meaningful in some patients. At 3 days immediately after the injection, all circulating $CD4^+$ cells were coated with mAbs, which offers the prospective that a state of tolerance might be achieved [19]. Several studies using nondepleting CD4 mAbs are being planned. Obviously, if treatment with anti-CD4 mAbs could induce a state of tolerance, this would be the preferred mechanism for the treatment of human autoimmune disease.

B. Other Monoclonal Antibodies Against T Cells

An immunoconjugate of murine IgG1 mAb against CD5 antigen coupled to ricine (a ribosomal inhibitory protein) was investigated in RA. CD5 is present on the majority of T cells and a subset of B cells. Following two positive open-label trials, a placebo-controlled randomized trial of 104 patients failed to show efficacy [20]. The responses in the placebo cohort exceeded the active treatment group. This agent is no longer under development. Monoclonal antibodies against the CD7 and CDw52 (Campath-1H) proteins, both present on the majority of T cells, have been investigated for antirheumatic properties in open studies [21,22]. Despite the induction of T lymphocytopenia by both antibodies, there was only modest and short-lived improvement in the clinical state and no significant change in the acute phase response. Campath-1H fixes complement effectively, and hence it is very lytic for CDw52-positive cells. Following infusions, severe lymphokine release syndromes have been reported. In addition, after Campath-1H treatment, several patients were found to develop life-threatening infections and malignant lymphomas, indicating that clinical experiments with mAbs against components of the immune system should be performed with great caution [23].

C. Interleukin-2 Fusion Toxin

Another strategy employed DAB interleukin-2 (IL-2), which is a fusion protein of the enzymatically active fragment of diphtheria toxin, the membrane-translocating portion, and sequences for human IL-2, produced by recombinant expression in *Escherichia coli*. DAB IL-2 binds specifically to the high-affinity IL-2R and is rapidly internalized via receptor-mediated endocytosis. Once internalized into an acidic vesicle, the enzymatically active fragment is released into the cytosol and inhibits protein synthesis, resulting in cell death. Only activated T cells express IL-2 receptors and will therefore be killed in particular. DAB IL-2 has been evaluated in short-term placebo-controlled trials in patients with long-standing refractory RA [24,25]. In an initial blinded study, a 5-day course of DAB IL-2 was compared with placebo. No responders were observed in the placebo group ($n = 23$) compared with 4 of 22 in the treatment group ($P = .05$) as defined by $\geq 25\%$ improvement in both swollen and tender joint count. In another placebo-controlled study of DAB Il-2, no difference was observed between the active ($n = 33$) and placebo ($n = 32$) treatment at 1 month.

D. Monoclonal Antibodies Against Adhesion Molecules

The strategy of targeting adhesion molecules is attractive, since these molecules are used by circulating immunocompetent and inflammatory cells to enter the site of inflammation. In addition, disease improvement may be obtained, because adhesion molecules are involved in the activation of many cells that participate in inflammation, T cells in particular [26]. Although T cells possess a repertoire of adhesion receptors, several studies have demonstrated a predominant role for lymphocyte function-associated antigen-1 (LFA-1), which binds to its ligand intracellular adhesion molecules 1–3 (ICAM1–3). A murine IgG2 anti–ICAM-1 mAb has been investigated as a treatment for RA in a open-label dose-escalating study [27].

The investigators conclude that anti–ICAM-1 mAb therapy is well tolerated and effective in at least some RA patients. Most patients relapsed 3 months after treatment. Transient lymphocytosis was noted in all patients, which was interpreted as suggesting that ICAM-1 mAb was blocking migration of lymphocytes from the circulation into inflammatory sites. This idea was further supported by the observation that cutaneous delayed-type hypersensitivity reactions were diminished during treatment. However, further placebo-controlled trials are necessary really to assess the role of this therapeutic principle in RA.

IV. POSSIBILITIES FOR LONG-TERM TREATMENT

Some of the observations discussed so far show promise but also suggest that long-term treatment may be necessary to control RA. This raises particular problems with the use of mAbs because anti-mAb responses occur frequently. After a single treatment cycle with murine CD4 mAbs, most patients developed human antimouse antibodies (HAMA). HAMA activity of most patients was also directed against the specific antigen-binding site [6]. In an attempt to lower the immunogenicity of mAb and thereby decrease HAMA formation chimeric antibodies with murine variable regions and human constant regions have been produced as well as humanized antibodies where only the antigen-binding site remains of murine origin. This indeed lowers the antiglobulin responses [22,28]. However, after repeated monthly treatments during 9 months with a chimeric CD4 mAb, most patients were found to have developed anti-mAb responses that block CD4 mAb–binding in vitro [29]. Antibodies against DAB IL-2 were also reported in the majority of patients treated as such. The antiglobulin responses may lead to allergic reactions and are likely to block the functional activity of the mAbs. The possible problems created by antiglobulin responses could conceivably be obviated by using completely human antibodies. Although completely human antibodies may be available in the future, the difficulty of generating human mAbs with high-activity specificities of interest has dictated that most mAbs are in part of mouse origin.

V. SPECIFIC IMMUNOTHERAPY

A. T-Cell and T-Cell Receptor Peptide Vaccination

A novel approach for the treatment of autoimmune diseases was suggested by Cohen and co-workers, who demonstrated in experimental autoimmune disease models that disease-inducing T-cell clones could be employed to induce resistance against autoimmune disease following attenuation of the T cells being employed as a vaccine. This procedure, designated T-cell vaccination (TCV), was assumed to be based on the interference in a network of T cells that recognize cell surface structures expressed by certain other T cells. The inoculation of rats with antigen-specific T cells that had been activated in vitro and subsequently attenuated yielded an anti–T-cell response consisting of T cells that were shown to recognize idiotypic or activation markers on the target T-cell clone. Rats that had been "vaccinated" with these T cells were resistant to active and passive disease induction. Protection could be transferred with these so-called "anti-idiotypic" T cells [30,31]. These experiments opened up new pathways for the treatment of human autoimmune disease. RA was a logical choice, since the T-cell population present in the joint was supposed to contain disease-relevant T-cell clones and since these cells were easily accessible for removal. In addition, analysis of the central portions of the antigen-binding site of TCR (CDR3 region) revealed an altered composition of amino acids in the CDR3 regions of TCRs derived from the site of inflammation compared with those of the periphery, suggesting that these T cells selectively accumulated in the synovium [32].

In an open study, 13 RA patients have been treated by means of a subcutaneous inoculation with attenuated autologous T cells [33]. None of the patients developed a clear cellular or humoral immune response to the vaccine. Responses of peripheral blood mononuclear cells (PBMCs) cells against irradiated, activated T cells from the inoculum could be detected but, with the possible exception of one patient, did not differ from pretreatment levels. Both before and after treatment, skin reactions against the intracutaneous administered vaccine T cells occurred and, although histology did show characteristics of a DTH reaction, the rapid onset and marginal induration were not typical. Finally, no anti–T-cell antibodies were detected in postvaccination sera. Nevertheless, several findings suggested immunomodulatory effects of the procedure. Interestingly, this was most pronounced in the patient with recent-onset disease, who was inoculated with the *Mycobacterium tuberculosis*-reactive T-cell clone. Apart from a beneficial clinical response within 2 weeks after treatment and lasting for 3 months, mitogen reactivity of PBMCs was reduced for 3 months, and the increased titers of rheumatoid factor (RF) of the IgM isotype returned to normal levels after treatment. In two other patients who were vaccinated, a strong decrease of serum rheumatoid factor (RF) levels was also noted.

Although the study was not designed to evaluate the clinical effectiveness of the treatment, a preliminary impression of the influence on disease activity could be obtained. Disease activity was determined by monitoring of the Ritchie index, grip strenght, morning stiffness, number of swollen joints, and laboratory parameters of disease activity. Taken as a group, mean values of all parameters indicated an improvement of disease activity during the first 2 months after treatment. However, variability of the responses among the individual patients was high, and a remission of disease was not observed in any of the patients.

Other investigators employing a similar protocol in multiple sclerosis reported a decrease in the frequency of circulating myelin basic protein (MBP) reactive T cells on vaccination with MBP-specific T cells [35]. The experience obtained now shows that this technique is feasible and safe. Another approach to eliminate putative pathogenic T cells is vaccination with peptides derived from portions of T-cell receptors. Since several studies have reported overrepresentation of Vβ14 and Vβ17 T-cell receptor utilization in synovial T-cell populations, the first open-label studies have been conducted in RA patients using immunization of Vβ14 and Vβ17 peptides with incomplete Freund's adjuvant. After 6 weeks, a cellular immune response against the peptide was detected in ±50% of the patients [36]. This approach will be studied more extensively in RA.

B. Oral Tolerance

Although the role of immune responses to collagen in the pathogenesis of RA has not been elucidated, anticollagen antibodies and anticollagen T-cell reactivity are present in patients with RA. Collagen has been suggested to be one of the inciting antigens in the initiation and/or perpetuation of synovitis. Oral administration of an antigen has been demonstrated to induce a state of specific immune unresponsiveness to the antigen; a procedure termed oral tolerance. Feeding of collagen type II was shown to be effective in the prevention and treatment of the adjuvant and collagen models of arthritis. A placebo-controlled randomized controlled trial utilized oral doses of chicken collagen type II in 60 patients with active RA [34]. Results revealed a greater reduction in the mean number of tender and swollen joints in collagen-treated patients compared with controls. At 3 months, 14% of the active group and 13% of the placebo group were considered responders. No toxicity was reported and no biological effect was apparent. This study has been criticized for its short duration and the absence of a wash-out period from dosing with second-line agents prior to initiating oral treatment. In addition, an asymmetrical distribution of patients with increased disease severity may have influenced the results. Recently, the results of a second study on oral administration of collagen have been presented [38]. In this study, 90 RA patients were treated over 12 weeks with bovine collagen type II in a dosage of 1 mg, 10 mg, or placebo in a double-blind randomized study. In this study, there was no significant difference in the response rate between the three groups. However, a strong clinical improvement was found in three patients of the 10-mg group and one patient of the 1-mg group. Further work will be necessary to elucidate better the potential clinical role of this well tolerated therapy.

VI. CONCLUSIONS

The initial clinical interventions with T-cell–targeted biological agents or immune-specific interventions have been met with great enthusiasm which has not been confirmed in subsequent controlled clinical trials. With the possible exception of therapy with CDw52 mAb therapy, major toxic side effects have not been observed. Despite the prolonged peripheral blood lymphocytopenia observed after treatment with chimeric CD4 mAbs, no clear evidence of an immune-compromized state has been obtained. It might be that more selectively targeted therapies may offer more benefit. However, for the further development of targeted therapies, several fundamental questions still need to be answered. These include: How does one define and select disease-inducing T cells or the immune reaction that drives the chronic inflammation in RA? What is an efficient way to block T-cell functions or to induce an immune response against those T cells that are relevant for the disease? How can one reliably measure the effect of a particular intervention on the pivotal immune mechanisms of the rheumatoid inflammation? Some of these questions may be addressed in animal models, but it has become quite clear during the studies discussed above that it is a long way from an experimental rodent model to the treatment of a patient.

REFERENCES

1. Pincus T, Callahan LF, Sale WG, et al. Severe functional declines, work disability, and increased mortality in seventy-five rheumatoid arthritis patients studied over nine years. Arthritis Rheum 1984; 27:864–872.
2. Pitzalis C, Kingsley G, Lanchbury JSS, et al. Expression of HLA-DR, DQ and DP antigens and interleukin-2 receptor on synovial fluid T lymphocyte subsets in rheumatoid arthritis: evidence for "frustrated" activation. J Rheumatol 1987; 14:662–666.
3. Zeben van D, Hazes JMW, Zwinderman AH, et al. Association of HLA-DR4 with a more progressive disease course in patients with rheumatoid arthritis. Arthritis Rheum 1991; 34:822–830.
4. Bijlsma JWJ, Derksen RWHM, Huber-Bruning O, Borleffs JCC. Does AIDS cure rheumatoid arthritis? Ann Rheum Dis 1988; 47:350–352.
5. Firestein GS, Zvaifler NJ. How important are T cells in chronic rheumatoid synovitis? Arthritis Rheum 1990; 33:768–773.
6. Horneff G, Burmester GR, Emmerich F, Kalden JR. Treatment of rheumatoid arthritis with an anti-CD4 monoclonal antibody. Arthritis Rheum 1991; 34:129–140.
7. Wendling D, Racadot E, Morel-Fourrier B, Wijdenes J. Treatment of rheumatoid arthritis with anti-CD4 monoclonal antibody. Open study of 25 patients with the B-F5 clone. Clin Rheumatol 1992; 11:542–547.
8. Goldberg D, Morel P, Chatenoud L, et al. Immunological effects of high dose administration of anti-CD4 antibody in rheumatoid arthritis patients. J Autoimmun 1991; 4:617–630.
9. Reiter C, Kakawand B, Rieber EP, et al. Treatment of rheumatoid arthritis with monoclonal CD4 antibody M-T151. Arthritis Rheum 1991; 34:525–536.
10. Herzog C, Walker C, Müller W, et al. Anti-CD4 antibody treatment of patients with rheumatoid arthritis: I Effect on clinical course and circulating T cells. J Autoimmun 1989; 2:627–642.
11. Van der Lubbe PA, Reiter C, Breedveld FC, et al. Chimeric CD4 monoclonal antibody cM-T412 as a therapeutic approach to rheumatoid arthritis. Arthritis Rheum 1993; 36:1375–1379.
12. Moreland LW, Bucy RP, Tilden A, et al. Use of a chimeric monoclonal anti-CD4 antibody in patients with refractory rheumatoid arthritis. Arthritis Rheum 1993; 36:307–318.
13. Choy EHS, Pitzalis C, Bijl JA, et al. The importance of dose and dosing regimen on anti-CD4 monoclonal antibody in the treatment of rheumatoid arthritis [abstr]. Arthritis Rheum 1993; 36:S129.
14. Moreland L, Pratt P, Mayes M, et al. Minimal efficacy of a depleting chimeric anti-CD4 (cM-T412) in treatment of patients with refractory rheumatoid arthritis receiving concomitant methotrexate [abstr]. Arthritis Rheum 1993; 36:S39.
15. Choy EHS, Chikanza IC, Kingsley GH, et al. Treatment of rheumatoid arthritis with single dose or weekly pulses of chimeric anti-CD5 monoclonal antibody. Scand J Immunol 1992; 36:291–298.
16. Lubbe van der PA, Dijkmans BAC, Markusse HM, et al. A randomized, double-blind, placebo-controlled study of CD4 monoclonal antibody therapy in early rheumatoid arthritis. Arthritis Rheum 1995; 38:1097–1106.
17. Tak PP, van der Lubbe PA, Cauli A, et al. Reduction of synovial inflammation after anti-CD4 monoclonal antibody treatment in early rheumatoid arthritis. Arthritis Rheum 1995; 38:1457–1465.
18. Benjamin KJ, Waldmann H. Induction of tolerance by monoclonal antibody therapy. Nature 1986; 320:449–451.

19. Yocum DE, Nordensson K, Solinger AM. Immunomodulatory effect of IDEC-CE9.1 on anti CD4 monoclonal antibody in rheumatoid arthritis. Arthritis Rheum 1994; 37(Suppl):S336.
20. Olsen NJ, Cush JJ, Lipsky PE, et al. Multicentre trial of an anti CD5 immunoconjugate in rheumatoid arthritis. Arthritis Rheum 1994; 37:S295.
21. Kirkham BW, Thien F, Pelton BK, et al. Chimeric CD7 monoclonal antibody therapy in rheumatoid arthritis. J Rheumatol 1992; 19:1348–1352.
22. Isaacs JB, Watts RA, Hazleman BL, et al. Humanized monoclonal antibody therapy for rheumatoid arthritis. Lancet 1992; 340:748–752.
23. Isaacs JB, Manna VK, Hazelman BL, et al. Campath 1H in rheumatoid arthritis. Arthritis Rheum 1993; 36:S40.
24. Sewell KL, Parker KP, Woodworth TG, Reuben J, Swartz W, Trentham D. DAB_{486}IL-2 fusion toxin in refractory rheumatoid arthritis. Arthritis Rheum 1993; 26:1223–1233.
25. Moreland LW, Sewell KL, Sullivan WF, et al. Double-blind placebo-controlled phase II trial of diphtheria-interleukin-2 fusion toxic (DAB486IL2) in patients with refractory rheumatoid arthritis (RA). Arthritis Rheum 1993; 36:S39.
26. Gearing AJH, Newman W. Circulating adhesion molecules in disease. Immunol Today 1993; 14:506–512.
27. Kavanaugh AF, Davis LS, Nichols LA, et al. Treatment of refractory rheumatoid arthritis with a monoclonal antibody to intercellular adhesion molecule 1. Arthritis Rheum 1994; 37:992–999.
28. Riethmüller G, Rieber EP, Kiefersauer S, et al. From antilymphocyte serum to therapeutic monoclonal antibodies: first experiences with a chimeric CD4 antibody in the treatment of autoimmune disease. Immunol Rev 1992; 129:81–104.
29. Lubbe van der PA, Miltenburg AMM, Tak PP, et al. Immunological effects of chimeric CD4 monoclonal antibody (cM-T412) in patients with early rheumatoid arthritis. Arthritis Rheum 1995; 38(Suppl):S185.
30. Ben-Nun A, Wekerle H, Cohen IR. Vaccination against autoimmune encephalomyelitis with T lymphocyte line cells reactive against myelin basic protein. Nature 1981; 292:60.
31. Cohen IR. Physiological basis of T cell vaccination against autoimmune disease. Cold Spring Harbor Symp Quant Biol 1989; 154:879.
32. Struyk L, Hawes GE, Dolhain RJEM, et al. Evidence for selective in vivo expansion of synovia tissue infiltrating $CD4^{+}CD45RO^{+}$ T-lymphocytes on the basis of CDR3 diversity. Int Immunol 1994; 6:897–907.
33. Laar van JM, Miltenburg AMM, Verdonk MJA, et al. Effects of inoculation with attenuated autologous T cells in patients with rheumatoid arthritis. J Autoimmun 1993; 6:159–167.
34. Lohse AW, Bakker NPM, Hermann E, Poralla T, Jonker M, Meyer zum Buschenfelde KH. Induction of an anti-vaccine response by T cell vaccination in non-human primates and humans. J Autoimmun 1993; 1:121–130.
35. Zhang J, Medaer R, Stinissen P, Hafler D, Raus J. MHC-restricted depletion of human myelin basic protein–reactive T cells by T cell vaccination. Science 1993; 261:1451.
36. Moreland LW, Heck LW Jr, Koopman WJ, Saway PA. Vβ17 T-cell receptor peptide vaccine: results of a phase I dose finding study in patients with rheumatoid arthritis. Arthritis Rheum 1994; 37:S337.
37. Trentham DE, Dynesius-Trentham RA, Orav EJ, et al. Effects of oral administration of type II collagen on rheumatoid arthritis. Science 1993; 261:1727–1730.
38. Sieper J, Kay S, Eggens U, Zink A, Michison NA. Treatment of rheumatoid arthritis with oral collagen type II: results of a double-blind placebo-controlled randomized trial. Arthritis Rheum 1995; 38(Suppl):S957.

18

The Clinical Application of Cytokine Blockade in the Therapy of Rheumatoid Arthritis

Diana Davis, Michael J. Elliott,* and Ravinder N. Maini
The Kennedy Institute of Rheumatology, London, United Kingdom

I. INTRODUCTION

The cytokine network comprises a complex system of interacting chemical mediators which act principally on the cells mediating immune and inflammatory responses, thereby controlling their synthetic and proliferative properties. Many cytokines also exert systemic effects which may involve distant organs; for example, the modulation of acute phase protein synthesis by hepatocytes or hemopoiesis in the bone marrow. There is growing evidence that an imbalance in cytokine production at the level of the synovium plays a major role in the pathogenesis of rheumatoid arthritis (RA) both in terms of the initiation and the perpetuation of the disease process.

RA is a chronic disease characterized by pannus formation and associated with progressive destruction of articular cartilage. The precise etiology of RA is unknown, but a likely mechanism involves the triggering of arthritis by an unknown antigen against a background of genetic susceptibility. The resulting immune response is not controlled by normal damage-limiting mechanisms but instead leads to progressive joint destruction and chronic disease. The cellular interactions involved in this process are complex and varied, with cytokines playing a prominent role. For example, cytokines are involved in the multistep interaction between circulating leukocytes and the endothelium, which under the influence of chemokines, leads to leukocyte accumulation in the synovium. Cytokines are also involved in the interplay between immune and inflammatory cells, and at the pannus-cartilage and bone junction, they induce tissue-damaging molecules.

Of the numerous cytokines detected within the synovium and the synovial fluid of RA patients, several have been implicated in the pathogenesis of RA and so represent potential targets for cytokine-blocking therapy. They include interleukin-1 (IL-1),

**Current affiliation*: SmithKline Beecham Pharmaceuticals, Harlow, United Kingdom

tumor necrosis factor-α (TNF-α), IL-8, IL-6, and granulocyte-macrophage colony-stimulating factor (GM-CSF). Natural inhibitors of these proinflammatory cytokines have also been shown to be locally produced within the synovial joint, such as IL-10, transforming growth factor-β (TGF-β), and the IL-1 receptor antagonist (IL-1ra), as well as the soluble receptors for IL-1 and TNF-α (cleavage products of the cell surface receptors). In rheumatoid arthritis, the normal balance between inflammatory cytokines and their natural inhibitors appears to be disturbed. Reestablishing this equilibrium, for example, by increasing the concentration or effectiveness of such physiological inhibitors, provides another attractive approach to the therapy of rheumatoid arthritis.

This chapter focuses on the effects of biological cytokine-blocking agents in the treatment of RA where clinical trials have been published.

II. TARGETS FOR CYTOKINE BLOCKING THERAPY IN RA

A. Tumor Necrosis Factor-α

TNF-α is a 17-kD protein produced predominantly by activated monocytes-macrophages as well as some T cells and fibroblasts. It is processed from a bioactive 26-kD membrane-bound molecule [1] and circulates as a trimer. Although a polymorphism has been discovered within the TNF-α gene [2] which might affect TNF-α production, different alleles have not so far been associated with either susceptibility to, or disease severity in, RA [3]. Two TNF cell surface receptors (TNFRs) have been identified, the p55 (~55 kD) and the p75 (~70–80 kD) receptors, which exist in varying amounts on most cell types. They belong to the TNFR superfamily whose nine other members include nerve growth factor receptor and Fas and which share homology of a cysteine-rich extracellular domain [4]. The surface receptors are shed to form soluble TNFRs which bind to and neutralize circulating TNF-α. The proteolytic cleavage of these surface TNF receptors can be inhibited by synthetic metalloproteinase inhibitors [5].

TNF-α has been detected in RA synovial fluid [6], and both TNF-α and its messenger ribonucleic acid (mRNA) have been identified within the RA synovium and localized to the cartilage-pannus junction [7,8]. Many of the cells found to synthesize TNF-α have also been shown to express TNFRs [9] showing potential for autocrine and paracrine roles for TNF-α in the synovial joint. Circulating TNF-α is often difficult to detect, but it has been found by some investigators to reflect RA disease activity [10]. However, the soluble TNF receptors may give a more reliable indication of the degree of RA joint inflammation, being raised in active RA compared with osteoarthritis patients and normals in both the synovial fluid and the serum. Levels fall as disease becomes less active and are higher in synovial fluid than serum, suggesting local production within the joint [11].

Animal studies have strengthened the view that TNF-α plays a key role in the pathogenesis of RA. For example, if TNF-α is injected into a rabbit knee joint, an acute, although temporary, synovitis develops with neutrophil infiltration into the joint. Similarly, in collagen-induced arthritis, TNF-α administered before or during the development of arthritis leads to a more severe form of joint inflammation [12], whereas mice receiving neutralizing antibodies to TNF-α either prior to or after the development of arthritis show significant amelioration of the disease process [13]. The importance of TNF-α in the development of arthritis has been confirmed by the development of mice carrying a 3′-modified human TNF-α gene. Such mice overproduce TNF-α and develop a symmetrical, destructive, and erosive arthritis which is prevented if anti–TNF-α antibodies are administered from birth [14].

TNF-α has been shown directly to induce many proinflammatory cytokines including IL-1 [15], GM-CSF [16], and chemotactic factors, including IL-8 [17]. TNF-α, IL-1, and GM-CSF (as well as several other proinflammatory cytokines) are produced spontaneously by cultured RA synovial cells, but adding neutralizing TNF-α antibodies to the culture medium inhibits production of both IL-1 [18] and GM-CSF [19] as well as TNF-α itself. These findings suggest that TNF-α is produced at a more proximal level in the RA inflammatory cytokine cascade than other cytokines.

TNF-α has a variety of biological actions which may contribute toward the development of arthritis. Among these are a synergistic effect with IL-1 in the induction of proteolytic enzymes such as metalloproteinases and stromelysin, which in combination with inhibition of matrix protein synthesis results in cartilage degradation [20]. TNF-α has been shown to stimulate osteoclastic activity, leading to bone resorption, possibly in synergy with IL-1 [21]. TNF-α also activates leukocytes and increases chemotaxis into the synovial joint via induction of IL-8 and other chemokines as well as the upregulation of adhesion molecules on vascular endothelium, particularly E-selectin, intracellular adhesion molecule-1 (ICAM-1), and vascular cellular adhesion molecule-1 (VCAM-1) [22]. Activated neutrophils at the site of inflammation may contribute to cartilage degradation by superoxide generation and elastase release, whereas activated macrophages show increased phagocytic ability and are able to amplify the cytokine cascade by further production of cytokines. TNF-α may cause further inflammation in the joint by stimulating synovial cell prostaglandin E_2 production [23] and stimulating fibroblast growth by increasing platelet-derived growth factor (PDGF) production [24]. TNF-α may also contribute to systemic features of RA; for example, by stimulating acute phase protein synthesis probably via induction of IL-6 and inhibiting erythropoiesis [25], thereby leading to the chronic anemia frequently seen in RA.

B. Interleukin-1

IL-1 is a 17.5-kD protein produced predominantly by macrophages and has a wide range of biological activities. It is secreted in two forms; IL-1α and IL-1β, which have different structures but are able to bind to either of the two IL-1 receptors. IL-1β is the major extracellular form of IL-1 and is cleaved from a biologically inactive larger precursor by the enzyme IL-1β convertase (ICE) [26], with most IL-1α remaining within the cytosol. Genetic polymorphism has also been identified at the IL-1α gene locus [27] and an association has been found between one particular allele and a subset of juvenile rheumatoid arthritis [28], which further emphasizes the importance of IL-1 in arthritis. In common with TNF-α receptors, the two forms of IL-1 receptors (type I and type II IL-1Rs) can be shed from the cell surface and antagonize the effects of IL-1. Studies on the type II soluble IL-1R suggest that it inhibits IL-1β at two steps; by preventing the processing of the IL-1β precursor and by blocking interaction of mature IL-1β with the type I IL-1R [29]. A further circulating inhibitor of IL-1 has been identified; the IL-1 receptor antagonist (IL-1ra), which shares 30% homology with IL-1β and 19% homology with IL-1α [30]. It binds competitively to the surface receptors but without producing a biological response, thus inhibiting the action of IL-1. Data from the use of IL-1ra in endotoxin-induced shock in animals suggest that IL-1ra needs to be present at concentrations 10- to 500-fold higher than IL-1β in order to block all IL-

1 effects [31]. IL-1ra is secreted predominantly by cells of the macrophage lineage and to a lesser extent by synovial fluid neutrophils [32].

There is considerable evidence that IL-1 is a major factor in the pathogenesis of RA, with studies using animal models providing useful insights into its role. For example, a single intra-articular injection of IL-1 into an animal leads to an acute but transient arthritis, with an infiltration of neutrophils and monocytes [33]. The arthritis becomes destructive if repeated injections are administered but does not become chronic. This suggests that IL-1 alone is not an adequate stimulus for the development of chronic arthritis [34], but it may initiate arthritis, possibly in combination with other cytokines, such as TNF-α, with which it has been shown to have a synergistic effect [35]. IL-1 administered systemically can exacerbate some of the effects of murine collagen-induced arthritis (CIA) [36] and greatly increases the severity of antigen-induced arthritis in mice, converting a transient arthritis into aggressive, destructive disease [37]. In murine antigen- and collagen-induced arthritis, IL-1 suppresses proteoglycan synthesis to a greater degree than TNF-α [20], suggesting that IL-1 may have the greater potential for cartilage destruction.

Animal studies investigating the effects of neutralizing IL-1 antibodies demonstrated an amelioration of murine CIA and were also able to prevent its onset if administered early enough [38,39]. Similar results were obtained with a blocking antibody to IL-1 receptor in mice, which also led to substantial alleviation of established CIA on a par with that seen after the administration of antibodies to TNF-α and CD4 in combination [40]. The administration of IL-1ra to mice with CIA [41] or rabbits with lipopolysaccharide (LPS)–induced arthritis [42] also prevented the onset of disease, but it was unable to halt the disease process in animal antigen-induced arthritis [43], although it is possible that far higher concentrations of IL-1ra need to be used to fully inhibit all IL-1 activity.

IL-1, IL-1R, and IL-1ra have all been detected at the cartilage-pannus junction [44]. High levels of both IL-1 [45] and IL-1ra [32] have been reported in RA synovial fluid. However, measurements of IL-1 in RA body fluids by different investigators have given conflicting results; possibly due to the presence of naturally occurring IL-1 inhibitors or autoantibodies interfering with immunoassays. Taking these confounding factors into account, immunoreactive IL-1 was found in less than one-quarter of RA synovial fluid samples with bioactive IL-1 in less than one-tenth [46]. Rheumatoid synovial fluid contains a high concentration of neutrophils which have the potential to produce IL-1ra, and these neutrophils may contribute to the raised level of IL-1ra in RA synovial fluid [32]. Studies also suggest that despite this abundance of IL-1ra, the ratio of IL-1ra to IL-1 in RA synovial tissue may not be high enough (10–500 times in excess) to inhibit completely IL-1 activity [47].

IL-1 is produced spontaneously in RA but not in osteoarthritis synovial cell cultures, and as described earlier, it may be regulated by TNF-α in this disease [18]. Many of the functions of IL-1 overlap with both TNF-α and IL-6 (Table 1). For example, like TNF-α, IL-1 is able to upregulate adhesion molecules and chemotactic factors as well as stimulate lymphocyte proliferation and increase the production of acute phase proteins by hepatocytes either directly or by induction of IL-6. IL-1 can also induce the synthesis of other proinflammatory cytokines such as GM-CSF and granulocyte colony-stimulating factors (G-CSF) and can induce fibroblast proliferation [48]. With TNF-α, IL-1 causes cartilage degradation via collagenase and prostaglandin E_2 induction in synovial cells [49] and can upregulate stromelysin production.

Table 1 Relative Importance of Different Cytokines in the Pathogenesis of RA

Putative action	Cytokine TNF-α	IL-1	IL-6
Cartilage/bone destruction	++	+++	+?
Fibroblast proliferation	++	++	+
Endothelial activation	+++	+++	–
Cytokine production	+++	++	+
Liver:			
acute phase protein synthesis	+	++	+++
T-cell activation	+	+++	++
B-cell activation	+	+	+++
Bone marrow:			
inhibition of erythropoiesis	++	++	–
thrombopoiesis	?	+	++

+++, major effect; ++ moderate effect; +, minor effect; ?, role unclear.

C. Interleukin-6

IL-6 is a 26-kD pleiotropic glycoprotein produced by many different activated cell types, including monocytes-macrophages, fibroblasts, chondrocytes, osteoblasts, bone marrow stromal cells, T and B cells, and granulocytes [50]. A variety of stimuli can effect IL-6 production, of which the most important include upregulation by TNF-α and IL-1 as well as by GM-CSF, PDGF, and LPS. IL-6 binds to its specific receptor in association with the gp130 protein which is responsible for signal transduction and which IL-6 shares with other members of the cytokine receptor family, including receptors for leukemia-inhibitory factor (LIF) and oncostatin M. Naturally occurring soluble IL-6 receptors have also been identified which bind IL-6 and can mediate signals via the membrane-bound gp130 proteins [51].

Several of the actions of IL-6 overlap with those of IL-1 and TNF-α, such as the induction of acute phase protein production by hepatocytes and the ability to stimulate lymphocyte activation, growth, and differentiation. IL-6 plays a particular role in the regulation of B-cell terminal differentiation and has been shown to induce the production of rheumatoid factor by $CD5^+$ B cells [52]. IL-6 also has the ability to stimulate early hemopoietic progenitors and megakaryocytes in the bone marrow, and so it may contribute toward the thrombocytosis commonly observed in active RA. Interestingly, IL-6 may also play a role in macrophage differentiation [53].

IL-6 is produced spontaneously in synovial cell cultures but not in such high concentrations as IL-1 and TNF-α. IL-6 and its mRNA have been detected in the lining and sublining layers of the RA synovium as well as at the cartilage-pannus junction [8,54,55], and IL-6 is found in raised concentrations in both the synovial fluid and serum of rheumatoid patients. Synovial fluid levels are considerably higher than serum levels, reflecting local production within the joint [56,57]. Changes in synovial fluid and serum levels have been reported to correlate with clinical and laboratory parameters of disease activity [58,59], although changes in serial levels in individual patients need to be interpreted taking into account the pronounced circadian rhythm of IL-6 seen in

RA [60]. Synovial fluid IL-6 and its soluble receptor have been shown to increase osteoclast formation in vitro [61], and IL-6 has also been implicated in the pathogenesis of postmenopausal osteoporosis [62].

The evidence for the role of IL-6 in cartilage degradation is conflicting; for example, IL-1 is a potent inducer of IL-6 synthesis by chondrocytes, and IL-6 has been shown to act subsequently as a cofactor with IL-1 in the inhibition of proteoglycan synthesis in vitro [63]. IL-6 is also thought to increase the catabolism of connective tissue matrix through the stimulation of urokinase-type plasminogen activator [64]. However, the effects of IL-6 administration on the development of adjuvant arthritis in rats were of an improvement in disease activity, with a reduction in paw swelling and also in delayed-type hypersensitivity, probably reflecting the role of IL-6 in T-cell activation [65]. The same study failed to show any beneficial effects after the administration of neutralizing IL-6 antibodies in terms of stimulating chondrocyte proteoglycan synthesis. Similarly, in murine antigen- and zymogen-induced arthritis models, the destructive effects of IL-6 were not confirmed and intra-articular IL-6 at high dose resulted in stimulation of proteoglycan synthesis [20]. There is some evidence that IL-6 stimulates TGF-β1 release by chondrocytes and may therefore have a beneficial effect on chondrocyte growth and cartilage production [66,67]. IL-6 may also enhance the expression of inhibitors of enzymes involved in cartilage destruction such as tissue inhibitor of metalloproteinases in synovial fibroblasts [61] and so may have a protective effect on cartilage. It is difficult to draw firm conclusions as to the exact role of IL-6 in the pathogenesis of RA; however, it would appear that there is a critical balance between the proinflammatory effects of IL-6 and its role in cartilage protection.

III. BIOLOGICAL AGENTS AS CYTOKINE-BLOCKING THERAPY FOR RHEUMATOID ARTHRITIS

A. TNF-α–Blocking Therapy

With growing expertise in hybridoma technology, it has become possible to engineer monoclonal antibodies (mAbs) with specificity for human antigens in sufficient quantities to use as therapeutic agents. Initially, such antibodies were principally of murine origin and therefore potentially antigenic, however, techniques are being developed to maximize their human protein content, resulting in the production of chimerized (murine Fv fragment only) and, more recently, humanized (murine hypervariable region–only) mAbs.

1. TNF-α Monoclonal Antibodies

The beneficial effects of TNF-α blockade in vitro and in animal models of arthritis suggested that it might be effective treatment in human RA and there have now been several clinical trials using TNF-α mAbs to investigate this issue [68]. The first such trial was an early pilot study [69] using a chimeric mAb to TNF-α, cA2, which is known to bind to and antagonize circulating TNF-α and has an IgG1κ isotope. cA2 at a total dose of 20-mg/kg was administered to 20 patients with active disease who had failed therapy with standard disease-modifying antirheumatic drugs (DMARDs). Using the Paulus 20% response criteria (at least 20% improvement in comparison with baseline in four of the following size variables; erythrocyte sedimentation rate (ESR), duration of early morning stiffness, tender and swollen joint count, and a two-grade improvement in physician's and patient's assessment of disease severity [70], every patient showed a significant clinical response, as well as a substantial improvement in the level of acute phase protein synthesis. For example, patients showed a significant fall in C-reactive protein (CRP), serum amyloid A, and IL-6 levels, which correlated with disease activity. Although all patients eventually relapsed, the median duration of therapeutic response was 12 weeks after a single treatment cycle. The treatment was well tolerated and associated with only minor side effects. Retreatment of patients following relapse for up to three further cycles of cA2 was also well tolerated with maintenance of response magnitude [71], although there was some evidence that the length of response was shorter on retreatment, with a median response duration of 7.7 weeks after the fourth treatment cycle.

These encouraging results led to a double-blind, multicenter European trial of cA2 in the treatment of 73 patients with uncontrolled RA, who had failed treatment with at least one DMARD [72]. Patients were randomly assigned to single infusions of either placebo (human albumin), low-dose cA2 (1 mg/kg), or high-dose cA2 (10 mg/kg). A substantial number of patients from both treatment groups showed significant improvements in terms of clinical and laboratory parameters in comparison with the placebo group. For example, 44% of patients treated with low-dose cA2 and 79% of patients treated with high-dose cA2 showed a 20% Paulus response at 4 weeks after treatment compared with 8% of the 24 patients who had received placebo. This improvement was substantial as over 0.5% the patients in the high-dose cA2 group achieved the more stringent 50% Paulus response. Both treatment groups showed significant falls in ESR, pain score, and platelet counts (not below normal levels) as well as increased grip strength, with maximum benefit in the high-dose group; the response in those receiving low-dose cA2 declined after 2 weeks. Similarly, acute phase protein levels also showed impressive reductions during the trial period, with the CRP in both groups falling significantly compared with placebo at 2 weeks posttreatment. This reduction was maintained at 4 weeks in the high-dose group, with some patients achieving normal CRP levels for the 4 weeks of trial follow-up and beyond. Serum amyloid A as well as plasma haptoglobin and fibrinogen levels also fell significantly following cA2 treatment. Circulating IL-6 levels showed a rapid and significant reduction compared with the placebo group, with maximal responses at day 1 in both treatment groups, preceding the reduction of the other acute phase proteins and thus giving further evidence that TNF-α modulates the acute phase response by inhibiting IL-6 production [73]. Interestingly, patients who received high-dose cA2 also showed an increase in hemoglobin concentration compared with baseline despite repeated venesection, suggesting that TNF may have an important role in the anemia of chronic disorders.

In order to identify patients most likely to respond to cA2, the clinical characteristics of responders and nonresponders in the low-dose patient group were compared. (Only 2 of 24 high-dose patients failed to respond.) However, this failed to reveal any important clinical differences between the two groups except that disease activity was slightly milder in the nonresponders at trial onset (Table 2). Duration of response was related to the persistence of serum levels of cA2 and the original antibody dose, with those who received 10 mg/kg having a median response duration of 8 weeks [74]. The antibody was well-tolerated, with minor infections and rashes being the commonest side effects. Two severe adverse events were reported; an episode of pneumonia which responded to antibiotics and a pathological fracture diagnosed 1 week after treatment secondary to an occult carcinoma of the breast.

Table 2 Clinical Characteristics of Responders and Nonresponders to Low-dose cA2

	Sex (F/M)	Disease duration (years)	No previous DMARDs	RF	Anatomical Stage III[c] (%)	Functional class III[d] (%)	Number swollen joints	CRP (mg/L)
Responders[a] (n = 17)	14/3	8.4[b] (4.2–9.8)	3[b]	94%	59	35	23.08[b] (19–27)	64[b] (34–80)
Nonresponders[a]	6/2	5.1 (4.0–10.3)	2 (1.5–2.0)	100%	50	25	16.5 (7.5–19.0)	58 (33–120)

[a]Responder status defined by 20% Paulus response on at least one occasion during the 4 weeks after treatment with low-dose cA2. Eight of the 25 low-dose cA2 patients were nonresponders by this definition. Only 2 of 24 high-dose cA2 patients were nonresponders (not presented here).
[b]Median (interquartile range).
[c]One patient classified as anatomical stage I; remainder either stage II or III.
[d]All patients classified as functional class II or III.

A trial using a humanized TNF-α IgG4κ antibody (CDP571) has confirmed the effectiveness of TNF-α blockade in RA therapy [75]. This placebo-controlled randomized trial tested three different doses of mAb: 0.1, 1, and 10 mg/kg in a total of 36 patients. Again, there were significant improvements in a composite disease activity score, tender joint score, pain score, and CRP, with greatest benefit in the high-dose treatment group, maximal within the first 2 weeks of treatment. Side effects were mild and there were no serious adverse events related to treatment. Both this and the cA2 placebo-controlled trial were continued in order to allow retreatment of patients (not double blinded); this again was effective, with few reported side effects.

These trials confirm not only that TNF-α contributes in a major way to disease activity in RA but also that TNF-α blockade may be safe and effective in the treatment of this disease; at least on a temporary basis. However, several important issues have been raised by these results. The first is the potential immunogenicity of administering a murine-derived protein to a human patient. Measurements of human antichimeric cA2 antibody (HACA) levels in patients from the cA2 pilot trial showed that a number did develop HACA responses following retreatment (four of eight patients, all specific to the murine variable region), and this may contribute to the shortening of response seen after repeated administration. Information concerning the development of antibody responses following treatment with CDP571 are not currently available, but given the lower murine content of such a humanized antibody, they might be expected to be less frequent. However, the administration of a humanized antilymphocyte mAb, CAMPATH-1H, to RA patients on a trial basis [76] has been associated with the development of anti-idiotype antibodies in a significant number of cases.

A second feature of cA2 administration has been the temporary development of antinuclear antibodies in three patients from the cA2 pilot study [77]. Two of these patients developed significant titers of double-stranded DNA (dsDNA) antibodies, detected at 6 weeks postinfusion and reaching peak levels of 86 and 53 U/mL, respectively (normal range less than 7-U/mL). Neither patient had raised dsDNA antibodies prior to trial entry, and one also developed anticardiolipin antibodies (peak 58 U/mL, normal range less than 15 U/mL). Both patients showed evidence of complement activation with a fall in C4 levels below the normal range as well as a slight rise in immunoglobulin subsets. However, there were no clinical features of systemic lupus erythematosus (SLE), and in both cases, the serology returned to normal within 9 months of treatment, confirming that cA2 was the most likely cause of these abnormalities. A possible explanation for this transient production of antinuclear antibodies lies in a murine model of SLE, the NZB/W F_1 mouse, which has a genetic polymorphism resulting in low levels of TNF-α production. The development of an immune complex nephritis in such mice can be prevented by the administration of TNF-α. It might therefore be postulated that the lowering of TNF-α levels by TNF-α antibodies in combination with other risk factors for SLE (such as a shared genetic predisposition to both RA and SLE in one patient with the HLA DR3/DR4 haplotype) may increase the possibility of the development of serological abnormalities typical of SLE. However, the potentially antagonistic role for TNF-α in RA and SLE may be further complicated by the interaction of other cytokines such as IL-10 and interferon-γ.

Further insight into the pathogenesis of RA and the more precise role of TNF-α in rheumatoid disease has been gained following studies of serum and synovial specimens after cA2 administration. In particular, emerging data shows a reduction in the expression of the adhesion molecules ICAM-1 and VCAM-1 in the synovial sublining layer [78]. There was also a decrease in the expression of E-selectin at the vascular endothelium as well as reduced serum E-selectin levels, suggesting that control of cell trafficking at the level of the synovial vasculature may be a particular target site for the actions of cA2 [79].

2. Soluble TNF Receptors in the Treatment of RA

Trials are now underway investigating the therapeutic application of a TNFR construct comprising two recombinant p75 TNFR chains fused to the Fc portion of human IgG1 which binds strongly to TNF-α. This construct has been used in a placebo-controlled, dose-escalation trial in 16 patients with active RA [80], with the initial intravenous dose ranging from 4 to 32 g/m^2 followed by twice weekly subcutaneous maintenance doses for 4 weeks. Apart from a mild injection site reaction, the treatment was well tolerated. All treated patients showed a significant reduction in tender and swollen joint counts, ESR, and morning stiffness as well as patient's and physician's global assessments at 31 days posttreatment compared with baseline, with improvements in CRP and joint score superior in the treatment group compared with the placebo group, although this did not reach statistical significance. There were no differences in efficacy in the different dose regimens. A larger double-blind trial is needed to establish more clearly the effectiveness of this treatment. Similar studies are underway with a p55 soluble TNFR construct, but no publications on safety or efficacy have been released yet.

B. Interleukin-1-blocking Therapy

Two approaches to IL-1 blockade have been used on a trial basis in the treatment of RA. The first is the therapeutic application of a recombinant human IL-1 receptor, which has been administered intra-articularly in a double-blind, randomized phase I trial of 16 patients with active RA [81]. Four treatment doses were used, with one patient at each level receiving placebo. A dose-related reduction in knee circumferences was seen at 48 h compared with the placebo group, with a trend toward reduction in ESR and walking time in the higher dose groups. Side effects included bandage-induced contact dermatitis, and another treated patient showed an increase in size of the knee effusion at 24 h. Following this a randomized, double-blind trial of subcutaneous recombinant IL-1R was performed on 23 RA patients. Patients received daily subcutaneous injections of rIL-1R [82] according to four different dose levels for 28 days. No patient achieved the trial criteria for significant response, although there were trends toward improvement in individual disease activity parameters. Two patients developed injection site reactions and one required hospitalization for bowel obstruction.

The second approach to IL-1 blockade involves the use of recombinant IL-1ra, again by subcutaneous injection. In a preliminary trial, 25 RA patients were randomized to receive a single injection of IL-1ra at one of five different doses [83]. This resulted in a significant decrease in the mean tender joint in the high-dose group compared with placebo. Following this, an open label, non–placebo-controlled trial of 15 RA patients was performed, each receiving once daily injections of different IL-1ra doses for a total of 28 days. After 7 days of treatment, there were reductions in the mean tender joint count, ESR, and CRP compared with baseline, with 12 of 15 patients showing a greater than 50% reduction in CRP. However, all patients developed skin reactions, for which two withdrew from the study, a third patient withdrew following the development of Felty's syndrome. No patient developed IL-1ra antibodies. In a large double-blind, placebo-controlled multicenter trial of the same agent, 175 RA patients were randomized to self-administer either 20, 70, or 200 mg of rIL-1ra with dose intervals varying from daily to once a week for 3 weeks [84]. The greatest clinical response was seen in those who received rIL-1ra daily, independent of dose, with patients showing a 50% or more improvement in clinical outcome measures such as painful and swollen joint count and patient's and physician's assessments of disease severity. This improvement was maintained in most parameters when patients continued with rIL-1ra treatment once daily for 4 weeks, particularly in those who received the 70 mg dose. Although injection site reactions were common, they necessitated study withdrawal in only 5% of patients. Six serious adverse events were reported and include soft tissue infections, chest pain, a urinary tract infection, and prostate disease. Although these results are encouraging, they have so far only been published in abstract form, with little information given about response in the placebo group. When the full results of this and any follow-up studies are published, it may be possible to establish more clearly whether rIL-1ra will be of therapeutic benefit in RA.

C. IL-6–Blocking Therapy

Only one group has examined the effects of IL-6 blockade in the treatment of rheumatoid arthritis. In an open-label pilot study, an anti–IL-6 mAb (B-E8) was used to treat five rheumatoid patients [85]. Each patient was hospitalized and treated with a daily infusion of 10 mg of antibody for 10 consecutive days. There were no side effects, and each patient showed an improvement in clinical variables, such as morning stiffness, pain score, tender joint count, and Ritchie articular index, which occurred within 15 days and was maintained for a mean duration of 2 months, with improvements lasting over 6 months in one patient. Similarly CRP and ESR also fell, with a maximal response at 15 days after treatment. One patient developed transient hypercalcaemia. Paradoxically, IL-6 levels rose during the study, returning to baseline after 60 days, possibly due to the formation of complexes between IL-6 and the monoclonal antibody. The same antibody was subsequently administered to three further RA patients, with a similar clinical response and fall in CRP [86]. Although such results are encouraging, the numbers of patients involved were very small, and as the trial did not contain a placebo group, these findings must be interpreted with caution until the results of larger double-blind studies are known.

D. Cytokine Blockade by Conventional RA Therapies

The growing interest in the role of specific cytokine-blocking biological agents in the treatment of RA has led to a reexamination of traditional RA therapies for their potential to modulate the cytokine network. Although some of the disease-modifying antirheumatic drugs have been shown to be effective in slowing RA disease activity, their exact mechanisms of action have yet to be clearly established. However, there is growing evidence that these agents are able to modulate the cytokine network. For example, methotrexate has been shown to inhibit some of the effects of IL-1 and reduce TNF-α levels as well as increasing the ratio of IL-1ra to IL-1 [87,88]. Methotrexate and also sulfasalazine administration leads to the accumulation of adensoine, which has potent anti-inflammatory and immunomodulatory effects and has been shown to inhibit the production of TNF-α in a murine air pouch model of inflammation [89,90]. This mechanism may provide a unifying theory for the effects of other disease-modifying drugs in RA. Other agents which have been shown to reduce cytokine levels, such as TNF-α, and are therefore of potential benefit in RA, include fish oils [91], pentoxifyline [92], tenidap [93], and members of the recently synthesized family of bicyclic imidazoles [94].

IV. DIRECTIONS FOR FUTURE CYTOKINE-BLOCKING THERAPY

TNF-α blockade is now established as effective and, in most cases, safe therapy in the short-term management of rheumatoid disease. Other cytokines, such as IL-1 and IL-6, also show promise as therapeutic targets, although definitive proof of the efficacy of blocking these cytokines is still to be presented. However, certain problems need to be addressed before anticytokine treatment can become a mainstay in the management of the RA patient. For example, TNF-α blockade with mAbs, although extremely effective, only results in a temporary improvement in disease activity, whereas repeated therapy may increase the likelihood of the development of human antibody responses and a reduction in response duration. This problem might be overcome in the future by the development of increasingly more "humanized" antibodies or by using TNF receptor constructs, such as those currently under trial. Alternatively, inhibition of the T-cell response may prevent the development of sensitization; for example, by using anti-CD4 prior to administering TNF-α antibodies. Another approach to blocking TNF-α may be through pharmacological upregulation of the surface TNFR cleavage which results in the soluble TNFRs. IL-1β–converting enzyme inhibitors may also provide a therapeutic approach to IL-1 inhibition and are currently being investigated. Soluble IL-6 receptors, although potentially of therapeutic benefit may, like other soluble cytokine receptors, have too short a half-life when used alone to be of practical use and might also be able to activate cells by binding to the gp130 protein. Finally, the actions of anti-inflammatory cytokines such as IL-4 and IL-10 in animal models of arthritis point the way to future therapy for rheumatoid disease.

ACKNOWLEDGMENTS

We wish to thank the Arthritis and Rheumatism Council which supports the research of the authors at the Kennedy Instiitute of Rheumatology, London. We also thank Centocor Inc. for collaborative studies with anti–TNF-α (cA2) antibody.

REFERENCES

1. Tracey KJ, Cerami A. Tumour necrosis factor, other cytokines and disease. Ann Rev Cell Biol 1993; 9:317–343.
2. Wilson AG, de Vries N, Pociot F, di Giovine F, van de Putte L, Duff G. An allelic polymorphism within the human tumor necrosis factorα promoter region is strongly associated with HLA A1, B8, and DR3 alleles. J Exp Med 1993; 177:577–580.
3. Wilson A, de Vries N, van de Putte L, Duff G. A tumour necrosis factor α polymorphism is not associated with rheumatoid arthritis. Ann Rheum Dis 1995; 54:601–603.
4. Beutler B, van Huffel C. Unravelling function in the TNF ligand and receptor families. Science 1994; 264:667–668.

5. Brennan F, Williams L, Gibbons D, Maini R, Feldmann M. Proteolytic cleavage of the p55 and p75 TNF receptor is blocked by a synthetic metalloproteinase inhibitor: independent of its effect on TNFα processing. Arthritis Rheum 1995; 38.8:S344.
6. Saxne T, Palladino Jr MA, Heinegard D, Talal N, Wollheim FA. Detection of tumour necrosis factor α but not tumour necrosis factor β in rheumatoid synovial fluid and serum. Arthritis Rheum 1988; 31:1041–1045.
7. Buchan G, Barrett K, Turner M, Chantry D, Maini R, Feldmann M. Interleukin-1 and tumour necrosis factor mRNA expression in rheumatoid arthritis: prolonged production of IL-1α. Clin Exp Immunol 1988; 73:449–455.
8. Chu C, Field M, Allard S, Abney E, Feldmann M, Maini R. Detection of cytokines at the cartilage/pannus junction in patients with rheumatoid arthritis: implications for the role of cytokines in cartilage destruction and repair. Br J Rheumatol 1992; 31:653–661.
9. Deleuran BW, Chu CQ, Field M, Brennan FM, Mitchell T, Feldmann M, Maini RN. Localization of tumour necrosis factor receptors in the synovial tissue and cartilage-pannus junction in patients with rheumatoid arthritis. Implications for local action of tumour necrosis factor alpha. Arthritis Rheum 1992; 35.10:1170–1178.
10. Vreugdenhil G, Lowenberg B, Van Eijk HG, Swaak AJ. Tumour necrosis factor alpha is associated with disease activity and the degree of anemia in patients with rheumatoid arthritis. Eur J Clin Invest 1992; 22:488–493.
11. Cope A, Aderka D, Doherty M, Engelmann H, Gibbons D, Jones A, Brennan F, Maini R, Wallach D, Feldmann M. Increased levels of soluble tumour necrosis factor receptors in the sera and synovial fluid of patients with rheumatic disease. Arthritis Rheum 1992; 35.10:1160–1169.
12. Cooper W, Fava R, Gates C, Cremer M, Townes A. Acceleration of onset of collagen-induced arthritis by intra-articular injection of tumour necrosis factor or transforming growth factor-beta. Clin Exp Immunol 1992; 89:244–250.
13. Williams RO, Feldmann N, Maini RN. Anti-tumor necrosis factor ameliorates joint disease in murine collagen-induced arthritis. Proc Natl Acad Sci USA 1992; 89:9784–9788.
14. Keffer J, Probert H, Cazlaris H, Georgopoulos S, Kaslaris E, Kioussis D, Kollias G. Transgenic mice expressing human tumour necrosis factor: a predictive genetic model of arthritis. EMBO 1991; 10.13:4025–4031.
15. Philip R, Meager A. Cytokines in synovial fluid: II The presence of tumour necrosis factor and interferon. Clin Exp Immunol 1988; 73:88–92.
16. Seelentag WK, Mermod JJ, Montesano R, Vassalli P. Additive effects of interleukin 1 and tumour necrosis factor alpha on the accumulation of the three granulocyte and macrophage colony-stimulating factor mRNAs in human endothelial cells. EMBOJ. 1987; 6.8:2261–2265.
17. Larsen CG, Anderson AO, Oppenheim JJ, Matsushima K. Production of interleukin-8 by human dermal fibroblasts and keratinocytes in response to interleukin-1 or tumour necrosis factor. Immunology 1989; 68.1:31–6.
18. Brennan F, Chantry D, Jackson A, Maini R, Feldmann M. Inhibitory effects of TNFα antibodies on synovial cell interleukin-1 production in rheumatoid arthritis. Lancet 1989; 1:244–247.
19. Haworth C, Brennan F, Chantry D, Turner M, Maini R, Feldmann M. Expression of granulocyte-macrophage colony stimulating factor (GM-CSF) in rheumatoid arthritis: regulation by tumour necrosis factor α. Eur J Immunol 1991; 21:2575–2579.
20. Van de Loo F, Joosten L, van Lent L, Arntz O, van den Berg W. Role of interleukin-1, tumor necrosis factorα, and interleukin-6 in cartilage proteoglycan metabolism and destruction: effects of in situ blocking murine antigen- and zymosan-induced arthritis. Arthritis Rheum 1995; 38.2:164–172.
21. Pfeilschifter J, Chenu C, Bird A, Mundy GR, Roodman GD. Interleukin-1 and tumour necrosis factor stimulate the formation of human osteoclastic cells in vitro. J. Bone Mineral Res 1989; 4.1:113–118.

22. Carlos TM, Harlan JM. Leukocyte-endothelial adhesion molecules. Blood 1994; 84:2068–2101.
23. Dayer JM, Beutler B, Cerami A. Cachectin/tumor necrosis factor stimulates collagenase and prostaglandin E2 production by human synovial cells and dermal fibroblasts. J Exp Med 1985; 126.6:2163–2168.
24. Vilcek J, Palombella VJ, Henriksen-DeStefano D, Swenson C, Feinman R, Hirai M, Tsujimoto M. Fibroblast growth enhancing activity of tumour necrosis factor and its relationship to other polypeptide growth factors. J Exp Med 1986; 163:632–643.
25. Roodman GD, Johnson RA, Clibon U. Tumor necrosis factor alpha and the anemia of chronic disease: effects of chronic exposure to TNF on erythropoiesis in vivo. Adv Exp Med Biol 1989; 271:185–196.
26. Kostura MJ, Tocci MJ, Limjuco G, Chin J, Cameron P, Hillman AG, Chartrain NA, Schmidt JA: Identification of a monocyte specific pre-interleukin-1 beta convertase activity. Proc Natl Acad Sci USA 1989; 86:5227.
27. Bailly S, di Giovine F, Blakemore A, Duff G. Genetic polymorphism of human interleukin-1α. Eur J Immunol 1993; 23:1240–1245.
28. McDowell T, Symons J, Ploski R, Forre O, Duff G. A genetic association between juvenile rheumatoid arthritis and a novel interleukin-1α polymorphism. Arthritis Rheum 1995; 38.2:221–228.
29. Symons J, Young P, Duff G. Soluble type II interleukin 1 (IL-1) receptor binds and blocks processing of IL-1β precursor and loses affinity for IL-1 receptor antagonist. Proc Natl Acad Sci USA 1995; 92:1714–1718.
30. Eisenberg S, Evans R, Arend W, Verderber E, Brewer M, Hannum C, Thompson R. Primary structure and functional expression from complementary DNA of a human interleukin-1 receptor antagonist. Nature 1990; 343:341–346.
31. Ohlsson K, Bjork P, Bergenfeldt M, Hageman R, Thompson R. Interleukin-1 receptor antagonist reduces mortality from endotoxin shock. Nature 1990; 348:550–552.
32. Malayak M, Swaney R, Arend W. Levels of synovial fluid interleukin-1 receptor antagonist in rheumatoid arthritis and other arthropathies: Potential contribution from synovial fluid neutrophils. Arthritis Rheum 1993; 36.6:781–789.
33. Henderson B, Pettipher E R. Comparison of the in vivo inflammatory intra-articular injection of natural and recombinant IL-1 alpha and IL-beta in the rabbit. Biochem Pharmacol 1988; 37:4171–4176.
34. Chandrasekhar S, Harvey AK, Hubrey PS, Bendele AM. Arthritis induced by interleukin-1 is dependent on the site and frequency of intraarticular injection. Clin Immunol Immunopathol 1990; 55:328–400.
35. Henderson B, Pettipher ER. Arthritogenic actions of recombinant IL-1 and tumour necrosis factor α in the rabbit: evidence for synergistic interactions between cytokines in vivo. Clin Exp Immunol 1989; 75:306–310.
36. Hom JT, Bendele AM, Carlson DG. In vivo administration with IL-1 accelerates the development of collagen-induced arthritis in mice. J Immunol 1988; 141:834–841.
37. Staite N, Richard K, Aspar D, Franz K, Galinet L, Dunn C. Induction of an acute erosive arthritis in mice by interleukin-1 and methylated bovine serum albumin. Arthritis Rheum 1990; 33:253–260.
38. Geiger T, Towbin H, Cosenti-Vargos A, Zingel O. Arnold J, Rordorf C, Glatt M, Vosbeck K. Neutralization of interleukin-1 beta activity in vivo with a monoclonal antibody alleviates collagen-induced arthritis in DBA/1 mice and prevents the associated acute-phase response. Clin Exp Immunol 1993; 1:515–522.
39. Van den Berg W, Joosten L, Helson M, Van de Loo F. Amelioration of established murine collagen-induced arthritis with anti-IL-1 treatment. Clin Exp Immunol 1994; 95:237–243.
40. Williams RO, Mason L, Feldmann M, Maini RN. Synergy between anti-CD4 and anti-tumour necrosis factor in the amelioration of established collagen-induced arthritis. Proc Natl Acad Sci USA 1994; 91.7:2762–2766.

41. Wooley PH, Whalen J, Chapman D, Berger A, Richard K, Aspar D, Staite N. The effect of an interleukin-1 receptor antagonist protein on type 11 collagen-induced arthritis and antigen-induced arthritis in mice. Arthritis Rheum 1993; 36:1305–1314.
42. Matsukawa A, Ohkawara S. Maeda T, Takagi K, Yoshinaga M. Production of IL-1 and IL-1 receptor antagonist and the pathological significance of lipopolysaccharide-induced arthritis in rabbits. Clin Exp Immunol 1993; 93.2:206–211.
43. Lewthwaite J, Blake S, Hardingham T, Warden P, Henderson B. The effect of recombinant human interleukin-1 receptor antagonist on the induction phase of antigen-induced arthritis in the rabbit. J Rheumatol 1994; 21.3:467–472.
44. Deleuran BW, Chu CQ, Field M, Brennan F, Katsikis P, Feldmann M, Maini R. Localisation of interleukin-1α, type 1 interleukin-1 receptor and interleukin-1 receptor antagonist in the synovial membrane and cartilage/pannus junction in rheumatoid arthritis. J Rheumatol 1992; 31:801–809.
45. Hopkins SJ, Humphreys M, Jaysen MI. Cytokines in the synovial fluid.1. the presence of biologically active and immunoreactive IL-1. Clin Exp Immunol 1989; 72:422–427.
46. Holt I, Cooper R, Denton J, Meager A, Hopkins S. Cytokine inter-relationships and their association with disease activity in arthritis. Br J Rheumatol 1992; 31:725–733.
47. Firestein G, Boyle D, Yu C, Paine M Whisenand T, Zvaifler N, Arend W. Synovial interleukin-1 receptor antagonist and interleukin-1 balance in rheumatoid arthritis. Arthritis Rheum 1994; 37:644–652.
48. Schmidt IA, Mizel SB, Cohen D, Green I. Interleukin 1. A potent regulator of growth. J Immunol 1982; 128:2177–2182.
49. Dayer JM, de Rochemonteix B, Burrus B, Demzuk S, Dinarello CA: Human recombinant interleukin 1 stimulates collagenase and prostaglandin E2 production by human synovial cells. J Cell Invest 1986; 77:645–652.
50. Akira S, Taga T, Kishimoto T. Interleukin-6 in biology and medicine. Adv Immunol 1993; 5:1–78.
51. Novick D, Engelman H, Revel M, Leitner O, Rubenstein M. Monoclonal antibodies to the soluble human IL-6 receptor: affinity purification, ELISA and inhibition of ligand binding. Hybridoma 1991; 10:137–146.
52. Nawata Y, Eugui EM, Lee SW, Allison AC. Il-6 is the principal factor produced by synovia of patients with rheumatoid arthritis that induces B-lymphocytes to secrete immunoglobulins. Ann NY Acad Sci 1989; 557:230–239.
53. Shabo Y, Lotem J, Rubenstein M, Revel M, Clark SC, Wolf SF, Kamen R, Sachs L. The myeloid blood cell differentiation-inducing protein MGI-2A is interleukin 6. Blood 1988; 72:2070–2073.
54. Field M, Chu M, Maini RN. Interleukin-6 localisation in the synovial membrane in rheumatoid arthritis. Rheumatol Int 1991; 11:45–50.
55. Firestein GS, Alavro-Garcia JM, Maki R. Quantitative analysis of cytokine gene expression in rheumatoid arthritis. J Immunol 1990; 144:3347–3353.
56. Swaak AJ, Van Rooyen A, Nieuwenhuis E, Aarden LA. Interleukin6 (IL-6) in synovial fluid and serum of patients with rheumatic diseases. Scand J Rheumatol 1988; 17:469–474.
57. Hirano T, Matsuda T, Turner M, Miyasaka N, Buchan G, Tang B, Sato K, Shimuzu M, Maini R, Feldmann M, Kishimoto T. Excessive production of interleukin 6/B cell stimulatory factor-2 in rheumatoid arthritis. Eur J Immunol 1988; 18:1797–1801.
58. Miltenburg AM, van Laar JM, de Kuiper R, Daha MR, Breedveld FC. Interleukin-6 activity in paired samples of synovial fluid. Correlation of synovial fluid interleukin-6 levels with clinical and laboratory parameters of inflammation. Br J Rheumatol 1991; 30:186–189.
59. Madhok R, Crilly A, Watson J, Capell HA. Serum interleukin 6 levels in rheumatoid arthritis: correlations with clinical and laboratory indices of disease activity. Ann Rheum Dis 1993; 52:232–234.
60. Arvidson NG, Gudbjornsson B, Elfman L, Ryden A, Totterham T, Hallgren R. Circadian rhythm of serum interleukin-6 in rheumatoid arthritis. Ann Rheum Dis 1994; 53:521–524.

61. Kotake S, Sato K, Kim KJ, Takahashi N, Udagawa N, Nakamura I, Yamaguchi A, Kashiwazaki S, Suda T. Interleukin-6 and soluble interleukin-6 receptors present in synovial fluids from rheumatoid arthritis patients are responsible for osteoclast-like cell formation. Arthritis Rheum 1994; 37:S309.
62. Jilka RL, Hangoc G, Girasole G, Passeri G, Williams DC, Abrams JS, Boyce B, Broxmeyer H. Manolagas SC. Increased osteoclastic development after estrogen loss: mediation by interleukin-6. Science 1992; 257:88–91.
63. Nietfeld JJ, Wilbrink B, Helle M, van Roy JL, den Otter RW,Swaak AJ, Huber-Bruning O. Interleukin-1 induced interleukin-6 is required for the inhibition of proteoglycan synthesis by interleukin-1 in human articular cartilage. Arthritis Rheum 1990; 33:1695–1701.
64. Ito A, Itoh Y, Sasaguri Y, Morimatsu M, Mori Y. Effects of interleukin-6 on the metabolism of connective tissue components in rheumatoid synovial fibroblasts. Arthritis Rheum 1992; 35.10:1197–1201.
65. Mihara M, Ikuta M, Koshihara Y, Oshugi Y. Interleukin 6 inhibits delayed-type hypersensitivity and the development of adjuvant arthritis. Eur J Immunol 1991; 21:2327–2331.
66. Allard SA, Bayliss MT, Maini RN. The synovium-cartilage junction of the normal human knee. Implications for joint destruction and repair. Arthritis Rheum 1990; 33:1170–1179.
67. Guerne PA, Villiger P, Lotz M. Unique synergy and interactions between IL-6 and TNF-β in the regulation of chondrocyte function [abstr]. Clin Rheumatol 1990; 9:527.
68. Maini RN, Elliott MF, Brennan FM, Williams WO, Chu CQ, Paleolog E, Charles PJ, Taylor PC, Feldmann M. Monoclonal anti-TNFα antibody as a probe of pathogenesis and therapy of rheumatoid disease. Immunol Rev 1995; 144:195–223.
69. Elliott MJ, Maini RN, Feldmann M, Long-Fox A, Charles P, Katsikis P, Brennan F, Walker J, Bijl H, Ghrayeb J, Woody J. Treatment of rheumatoid arthritis with chimeric antibodies to tumor necrosis factorα. Arthritis Rheum 1993; 36:1681–1690.
70. Paulus HE, Egger MJ, Ward JR, Williams HJ. group CSSoRD: Analysis or improvement in individual rheumatoid arthritis patients treated with disease-modifying antirheumatic drugs, based on the findings in patients treated with placebo. Arthritis Rheum 1990; 33:447–480.
71. Elliott MJ, Maini RN, Feldmann M, Long-Fox A, Charles P, Bijl H, Woody J. Repeated therapy with monoclonal antibody to tumour necrosis factorα (cA2) in patients with rheumatoid arthritis. Lancet 1994; 344:1125–1127.
72. Elliott MJ, Maini RN, Feldmann M, Kalden JC, Antoni C, Smolen J, Leeb B, Breedveld FC, Macfarlane JD, Bijl H. Randomised double-blind comparison of chimeric monoclonal antibody to tumour necrosis factorα (cA2) versus placebo in rheumatoid arthritis. Lancet 1994; 344:1105–1110.
73. Charles P, Elliott M, Davis D, Potter A, Kalden J, Antoni C, Breedveld F, Smolen J, Eberl G, Woody J, Feldmann M, Maini R. Regulation of cytokines and acute phase proteins following TNFα blockade in rheumatoid arthritis. Submitted for publication.
74. Maini RN, Elliott MJ, Long-Fox A, Feldmann M, Kalden J, Antonio C, Smolen J, Leeb B, Breedveld FC, Macfarlane JD, Bijl H, Woody JN. Clinical response to rheumatoid arthritis (RA) to anti-TNFα (cA2) monoclonal antibody (mab) is related to administered dose and persistence of circulating antibody. Arthritis Rheum 1995; 38:S186.
75. Rankin EC, Choy EH, Kassimos D, Kingsley GH, Sopwith AM, Isenberg DA, Panayl GS. The therapeutic effect of an engineered human anti-tumour necrosis factor alpha antibody (CDP571) in rheumatoid arthritis. Br J Rheum 1995; 34:334–342.
76. Matteson E, Yocum D, St. Clair W, Achkar A, Thakor M, Jacobs M, Hays A, Heitman C, Johnston J. Treatment of active refractory rheumatoid arthritis with humanized monoclonal antibody CAMPATH-1H administered by daily subcutaneous injection. Arthritis Rheum 1995; 38:1187–1193.
77. Maini R, Elliott M, Charles P, Feldmann M. Immunological intervention reveals reciprocal roles for tumour necrosis factor-α and interleukin-10 in rheumatoid arthritis and systemic lupus erythematosus. Springer Semin Immunopathol 1994; 16:327–336.

78. Tak P, Taylor P, Breedveld F, Macfarlane J, Smeets T, Daha M, Kluin P, Meinders A, Maini R. Infiltrate analysis of rheumatoid synovial tissue before and after anti-TNFα monoclonal antibody treatment. Arthritis Rheum 1996; 39:1077–1081.
79. Paleolog E, Taylor P, Tak P, Elliott M, Feldmann M, Breedveld F, Maini R. Treatment of rheumatoid arthritis with antibody to TNFα decreases expression and shedding of E-selectin. Arthritis Rheum 1996; 39:1082–1091.
80. Moreland L, Margolies G, Heck L, Saway P, Jacobs C, Beck C, Blosch C, Koopman W. Soluble tumour necrosis factor receptor (sTNFR): results of a phase I dose-escalation study in patients with rheumatoid arthritis. Arthritis Rheum 1994; 37:S813.
81. Drevlov B, Capezio J, Lovis R, Jacobs C, Landay A, Pope R. Phase 1 study of recombinant human interleukin-1 receptor (RHUIL-1R) administered intra-articularly in active rheumatoid arthritis. Arthritis Rheum 1993; 36:S39.
82. Dreslow B, Lovis R, Haag M, Sinacore J, Jacobs C, Blosch C, Beck D, Landay A, Moreland L, Pope R. Phase 1 study of recombinant interleukin-1 receptor (RHUIL-1R) administered subcutaneously in patients with active rheumatoid arthritis. Arthritis Rheum 1994; 37:S339.
83. Lesback M, Paul C, Bloedow D, Burch F, Sack M, Chase W, Catelano M. Subcutaneous IL-1 receptor antagonist in patients with rheumatoid arthritis. Arthritis Rheum 1991; 34:S45.
84. Lesback M, Paul C, Martindale J, Catalano M. A dose and regimen-ranging study of IL-1 receptor antagonist in patients with rheumatoid arthritis. Arthritis Rheum 1993; 36:S39.
85. Wendling D, Racadot E, Wijdenes J. Treatment of severe rheumatoid arthritis by anti-interleukin 6 monoclonal antibody. J Rheum 1993; 20:259–262.
86. Wendling D, Racadot E, Wijdenes J. Serum levels of IL 6, CRP, IL 6 receptor and cortisol after anti IL6 monoclonal antibody therapy in rheumatoid arthritis. Arthritis Rheum 1994; 37:S382.
87. Chang DM, Weinblatt ME, Scur PH. The effects of methotrexate on interleukin1 in patients with rheumatoid arthritis. J Rheumatol 1992; 19:1678–1682.
88. Seitz M, Loetscher P, Dewald B, Towbin H, Rordorf C, Gallati H, Baggiolini M, Gerber NJ. Methotrexate action in rheumatoid arthritis: stimulation of cytokine inhibitor and inhibition of chemokine production by peripheral mononuclear cells. Br J Rheumatol 1995; 34:602–609.
89. Cronstein B, Naime D, Firestein G. Adenosine mediates the anti-inflammatory effects of the adenosine kinase inhibitor GP-1-515 in the murine air pouch model of inflammation. Arthritis Rheum 1993; 36:S200.
90. Gadangi P, Longaker M, Naime D, Cronstein B. The antiinflammatory action of sulfasalazine (SSA) is mediated by adensoine (ADO). Arthritis Rheum 1995; 389:S1308.
91. Endres S, Ghorbani R, Kelley V, Georgilis K, Lonnemann G, van der Meer J, Cannon J, Rogers T, Klempner M, Weber P, Schaefer E, Wolff S, Dinarello C. The effect of dietary supplementation with n-3 polyunsaturated fatty acids on the synthesis of interleukin-1 and tumour necrosis factor by mononuclear cells. N Engl J Med 1989; 320:265–271.
92. Strieter R, Remick D, Ward P, Spengler R, Lynch J, Kunkel S. Cellular and molecular regulation of tumour necrosis factor-alpha production by pentoxifylline. Biochem Biophys Res Commun 1988; 15:1230–1236.
78. Otterness IG, Bilven ML, Downs JT, Natoli EJ, Hanson DC. Inhibition of interleukin 1 synthesis by tenidap: a new drug for arthritis. Cytokine 1991; 3:277–283.
94. Young P, McDonnell P, Dunnington D, Hand A, Layden J, Lee L. Pyridinyl imidazoles inhibit IL-1 and TNFα production at the protein level. Agents Actions 1993; 39:C67–C69 (conference issue).

19
Local Therapy for Inflammatory Arthritis

John Edmonds
St. George Hospital, and University of New South Wales, Sydney, New South Wales, Australia

I. INTRODUCTION

Other chapters in this book detail just some of the many excellent therapies prescribed by rheumatologists, yet most would concede that local steroid injections join the small list of therapies, unarguably within the special domain of the rheumatologist, that predictably help patients with inflammatory arthritis—sometimes dramatically and often for significant periods. Indeed, practicing rheumatology without the aid of local steroids would be painful both for patients and, to a lesser degree, their physicians, which is an experience we can now avoid. In a survey of four practices in the United Kingdom [1], corticosteroids were injected locally to joints and soft tissues in 10–16% of patients; with a similar frequency of use in the United States [2], this is surely the commonest procedure in rheumatological practice.

It is puzzling then, that such a central rheumatological procedure and therapy has been subjected to so little recent rigorous testing and that, with regard to practice and procedures, rheumatologists continue to combine "total dogmatism with a complete lack of consistency" [3]. Is it a lack of intellectual interest, inadequate published data, or the view that local therapy is of little real importance which accounts for the omission of any reference to intra-articular corticosteroids and only brief mention of chemical and radiation synovectomy in an otherwise comprehensive recent volume on rheumatoid arthritis [4]?

This chapter examines the literature on the principles and practice in the areas of arthrocentesis procedures, intra-articular corticosteroids, and chemical and radioactive synovectomy as they relate to rheumatoid arthritis and, where information is available, to other inflammatory arthropathies.

Other forms of local treatment, such as physiotherapy in its various forms, tidal joint lavage, and topical nonsteroidal anti-inflammatory drugs (NSAIDs), are not considered.

II. ARTHROCENTESIS

Arthrocentesis means needle puncture or aspiration of the joint. Strictly, the term *synoviocentesis* may be the more correct one to cover the process of needle entry to the synovial lined joint, tendon sheath, or bursa—the starting point for synovial fluid examination or intrasynovial therapy in any form.

The approach to synoviocentesis has developed empirically and uncritically, and it has been influenced by two fears: damage to local structures and iatrogenic infection. As a result, basic principles are fairly standard [5–8,71], whereas individual practices vary [3,9]. Only recently has science been brought to bear on the way we do things [10–13].

A. Variability

Surveys in the United Kingdom and Australia reveal variability in the use of local anesthetic, skin and operator preparation, and the environment in which arthrocentesis is performed.

In a postal survey of 64 Australian rheumatologists, Lawford et al. [9] reported 75% used a simple soap wash; 20% used a full surgical wash; 56% used a spirit swab, 42% used iodine; about 25% used gloves, unless there was a known biohazard; only 40% discouraged conversation during the procedure; and 70% warned patients about potential complications.

Haslock and his colleagues [3] surveyed 172 consultant rheumatologist members of the British Society for Rheumatology by postal questionnaire and found "wide diversity of opinion . . . regarding almost every aspect of intra-articular and soft tissue injection technique." Most of those responding were prepared to undertake arthrocentesis and joint injection in any standard environment—theatre, ward, outpatients, or patient's home. A few less than 10% used gloves or a "surgical scrub"; a few more than 10% shaved hairy skin or wore a mask. Over 50% cleaned the site with an alcohol or Hibitane swab, whereas about 16% used iodine. About 30% used local anesthetic before joint injection, but only 17% used it before soft tissue injection, whereas one in four used no local anesthetic in either situation. It was surprising that in such a recent survey, just under 50% still had a nurse assistant at joint injection. Haslock et al. drew attention to a brief report [14] indicating that 12% of rheumatology nurse specialists in the United Kingdom routinely perform joint injections, foreshadowing, perhaps, a significant future trend.

B. Scrutiny of Practice Variables

Does this variability matter? Reports on infection and other adverse events come mainly from series on the intra-articular administration of chemicals, so it is difficult to glean data on morbidity arising from arthrocentesis alone. But given the rarity of sepsis following steroid, chemical, or radiation synovectomy, simple arthrocentesis must have a very low risk indeed, probably because the technique, as it has evolved, provides a broad measure of patient safety. Variability in approach may be more relevant to issues of cost and efficiency.

In a study of patients requiring bilateral knee aspiration, Kirwan et al.. [10], showed no overall patient preference for or against the administration of 1 mL 2% lignocaine injected intradermally and then subcutaneously 2–3 min before arthrocentesis. No comment was made on the relationship between patient preference for local anesthetic and the ease of joint puncture; difficult access, synovial fluid requiring a larger bore needle for aspiration, and the nervous patient may have altered the conclusion.

Cawley and Morris [12] compared skin preparation for arthrocentesis using an isopropyl alcohol swab applied for a few seconds (Mediswab swipe method) with the use of chlorhexidine in spirit-soaked cotton wool balls for 1 min (full aseptic technique) in terms of the effect on bacteriological culture of the used needles. Control needles, cultured after venipuncture or intramuscular injection without skin preparation, were generally culture positive. Although neither skin preparation method produced sterile needles on all occasions, the frequency of positive culture was markedly reduced but without a significant difference between methods. The alcohol swab "swipe" method had a clear advantage in terms of cost. Critics [13] noted the small study numbers, the trend in favor of the aseptic technique, and the possibility of a type II error.

C. Main Points in Approach to Arthrocentesis

Major rheumatology texts [4–7] include chapters on joint aspiration and injection techniques, often with photographs or line drawings of variable quality illustrating methods of access to individual joints. The EULAR Monograph No. 4 on Local Injection Therapy in Rheumatic Diseases [8], published in 1983, remains a useful and comprehensive guide. Videos may offer the novice more help than a drawing in the early approaches to an unfamiliar locomotor landscape. Unfortunately, patients, their articulations, and integumentary blankets vary enough to cause even experienced operators occasional difficulty entering an area as familiar as the knee or subacromial space. A second problem is the degree to which satisfactory injection technique is dependent on "feel"—the basis for the recommendation that the injector develop familiarity with a limited range of syringe and needle sizes.

For these reasons, anyone with a serious interest in joint aspiration and injection will do better to review the relevant anatomy and then learn the technique from an experienced practitioner. It is important to get the injection in the right spot, and acquiring this ability, like most other skilled procedures, is an apprenticeship task. However, to reinforce common practice, which has proved so generally safe and effective, it seems worthwhile to restate the main points of advice from standard reference texts [4–8]. Precautions and warnings on specific injections, such as corticosteroids and radiopharmaceuticals, will be detailed under those heading.

The following are commonly advised points of technique related to synoviocentesis in general:

Inform the patient about the procedure, its purpose, and its possible adverse effects and obtain at least verbal consent.

Mark the planned injection site; some practitioners make an impression on the skin with the point of a retracted ballpoint pen, whereas others use their thumb nail for this purpose.

Use once-only prepacked sterilized disposable syringes and needles, which should not be opened until immediately before use.

Use single-dose ampules of local anesthetic and other injectables.

Ensure that all necessary equipment, including specimen bottles for synovial fluid examination and culture, are available before starting.

Wash and dry the hands so that water will not drip onto the injection site.

Use gloves to reduce the risk of body fluid–borne viral infections; although now a standard recommendation, some authorities doubt their value in protecting either the patient or the therapist [15].

Avoid talking during the procedure to avoid droplet infection of the injection site or wear a mask.

Clean the site carefully—an alcohol swab is probably as satisfactory as a more formal aseptic scrub [12], although some may opt for the latter.

Avoid injection into the joint through overlying infection such as cellulitis.

Use a no-touch technique.

Use a 23-gauge needle for most large joints such as the knee or shoulder; a 25-gauge needle for small joints in the hand; a 16- or 19-gauge needle for aspiration of hemarthroses or thick synovial fluid.

Use of local anesthetic is a matter of patient and practitioner preference, since in many instances the local anesthetic itself is as painful as the injection; it is warranted when the patient is especially nervous, access is judged likely to be difficult, or when a needle larger than 23 gauge is needed; the skin and the joint capsule are the main pain-sensitive structures, so that alternative approaches are topical refrigerant spray to deaden the skin and/or infiltration of 1 or 2% lignocaine intradermally and then down to the joint capsule, allowing 3–5 min for it to take effect.

In general, the site for joint puncture is the extensor surface, where the synovial pouch is closest to the skin, and as remote as possible from major nerves, arteries, and veins [16].

Confirm that the needle is in the right place by

- Aspiration of synovial fluid; often possible only in larger joints such as the knee
- The "feel" of injection into the site, a skill obtained only with experience
- Use of radiocontrast material and radiographic control

Avoid injection against resistence; different sized syringes, needles, joints, and spaces each produce a different degree of resistence which is learned with experience.

- Injecting a proximal interphalangeal (PIP) joint produces a very different "feel" to injecting a knee joint, but the same principle applies.
- It is recommended by some [8] that injection for tennis elbow must be made under considerable pressure, but in my experience, the result is as satisfactory when the area is infiltrated without force.
- Injection against resistence in the shoulder region seems the usual explanation for those memorably painful experiences sometimes reported by unfortunate patients.

Always examine aspirated synovial fluid and routinely send it for culture [17,18].

Difficult joint access becomes easier with the use of a stiff needle of larger size such as gauge 21 or less; a thicker needle is also necessary when synovial fluid contains much debris.

Take care not to impale or damage joint cartilage.

After the needle is withdrawn, cover the site with a sterile dressing; if much fluid has been aspirated, an elastic bandage reduces the feeling of instability. Dispose of needles and syringes safely.

Advise the patient about postinjection care and, most importantly, advise immediate return should adverse events occur.

III. CORTICOSTEROIDS

A. History

Joseph Hollander and later Daniel McCarty are the two people especially responsible for the development and use of intra-articular and intralesional corticosteroids.

G. W. Thorn is credited by Hollander [19] with the first use of intra-articular steroid. Early in 1950, Thorn injected compound F, or hydrocortisone, into the inflamed knee of a patient with rheumatoid arthritis, but because local improvement was accompanied by general improvement, he attributed the former to the latter and did not pursue this therapy further.

Hollander and his colleagues were not so easily deterred even by the minimal, inconsistent, and transient benefit following their initial use of intra-articular cortisone. However, when Merck and Company made hydrocortisone available in January 1951, a comparative study of intra-articular cortisone and hydrocortisone demonstrated the clear advantage of hydrocortisone with symptomatic improvement over days to weeks, reduced joint temperature, and in some cases reduced synovial fluid cell counts. This therapy was immediately extended to conditions other than rheumatoid arthritis (RA), with the claim that despite the absence of inflammation in most cases, the duration of symptomatic improvement in patients with osteoarthritis of the knee was "several times as great as in cases of rheumatoid arthritis and often persisted until the patient abused the affected joint in some way." By the end of 1951, they presented [19] results on almost 700 injections to 129 patients, mostly with RA but also osteoarthritis (OA), bursitis, systemic lupus erythematosus (SLE) (with injections into both the pleural cavity and a knee), acute gouty arthritis, and acute traumatic arthritis—with little systemic and no other untoward effects.

By 1953, Hollander [20] had injected hydrocortisone on 8693 occasions to the knee, ankle, wrist, hip, shoulder, phalangeal and other joints, bursas, or tendon sheaths in 852 patients; "success" was related to placing the hydrocortisone within the synovial space and therefore the more difficult the joint to aspirate and inject, the poorer the results. Adverse reactions occurred in 2.3% of injections, with the most common being a postinjection flare, lasting 2–72 h and occurring in 1.9% cases; infection occurred in two patients, an incidence of 0.02% and local urticaria, possibly related to local anesthetic or the suspending agent, developed in four patients. Attention was drawn to one patient with tuberculosis of the ankle, injected in error, who initially improved but then suffered severe relapse.

In 1961, Hollander presented the results of "a decade of use" of corticosteroids [21]: >100,000 injections to ~4000 patients.

In the 1972 edition of *Arthritis and Allied Conditions*, Hollander [16] reported on >250,000 injections to >8000 patients—a formidable experience—throughout which he stressed the adjunctive role of local steroid therapy as one component in overall management. In the same year, McCarty [22] published the results of a controlled, long-term study on intrasynovial triamcinolone hexacetonide followed by joint rest, which showed sufficient promise for him to raise the possibility of its use, not simply as adjunctive therapy, but as a method of "medical synovectomy." His most recent report [15] returns to the notion of local steroid as "adjunctive to systemic therapy, but . . . a very important adjunct"—a view widely shared in practice.

B. Efficacy

Is intra-articular corticosteroid really effective in inflammatory synovitis?

Most of Hollander's vast experience [16] was uncontrolled and observational, with some early comparative evaluation of different preparations [19]. He claimed that following his customary use of hydrocortisone, nearly 90% of injections were followed by definite improvement in the local condition for days to weeks. Poor results he considered mainly to be due to failure to enter the joint space.

McCarty's original study [22] on triamcinolone hexacetonide followed by 3 weeks joint rest in patients with inflammatory arthritis of the hand or wrist used the symmetrically involved but uninjected (or rested) joints as controls. In 12 patients followed for 14–27 months, 88% of small hand joints and tendon sheaths were still in remission on average almost 22 months after injection; synovitis recurred in only 6 of 70 injected joints but in 28 of 59 joints which were not treated locally. Measured joint size, grip strength, and hand function all improved and radiological progression, although evident, he thought to be less on the treated side.

1. Rheumatoid Arthritis

In 1995, McCarty presented the results of an observational study [15] on 956 triamcinolone injections (again with strict enforcement of upper limb joint rest for 3 weeks and lower limb rest for 6 weeks) to 140 patients with seropositive RA followed for a mean period of 7 years. Over that long follow-up period, ~75% of injected synovial structures remained in remission. There was a failure rate, defined as the need for a further injection, of only 23%, which more usually involved the knee (37%) than hand and wrist structures (12.8%). Since 1965, when triamcinolone hexacetonide became available for clinical studies, none of his patients has undergone surgical synovectomy. The effect of local steroid injection on radiological progression was not mentioned.

In comprehensive reviews [2,23] Gray, Gottlieb, and Tenenbaum summarized the literature on local corticosteroid use up to the early 1980s. Citing numerous references, they claimed that "the efficacy of intra-articular steroids in rheumatoid arthritis has been well established by controlled studies and extensive clinical experience." Although it is true that the literature contains numerous persuasive reports on the efficacy of local steroid in rheumatoid synovitis together with data on the relative benefits of different preparations and even some placebo-controlled, double-blinded studies, [24] much of that work is old, many reports relate to preparations not much in current use [25], or they describe large numbers in observational studies and only small numbers in controlled studies with variable endpoint measures.

It is noteworthy that in OA of the knee, there were also enthusiastic reports [19–21] of symptomatic benefit from intra-articular corticosteroids; at least until two small, double-blind, placebo-controlled trials showed only transient benefit little better than placebo [26,27]. In a more recent placebo-controlled study on 84 patients, triamcinolone hexacetonide provided only short-term pain relief in patients with OA of the knee, and even then most benefit was related to aspiration of a knee effusion prior to knee injection [28]. Supraspinatus tendinitis, a condition most clinicians think ideally suited to treatment with local steroid, failed to respond more convincingly to methylprednisolone injection than to placebo in two controlled trials [29,30]. Nonetheless, recent studies in rheumatoid arthritis [31–35] seem to have accepted the basic symptomatic efficacy of intra-articular steroids in order to focus on other issues.

The advent of bufexamac, an anti-inflammatory drug with specific topical activity on mucosa, encouraged Mielants and his colleagues to determine whether its intra-articular use would compare favorably with methylprednisolone acetate in inflammatory arthritis [31]. Intra-articular steroid remained convincingly superior.

Uncontrolled studies of chemical synovectomy with sodium morrhuate (Varicocid) [36] prompted Menninger et al. [34] to subject it to a controlled, but apparently unblinded, comparative study with triamcinolone hexacetonide. Again, the steroid was clearly superior.

Luukainen et al. [32] tried to determine whether certain blood and synovial fluid characteristics would predict responsiveness to intra-articular triamcinolone hexacetonide. At 6 months' follow-up, only an initially high percentage of synovial fluid polymorphonuclear leukocytes related to a better result. In general, the predictive value of synovial fluid analysis was low.

Because earlier publications reported rather different durations of reponse following injections of the same agent, Blyth et al. [4] reasoned that this may have been related to variability in concurrent control of systemic disease. In 1994, they returned to the issue of pain relief duration following different steroid preparations. In a single blind, controlled study on 300 patients with RA comparing hydrocortisone succinate 100 mg, triamcinolone acetonide 40 mg, and triamcinolone hexacetonide 20 mg injections to the knee, the benefits of intra-articular triamcinolone hexacetonide exceeded those of triamcinolone acetonide, whereas hydrocortisone succinate, quite a soluble preparation, was substantially less effective. At the final 12 week follow-up, almost 60% of the triamcinolone hexacetonide group but only 44% of the triamcinolone acetonide–treated patients were improved—all without adverse events. This perhaps reaffirms, in a more contemporary setting, that intra-articular steroids provide useful, safe palliation for rheumatoid synovitis and that triamcinolone hexacetonide is the preferred preparation.

If we accept that intra-articular steroids are better than placebo, the next issue is whether simple modifications in administration can increase their efficacy. Srinivasan et al. [35] studied the effect of knee lavage. In a single blind, controlled trial in 60 patients with RA of the knee, 20 mg triamcinolone hexacetonide was compared with knee lavage alone or combined lavage and steroid administration. Perhaps it is relevant that lavage consisted of instillation and aspiration of only 20 mL normal saline on two occasions, but alone or in combination with steroid, it conferred no benefit over conventional joint aspiration and triamcinolone injection.

A period of joint rest after injection appears to be much more useful in extending efficacy. McCarty [15,22] has always stressed the importance of this step; arbitrarily choosing 3 weeks of splinting for upper limb joints and 6 weeks of crutch walking for lower limb joints. In their review, Gray and Gottlieb [2] include data from Neustadt showing that 3 days of bed rest followed by 3 weeks of limited ambulation extended the mean duration of response to prednisolone TBA from 5.5 to 9.5 weeks and triamcinolone hexacetonide from 21 to 35 weeks. Chakravarty and his colleagues [37] recently compared standard outpatient discharge with 24-h inpatient non–weight-bearing bed rest following injection to the knees of 91 patients with inflammatory arthritis using 40 mg triamcinolone hexacetonide and 2 mL 2% lignocaine. Surprising perhaps, but even such a brief period of rest had a marked effect on outcomes: Pain was significantly improved in both groups at 3 weeks, but the benefit was maintained in the rested group at the final 24 weeks of follow-up. Judging by the median area under the curve of different response variables, rest doubled the improvement in pain and the C reactive protein (CRP) and increased walking time by 50%.

The rationale for postinjection rest is fourfold: to prevent leakage of steroid into lymphatics or along the needle track; to minimize loss into the systemic circulation; to allow time for the steroid to exert its effect on the inflamed synovium; and to reduce the exacerbating effect of overuse of a joint rendered relatively painless. The next step will be to determine the optimal period of postinjection rest.

Nonarticular problems in rheumatoid arthritis for which local corticosteroid therapy may be appropriate include tenosynovitis, nerve entrapment syndromes, and rheumatoid nodules. The technique of injection and results of therapy in flexor tenosynovitis of the hand (trigger finger) are discussed by Anderson and Kaye [38]. Local steroid injection is usually mentioned among the therapeutic options for carpal tunnel and tarsal tunnel syndromes, although there is no convincing evidence of long-term benefit [2], and justification for its use seems more based on tradition than on supporting documentation, much of which is rather old [39] or thin [40]. It is fairly standard advice that carpal tunnel injection should be avoided by the inexperienced, since good technique [41] is necessary to avoid injury [42]. Control of wrist synovitis and improved wrist stability are important measures in the long-term management of carpal tunnel syndrome, and when those measures fail, surgery may be the best next step. Rheumatoid nodules are sometimes injected directly with steroid and may undergo involution [192].

2. *Other Types of Inflammatory Arthritis*

Some of the early reports include all types of inflammatory arthritis [19,21,22], whereas more recent studies, such as those discussed above, provide data specifically on rheumatoid arthritis. Juvenile chronic arthritis has generated a number of publications but otherwise good data are scarce.

Juvenile Chronic Arthritis. Although there is a growing literature on the apparent value of triamcinolone hexacetonide, particularly in juvenile-onset oligoarthritis, placebo-controlled data are wanting.

In 1986, Allen et al. [43] reported an uncontrolled study on the use of 20–40-mg triamcinolone hexacetonide injections to 49 knees of 40 children with chronic arthritis. Most had pauciarticular-onset chronic arthritis but there were 11 children with spondylarthropathies—psoriatic arthritis, the enthesopathy-arthropathy syndrome, and a patient with juvenile-onset ankylosing spondylitis. At the 6-month follow-up, ~68% of the pauciarticular juvenile chronic arthritis (JCA) group and 50% of the spondylarthropathy group had responded; at 12 months, the percentages were 50 and 30, and at 2 years, they were 17.4 and 12.5, respectively. Response to a second injection for relapse was usually satisfactory. In general, the response rate was highest in young children with disease of shorter duration and those who had received higher doses. The only recognized complication was a small area of subcutaneous fat atrophy in one patient.

Slightly better results were reported by a British group [44], who found that 12 months after 20–40-mg triamcinolone hexacetonide injectinos to 83 knees of 60 children with pauciarticular-onset JCA, 77% were considered good or excellent; 11 knees which had relapsed reponded to a second injection and to a third injection in two cases; two patients had small areas of subcutaneous atrophy. They saw no evidence of cartilage damage following injection.

Balogh and Ruzsonyi [45] confirmed the efficacy of triamcinolone hexacetonide and its superiority to betamethasone in a double-blind controlled trial on 23 children with knee involvement in pauciarticular-onset JCA. Further support came from a Dutch group [46] using 10–20 mg triamcinolone hexacetonide in 27 knees of 21 children with pauciarticular JCA type 1; that is, typically ANA positive with a high incidence of chronic uveitis. A single injection proved effective in suppressing all signs of active arthritis for at least 6 months in 70% of the patients, with more extended benefit being related to disease of shorter duration. No other determinants of outcome were identified. Two patients had small atrophic lesions at the site of injection and one had a transiently red, painful knee but no increase in joint damage was seen on radiographic follow-up.

In a subsequent paper, Hertzberger-ten Cate et al. drew attention to ultrasound-detected, intra-articular septa preventing dispersal of the steroid as a cause for the failure of local therapy in pauciarticular JCA [47].

In a discussion of the surgical management of the hip in JCA, McCullough [48] refers to the proceedings of a Workshop on JCA in Garmisch-Partenkirchen in which hip involvement without ischemic or major erosive change was treated with triamcinolone hexacetonide injections "with good results reported in 20 such hips within the first few months . . . and successful results maintained in 15 of 20 hips over a mean period of follow-up of 3 years."

Job-Deslandre and Menkes [49] warned about side effects following injection of 10–40 mg triamcinolone hexacetonide to 144 joints of 48 children with various types of juvenile-onset arthritis; most had pauciarticular type 1, but 13 had B27-related arthritis and 6 had polyarticular disease. After treatment, joints were immobilized for 48 h; multiple injections were performed in 27 joints. Subcutaneous tissue atrophy developed near 12 joints (8.2%), appearing in the first few months following injection and not resolving over 2–4 years. Small joint size, and presumably the predisposition to backflow of the steroid along the needle track, seemed the main determinant, since the problem occurred in <6% of knees but in 16% of ankles, 22% of wrists, and 50% of metatarsophalangeal (MTP) joints. Articular and periarticular calcification, appearing after 6–12 months, was seen in just under 5% of injected joints, although never in the B27-associated arthritis. While stressing the need to ensure intra-articular delivery of the steroid in a volume appropriate to the joint size, the authors reaffirmed the value of this therapy.

In older children, especially for injection of easily accessible joints, local anesthesia is usually appropriate, with general anesthetic or midazolam sedation being reserved for younger children, hip joint injection, children in whom flexion deformities require casting, or those not expected to cooperate. As in adult disease, dosage remains fairly arbitrary, with some concensus that triamcinolone 1 mg/kg up to 20 mg is a reasonable dose for small joints and 2 mg/kg up to 40 mg for large joints [50].

Spondylarthropathy. Gray and Gottlieb [2,23] suggest that, although controlled trial data are lacking, clinical experience indicates that the spondylarthropathies respond to intra-articular steroid with benefits comparable to those in RA. This attitude of "accepting the obvious" is certainly the impression given by the major rheumatology texts. Haslock [51] and Wollheim [52] provide no references, but they assert the benefit of local steroid for synovitis of peripheral joints and enthesopathy in patients with ankylosing spondylitis. Bennett [53], Michet [54], and Espinoza and Cuellar [55] provide similar unreferenced recommendations in the management of psoriatic arthritis. In patients with reactive arthritis, Yu and Peng Thim Fan [56], reflecting my own skepticism, state that "repeated aspiration and injection of chronically inflamed joints with glucocorticoids in combination with a sequence of NSAIDs at full dosage are only occasionally effective." Cush and Lipsky [57] apply no qualifications to the benefits of local steroids, and Toivanen [58] asserts that "in many cases, intra-articular administration (of steroids) gives prompt relief." As we approach the end of the 20th century, it would be good to have better data on the efficacy of local corticosteroids in this important group of conditions in which oligoarthritis is such a common feature.

In uncontrolled trials, two European groups have reported benefit of steroid injection to the sacroiliac joints: Maugars et al. [193] first injected contrast medium to establish correct positioning of the needle; Braun et al. used computed tomography for the injection of triamcinolone acetonide and evaluated the response both clinically and by its effect on enhancement following gadolinium [194].

In our experience, steroid injections to the cervical zygoapophyseal joints, performed by an experienced radiologist under radiographic control, sometimes give enough temporary benefit to facilitate physiotherapy and help patients through the very difficult problem of late-onset neck pain in ankylosing spondylitis (D. Macauley, personal communication).

Connective Tissue Diseases. Various reviews and early studies [2,19,23] report benefit in the synovitis of SLE and other connective tissue diseases (CTDs) but basic data are vanishingly scarce. In an abstract to the ACR, Dorwart reported improved hand function of puffy hands in mixed connective tissue diseases (MCTD) following palmar flexor tendon sheath steroid injection [59].

Well-designed, placebo-controlled trials of intra-articular steroid using clear outcome measures, in defined groups of inflammatory arthritis, with sufficient numbers of patients to provide good statistical power would not be redundant.

C. Pharmacology and Mechanism of Action

Derendorf et al. [67] have undertaken pharmacokinetic and pharmacodynamic studies on intra-articular triamcinolone acetonide, triamcinolone hexacetonide, and betamethasone. They showed that both triamcinolone acetonide and hexacetonide are fully absorbed but at quite different rates, with the latter being less soluble and absorbed much more slowly, thereby producing a more prolonged local effect and less endogenous hydrocortisone suppression. By contrast, betamethasone is absorbed rapidly, since the phosphate is very water soluble, resulting in effective endogenous hydrocortisone suppression during the first day. Armstrong et al. [104] studied serum methylprednisolone and cortisol levels following intra-articular administration of the former. The quantity of steroid absorbed from the joint bore a close relationship with the amount injected, but because a given dose injected simultaneously into two knees resulted in greater absorption than when given as a single injection, they considered absorption to be influenced not only by the solubility of the preparation and the dose but by the total surface area of inflamed synovial membrane to which the steroid is exposed. Studying patients with both OA and RA, Bertouch et al. [190] were unable to demonstrate any difference in the rate or extent of absorption, and they concluded that the dose and formulation rather than the characteristics of the synovial membrane control absorption. Bird et al. [68] compared the effects of prednisolone t-butyl acetate, methylprednisolone acetate, and triamcinolone hexacetonide and found that all three drugs produced adrenal suppression, which was maximal by 2–4 days but was most pronounced in patients receiving methylprednisolone.

So there is no lack of data on the significant systemic absorption of corticosteroid, and it is clear that intra-articular steroids produce benefit from a systemic effect, but there is a more marked local effect, and it is the mechanism of this effect that is still unclear.

We know that systemically glucocorticoid hormones bind to a cytoplasmic receptor to form a complex which moves to the nucleus, binding reversibly to nuclear DNA to induce the transcription of mRNAs which then code for the proteins or enzymes that cause the hormonal effects. One of those products, at least in some cell lines, lipocortin-1 (annexin-1), may have an important role in suppression of inflammation through inhibition of phospholipase A^2. Translational and posttranslational processes also affect protein synthesis, secretion, cell growth, division, and apoptosis. Lymphocytes and cells of the monocyte-macrophage series, as particular targets of corticosteroids, show many changes in function, including cell trafficking, Ig and cytokine production. Suppression of interleukins (IL-2, IL-3, IL-6) and interferon-γ from T cells and of granulocyte-monocyte colony-stimulating factor (GM-CSF), TNF-α, and tumor necrosis factor-α and IL-1 from monocyte-derived cells constitute important mechanisms by which steroids suppress immune and inflammatory reponses [60].

Information is beginning to emerge that similar mechanisms are operating at the local level following intra-articular steroids. The fate of corticosteroid ester crystals has never been clearly established [15], but like other crystals of similar size and shape, such as CPPD, they are probably taken up by synovial cells and digested in phagolysosomes. Firestein et al. [61], using in situ hybridization, localized and quantified mRNA expression in synovial tissue for collagenase, TIMP, HLA-DR, and complement components C2 and C3. Using serial percutaneous biopsy, they were able to study the effect of intra-articular triamcinolone 1–2 weeks after injection. mRNA for collagenase had become almost undetectable and there was decreased gene expression for TIMP, HLA-DR, and to a lesser extent C2 and C3. Easier access to synovial sampling and the use of quantitative molecular techniques in studies such as this should begin to provide some answers.

D. Indications

In inflammatory arthritis, current indications for intra-articular steroids are very much the same as those proposed initially by Hollander [19]:

- Involvement of only one or two peripheral joints
- Patients in whom systemic therapy has helped all but a few joints
- Patients in whom systemic therapy is contraindicated
- As an adjunct to correction of flexion deformities
- For control of a sudden exacerbation of synovitis in one or two joints (provided infection is excluded)

In inflammatory arthritis, it is always recommended that local steroid be used together with systemic anti-inflammatory medication, joint rest, and physical therapy.

McCarty's recommendation [15] that intra-articular steroid be used for "the initial debulking of the burden of inflammation" may well be reasonable, particularly if administered according to his technique, but I find no evidence that is has become a widely used tactic.

E. Contraindications

There are a few absolute and many relative contraindications to local steroid injection that are mostly related to concerns about introducing or worsening infection and causing bleeding or local damage to cartilage and bone. Some contraindications are based on common sense, some on clinical experience, and others seem to be untested assertions strengthened by repetition [2,16].

1. Infection in or near the joint:

Known or suspected infection with pyogenic, mycobacterial, or other organisms is a clear contraindication to local steroid injection.

Previous infective arthritis would be considered an absolute contraindication by most rheumatologists.

Cellulitis or a psoriatic plaque contraindicates arthrocentesis unless septic arthritis is suspected to be the underlying problem and there is no other access.

Bacterial endocarditis, pneumonia, and other conditions likely to cause bacteremia are generally regarded as contraindications to local steroid injection and also to arthrocentesis (unless septic arthritis is suspected when joint aspiration becomes mandatory).

Other sources of local or systemic infection require careful evaluation.

Immunosuppression through systemic corticosteroids and immunosuppressives increases vulnerability to septic arthritis, especially in damaged rheumatoid joints [62], and although not a contraindication, it requires risk evaluation.

2. Damaged and prosthetic joints:

Severely damaged or unstable joints are regarded by some as a contraindication [2,16] either because local steroid is unlikely to be of help in that situation or, if the joint has been injected on multiple occasions in the past, for fear of worsening so-called "steroid arthropathy."

Prosthetic joints are generally considered [2] an absolute contraindication to local steroid injection, since "spontaneous" early and late infection is an unusual but well-recognized disaster and most therapists have judged it prudent to avoid even apparent liability. However, synovitis does recur following total joint arthroplasty, and Owen [6] reports on >400 replaced joints injected with glucocorticoids with benefit and without sequelae, although he recommends prior synovial fluid analysis and culture before injection, and presumably the procedure should be carried out with as much attention to asepsis as occurred at the insertion of the prosthesis.

Osteochondral fracture, internal derangements of the joint, and other such mechanical problems are inappropriate conditions for local steroid therapy.

3. Bleeding disorders and anticoagulant therapy:

Uncontrolled bleeding or coagulation disorders clearly increase the risk of hemarthrosis from joint injection.

Hemarthrosis is often listed as a contraindication to local steroid therapy mainly because of concern about the introduction of infection or because bleeding may indicate an osteochondral fracture; otherwise local steroid may help reduce the synovial irritation provoked by intrasynovial blood. In a small pilot study in patients with hemophilic arthropathy, Shupak et al. [63] reported symptomatic improvement and fewer further bleeds in injected joints, although York did not consider it helpful in this situation [64].

Anticoagulant therapy must increase the risk of bleeding, although Owen [6] suggests that arthrocentesis can be performed on patients receiving anticoagulants if the joint is subsequently immobilized for 24–48 h; the literature provides no data on relative risks, but I consider it unwise to perform elective arthrocentesis with an INR > 2, preferring, if possible, to stop anticoagulation for a day or two.

4. Other contraindications and precautions:

The absence of a diagnosis is a good reason to undertake a diagnostic arthrocentesis but a poor reason to inject steroid.

Failure to respond to previous injections should prompt a reevaluation of the underlying diagnosis, contraindicate further local steroid, and promote the development of an alternative management plan.

Poorly controlled diabetes may be worsened by the systemic effect of steroids.

Severe juxta-articular osteoporosis is listed by Hollander [16] as a concern, but since this is a regular consequence of active, established synovitis, it may as well be argued that therapy which moderates synovitis is more likely to help this problem than to worsen it.

Difficult joint access was a reasonable contraindication to the attempt in the past, solved now by imaging control, which in experienced hands provides access to almost every joint. Hollander [20] seemed to regret his inability to inject the spinal zygapophyseal joints, but now that we can do so readily, benefit, at least in noninflammatory pain, has not been supported by controlled trials examining the cervical [65] or the lumbar spine [66]; the situation in inflammatory spinal disease remains untested.

F. Formulations

The pharmaceutical industry has generated a number of different preparations of steroids for local use in an attempt to improve the efficacy and duration of effect of hydrocortisone, the physiologically active form of cortisone. The addition of fluorine and a hydroxyl group to produce triamcinolone enhances pharmacological potency; its formulation with acetate reduces solubility and thereby enhances its duration of local efficacy. Triamcinolone hexacetonide is the 21-t-butylacetate of triamcinolone acetonide [67] and has been shown repeatedly to have the most marked and sustained effect [33,68] of the commonly available preparations (trade names and usual concentrations are shown in Table 1).

In the 1970s, attempts were made to increase joint retention and duration of response to steroid and to minimize systemic effects by incorporating the steroid ester into liposomes. Initial studies in animals [69] and humans [70] looked promising but have not been further developed.

Table 1 Commonly Available Steroid Preparations

Generic name	Trade name	Concentration (mg/mL)
Hydrocortisone acetate	Hydrocortistab	25
Hydrocortisone tertiary butylacetate (TBA)		
Prednisolone acetate	Meticortelone	
	Deltacortril	25
Prednisolone TBA	Hydeltra-TBA	
	Codelcortone	20
Methylprednisolone acetate	Depomedrol	40
	Depomedrone	
Dexamethasone phosphate	Decadron (Phos)	4
Dexamethasone TBA	Decadron	
Betamethasone acetate	Celestone	5.7
and	Chronodose	
Betamethasone sodium phosphate		
Triamcinolone diacetate	Aristocort Forte	
Triamcinolone acetonide	Kenacort A10	10
	Kenacort A40	40
	Kenalog	
Triamcinolone hexacetonide	Aristospan	20
	Lederspan	

G. Administration and Dosage

The choice of steroid formulation depends on the condition. Acute problems such as bursitis may be treated effectively with a short-acting preparation; for rheumatoid synovitis, it is better to use a potent, longer acting prepation such as triamcinolone hexacetonide. In more superficial situations where leakage from the joint capsule is likely to produce skin and subcutaneous tissue atrophy, hydrocortisone or methylprednisolone are less liable to cause this problem and may be preferable.

Dosage seems to have been determined empirically, and it is hard to know whether the rationale has been injection volume relative to joint capacity, steroid dose relative to synovial area, or something more intuitive. Tables listing different preparations sometimes provide an indication of relative steroid potency [71], but as Gray and Gottlieb point out [2], these are based largely on the relative effect on hypothalamic-pituitary-adrenal axis suppression which may have little relevance to intrasynovial anti-inflammatory potency. Until we have a method to measure the level of inflammation in a given joint and considerably more synovial dose-response data, current arbitrary recommendations will prevail.

McCarty [15] uses the following doses of triamcinolone hexacetonide: knee or hip, 40 mg; ankle, subtalar joint, peroneal or posterior tibial tendon sheath, shoulder or elbow, 30-mg; wrist or carpus, 20 mg; distal radioulnar joint, 15 mg; MCP and PIP joints, flexor carpi radialis, extensor carpi ulnaris, common flexor tendons, or extensor digitorium sheath, 10 mg; distal interphalangeal (DIP) joint 5 mg.

The manufacturers provide guidelines to dosage and administration but give no references: hydrocortisone acetate 50–75 mg for smaller joints, up to 125 mg for larger joints; methylprednisolone acetate 4–10 mg for smaller joints, 10–40 mg for elbows and wrists, and 20–80 mg for larger joints, such as knees, ankles, and shoulders; triamcinolone acetonide up to 10 mg for smaller joints and up to 40 mg for larger joints.

Depomedrol should not be mixed with other solutions, including local aneasthetic, since this can result in flocculation of the steroid. Provided paraben preservative containing formulations of local anesthetic are avoided, this problem is not seen with Celestone Chronodose or triamcinolone acetonide. Although a common practice [7], the addition of lignocaine to injected steroid has been questioned by Jenkinson [11], who contends that the acid pH of the local anesthetic may not be adequately offset by the neutral pH of the steroid and synovial fluid, inducing an acid environment which could promote activation of proteolytic enzymes. There is, however, no clinical evidence that articular cartilage is adversely affected by lignocaine solutions.

The use of local steroid injections in pregnancy and lactation is endorsed with the usual warnings by the manufacturers, although I am not aware of problems reported in the literature, and flares in the postpartum period are often more easily managed with local than systemic therapy.

How often can steroid be injected safely into any one joint? A common question on which opinion is plentiful but data scarce. Hollander considered that intra-articular steroid could be "repeated apparently indefinitely" [16], and he gave as many as 142 injections into a single joint [21]. The period over which these injections were given is not clear, although he indicates that they were not repeated more often than once a month. The reports of Chandler et al. in 1959 [72,73] describing a Charcot-like arthropathy following repeated injections caused great concern and led to the view that intra-articular steroid injections should be "used sparingly, that is, preferably no more than two or three injections in the one joint over a 12 month period" [74]. Although a recommendation within this range seems reasonable [5,8,9], we know that patients have received >150 injections over periods up to 15 years without evidence of radiographic deterioration [75], so that current guidelines should provide a satisfactory safety margin unless there are other risk factors of which we are currently unaware. Certainly repeating a steroid injection assumes that a good response has occurred initially. In my experience, repetition is often accompanied by a diminishing response, which is a clear indication to consider an alternative approach.

How many joints can safely be injected at the one time? Again, the answer must be guided more by common sense than evidence-based information. Limitations include patient tolerance [8] and the systemic effect of multiple steroid injections. McCarty, at least in his initial study [22], apparently injected multiple hand and wrist joints at the one sitting, but Hollander [16] advocated that no more than two or three joints be injected at any one visit, and Owen [6] endorses this advice.

H. Adverse Effects

If local corticosteroid injections are given for appropriate indications, using proper techniques with appropriate formulations and doses and avoiding situations which are contraindicated, then significant adverse effects are extremely rare.

Hollander maintained that he kept accurate records of all adverse effects throughout his 20-odd years of local steroid therapy use [16]. He used hydrocortisone acetate principally but not exclusively and found postinjection flares to be the commonest problem, with an incidence of ~2% of 250,000 injections; infection was the most serious problem, with an incidence of 1 in 14,000 injections; <1% showed enough deterioration in joint structure to result in instability, whereas aseptic necrosis occurred after ~1 in 25,000 injections.

In his recent report on 956 triamcinolone hexacetonide injections in 140 patients treated over 18 years, McCarty [15] encountered postinjection flares after 6% of injections and rupture of one extensor tendon and of one peroneal tendon many months after local therapy, but he had no problem with infections.

Despite this fairly remarkable record of nontoxicity, the adverse effects of local steroid injection have been analyzed and documented in an extensive literature and well summarized in the reviews of Gray, Gottlieb, and Tenenbaum [2,23].

1. Infection

Most large series support an incidence of infection of an order similar to that reported by Hollander. In 1957, Kendall [76] reported on 6700 injections to 2256 patients at Guy's Hospital where sepsis had occurred in four patients, or 0.06%; two had subcutaneous abscess associated with a soft tissue injection; two patients, a physician's wife and another relative of the medical staff, developed septic arthritis. According to Fitzgerald [77], ~3000 local steroid injections were being administered annually at the Mayo Clinic "under rigid aseptic technique," none of which was complicated by infection. Gray et al. [23] estimated that nearly 100,000 intra-articular injections had been administered without gloves or gowns by medical students, house officers, and faculty members attending outpatient clinics at the University of Miami Medical School with only two instances of infection. In a recent survey of New South Wales rheumatologists, Lawford [9] found 12 cases of sepsis associated with an estimated 350,000 injections: an incidence of 1 in ~30,000.

McCarty [78] considers it likely that some bacteria are carried into the joint every time arthrocentesis is performed but in a dose too small to initiate sepsis. He noted that he "had never seen a joint infected from the skin by arthrocentesis but . . . had seen five joints infected from the blood by needling that was performed when the patient had bacteremia." The report of a child who developed a *Haemophilus influenzae* septic arthritis in an ankle following an injection of steroid to a knee during an apparently mild upper respiratory tract infection [79] is presumably a variation on this theme.

In a brief review, von Essen and Savolainen [80] assembled a number of case reports of postinjection bacterial arthritis which confirmed that *Staphylococcus aureus* is the usual organism responsible for sepsis in almost 50% of cases. Their report also highlighted the dangers of multidose containers in transmitting infection, particularly with unusual bacterial culprits: *Pseudomonas cepacia* in one case, *Serratia marcescens* in another. They had themselves reported the only case they found of a skin resident, *Propionibacterium acnes*, responsible for postinjection sepsis. About 20% of their collected cases identified mycobacterial infection, initiated or reactivated following steroid infection, a problem well recognized and noted for its seriousness by Hollander [20]. Two cases of fatal gas gangrene following intra-articular steroid have been reported [80,81].

However rare it may be, most would agree with Fitzgerald [77] that "sepsis after a therapeutic injection is a disaster." The key to damage control is prompt diagnosis and appropriate treatment. The first requires that patients are warned to return immediately for evaluation should the injection be followed by worsening symptoms. The rest should be standard: arthrocentesis, immediate bacteriological examination and culture of synovial fluid, and initiation of antibiotics pending culture results if there is any reasonable suspicion of infection.

2. *Articular Problems*

Steroid Arthropathy. I was once told by a student that "cortisone kills chondrocytes" which echoed the warning of his orthopedic tutor. Oversimplification and poetic licence aside, is there any truth in this assertion? Or put another way, why do we advise that any one joint be injected no more often than two to four times per year?

The term *steroid arthropathy* refers here to accelerated joint damage or articular disorganization occurring after repeated intra-articular corticosteroid injections—a concept for which clinical, laboratory, and animal studies provide both support and rebuttal.

The alarm was first sounded in 1958 when Chandler and Wright [73] reported radiographic deterioration, sometimes considerable, in the knees of 13 of 25 patients after each knee was injected at 2-week intervals with four injections each of three preparations—hydrocortisone acetate, hydrocortisone TBA, and placebo—with an interval of 8 weeks between treatments; that is, each knee was injected 12 times over a period of 48 weeks. They thought it unlikely that this represented the natural history of the disease but were drawn to the conclusion that the very success of the treatment in relieving pain "encourages a degree of weight bearing and mobility which is inherently traumatic." The following year, they reported the case of a physician's wife whose osteoarthritic hip showed clinical, radiographic, and histological changes consistent with Charcot's arthropathy following monthly injections of hydrocortisone acetate 50 mg over a period of 18 months [72].

Several other case reports followed over the next decade [23,188]. Even in recent years, Parikh et al. [82] reported Charcot's arthropathy of the shoulder following 18 intra-articular injections of triamcinolone acetonide 40 mg over the preceding 4 months with intermittent injections previously. At shoulder arthroplasty, there was necrotizing destruction of the cartilage, necrosis, and regenerative changes of underlying bone and proliferative synovitis.

Experience suggests that the high incidence of accelerated joint damage noted in Chandler's trial [73], although useful in bringing the problem to attention, was surely atypical. Although a distressing and memorable experience which deserves to be publicized, most cases are anecdotal, and the incidence of this problem in larger trial or observational series has been consistently low. Hollander [16] recognized it in $<1\%$ of his vast series, and McCarty seems not to have encountered it in his patients.

Balch et al. [75] undertook a radiographic survey of 35 patients with RA and 30 with OA who had a minimum of 15 injections over 4 years and a maximum of 167 injections over 12 years, although not more often than monthly. Only two knees (in the same patient) showed gross radiographic change after 82 and 85 injections over 7 years. In 80,000 injections over a period of 20 years, the incidence of rapid joint damage remained at $<1\%$. Similar figures from the series of Stolzer and Keagy and Keim were reported by Gray et al. [23], who, perhaps to provide some balance, presented their own case of a 51-year-old woman with long-standing inflammatory arthritis, primarily involving the knees, who had 100 steroid injections into each knee over 10 years without evidence of radiographic deterioration and had been able to continue work as a door-to-door sales representative.

The pediatricians were concerned about steroid arthropathy, because, after demonstrating long-lasting benefit in pauciarticular disease involving the knee [43–45], they had extended the use local steroid injection to other joints, injecting several joints at once and the same joint more than once. In 1990, Sparling et al. [83] presented a radiographic review of 145 joints of 55 children at 1–9 years of follow-up. Following injection of 18 hips, 75 knees, 22 ankles, 4 subtalar joints, 4 shoulders, 11 elbows, and 11 wrists, the only symptomatic and serious abnormality was avascular necrosis of 1 hip, which had already shown rapid changes prior to injection. In 76 joints of 30 children for whom serial radiographs were available from the date of the first injection, deterioration was unusual and mild except in the hip where 4 of 12 joints showed two or more grades of change for the worse. A number of joints had been injected two, three, or even four times, but these showed no special radiographic features. Overall, some change, possibly attributable to steroid injection, was seen in 16 joints of 11 patients: small patella in 2; periarticular calcification in 9; osteochondritis dissecans of the patella in 1; a tibial spur in 1; avascular necrosis of the distal radial epiphysis in 2; and the previously mentioned symptomatic hip change in 1. A number of the abnormalities could have been due to the disease rather than its treatment. The investigators found that intra-articular triamcinolone hexacetonide was not associated with significant joint damage but raised a caution regarding its role in hip disease.

Do animal studies help? Initial work in rabbits appeared to indict local steroid, particularly as a cause of cartilage damage. This extensive early work, largely on rabbit cartilage, has been well summarized by Gray and Gottlieb [2]. Mankin [84,85], Moskowitz [86], Behrens [87], and others showed impairment of protein, proteoglycan, and collagen synthesis and reported fibrillation, fissures, and cyst formation in rabbit cartilage following substantial weekly doses of hydrocortisone acetate. But the problem was not a simple one: Longer term studies with less frequent injection showed that acute changes did not necessarily progress [88], and Gibson et al. [89] found no damage to primate cartilage following injections of methylprednisolone. They asked whether the earlier rabbit work was relevant to humans.

In more recent experimental work, the tide seems to have turned even further. Williams and Brandt [90] found triamcinolone hexacetonide protected against fibrillation and osteophyte formation following cartilage damage induced by sodium iodoacetate in guinea pigs. The Pelletiers [91], using the Pond-Nuki dog model of osteoarthritis, reported that both oral and intra-articular corticosteroid reduced early OA changes, with intra-articular triamcinolone hexacetonide having the greater protective effect on histological change in cartilage. Wollheim et al. [92] showed that triamcinolone hexacetonide, even when administered well after the onset of antigen-induced arthritis in New Zealand white rabbits, is able to control inflammation and protect joint structures from damage. It is clear that the story is far from ended.

In terms of possible mechanisms, the focus has been largely on cartilage, but it is interesting that dorsal dislocation of the second MTP joint in two patients 3–4 weeks after methylprednisolone acetate injections [93] was thought to result from weakening of the plantar capsule. Could the problem of steroid arthropathy primarily be due to the induction of ligamentous laxity in susceptible individuals?

On clinical and experimental evidence, it seems reasonable to conclude that steroid arthropathy is real but rare; most cases follow manifest abuse of this therapy. However, some patients seem especially sensitive, others quite resistent, and we have as yet no special clues to risk factors.

Avascular Necrosis. McCarty described a patient with recurrent knee synovitis, treated with brief courses of systemic steroids and several intra-articular injections of triamcinolone hexacetonide, who developed osteonecrosis of her distal femurs and proximal tibias with recurrence of inflammatory synovitis due to leakage of necrotic fat into the joint [94]. Hollander [16] had 10 patients with more typical avascular necrosis of the femoral head. Laroche et al. [95] reported two cases of multifocal osteonecrosis following intra-articular triamcinolone acetonide injections which had induced features of hypercortisolism in both patients; both suffered bilateral femoral head osteonecrosis, and one also had involvement of both shoulders.

Postinjection Flare. In about 2% of patients, Hollander [16] noted increased pain, swelling, and tenderness in the joint coming on within a few hours of injection and lasting from a few hours to 4 days. The problem was generally mild, responding to rest, ice packs, and oral analgesics. McCarty [15] recorded postinjection flares lasting 4–24 h after 6% of local injections.

This phenomenon is thought to be due to a steroid crystal–induced acute synovitis. In experiments with dogs and humans, McCarty and Hogan [96] found that the microcrystalline preparations of corticosteroid esters could induce a sterile inflammatory reaction, although much less intense than that caused by urate or calcium pyrophosphate crystals. Recently, Berger and Yount [97] described a patient who had rapid intense inflammation following intra-articular triamcinolone hexacetonide. Polarized microscopy revealed numerous negatively birefringent intra- and extracellular crystals in the synovial fluid, which are considered to be consistent with cellular ingestion of the microcrystalline steroid ester. It is not clear how they distinguished these crystals from urate crystals [23].

The use of well-mixed, newer steroid preparation has made postinjection flare less common than it was with hydrocortisone acetate. In my experience, when injecting mainly triamcinolone acetate with lignocaine, a postinjection flare is so rare that such a presentation would warrant immediate steps to exclude infection.

Periarticular Calcification. McCarty noted the appearance of capsular calcification appearing 1–2 years after injection of small joints of the hand [22]. He studied some of these at autopsy and concluded that they were calcium hydroxyapatite, probably representing dystrophic calcification caused by injecting small-volume joints under pressure. Many appeared at the site of the injection, probably as a result of leakage of steroid from the joint capsule. They often disappeared between the second and third years after treatment. No mention is made of this complication in McCarty's later paper [15].

Periarticular calcification was also noted in the radiographic follow-up of children [83].

3. Tendon Problems

Tendon rupture following local steroid injection is well recognized [2,15,23]. The most common sites are the Achilles tendon, the long head of the biceps, and tendons around the wrist in RA. It is sometimes difficult to know whether the steroid itself is responsible or was given to relieve the pain caused by the rupturing process. Gottlieb and Riskin reported bilateral digital flexor tendon rupture following carpal tunnel injection [98], but Gray [2] did not observe a similar problem following more than 300 injections into the flexor tendon sheaths in patients with RA. On the other hand, Weiss [99] contends that "this complication arises far more frequently than would be indicated from the few anecdotal reports in the literature." It is important to inject steroid into the tendon sheath and never into the tendon itself and to warn patients of this potential complication before the procedure.

4. Dermatological Problems

Skin atrophy, depigmentation, localized fat necrosis, and ecchymosis have all been observed following local corticosteroid injections [2,22,23,77,99,100]. McCarty reported skin changes after 28 of 124 injections of triamcinolone hexacetonide [22], but it is not mentioned in the review by Hollander, who used mainly hydrocortisone acetate over a period of 20 years [16]. The problem seems fairly clearly to be related to the leakage of steroid back along the needle track and probably to the use of longer acting formulations. Sometimes the changes resolve, and sometimes they persist [2].

5. Systemic Problems

Hypercortisolism. It has been known for some time that adrenal suppression can follow intra-articular corticosteroid therapy. As early as 1953, Ward and Mason reported clinical and biochemical evidence of the systemic effect from intra-articular hydrocortisone acetate [101], and Shuster and Williams showed in 1961 [102] that 50 mg or more of intra-articular triamcinolone effectively suppressed adrenal function for 4–5 days. Others [103,104] have confirmed a similar duration of plasma cortisol suppression, and Koehler et al. [103] demonstrated total suppression of the hypothalamic-pituitary-adrenal axis to insulin hypoglycemia for 48 h after 80 mg intra-articular methylprednisolone acetate in five of six patients. A single dose of triamcinolone acetonide, given by intramuscular injection on day 1 or 2 of the menstrual cycle inhibits ovulation [105], and Owen [6] draws attention to instances of steroid-induced postmenopausal bleeding. The benefit of a local steroid injection to joints other than the one injected and to an effect on general well-being is a well-recognized event in the patient with inflammatory arthritis [103].

Since intra-articular steroid absorption is related to the solubility of the formulation, it is not surprising that more potent preparations [68], in higher doses, administered repeatedly or simultaneously to multiple joints have been shown to induce acute and even chronic systemic steroid effects in some patients.

O'Sullivan et al. [106] present the case of a man with RA given 300 mg triamcinolone hexacetonide divided between four joints at 8-week intervals for 8 years, who had Cushing's syndrome with prolonged suppression of the hypothalamic-pituitary-adrenal axis requiring replacement steroid therapy. A similar patient with Cushing's features is reported by Gray et al. [23]. Patients with diabetes should be warned that a local steroid injection is likely to increase blood sugar levels for about 4 days, and those on insulin may need to adjust the dose as they would during an intercurrent infection. One would expect this occasionally to be of sufficient degree to cause problems in unstable diabetes, and I was surprised that the literature, so assiduous in its coverage of local steroid-induced problems, seems to lack an instance of a serious hyperglycaemic event precipitated by a local steroid injection.

Facial Flushing. Flushing of the face, neck, and sometimes the upper torso is common. In a study by Pattrick and Doherty [107], flushing occurred in 40% of patients 2–30 h after intra-articular triamcinolone acetonide of sufficient degree to be termed "unpleasant" in 15%. It generally lasted about 36 h, but in some, it lasted up to 96 h and it was more common in women. Flushing is seen more frequently after triamcinolone use [2] and may be more common after the acetonide than the hexacetonide [107], but it can occur after the use of other steroid preparations. Flushing may be accompanied by chilliness, shaking, and headache [98]. Although it is a benign and self-limiting event, flushing is sufficiently distressing for some patients to require use of an alternative preparation. The cause of this nitritoid-type reaction has not been determined.

Allergic and Anaphylactic Reactions. Kendall [76] was the first to report allergic reactions following intra-articular and intralesional corticosteroids. Some, but not all, of his steroid injections were accompanied by 2% procaine and 1000 units of hyaluronidase; one patient, following the administration of the cocktail, developed an anaphylactic reaction with severe bronchospasm, widespread urticaria, and edema of the face and larynx but recovered. Eight patients suffered generalized urticaria, appearing 30 min to 8 h after injection, whereas another 11 patients had urticaria and edema around the injection site. Hollander [16] commented that one patient developed local urticaria "due to allergy to the aqueous vehicle of the hormone suspension."

In 1988, Larsson [108] observed an anaphylactic reaction in a patient following triamcinolone acetonide and lignocaine to both shoulders and two PIP joints a few weeks after an earlier injection of triamcinolone hexacetonide without local anesthetic to her knees. Recently, a Dutch group [109] reported a prolonged urticarial type rash following an intra-articular injection of triamcinolone acetonide and procaine; delayed-type hypersensitivity to triamcinolone was observed after patch and intradermal testing. Patterson et al. [110] reported an anaphylactic response to intracutaneous lignocaine, epinephrine, and triamcinolone acetonide due to the suspending agent carboxymethylcellulose in the steroid formulation. They report that others have found the same component responsible for an allergic reaction.

Allergic reactions to corticosteroid and to local anesthetic are rare but can be serious; now that techniques are available to do so, it is important to determine the responsible component.

Other Rare and Unusual Problems. "A peculiar local weakness" in the injected limb lasting 1–3 days was prominent in Hollander's list of adverse events [16]. Interestingly, Kendall [76] also reported this in 24 of his patients, especially after injection for tennis elbow and when using hydrocortisone without local anesthetic. The weakness was objective but without sensory loss or electromyographic abnormalities and all patients recovered spontaneously. I am not familiar with the problem among my patients and have seen no references to it in the recent literature. Is this because we have changed our technique or because we no longer ask about it?

Sickle cell crisis was apparently precipitated in two patients by intra-articular methylprednisolone acetate; no mechanism was proposed [111]. Nausea, vertigo, and malaise are reported but probably at an incidence similar to placebo.

I. Summary

If others using McCarty's methods, could obtain his impressive results [15], then many rheumatologists are using local corticosteroids suboptimally. That being the case, it is even more important to begin acquiring important missing data: Just what conditions provide optimal use of local steroid; how should doses be calculated and does it make a difference; what is the effect, for example, of local steroid/rest/local anesthetic on the synovium, the cartilage, and the capsule; how long do those effects persist and what is the interaction with systemic therapy; is benefit reflected radiologically; is response different in different types of inflammatory arthritis? These and many more questions. . . .

After almost half a century of enthusiastic use and millions of local steroid injections, there is abundant evidence that, given the administration protocol and precautions which have become standard practice within rheumatology, this is an acceptably safe form of therapy—safer than NSAIDs or second-line agents and much safer and easier than surgery. There is little persuasive evidence that "chemical" or "radioactive synovectomy" are a better than intra-articular triamcinolone hexacetonide followed by a period of rest for the joint. Current preoccupations with the evaluation of combination and biological therapies notwithstanding, it seems worthwhile undertaking a little more work to define just how good this very important adjunct can become in inflammatory arthritis.

IV. CHEMICAL SYNOVECTOMY

Hollander [16] mentions chemicals that were injected into joints prior to the advent of corticosteroids: liquid petrolatum, lipiodol, procaine hydrochloride, penicillin, and lactic acid "to stimulate natural local tissue reactions."

Later, a variety of chemical agents, anti-inflammatory drugs, antibiotics, and immunosuppressive agents were tried in an attempt to suppress local synovitis. If mentioned at all, current Anglo-American rheumatology texts deal with the subject of chemical synovectomy or synoviorthesis in a cursory way, suggesting that osmic acid, orgotein, and intra-articular antimetabolites have only historical status. However, osmic acid remains in use, at least in Scandinavia [112], and, given the cyclical nature of therapies in rheumatology, it seems appropriate to review briefly agents which have often been used extensively in Europe [113]. In reviewing the data on these agents, the tests to be applied are whether there is evidence that (a) they provide better clinical benefit than optimally used corticosteroids and (b) they modify the inflamed synovium sufficiently to allow more normal tissue to regenerate.

A. Osmic Acid

Osmic acid is used as an aqueous solution of osmium tetroxide, a vigorous oxidizing agent which on contact with tissue causes cell destruction and is immediately reduced to insoluble oxides.

In the early 1950s, von Reis and Swensson [114] were trying not to ablate the inflamed synovium but to "eliminate the nerve endings in the synovial membrane . . . by injecting into the joint cavity a substance that coagulates the entire inner surface." They considered osmic acid suitable, because it penetrated tissue very slowly, and caused no evidence of cartilage damage and no general toxicity. Following initial animal studies, they treated the knees of 35 patients with OA and RA with 1% osmic acid. Despite first injecting local anesthetic into the joint, patients generally experienced intense burning knee pain 3–4 h after injection and lasting 1–3 days with marked joint swelling, fevers, and leukocytosis. About two thirds of the patients ultimately reported improvement over periods up to 12 months; they also noted improvement in uninvolved joints—or perhaps the patients feared the consequences of continued complaints.

Undeterred by this rather ferocious therapy, Scandinavian workers continued to use osmic acid, learning that the addition of corticosteroid and lignocaine ameliorated the adverse reactions and that responses were best when inflammation was prominent and structural damage minimal. In general, satisfactory results were obtained in >50% of patients at 6–12 months. Following extensive use in the 1960s, controlled trials were undertaken in the 1970s, although strangely not in an especially logical order.

In 1975, Anttinen and Oka [115] compared osmic acid 100 mg plus triamcinolone hexacetonide 40 mg and 2 mL 2% lidocaine with the steroid and local anesthetic alone in 43 knees of patients with RA. At 12 months, clinical improvement was similar in both groups, although some objective measurements of local disease were better in the osmic acid group. There followed trials setting osmic acid against weaker competition, demonstrating its superiority to placebo [116] and methylprednisolone [117].

Sheppeard et al. [118] then compared osmic acid plus methylprednisolone 80 mg and lidocaine with 5 mCi yttrium silicate without steroid, reporting that osmic acid appeared more effective throughout the follow-up period, but this reached significance only at 3 years. Progression of radiographic change occurred in about 30% of each group. Following osmic acid, some patients had dark discoloration of the urine, several had a fever, and one developed a fistula along the needle track which healed after surgical excision. Either treatment was considered a suitable alternative to surgical synovectomy. In 1978, Nissila et al. [119] reported on 66 patients with RA knee synovitis randomly assigned to treatment with osmic acid, yttrium, or surgical synovectomy. Swelling was best helped by surgery, whereas pain was a little better in patients treated with osmic acid or surgery than in those receiving yttrium; over all, good results were achieved in slightly over half the cases. At 1-year follow-up radiographic osteoarthritis had progressed more often in the knee joints treated surgically. In discussing the pros and cons of the various treatments, they concluded that "osmic acid is in first place" because "it is simple to inject and has not been found to have any unpleasant immediate or late side effects."

In 1980, Sheppeard and Ward [120] summarized 5 years' experience of osmic acid injections to 305 knees of 201 paitents with "satisfactory results" in 61% at 1 year and falling to 22% at 5 years. Only two patients had developed acute knee effusions on the day of injection and two developed fistulas, whereas transient fever and leukocytosis occurred in 15.

Concern had arisen over reports of osmic acid–induced cartilage damage in rabbits and in humans. Menkes showed that osmic acid severely affected growth cartilage and epiphyseal growth in young rabbits but not those over 12 weeks of age [121]. In 1973, Mitchell et al. [122] found that both osmic acid and nitrogen mustard caused early and extensive chondrocyte necrosis in rabbits and that within 3 to 7 months, the cartilage surface began to disintegrate. He concluded that these agents were not suitable for chemical synovectomy. Niculescu et al. [123] found ultrastructural change in the cartilage of two RA patients biopsied after the use of osmic acid. Nissila [124] agreed that osmic acid caused cartilage changes but considered these superficial and of questionable clinical significance. Sheppeard [120] found no clinical evidence that osmic acid increased the rate of joint surfaces damage, confirming the clinical experience of Nissila et al. [116], who claimed that after 4000 osmic acid injections since the early 1950s, no unfavorable destructive effects were observed. He looked specifically at this issue [124] in 52 adults and 31 children treated with osmic acid, observed for 8–18 years, again concluding that such cartilage damage as may occur is not clinically significant and even on long-term follow-up, degenerative joint changes were not increased. In juvenile patients who had received osmic acid before the age of 10 years, there was evidence of more osteoarthritic change in the treated than the untreated knee, but perhaps it occurred as a result of asymmetrical disease.

Lagier and his colleagues [125] had the opportunity to study at autopsy the knee of a patient with RA treated 32 months previously with osmic acid. They observed deposits of osmium in fat lobules and some histiocytes with a fibrotic synovial membrane. They assumed the osmic acid had caused necrosis of the inflamed synovium and then stimulated an intense fibroblastic reaction. Much more recently, Ostergaard et al. [112], using magnetic resonance imaging (MRI) for the first time to evaluate therapy-induced changes in the synovial membrane, showed that 1 month after osmic acid to the knees of adults and children with various inflammatory arthropathies, the synovial membrane volume was reduced by a mean of 52% in those with a good clinical response but unchanged in those whose knees had relapsed or failed to respond.

It is possible then that osmic acid effects an important change in the synovial membrane with a clinical response as good as triamcinolone hexacetonide. But despite reassurances about long-term safety from the Scandinavian literature, its continued use in inflammatory arthritis [112], and even a recent report of its value in persistent arthritis after controlled septic arthritis [126], osmic acid remains a strictly regional local therapy.

B. Orgotein

Orgotein, a copper-zinc superoxide dismutase, is a metalloprotein widely distributed in the cells of a number of tissues which inhibits detrimental molecular oxygen radicals. Since free-radical oxidation products are present in larger quantity in RA than in degenerative or normal synovial fluid [127], it was assumed that a substance acting as a powerful free-radical inhibitor should prove beneficial.

Goebel et al. undertook two trials on RA knee synovitis. First they compared intra-articular orgotein 4 mg/week for 6 weeks with intra-articular aspirin 4 mg/week for 6 weeks and at 12 weeks showed clinical and biochemical superiority of orgotein, although more than 50% of patients in the orgotein group experienced local painful subcutaneous reactions [128]. Then they compared the same dose and regimen of orgotein with six weekly injections of 4 mg (sic) methylprednisolone acetate; both groups had improved equally at 6 weeks, but at 24 weeks, orgotein was clinically superior [129]. The effect of orgotein on the synovial membrane itself was not assessed.

Despite reports of prolonged benefit in osteoarthritis, in trials comparing it with placebo [130] and with intra-articular steroid [131], orgotein does not appear to have stimulated the additional studies needed to clarify better its role in local RA therapy.

C. Other Agents

Aspirin was used as a control for intra-articular orgotein [128], and in 1980, Rylance [132] compared intra-articular acetylsalicylic acid with hydrocortisone acetate 50 mg and normal saline in the knees of patients with RA. All three preparations were found equally effective in relieving pain and improving the range of motion.

Intra-articular injections of nitrogen mustard in variable doses, usually with corticosteroid, was given initially to dogs and later to humans by Scherbel et al. [133] in an uncontrolled study which claimed to provide benefit over periods of up to 2 years. There was no significant hemopoietic depression and follow-up radiographs showed no evidence of injury to cartilage or bone, but nausea and vomiting were frequent. Extra-articular administration caused crusted induration which disappeared over months. Studies on the synovial membrane of one patient before and 1 month after treatment were said to show "alterations . . . resulting in eventual regeneration," although documented support for this contention was slim.

Thiotepa, a related alkylating agent, failed to show significant benefit in a saline placebo–controlled trial of intra-articular therapy in RA but caused local pain on a number of ocassions [134]. In a further study comparing thiotepa with methylprednisolone and procaine, Gristina et al. [135] showed slight superiority of thiotepa but considered its use unwarranted given the potential for adverse effects. Their histological studies did not support the idea that thiotepa achieves medical synovectomy.

Methotrexate given by intra-articular injection to patients with various arthropathies gave sufficient benefit to convince Hall et al. [136] to undertake a controlled double-blind trial comparing 2.5 and 10.0 mg methotrexate with saline following joint lavage at arthroscopy. Clinical improvement was equal in the methotrexate and saline groups, although, judging by synovial fluid cell count, there was some short-term advantage of methotrexate over saline in patients with psoriatic arthritis. No toxicity was recorded. The authors were aware of the strong confounding influence of joint lavage on their assessment. In a group of RA patients resistent to other forms of intra-articular therapy, Marks et al. [137] failed to show any advantage of intra-articular methotrexate 5 mg with hydrocortisone 50 mg over hydrocortisone alone. In an abstract, Tiliakos et al. [138] reported significantly more benefit from intra-articular methotrexate 0.035 mg/kg with dexamethasone and lidocaine than the steroid and local anesthetic alone. It is difficult to interpret the results of Franchi et al. [139], who claimed to show support for the benefit of intra-articular methotrexate on the basis of a study of five patients given only 0.05–0.1 mg methotrexate with 8 mg orgotein in courses of 3 to 5 weekly injections.

Rifamicin, from which the commonly used antituberculous drug rifampicin is derived, was first used by Caruso et al. [140] because the drug had inhibited the uptake of labeled precursors of RNA and DNA by inflammatory cells and hyperplastic lining cells without evidence of cell necrosis in an animal model. In 34 of 35 RA patients treated with 500 mg rifamicin SV by daily intra-articular injection for variable periods, joint effusions completely resolved. In a subsequent double-blind study on 30 patients with RA knee synovitis comparing rifamicin SV 500 mg weekly with saline over periods up to 12 weeks, the same group [141] reported "impressive clinical improvement" in the antibiotic-treated group and attributed this to a possible antimitotic effect. After a follow-up of 5 years, only one patient had experienced relapse of effusion.

These results prompted another Italian group [142] to compare rifamicin SV 250 mg weekly (up to a maximum of 10 injections) with triamcinolone acetonide 40 mg given on one ocassion only, in 87 patients with knee effusion due to RA. Unfortunately, rifamicin did not prove to be a serious contender as a new form of local therapy: it was significantly less effective but more expensive than triamcinolone and was uniformly responsible for an acute local reaction with pain and swelling that subsided over 2–4 days but became worse with each successive injection.

Sodium morrhuate (Varicocid) [34,36] and bufexamac [31] were discussed in the section on corticosteroids.

D. Summary

In a recent review of nonsurgical synovectomy, Cruz-Esteban and Wilke [143] make the point that these agents are yet to show that they really modify the pathological synovium in a way which allows regeneration of normal synovium. They consider chemical synoviorthesis comparable to corticosteroid injection in providing only short-term relief and believe that the potential of osmic acid and alkylating agents to cause adverse effects remains of concern. They concede that some of these agents may benefit subsets of patients, but as yet those subsets are undefined. The Europeans [113], on the other hand, see chemical or radioactive synoviorthesis as a satisfactory alternative or preliminary step to surgery, with osmic acid being preferable to radiation synovectomy, particularly in the young.

V. RADIATION SYNOVECTOMY

Ansell, Crook, Mallard, and Bywaters may not have been the first to use radiolabeled colloids to treat arthritis [145], but their report [144] on the injection of colloidal Au-198 to treat persistent knee effusions by radiation-inducted destruction of the superficial layers of the synovial membrane, initiated the widespread adoption of this new form of local treatment, at least outside the United States.

Menkes, with the group at the Hôpital Cochin, Paris, France, has treated >20,000 joints with radioisotopes [121], and in their recent survey of radiation synovectomy in Europe over the period 1991–1993, Clunie and Ell [146] reported on 13,450 joint injections in 8578 patients.

Radiation synovectomy has proved attractive, because it is generally effective [145], has a low incidence of obvious adverse effects [113], and is said to be as effective as surgical synovectomy over a 2-year follow-up [147] without the risks of general anesthetic or the cost, pain, and rehabilitation of surgery. As in the case of chemical synovectomy, the important issues are whether radioisotopes really modify inflamed synovium without affecting cartilage, whether this procedure is as safe as we think, and, most cogently, whether radiation synovectomy is really any better than the optimal use of corticosteroids.

A. Radiation Synovectomy Agents: Requirements, Characteristics, Formulations

Material injected to achieve radiation synovectomy consists of a radioisotope attached to a carrier particle which retains the radioisotope within the joint and promotes synovial irradiation following its phagocytosis by synoviocytes. The ideal agent requires the radioisotope, the carrier, and the link between them to have certain characteristics, which has been clearly ennunciated by Deutsch et al. [145]:

The radionuclide should emit sufficient β energy to penetrate and ablate inflamed synovial tissue without damaging cartilage or overlying skin.

The carrier should be small enough to allow synoviocyte phagocytosis but large enough to minimize leakage from the synovial cavity; 2–5 μm is considered ideal.

Binding between the carrier and the isotope must be irreversible throughout the course of radiotherapy, a period determined by the half-life of the isotope; thereafter, the carrier should be degraded in a way which releases the radionuclide in a chemical form that allows rapid elimination from the body.

1. *Radioisotopes*

It is clear that a number of clinical and logistic considerations influence the choice of radioisotope. Large joints with relatively thick synovium, such as the knee, require an isotope with greater energy and range of penetration than a joint such as the MCP joint. The longer the half-life, the longer the joint (and the patient) needs to be immobilized. The more γ emission, the more widespread the radiation, hence the requirement that the radionuclide emits predominantly β energy. Some suitable isotopes, such as Y-90 and Re-188 can be generator produced, whereas Dy-165 requires a reactor temporally close to the site of administration.

A large number of radioisotopes have been tested [145], but Clunie and Ell [146] and Menkes [121] indicate that yttrium-90, erbium-169, rhenium-186, and to a lesser extent dysprosium-165, gold -198, and phosphorus-32 remain in current use for radiation synovectomy. The characteristics of these radioisotopes [113,143,145] are shown in Table 2.

2. *Carrier Particles*

Smaller particle size results in more homogeneous spread of the radioisotope but also increased joint leakage and lymphatic spread. Most carrier particles used for radiation synovectomy are colloidal suspensions, their size varying with chemical composition. Yttrium has been complexed with citrate, silicate, ferric hydroxide, and resin colloids, whereas rhenium has been made available as a sulfur colloid and erbium as citrate colloid. Although particle size is homogeneous in some preparations, in others there is considerable variation; for example, Y-90 and Er-169 citrate preparations have as many as 60% of particles <10 nm and 10% >1000 nm [148]. Gumpel [149] compared retained knee activity and lymph node uptake following four Y-90 radiocolloid preparations and found the resin to be superior to the silicate, ferric hydroxide, or the citrate. Since the biodegradability of the resin is poor [148] with immunogenic potential and because of problems in manufacture, this formulation was withdrawn. Sledge et al. [150] addressed the problem by developing a macroaggregate of ferric hydroxide as a car-

Table 2 Characteristics of Radioisotopes in Current Use for Radiation Synovectomy

Isotope	Half-life (days)	β energy MeV	β energy (%)	γ energy κeV	γ energy (%)	Penetration range (mm) Mean	Penetration range (mm) Max
Y-90	2.7	2.28	(100)	0	0	3.6	11
P-32	14	1.71	(100)	0	0	2.6	7.9
Er-169	9.4	0.34	(45)	0	0	0.3	1
Dy-165	0.1 (2.3 h)	1.29	(83)	95	(4)	-	5.7
Au-198	2.7	0.96	(99)	411	(96)	1.2	3.6
Re-186	3.7	1.07	(74)	137	(10)	1.2	3.6

rier for Dy-165, which gave particles 1–5 μm in diameter, approximately 100 times larger than previously used colloids, although still with 1.4–2.0% of particles <0.45 μm in size. McLaren et al. [151] produced Dy-165 hydroxide macroaggregate which maintains a particle size of 2–5 μm at pH 10.5 with <0.01% of particles passing through a 0.45-μm filter. The use of these larger, homogeneous carriers of the radionuclide appears to be rewarded by comparable efficacy but better joint retention and less extra-articular leakage than traditional radiocolloids [150,152].

Some basic and animal work has been done to explore the use of liposomes as carriers in radiation synovectomy [145].

According to the survey of Clunie and Ell [146], centers around Europe continue commonly to use Er-169, Re-186, and especially Y-90 as the citrate or silicate colloid.

B. Administration and Dosage

1. Practical Considerations

Intra-articular administration of a radioactive material requires a range of precautions to protect the patient, the operator, and the environment.

Arthrocentesis is performed in the usual way with standard antiseptic measures. To minimize subsequent leakage, the synovial cavity should be punctured only once. If local anesthetic is used, the skin and subcutaneous tissue are infiltrated, the synovial cavity entered, and the joint aspirated, leaving the needle in place to inject the radionuclide. The needle is best fitted with a three-way stopcock so that it can be flushed without leakage.

It is essential that the needle is within the synovial space at the time of the radionuclide injection, since extravasation of radioactive material will cause local tissue damage. For knee injection, operators generally rely on their clinical judgment aided by aspiration of synovial fluid, but for other joints, arthrocentesis is confirmed by distribution of contrast under radiographic control.

The use of a syringe shield will minimize physician exposure to irradiation. Following injection of the radionuclide and using the other port of the three-way stopcock to prevent backflow of the radioactive material, the syringe should be flushed through. Clunie and Ell [146] found that 60% of centers coinject corticosteroid, usually triamcinolone hexacetonide, and this and/or 1% lignocaine can be used to flush the needle.

Following injection, the joint should be immobilized, preferably in a bandaged splint, and the patient hospitalized, with the duration being determined by the half-life of the injected material [152,153].

At the conclusion of the procedure, all materials potentially contaminated with radioactivity should be disposed of according to approved methods.

2. Choice of Radiopharmaceutical

Selection of a particular radiopharmaceutical for a particular joint is governed by the characteristics of the radionuclide. For large joints with thick synovium, the most suitable agent will have higher energy β emission with a greater depth of penetration; for a small, superficial joint, such as those in the hand, lower energy with less penetration is required.

Clunie and Ell [146] found that yttrium-90 is commonly used for the knee and occassionally the shoulder, elbow, and ankle; rhenium-186 for the shoulder, elbow, wrist, and ankle; and erbium-169 for finger joints and occassionally the wrist. Along with others [145], they point out that this approach is rational so long as the radiopharmaceutical remains in the synovial lining and does not migrate into deeper layers of the synovium.

3. *Dosage*

Deutsch et al. [145] conclude that the rationale for choosing a particular dose of a given isotope for a given joint is "obscure," since very few studies have tried to determine the dose required to ablate inflamed synovial tissue. In 1988, van Soesbergen et al. [154] undertook a double-blind, controlled trial of 1 mCi versus 5 mCi of Au-198 in 60 knees of 46 patients with RA, but on follow-up at 12 months, both groups had improved and they were unable to show a statistically significant difference in effectiveness, with a trend favoring the higher dose. Studies with yttrium have used 3–6 mCi, generally 5 mCi, for treatment of the knee [155], and for other radioisotopes, the dose has been adjusted to provide a similar degree of radiation [150,152]. Menkes [121] admits that the appropriate radiation dose for each clinical situation is "difficult to define"; he found that, for the knee, the results following 3 or 6 mCi of yttrium did not differ significantly [113]. Based on clinical experience, the doses used at the Hôpital Cochin [121] are:

Y-90 knee		4 mCi limiting the total dose/patient to 15 mCi
Re-186 wrist		1–2 mCi
Ankle, elbow, shoulder		2 mCi
Hip		3 mCi
Er-169	PIP	0.5 mCi
	MCP	1 mCi

C. Indications and Contraindication

Indications

1. Inflammatory synovitis, particularly when localized, is the major indication

Conventional medical treatment, including long-acting local steroid, should have been found unsuccessful.

Significant articular damage should not be present. It has been possible to define clear histological characteristics which predict outcome, although Menkes [113] found failure more likely when necrosis was evident and synovial lining cell proliferation absent.

Joints treated in the European survey [146]:

- Knee 46%
- Finger joints 20%
- Wrist 11%
- Ankle 8%
- Shoulder 6%
- Elbow 5.5%

Inflammatory arthropathies treated [146]:

- Rheumatoid arthritis 71%
- Psoriatic arthritis 11.5%
- Reactive arthritis 5%
- Ankylosing spondylitis 0.6%
- Juvenile chronic arthritis $<0.1\%$

2. Other conditions:
Osteoarthritis [146,152,156,157] where recurrent effusion is prominent
Chronic pyrophosphate arthropathy [158]
Pigmented villonodular synovitis [159,160]
Hemophilic arthropathy [161–163]

Contraindications:

Significant mechanical joint damage, especially with instability.
Pregnancy, lactation, and women of childbearing age [121].
Young patients: clearly some physicians do not observe this precaution, since radiation synovectomy was performed on a small number of patients with JCA in the European survey [146] and in those with hemophilic arthropathy. No specific age limit has been defined, although some [164] have recommended that radiation synovectomy be avoided in those below middle age.
Septic arthritis and postinfectious synovitis would seem to be contraindications, although I am unaware of data bearing on this assumption.

D. Mechanism of Action

According to Deutsch [145], the "accepted" mechanism by which radiopharmaceuticals function "involves their rapid phagocytosis by synoviocytes which then distribute evenly over the surface of the synovium." Many years ago, Ingrand [148] showed on autoradiography after injection of Er-169 to rabbit knees that the radioactivity was concentrated in the synovium but spared the cartilage. In humans, the radioactive colloid distributed through the joint in the shape of the synovium so that a scintigram looked similar to an arthrogram.

In Finland, Isomäki and his colleagues [165] examined synovial fluid at 10 min, 30 min, 24 h, and 1 week and synovial biopsy at 3 days and 1 week after injection to the knee of 6 mCi Y-90. Within 24 h, most of the Y-90 had became bound, probably to synovial membrane, since it was no longer present in any synovial fluid protein fraction. Radioautographs of synovial biopsies showed aggregates of radioactive particles in the cytoplasm of the cells lining the synovial cavity with some activity in the subsynovial tissue, apparently in endothelial cells and macrophages. Not surprisingly, no distinct radioactivity could be seen in the synovium 1 week after injection. On electron microscopy, the cytoplasmic ultrastructure of synovial lining cells showed severe damage at 3 days, but in specimens taken after 1 week, cellular changes were considered to be sublethal, especially in the subsynovial cells. Y-90 particles accumulated in the intercellular substance, and it was assumed that penetration of the radiopharmaceutical to deeper layers of the synovium and perhaps into the lymphatic system occurs via this route.

Yates [166] performed arthroscopy and synovial biopsy 10 days before and 4 weeks after 5 mCi Y-90 silicate injections to the knee. Treatment caused a considerable increase in synovial lining layer thickness with more fibrin deposition but no appreciable changes in the deeper synovial structures and no change in mononuclear cell infiltration.

Onetti et al. [167] studied synovial biopsies from the knee of eight patients with RA before and 2–12 months after injection of 6 mCi colloidal chromic P-32. On light microscopy, there were fewer lining layer cells and reduced cellular infiltration and fibrinoid deposits. Electron microscopy showed changes of cytoplasmic disruption most marked in the type A cells. Unfortunately, there was no comment regarding synovial regeneration nor any description of changing appearances over the longer follow-up periods.

The general concept put forward by Deutsch appears to be supported by the evidence available but leaves significant gaps in our understanding of the serial effects of intra-articular radioactivity in the doses and forms commonly used.

E. Efficacy

1. Rheumatoid Arthritis

In their 1993 review, Deutsch et al. [145] did a fine job tabulating over 50 trials and studies of radiopharmaceutical treatment of rheumatoid synovitis, referencing each study and listing the types and numbers of joints injected, the isotope, vehicle, activity range, and overall response; where possible, they also showed the degree of response related to the Steinbrocker stage of disease. Although it is probably specious to average figures from so many sources, different joints, different isotopes, and follow-up periods, nonetheless, clinical benefit was judged fair to excellent in ~66%, ranging from 35 to 100%, with less benefit linked to increasing joint damage. This is a reasonably satisfactory response, but does it represent a significant gain over intra-articular steroids?

In the extensive experience of the Hôpital Cochin, Menkes [121] achieved good or very good results in 64% of RA knees between 1 and 2 years posttreatment. He also made the point [113] that response can increase over time and be maintained. In 547 patients seen 6 months after yttrium synovectomy for RA of the knee, 46% were good or very good; at 1- to 2-year follow-up, 64% were judged to be good or very good. In 21 patients followed for 5 years without other modification in their treatment, excellent results were maintained in 38%. In general, however, long-term follow-up [168,191] has shown the failure rate of radiation synovectomy, like surgical synovectomy, increases with time.

Even passing acquaintance with modern clinical epidemiology engenders deep suspicion of composite results from trials with relatively small patient numbers and variable endpoint measures. In the attempt to increase statistical power and resolve this uncertainty, Jones [155] undertook a meta-analysis on results from eight trials reported in the English literature to determine whether yttrium synovectomy of the knee is superior to placebo, triamcinolone, or chemical or surgical synovectomy. Yttrium was shown to be superior to placebo, with an odds ratio of 2.4 but not to either triamcinolone or other modalities.

The issue of the benefit of radiation synovectomy over steroid alone is especially important, because in so many of the positive reports [113,156], patients receiving a radiopharmaceutical also enjoy the benefits of coinjection of steroid followed by a period of bedrest. In a trial published as an abstract, Yates et al. [169] compared radioactive and nonradioactive yttrium and failed to show either clinical or arthroscopic benefit of one over the other. In the early 1980s, the British Arthritis and Rheumatism Council tried to undertake a well-designed multicenter controlled trial of yttrium-90 alone against triamcinolone hexacetonide alone [170]. Unfortunately, the trial had to be discontinued because of recruitment difficulties and the result was inconclusive. From 20 matched pairs of patients on whom results could be analyzed, the results failed to support the notion that yttrium-90 is superior to the steroid.

When dysprosium-165, with its very short half-life of 2.3 h, was shown to be a useful agent for radiation synovectomy [150] and to be as effective and as safe as yttrium-90 [152], it seemed feasible to take advantage of the short postinjection immobilization during day-only admission and to attempt a further comparative trial. Unfortunately, the Australian manufacturer decided that such a short half-life jeopardized commercial viability and discontinued supply of Dy-165.

Finger joints treated with erbium-169 were shown by Menkes et al. [171] to have done very much better than those injected with steroid alone, but Gumpel et al. [172] could show no advantage of the radioactive preparation, and Ruotsi and his colleagues [173] report significant benefit at 1, 3, and 6 months of triamcinolone hexacetonide over Er-169.

Chemical synovectomy is not clearly inferior to radioactive synovectomy [118,119,155,174], although different trials have marginally favored one or the other.

The other important comparison for radiation synovectomy is surgical synovectomy with all its attendant problems of anesthetic risk, pain, postoperative rehabilitation, hospitalization, and cost. In a small controlled trial with 2-year follow-up, Gumpel and Roles [147] reached the conclusion that clinical results were similar, but yttrium was clearly better in terms of side effects, hospital stay, and rehabilitation. It is this report which gives particular weight to the view that radiation synovectomy should be tried first [113], especially in the elderly, when RA synovitis has proved resistent to systemic therapy and local steroid and when surgical synovectomy is being considered.

Failure to respond fully to initial radiation treatment is not a barrier to a repeat injection of either yttrium [175] or dysprosium [176], nor does it preclude subsequent successful surgical synovectomy [177].

2. Other Inflammatory Arthropathies

Given the oligoarticular pattern of spondylarthropathy, it is hardly surprising that patients with these conditions are commonly included in the published series of radiation synovectomy [113,144,156,172]. In their European survey, Clunie and Ell [146] found that about 13% of the 8578 patients treated by radiation synovectomy had psoriatic arthritis, reactive arthritis, or ankylkosing spondylitis. They went on to add that despite these numbers, there are "few, if any reports in the literature studying outcome in this particular group of patients." In numbers far too small to draw conclusions, Stucki et al. [156] had a lot of success in ankylosing spondylitis but little in psoriatic arthritis. Menkes [113] found that Y-90 synoviorthesis of the hip showed considerably better results at 1–2 years in RA patients than in those with ankylosing spondylitis. Perhaps there are real differences in different types of inflammatory arthritis and, as in the case of intra-articular corticosteroids, it is time we knew.

3. Other Conditions

It is not within the scope of this review to consider in detail the role of radiation synovectomy in noninflammatory conditions. Deutsch et al. [145] tabulate results of reported studies in patients with osteoarthritis, pigmented villonodular synovitis, and hemophilic arthritis, with high levels of success, particularly in the last. The reduced number of bleeding episodes, even long term [161], seemed to outweigh the disadvantages of radiation synovectomy in this relatively youthful age group [162,163]. It is possible that it is in some of these other conditions, PVNS [159,160], CPPD [158], and hemophilia [161–163] that radiation synovectomy has a role which cannot be as well served by intra-articular steroid.

F. Adverse Effects

Quite reasonably, the administration of a radioactive material to the joint has generated intense concern about possible adverse effects, both overt and, more particularly, covert. The former seem remarkably uncommon.

1. Postinjection Flare

Increased joint discomfort and effusion may occur [150,167] but are uncommon if steroid is injected with the radiopharmaceutical.

2. Local Radiation Damage

If injected radioactive material leaks back along the needle track, it can cause a radiation burn. Attempts to minimize this possibility include flushing the needle with steroid and/or local anesthetic following the radiopharmaceutical, maintaining firm pressure over the injection site, and some even move the skin over the underlying tissue before injection to create an indirect track following needle removal, the so-called Z technique. Perhaps because of precautions taken, radiation burns are uncommon [150,152,156,158,162]. Menkes reports just two cases of skin necrosis with Y-90 and osmic acid [113]; following finger joint injection, Ruotsi [173] noted a bullous eruption in two patients and erythema in another; Onetti [167] sometimes found melanotic pigmentation following P-32 synovectomy and, more worrying, had three cases of radiation osteonecrosis which went on to spontaneous healing.

3. Septic Arthritis

As expected from experience with intra-articular corticosteroid injection, septic arthritis following radiation synovectomy is very rare. Menkes [113] reports three cases in his experience of 9000 joints injected with radioisotopes. Gumpel [178], the rheumatologist in the United Kingdom with most experience of this form of therapy, has reported a single case of *Listeria monocytogenes* septic arthritis following a Y-90 injection to the knee of a patient who, on the day after injection, visited a farm and rested on a manure heap!

4. Leakage of Radioactivity

It is well recognised that radiopharmaceuticals can leak from the joint into lymphatics [149,153,179,180]. The important questions are the levels of radiation delivered to organs and tissues outside the joint, the biological significance of this level of irradiation, and the extent to which leakage can be reduced by modifications of the isotope, the carrier, and the method of therapy delivery.

Direct measurement of leakage, by calculation of retained knee activity or uptake in the regional lymph nodes and liver, is more difficult when the pure β emitters, P-32 or Y-90 are used, since these allow only bremsstrahlung imaging, a technique subject to some degree of error. Gold-198, R-186, and Dy-165, with both β and γ emission, can be scanned more directly.

In the 1970s, Gumpel et al. [180] showed that following injection of Y-90 colloid resin to the knee, retention after 5 days varied from 52 to 91% (averaging 78%). In all but one patient, lymph node activity was $<5\%$ of the injected dose. By way of comparison, he quoted some of the earlier studies in which almost 40% of patients showed $>10\%$ of the injected dose of Au-198 in the regional lymph nodes. It was soon appreciated that immobilization of the joint following injection increased the retention of activity. A direct relationship could be demonstrated between early mobilization and percentage Y-90 retention, on the one hand [180], and increased chromosome damage on the other [181]. Gumpel and his colleagues went on to show that strict bedrest is not necessary if the knee is immobilized in a rigid splint [182,183]. Coinjection of corticosteroid was reported by Goode and Howey to prevent leakage of radioactive gold to the lymph nodes [184], but Jaworski et al. [153] could find no effect, in addition to strict immobilization, of coinjected steroid on either retained joint activity or leakage to regional lymph nodes. They found that these measurements were influenced by underlying pathology in that retained radioactivity was reduced and lymph node and liver uptake increased after injection of more inflamed joints, at least as judged by radionuclide blood pool scan. They considered that it is this group for whom strict postinjection joint rest is particularly necessary.

This work is important because it has resulted in a careful, widely adopted protocol which, in recent studies, generally provides acceptable levels of retained activity and infrequent regional lymph node uptake. Will et al. [157] showed only minimal lymph node activity from 1 of 37 injected joints; Stucki et al. [156] detected no leakage of Y-90 over the groin, the aortic lymph nodes, or the liver; and Sledge [150], using Dy-165 ferric hydroxide macroaggregates, reported minimal leakage with negligible lymph node activity. In a study using both Y-90 silicate colloid and Dy-165 hydroxide macroaggregates, Edmonds et al. [152] found 90–100% retained activity following Dy-165 and 83–100% after Y-90, with lymph node uptake of 0.4–8.9% of the injected dose in 6 of 29 patients after Y-90 and 0.02–1.1% of Dy-165 in 7 of 41 patients.

Just what these degrees of leakage mean in terms of clinical effect is uncertain. The fear is the potential to cause neoplasia. A measurable biological endpoint of irradiation is chromosome damage.

5. Chromosome Damage

Metaphase analysis of peripheral blood lymphocytes has shown radiation-induced chromosomal aberrations such as structural rearrangements, fragments, and dicentrics to be more common after radiation synovectomy, particularly if the patient is not immobilized [164,181,185,186]. De la Chapelle et al. [181] found the control frequency of chromosomal aberrations to be 0.47%; following Y-90 knee synovectomy, chromosomal abnormalities were found in 1.67% of lymphocytes from patients immobilized for 3 days after injection but rose to 2.99% in patients mobilized early. Even so, the frequency of damage in this study was considerably less than that reported by Stevenson et al. [164], who initially found that 8.5% of cells showed abnormalities after intra-articular radioactive gold. In a later study which included patients who had also received both Y-90 and Au-198, the frequency of dicentrics rose from 0.07% to 1.77% after treatment. Jalava and Salonius [218] studied patients after Y-90 and found damaged cells rose from 0.31 to 1.31% 1 week after injection and remained at about 1.18% during a 6- to 12-month follow-up.

De la Chapelle [181] thought that damage occurred to cells circulating through the knee region as well as in the regional lymph nodes, but subsequent opinion [185] favored the latter as the main site of irradiation.

Because metaphase analysis is such a tedious and expensive process, Prosser et al. [187] used the frequency of micronucleus formation in peripheral blood lymphocytes before and after knee radiation synovectomy with Y-90 and Dy-165 to reflect radiation-induced damage. Overall no significant increase in micronucleus frequency was observed in this group of patients, all of whom were immobilized following therapy. It was of interest that of the 42 patients, 13 showed measurable uptake of radiation in regional lymph nodes, and four of these had an increase in the frequency of micronuclei. Since the level of damage, albeit judged by a different method, was lower than that observed in studies undertaken in the 1970s, the authors drew the conclusion that current materials and methods do not result in significant leakage of radioactive material from the injection site irrespective of the choice of radiopharmaceutical. Similar conclusions have been reached by others [163]. The clinical significance of observed chromosome damage following radiation synovectomy is not clear, since there is no evidence, to date, that it translates to a cancer risk.

6. *Neoplasia*

In his brief 1992 review, Menkes [17] stated that he was unaware of an increased incidence of cancer among patients treated with radiation synovectomy. He mentioned a case of leukemia and one case of lymphoma in elderly patients but did not consider them linked explicitly to the therapy. He had previously reported [82] a patient aged 70 years, who had developed a sarcoma of the inguinal lymph nodes 2 years after Y-90 injection to both knees. Stevenson et al. [153] mention the occurrence of sarcomas after tracer doses of Au-198 were injected into the toe web space in two patients, a reticulum cell sarcoma in one patient, and an anaplastic bronchial carcinoma in another patient following knee synovectomy with Au-198. I can find no reference to the development of leukemia in patients following radiation synovectomy. In a long-term follow-up of 164 injections in 82 patients, Stucki [16], reported no local or systemic malignancy over 307 patient years. Given more than 40 years of use, together with the intense concern over this possibility, it seems likely that an increased frequency of neoplasia would now be at least suspected in units commonly performing radiation synovectomy. However, a definite answer may perhaps require a study like that of Court-Brown and Doll [189] on patients treated with radiotherapy for ankylosing spondylitis. Until that time, the strictest precautions to prevent and monitor leakage of radioactive material must continue.

G. Summary

The role of radiation synovectomy in inflammatory synovitis depends on whether it can be shown clearly to do more good than harm. To date, after many thousands of radiation synovectomies, the amount of demonstrated harm appears very little, perhaps because the procedure has always been treated with the most careful respect. It certainly appears a more benign procedure than surgical synovectomy and, in older patients, warrants consideration first. The persisting doubt is whether it is really any better than triamcinolone hexacetonide followed by an adequate period of joint rest.

REFERENCES

1. Bamji AN, et al. Clinical Practice. What do rheumatologists do? A pilot audit study. Br J Rheumatol. 1990; 29:295–298.
2. Gray RG, Gottlieb NL. Intra-articular corticosteroids. An updated assessment. Clin Orthop 1983; 177:235–263.

3. Haslock I, et al. Clinical Practice. Intra-articular and soft tissue injections: a survey of current practice. Br J Rheumatol 1995; 34:449–452.
4. Wolfe F, Pincus T. Rheumatoid Arthritis. New York: Marcel Dekker, 1994.
5. Gatter RA. Arthrocentesis technique and intrasynovial therapy. In: McCarty DJ, Coopman WJ, eds. Arthritis and Allied Conditions. 12th ed. Philadelphia: Lea & Febiger, 1993:711–720.
6. Owen DS. Aspiration and injection of joints and soft tissues. In: Kelly WN, Harris ED, Ruddy S, Sledge CB, eds. Textbook of Rheumatology. 4th ed. Philadelphia: Saunders, 1993:545–561.
7. Clarke AK. Non-surgical rehabilitation of adults with rheumatic diseases. In: Maddison PJ, Isenberg DA, Woo P, Glass DN eds. Oxford Textbook of Rheumatology. Oxford, England: Oxford University Press, 1993:1124–1135.
8. Dixon AStJ, Graber J. Local Injection Therapy in Rheumatic Diseases. Ed. Dürriglt, eds. Monograph Series 1983 No. 4. Basle, Switzerland. EULAR Publishers.
9. Lawford R, et al. Intra-articular and soft tissue steroid injections: theory versus practice. Proceed Aust Rheumatol Assoc Ann Scientific Meeting 22–24/5/94.
10. Kirwan JR, et al. The use of sequential analysis to assess patient preference for local skin anaesthesia during knee aspiration. Br J Rheumatol 1984; 23:210–213.
11. Jenkinson ML. A reason to use lignocaine-containing solutions with circumspection in arthrocentesis (letter). Br J Rheumatol 1987; 26, 6:471–472.
12. Cawley PJ, Morris IM. A study to compare the efficacy of two methods of skin preparation prior to joint injection. Br J Rheumatol 1992; 31:847–848.
13. Smith RW, et al. Methods of skin preparation prior to intra-articular injection (letter). Br J Rheumatol 1993; 32:648.
14. Phelan MJI, et al. A profile of the rheumatology nurse specialist in the United Kingdom. Br J Rheumatol 1992; 31:858–859.
15. McCarty DJ, et al. Treatment of rheumatoid joint inflammation with intrasynovial triamcinolone hexacetonide. J Rheumatol 1995; 22:1631–1635.
16. Hollander JL. Intrasynovial corticosteroid therapy. In: Hollander JL, McCarty DJ. eds. Arthritis & Allied Conditions. 8th ed. Philadelphia: Lea & Febiger, 1972:517–534.
17. Gray RG, Poppo MJ. Comment on the article by Goldenberg. Arthritis Rheum 1989; 32,11:1487.
18. Goldenberg DL. Reply. Arthritis Rheum 1989; 32,11:1487.
19. Hollander JL, et al. Hydrocortisone and cortisone injected into arthritic joints. comparative effects of and use of hydrocortisone as a local antiarthritic agent. JAMA 1951; 147:1629–1635.
20. Hollander JL. Intra-articular Hydrocortisone in the treatment of Arthritis. Ann Intern Med 1953; 39:735–746.
21. Hollander JL, et al. Intra-synovial corticosteroid therapy: a decade of use. Bull Rheum Dis 1961; 11:239–240
22. McCarty DJ. Treatment of rheumatoid joint inflammation with triamcinolone hexacetonide. Arthritis Rheum 1972; 15:157–173.
23. Gray RG, et al. Local Corticosteroid injection treatment in rheumatic disorders. Semin Arthritis Rheum 1981; 10:231–254.
24. Chandler GN, et al. Intra-articular therapy in rheumatoid arthritis. Comparison of hydrocortisone tertiary butyl acetate and hydrocortisone acetate. Lancet 1958; 2:659–661.
25. Ziff M, et al. Effects in rheumatoid arthritis of hydrocortisone and cortisone injected intra-articularly. Arch Intern Med 1952; 90:774–784.
26. Friedman DM, Moore ME. The efficacy of intraarticular steroids in osteoarthritis: a double blind study. J Rheumatol 1980; 7:850–856.
27. Dieppe PA, et al. Intra-articular steroid in osteoarthritis. Rheumatol Rehabil 1980; 19:212–217.

28. Gaffney K, et al. Intra-articular triamcinolone hexacetonide in knee osteoarthritis: factors influencing the clinical response. Ann Rheum Dis 1995; 54:379–381.
29. Withrington RH, et al. A Placebo-controlled trial of steroid injections in the treatment of supraspinatus tendonitis. Scand J Rheumatol 1985; 14:76–78.
30. Vecchio PC, et al. A double-blind trial comparing subacromial methylprednisolone and lignocaine in acute rotator cuff tendonitis. Br J Rheumatol 1993; 32:743–745.
31. Mielants H, et al. Intra-articular treatment of inflammatory arthritis: double-blind trial comparing Bufexamac with methylprednisolone acetate. Clin Rheumatol 1987; 6:55–60.
32. Luukkainen R, et al. Predictive value of synovial fluid analysis in estimating the efficacy of intra-articular corticosteroid injections in patients with rheumatoid arthritis. Ann Rheum Dis 1992; 51:874–876.
33. Blyth T, et al. Pain relief in the rheumatoid knee after steroid injection. A single-blind comparison of hydrocortisone succinate and triamcinolone acetonide or hexacetonide. Br J Rheumatol 1994; 33:461–463.
34. Menninger H, et al. Intra-articular treatment of rheumatoid Knee-joint effusion with triamcinolone hexacetonide versus sodium morrhuate. Scand J Rheumatol 1994; 23:249–254.
35. Srinivasan A, et al. The effects of joint washout and steroid injection compared with either joint washout or steroid injection alone in rheumatoid knee effusion. Br J Rheumatol 1995; 34:771–773.
36. Kastner P, Wessel G. Chemical synovectomy with varicocid in rheumatoid arthritis—further results. Scand J Rheumatol 1977; 6:28–32.
37. Chakravarty K, et al. A randomized controlled study of post-injection rest following intra-articular steroid therapy for knee synovitis. Br J Rheumatol 1994; 33:464–468.
38. Anderson B, Kaye S. Treatment of flexor tenosynovitis of the hand ('trigger finger') with corticosteroids. Arch Intern Med 1991; 151:153–156.
39. Posch JL, Marcotte DR. Carpal tunnel syndrome: an analysis of 1201 cases. Orthop Rev 1976; 5:25–35.
40. Schuchmann JA, et al. Evaluation of local steroid injection for carpal tunnel syndrome. Arch Phys Med Rehab 1971; 51:253–255.
41. Kay NRM. A safe, reliable method of carpal tunnel injection. J Hand Surg 1992; 17A:1160–1161.
42. Linskey ME, Segal R. Median nerve injury from local steroid injection in carpal tunnel syndrome. Neurosurgery 1990; 26:512–515.
43. Allen RC, et al. Intraarticular triamcinolone hexacetonide in the management of chronic arthritis in children. Arthritis Rheum 1986; 29:997–1001.
44. Earley A, et al. Triamcinolone into the knee joint in juvenile chronic arthritis. Clin Exp Rheumatol 1988; 6:153–155.
45. Balogh Z, Ruzsonyi E. Triamcinolone hexacetonide versus betamethasone. Scand J Rheumatol 1988; 67(Suppl):80–82.
46. Hertzberger-ten Cate R, et al. Intra-articular steroids in pauciarticular juvenile chronic arthritis, type 1. Eur J Pediatr 1991; 150:170–172.
47. Hertzberger-ten Cate R, et al. Septa within the suprapatellar region blocking intra-articular steroids in pauciarticular juvenile chronic arthritis. Clin Exp Rheumatol 1992; 10:93–94.
48. McCullough CJ, et al. Surgical management of the hip in juvenile chronic arthritis. Br J Rheumatol 1994; 33:178–183.
49. Job-Deslandre C, Menkes CJ. Complications of intra-articular injections of triamcinolone hexacetonide in chronic arthritis in children. Clin Exp Rheumatol 1990; 8:413–416.
50. Petty R. The treatment of juvenile rheumatoid arthritis. In: McCarty DI, Coopman WJ, eds. Arthritis and Allied Conditions. 12th ed. Philadelphia: Lea & Febiger, 1993:1039–1050.

51. Haslock I. Ankylosing spondylitis: management. In: Klippel JH, Dieppe PA, eds. Rheumatology. St. Louis: Mosby, 1994:3.29.1–10.
52. Wollheim FA. Ankylosing spondylitis. In: Kelly WN, Harris ED, Ruddy S, Sledge CB, eds. Textbook of Rheumatology. 4th ed. Philadelphia: Saunders, 1993:943–960.
53. Bennett RM. Psoriatic arthritis. In: McCarty DJ, Coopman WJ, eds. Arthritis and Allied Conditions. 12th ed. Philadelphia: Lea & Febiger, 1993:1079–1094.
54. Michet CJ. Psoriatic arthritis. In: Kelly WN, Harris ED, Ruddy S, Sledge CB, eds. Textbook of Rheumatology. 4th ed. Philadelphia: Saunders, 1993:974–984.
55. Espinoza LR, Cuellar ML. Psoriatic arthritis: management. In: Klippel JH, Dieppe PA, eds. Rheumatology. St. Louis: Mosby, 1994:3.3.1–6.
56. Cush J, Lipsky PE. Reiter's syndome in reactive arthritis. In: McCarty DJ, Coopman WJ, eds. Arthritis and Allied Conditions. 12th ed. Philadelphia: Lea & Febiger, 1993:1061–1078.
57. Peng Thim Fan, Yu DTY. Reiter's syndrome. In: Kelly WN, Harris ED, Ruddy S, Sledge CB, eds. Textbook of Rheumatology. 4th ed. Philadelphia: Saunders, 1993:961–973.
58. Toivanen A. Reactive arthritis. In: Klippel JH, Dieppe PA, eds. Rheumatology. St. Louis: Mosby, 1994:4.9.1–8.
59. Dorwart BB. Improved function of puffy hands in mixed connective tissue disease after palmar flexor tendon sheath injection. Arthritis Rheum 1982; 25:S79.
60. Goulding NJ, Guyre PM. Glucocorticoids, lipocortins and the immune response. Current Opin Immunol 1993; 5:108–113.
61. Firestein GS, et al. Gene Expression (collagenase, tissue inhibitor of metalloproteinases, complement, and HLA-DR) in rheumatoid arthritis and osteoarthritis synovium. Arthritis Rheum 1991; 34:1094–1105.
62. Gumpel JM. Intra-articular therapy. In: Scott JE, ed. Copeman's Textbook of the Rheumatic Diseases. 6th ed. Edinburgh: Churchill Livingstone, 1986:584–591.
63. Shupak R, et al. Intraarticular methylpresnisolone therapy in hemophilic arthropathy. Am J Hematol 1988; 17:26–29.
64. York J. Hemophilia. In: Klippel JH, Dieppe PA, eds. Rheumatology. St. Louis: Mosby, 1994:7.21.1-4.
65. Barnsley L, et al. Lack of effect of intraarticular corticosteroids for chronic pain in the cervical zygapophyseal joints. N Engl J Med 1994; 330:1047–1050.
66. Carette, et al. Controlled trial of corticosteroid injections into facet joints for chronic low back pain. N Engl J Med 1991; 325:1002–1007.
67. Derendorf H, et al. Pharmacokinetics and pharmacodynamics of glucocorticoid suspensions after intra-articular administration. Clin Pharmacol Ther 1986; 39:313–317
68. Bird HA, et al. A Thermographic and clinical comparison of three intra-articular steroid preparations in rheumatoid arthritis. Ann Rheum Dis 1979; 38:36–39.
69. Dingle JT, et al. Novel treatment for joint inflammation. Nature 1978; 271:372.
70. de Silva M, et al. Liposomes in arthritis: a new approach. Lancet 1979; 1:1320–1322.
71. Bird HA. Intra-articular and intralesional therapy. In: Klippel HJ, Dieppe PA, eds. Rheumatology. St. Louis: Mosby, 1994; 16:1–6.
72. Chandler GN, et al. Charcot's arthropathy following intra-articular hydrocortisone. Br Med J 1959; 1:952–953.
73. Chandler GN, Wright V. Deleterious effect of intra-articular hydrocortisone. Lancet, 1958; 2:661–663.
74. Barraclough D. The use of corticosteroid agents in connective tissue disorders. Med J Aust 1986; 144:427–432.
75. Balch HW, et al. Repeated corticosteroid injections into knee joints. Rheumatol Rehabil 1977; 15:137–140.
76. Hume Kendall P. Untoward effects following local hydrocortisone injection. Ann Phys Med 1957; 8:170–175.

77. Fitzgerald RH. Intrasynovial injection of steroids. Uses and abuses. Mayo Clin Proc 1976; 51:655–659.
78. McCarty DJ. Joint sepsis: a chance for cure (editorial). JAMA 1982; 247:835.
79. Shore A, Rush PJ. Possible danger of intra-articular steroid injection in children with respiratory tract infections. Br J Rheumatol 1987; 26:73.
80. von Essen R, Savolainen HA. Bacterial infection following intra-articular injection. Scand J Rheumatol 1989; 18:7–12.
81. Seradge H, Anderson MG. Clostridial myonecrosis following intra-articular steroid injection. Clin Orthop 1980; 147:207–209.
82. Parikh JR, et al. Charcot's arthropathy of the shoulder following intraarticular corticosteroid injections. J Rheumatol 1993; 20:885–887
83. Sparling M, et al. Radiographic followup of joints injected with triamcinolone hexacetonide for the management of childhood arthritis. Arthritis Rheum 1900; 33:821–826.
84. Mankin HJ, Conger KA. The acute effects of intra-articular hydrocortisone articular cartilage in rabbits. J Bone Joint Surg 1966: 48(A):1383–1388.
85. Mankin HJ, et al. The effect of systemic corticosteroids on rabbit articular cartilage. Arthritis Rheum 1972; 15:593–598.
86. Moskowitz RW, et al. Experimentally induced corticosteroid arthropathy. Arthritis Rheum 1970; 13:236–243.
87. Behrens F, et al. Alteration of rabbit articular cartilage by intra-articular injections of glucocorticoids. J Bone Joint Surg 1975; 57(A):70–76.
88. Tenenbaum J, et al. The effects of intraarticular corticosteroids on articular cartilage. Semin Arthritis Rheum 1981; 11(Supp 1):140–141.
89. Gibson T, et al. Effect of intra-articular corticosteroid injections on primate cartilage. Ann Rheum Dis 1976; 36:74–79.
90. Williams JM, Brandt KD. Triamcinolone hexacetonide protects against fibrillation and oseophyte formation following chemically induced articular cartilage damage. Arthritis Rheum 1985: 28:1267–1274.
91. Pelletier JP, Martel-Pelletier J. Protective effects of corticosteroids on cartilage lesions and osteophyte formation in the Pond-Nuki dog model of osteoarthritis. Arthritis Rheum 1989; 32:181–193
92. Wollheim FA, et al. Prevention of joint destruction in antigen-induced arthritis. Clin Immunol Immunopathol 1994; 70:19–21.
93. Reis ND, et al. Metatarsophalangeal joint dislocation after local steroid injection. J Bone Joint Surg 1989; 71(B):864.
94. McCarty DJ, et al. Intraarticular corticosteroids possibly leading to local osteonecrosis and marrow fat induced synovitis. J Rheumatol 1991; 18:1091–1094.
95. Laroche M, et al. Osteonecrosis of the femoral and humeral heads after intraarticular corticosteroid injections. J Rheumatol 1990; 17:549–551.
96. McCarty DJ, Hogan JM. Inflammatory reaction after intrasynovial injection of microcrystalline adrenocorticosteroid esters. Arthritis Rheum 1964; 7:359–367
97. Berger RG, Yount WJ. Immediate "steroid flare" from intraarticular triamcinolone hexacetonide injection: case report and review of the literature. Arthritis Rheum 33:1284–1286.
98. Gottlieb NL, Riskin WG. Complications of local corticosteroid injections. JAMA 1980; 243:1547–1548.
99. Weiss MM. Corticosteroids in rheumatoid arthritis. Semin Arthritis Rheum 1989; 19:9–21.
100. Weinstein PS, et al. Long-term follow-up of corticosteroid injection for traumatic olecranon bursitis. Ann Rheum Dis 1984; 43:44–46
101. Ward LE, Mason HL. Systemic effects from hydrocortisone acetate administered intraarticularly to rheumatoid patients. J Lab Clin Med 1953; 42:961–962.

102. Shuster S, Williams IA. Adrenal suppression due to intra-articular corticosteroid therapy. Lancet 1961; 2:171–172.
103. Koehler BE, et al. The systemic effects of intra-articular corticosteroid. J Rheumatol 1974; 1:117–125.
104. Armstrong RD, et al. Serum methylprednisolone levels following intra-articular injection of methylprednisolone acetate. Ann Rheum Dis 1981; 40:571–574.
105. Cunningham GR, et al. The mechanism of ovulation inhibition by triamcinolone acetonide. J Clin Endocrinol Metab 1978; 46:8–14.
106. O'Sullivan MM, et al. Cushing's syndrome with suppression of the hypothalamic-pituitary-adrenal axis after intra-articular steroid injections. Ann Rheum Dis 1985; 44:561–563.
107. Pattrick M, Doherty M. Facial flushing after intra-articular injection of steroid. Br Med J 1987; 295:1380.
108. Larsson LG. Anaphylactic shock after i.a. administration of triamcinolone acetonide in a 35-year-old female. Scand J Rheumatol 1989; 18:441–442.
109. Ijsselmuiden OE, et al. Cutaneous adverse reactions after intra-articular injection of triamcinolone acetonide. Acta Derm Venereol 1995; 75:57–58.
110. Patterson DL, et al. Anaphylaxis induced by carboxymethylcellulose component of injectable triamcinolone acetonide suspension (Kenalog). Ann Allergy Asthma Immunol 1995; 74:163–166.
111. Gladman DD, Bombardier C. Sickle cell crisis following intraarticular steroid therapy for rheumatoid arthritis. Arthritis Rheum 1987; 30:1065–1068.
112. Østergaard M, et al. Effect of intraarticular osmic acid on synovial membrane volume and inflammation, determined by magnetic resonance imaging. Scand J Rheumatol 1995; 24:5–12.
113. Menkes CJ. Is there a place for chemical and radiation synovectomy in rheumatic diseases? Rheumatol Rehab 1979; 18:65–77.
114. von Reis G, Swennson A. Intra-articular injections of osmic acid in painful joint affections. Acta Med Scand 1952; S259:27–32.
115. Anttinen J, Oka M. Intra-articular triamcinolone hexacetonide and osmic acid in persistent synovitis of the knee. Scand J Rheumatol. 1975; 4:125–128.
116. Nissilä M, et al. Osmic acid in rheumatoid synovitis. Scand J Rheumatol 1977; 6:158–160.
117. Nissilä M, et al. Osmic acid in rheumatoid synovitis. Scand J Rheumatol 1977; 6:111–112
118. Sheppeard H, et al. Osmic acid versus yttrium-90 in rheumatoid synovitis of the knee. Scand J Rheumatol 1981; 10:234–236
119. Nissilä M, et al. Comparison of chemical, radiation and surgical synovectomy for knee joint synovitis. Scand J Rheumatol 1978; 7:225–228.
120. Sheppeard H, Ward DJ. Intra-articular osmic acid in rheumatoid arthritis: five years' experience. Rheumatol Rehabil 1980; 19:25–29.
121. Menkès CJ. Chemical and radiation synovectomy in rheumatic diseases. New Standards in Arthritis Care 1992; 3:8–11.
122. Mitchell N, et al. The effect of osmium tetroxide and nitrogen mustard on normal articular cartilage. J Bone Joint Surg 1973; 55(B):814–821.
123. Niculescu D. Ultra structural changes in cartilage after intra-articular administration of osmium tetroxide and the sodium salts of fish oil fatty acids. Scand J Rheumatol 1976; 5:133–140.
124. Nissilä M. Absence of increased frequency of degenerative joint changes after osmic acid injections. Scand J Rheumatol 1978; 7:81–84.
125. Lagier R, et al. Synovial deposit of osmic acid after intra-articular injection. Virchows Arch A Pathol Anat a Histol 1976; 372:237–244.
126. Järvinen P, et al. Intraarticular osmic acid in postinfectious arthritis persisting after treated bacterial arthritis. J Rheumatol 1990; 17:1704–1706.
127. Lunec J, et al. Free-radical oxidation (peroxidation) products in serum and synovial fluid in rheumatoid arthritis. J Rheumatol 198; 8:233–243.

128. Goebel K, et al. Intrasynovial orgotein therapy in rheumatoid arthritis. Lancet 1981; 1:1015–1017.
129. Goebel K, et al. Effect of intra-articular orgotein versus a corticosteroid on rheumatoid arthritis of the knees. Am J Med 1983; 74:124–128.
130. McIlwain H, et al. Intra-articular orgotein in osteoarthritis of the knee: a placebo-controlled efficacy, safety and dosage comparison. Am J Med 189; 87:295–300.
131. Mazieres B, et al. A French controlled multicenter study of inraarticular orgotein versus intraarticular corticosteroids in the treatment of knee osteoarthritis: a one-year followup. J Rheumatol 1991; 18:134–137.
132. Rylance HJ, Chalmers TM. Clinical trials of intra-articular aspirin in rheumatoid arthritis. Lancet 1980; 2:1099–1102.
133. Scherbel AL, Schuchter SL. II. Intraarticular administration of nitrogen mustard alone and combined with a corticosteroid for rheumatoid arthritis. Cleveland Clin Q 1957; 24:78–89.
134. Zuckner J, et al. Intraarticular administration of the alkylating agent, thio-tepa, in rheumatoid arthritis. Arthritis Rheum 1964; 7:355.
135. Gristina AG, et al. Intra-articular thio-tepa compared with depo-medrol and procaine in the treatment of arthritis. J Bone Joint Surg 1970; 52-A:1603–1610.
136. Hall GH, et al. Intra-articular methotrexate. Clinical and laboratory study in rheumatoid and psoriatic arthritis. Ann Rheum Dis 1978; 37:351–356.
137. Marks JS, et al. Intra-articular methotrexate in rheumatoid arthritis. Lancet 1976; 2:857–858.
138. Tiliakos NA, et al. Intra-articular methotrexate in intractable rheumatoid knees. Arthritis Rheum 1982; 25:S65.
139. Franchi F, et al. Intraarticular methotrexate in the therapy of rheumatoid arthritis. Rec Prog Med 1989; 80:261–262.
140. Caruso I, et al. Rheumatoid knee synovitis successfully treated with intraarticular rifamicin SV. Arthritis Rheum 1980; 23:518–519.
141. Caruso I, et al. Rheumatoid knee synovitis successfully treated with intra-articular rifamycin SV. Ann Rheum Dis 1982; 41:232–236.
142. Marchesoni A, et al. Rifamycin SV versus triamcinolone in local treatment of rheumatoid synovitis. Scand J Rheumatolatol 1993; 22:194–198.
143. Cruz-Esteban C, Wilke WS. Non-surgical synovectomy. Baillières Clin Rheumatol 1995; 9:787–801.
144. Ansell BA, et al. Evaluation of intra-articular colloidal Gold Au 198 in the treatment of persistent knee effusions. Ann Rheum Dis 1963; 22:435–439.
145. Deutsch E, et al. Radiation synovectomy revisited. Eur J Nucl Med 1993; 20:1113–1127.
146. Clunie G, Ell PJ. A survey of radiation synovectomy in Europe, 1991–1993. Eur J Nucl Med 1995; 22:970–976.
147. Gumpel JM, Roles NC. A controlled trial of intra-articular radiocolloids versus surgical synovectomy in persistent synovitis. Lancet 1975; 1:488–489.
148. Ingrand J. Characteristics of radio-isotopes for intra-articular therapy. Ann Rheum Dis 1973; 32:S3–S9.
149. Gumpel JM, et al. Yttrium-90 in persistent synovitis of the knee—a single centre comparison. The retention and extra-articular spread of four ^{90}Y radiocolloids. Br J Radiol 1975; 48:377–381.
150. Sledge CB, et al. Treatment of rheumatoid synovitis of the knee with intraarticular injection of dysprosium 165-ferric hydroxide macroaggregates. Arthritis Rheum 1986; 29:153–159.
151. McLaren AB, et al. The development of Dysprosium-165 hydroxide macroaggregates for radiation synovectomy. ANSTO E Report 1988; 673:1–21.
152. Edmonds J, et al. A comparative study of the safety and efficacy of dysprosium-165 hy-

droxide macro-Aggregate and yttrium-90 silicate colloid in radiation synovectomy—a multicentre double blind clinical trial. Br J Rheumatol 1994:33:947–953.
153. Jaworski R, et al. Re-evaluating the need for hospitalization following synovectomy using yttrium-90 silicate. Br J Rheumatol 1993; 32:1012–1017.
154. Van Soesbergen RM, et al. Radiosynoviorthesis of the knee: a doubleblind trial of 1 versus 5 mCi Gold-198. Clin Rheumatol 1988; 7:224–230.
155. Jones G. Yttrium synovectomy: a meta-analysis of the literature. Aust NZ J Med 1993; 23:272–275.
156. Stucki G, et al. Efficacy and safety of radiation synovectomy with yttrium-90: a retrospective long-term analysis of 164 applications in 82 patients. Br J Rheumatol 1993; 32:383–386.
157. Will R, et al. Comparison of two yttrium-90 regimens in inflammatory and osteoarthropathies. Ann Rheum Dis 1992; 51:262–265.
158. Doherty M, Dieppe PA. Effect of intra-articular yttrium-90 on chronic pyrophosphate arthropathy of the knee. Lancet 1981; 2:1243–1246.
159. Franssen MJAM, et al. Treatment of pigmented villonodular synovitis of the knee with yttrium-90 silicate: prospective evaluations by arthroscopy, histology and ^{99m}Tc pertechnetate uptake measurements. Ann Rheum Dis 1989; 48:1007–1013.
160. O'Sullivan MM, et al. Yttrium 90 synovectomy—a new treatment for pigmented villonodular synovitis. Br J Rheumatol 1987; 26,1:71–72.
161. Van Kasteren MEE, et al. Long term follow up of radiosynovectomy with yttrium-90 silicate in haemophilic haemarthrosis. Ann Rheum Dis 1993; 52:548–550
162. Dawson TM, et al. Yttrium synovectomy in haemophilic arthropathy. Br J Rheumatol 1994; 33:351–356.
163. Rivard G, et al. Synoviorthesis with colloidal ^{32}P chromic phosphate for hemophilic arthropathy: clinical follow-up. Arch Phys Med Rehabil 1985; 66:753–755.
164. Stevenson AC, et al. Chromosome damage in patients who have had intra-articular injections of radioactive gold. Lancet 1971; 1:837–839.
165. Isomäki AM, et al. Uptake of ^{90}Y resin colloid by synovial fluid cells and synovial membrane in rheumatoid arthritis. Scand J Rheumatol 1972; 1:53–60.
166. Yates DB. Arthroscopy of the knee after the Injection of ^{90}Y. Ann Rheum Dis 1973; 32:S48–S49.
167. Onetti CM, et al. Synoviorthesis with ^{32}P-colloidal chromic phosphate in rheumatoid arthritis—clinical, histopathologic and arthrographic changes. J Rheumatol 1982; 9:229–238.
168. Szanto E. Long-term follow-up of ^{90}yttrium-treated knee-joint arthritis. Scand J Rheumatol 1977; 6:209–212.
169. Yates DB, et al. Double-blind trial of yttrium-90 for chronic inflammatory synovitis of the knee. Ann Rheum Dis 1977; 36:481.
170. ARC Multicentre Radiosynoviorthesis Trial Group. Intra-articular radioactive yttrium and triamcinolone hexacetonide: an inconclusive trial. Ann Rheum Dis 1984; 43:620–623.
171. Menkes CJ, et al. Double-blind study of erbium 169 injection (synoviorthesis) in rheumatoid digital joints. Ann Rheum Dis 1977; 36:254–256.
172. Gumpel JM, et al. Synoviorthesis with erbium-169: a double-blind controlled comparison of erbium-169 with corticosteroid. Ann Rheum Dis 1979; 38:341–343
173. Ruotsi A, et al. Erbium-169 versus triamcinolone hexacetonide in the treatment of rheumatoid finger joints. Ann Rheum Dis 1979; 38:45–47.
174. Sheppeard H, et al. Osmic acid versus yttrium-90 in rheumatoid synovitis of the knees. Scand J Rheumatolatol. 1981; 10:234–236.
175. Winfield J, Gumpel JM. An evaluation of repeat intra-articular injections of yttrium-90 colloids in persistent synovitis of the knee. Ann Rheum Dis 1979; 38:145–147.
176. Vella M, et al. Repeat radiation synovectomy with dysprosium 165-ferric hydroxide macroaggregates in rheumatoid knees unresponsive to initial injection. Arthritis Rheum 1988; 31:789–792.

177. Combe B, et al. Treatment of chronic knee synovitis with arthroscopic synovectomy after failure of intraarticular injection of radionuclide. Arthritis Rheum 1989; 32:10–14.
178. Wilson APR, et al. Listeria monocytogenes septic arthritis following intra-articular yttrium-90 therapy. Ann Rheum Dis 1984; 43:518–519.
179. Williams ED, et al. Distribution of yttrium 90 ferric hydoxide colloid and gold 198 colloid after injection into knee. Ann Rheum Dis 1976; 35:516–520.
180. Gumpel JM, et al. Use of yttrium 90 in persistent synovitis of the knee. 1. Retention in the knee and spread in the body after injection. Ann Rheum Dis 1973; 32:223–227.
181. de la Chapelle A, et al. Chromosome damage after intra-articular injections of radioactive yttrium. Effect of immobilisation on the biological dose. Ann Rheum Dis 1972; 31:508–512.
182. Winfield J, et al. Evaluation of two regimens to immobilise the knee after injections of yttrium-90. Br Med J 1979; 1:986–987.
183. Williams PL, et al. Feasibility of outpatient management after intra-articular yttrium-90: comparison of two regimens. Br Med J 1981; 282:13–14.
184. Goode JD, Howey S. Effect of premedication with intra-articular hydrocortisone on the retention of ^{198}Au in the knee joint in rheumatoid arthritis. Ann Rheum Dis 1973; 32(Suppl):43–45.
185. Stevenson AC, et al. Cytogenetic and scanning study of patients receiving intra-articular injections of gold-198 and yttrium-90. Ann Rheum Dis 1973; 32:112–123.
186. Jalava S, Salonius A-L. Chromosomes of patients treated with yttrium-90. Lancet 1974; 1:807.
187. Prosser JS, et al. Induction of micronuclei in peripheral blood lymphocytes of patients treated for rheumatoid or osteo-arthritis of the knee with dysprosium-165 hydroxide macroaggregates or yttrium-90 silicate. Cytobios 1993; 73:7–15.
188. Bentley G, Goodfellow JW. Disorganisation of the knees following intra-articular hydrocortisone injections. J Bone Joint Surg 1969; 51-B:498–502.
189. Court-Brown WM, Doll R. Mortality from cancer and other causes after radiotherapy for ankylosing spondylitis. Br Med J 1965; 2:1327–1332.
190. Bertouch JV, et al. A comparison of plasma methylprednisolone concentrations following intra-articular injection in patients with rheumatoid arthritis and osteoarthritis. Aust NZ J Med 1983; 13:583–586.
191. Oka M, Hypén M. Radiation synovectomy. Results in rheumatoid knee effusions treated with radioactive yttrium. Scand J Rheumatol 1974; 3:33–38.
192. Ching DWT, Petrie. Injection therapy of superficial rheumatoid nodules. Br J Rheumatol 1992; 31:775–777.
193. Maugars Y, et al. Corticosteroid injection of the sacroiliac joint in patients with seronegative spondylarthropathy. Arthritis Rheum 1992; 35:564–568.
194. Braum J, et al. Computed tomography guided corticosteroid injection of the sacroiliitic joint in patients with spondylarthropathy with sacroiliitis: clinical outcome and follow up by dynamic magnetic resonance imaging. J Rheumatol 1996; 23:659–664.

20
Antibiotic Treatment of Rheumatoid Arthritis

Christopher G. Jackson
University of Utah and Veterans Affairs Medical Center, Salt Lake City, Utah

1. INTRODUCTION AND HISTORY

Interest in antibiotic treatment for rheumatoid arthritis has been long-standing and recently has received renewed attention. This interest arose initially from the observation that certain infections shared clinical similarities with rheumatoid arthritis which in turn gave rise to the supposition that an infectious process might be responsible for the induction or perpetuation of chronic inflammation in a susceptible host. Adequate treatment of such an infectious process, it was reasoned, might be expected to decrease inflammation and, thereby, produce clinical improvement.

This notion led to the investigation and eventual demonstration of gold salts as effective therapy for rheumatoid arthritis. Forestier postulated that tuberculosis and rheumatoid arthritis had a common infectious origin [1] and pursued the study of gold compounds which were considered antiseptic and beneficial in the treatment of tuberculosis and other infections.

Interestingly, other treatments with known efficacy in the treatment of rheumatoid arthritis also have demonstrated antimicrobial actions. Chloroquine, for example, is an effective treatment for malarial infections and also has an attenuating effect on the virulence of some bacteria and viruses [2], whereas sulfasalazine, comprised of a salicylate (5-amino salicyclic acid) and an antibiotic (sulfapyridine) moiety, may well owe its efficacy in rheumatoid arthritis to the antibiotic portion of the compound [3]. Gold, chloroquine, and sulfasalazine are discussed in greater detail elsewhere in this textbook. The focus of this chapter will be those antibiotic compounds, known and used clinically as antimicrobials, which have also been considered and studied as treatment for rheumatoid arthritis.

II. RATIONALE

The etiology and pathogenesis of rheumatoid arthritis remains unknown, and consequently the present rationale for using antibiotics as antirheumatic treatment is empiric. As previously noted, the origins of antibiotic therapy for rheumatic conditions can be traced to clinical and laboratory observations which hint at a relationship between infection and inflammatory arthritis. More recently, consideration of such therapy has been reinforced by studies demonstrating previously unrecognized antibiotic modulation of both the immune and inflammatory responses. These observations of "nonantimicrobial" antibiotic properties suggest a direction for future investigation which may eventually define a mechanism of action and produce an understandable rationale for antibiotic treatment. Important in this investigation will be the study of antibiotics which possess diverse spectrums of antimicrobial activity but lack any nonantimicrobial effect as well as antibiotics which have known nonantimicrobial effects but have been altered so as to modify or eliminate their antimicrobial activity. For the present, the significance and relative importance of these antimicrobial and nonantimicrobial properties are unknown and speculative, but these properties do provide a format for considering potential mechanisms of antibiotic effect in the treatment of rheumatoid arthritis.

A. Antimicrobial Considerations

A causative or facilitating role for infectious agents in the development of rheumatoid arthritis in a susceptible host has long been entertained. Germane to this concept are two examples of polyarthritis, rheumatic fever and Lyme disease, which are clinically similar to rheumatoid arthritis and are known to be secondary to specific infections. Additionally, some arthritides in animals, particularly rodents, follow specific infections. These phenomena are important in contemplating possible infectious mechanisms in the etiopathogenesis of rheumatoid arthritis and in constructing a credible antimicrobial basis for using antibiotics as antirheumatic therapy.

Rheumatic fever follows pharyngeal infection by group A β-hemolytic streptococci in susceptible hosts. Susceptibility to rheumatic fever, once one of the most common causes of polyarthritis, has been shown to have a genetic predilection, as demonstrated by the disease concordance which exists between identical twins as well as by an association with HLA-DR4 in white patients and HLA-DR2 allotypes in American blacks [4]. Additionally, evidence that B-cell allotypes confer an increased risk has also been reported [5]. The streptococcus does not actually invade the joint or other affected organs, rather immunological mimcry between microbe and host seems to account for many disease manifestations, including the inflammatory arthritis [6].

Until relatively recently, Lyme disease, as is presently true of rheumatoid arthritis, was an inflammatory arthritis of unknown etiology. Following years of elegant epidemiological, microbiological, and genetic study, it is now known to occur more commonly in individuals who are HLA-DR4 or HLA-DR2 positive following infection by the spirochete *Borrelia burgdorferi* [7]. In contrast to rheumatic fever, the microbe in Lyme disease is present within the joint space and produces a septic arthritis as demonstrated by both polymerase chain reaction and positive cultures [8]. The inflammatory damage to the joint is thought to occur from a direct toxic effect [9]. If diagnosed early, Lyme disease can usually be eradicated with a short course. of oral antibiotics

[10]; however, established disease is considerably more recalcitrant requiring sustained treatment and/or parenteral administration [11,12].

The most common infectious agents in animal arthritis are the *Mycoplasma* species [13]. For example, *M. arthritidis* infection in rodents produces a chronic arthritis which is characterized by synovial infiltration with lymphocytes, plasma cells, and macrophages followed by neovascularization, pannus formation, and ultimately joint destruction [14]. Many of these features are strikingly similar to rheumatoid arthritis. Although the mycoplasmal organism has been shown to invade the joint, much of the persistent immune and inflammatory activity is presently thought to be mediated by a superantigen, mycoplasma arthritidis mitogen, which is produced by the microbe [15].

Mycoplasma species are ubiquitous in humans, with certain strains being part of the normal flora, whereas others are clearly pathogenic. For instance, *M. salivarium* and *M. orale* have been cultured from 84% of normal patients [16], whereas *M. pneumoniae*, *M. hominis*, and *Ureaplasma urealyticum* have been shown to cause human disease. Of interest is the fact that these strains have also been associated with chronic arthritis in some human hosts. *M. hominis* is reported to cause a polyarthritis in renal transplant patients, whereas *U. urealyticum* has caused a Reiter's syndrome–like inflammatory arthritis [17]. In addition, *M. pneumoniae* is associated with autoimmune activity, specifically the production of autoantibodies and rheumatoid factor [18].

In summary, several infection-associated mechanisms may contribute to the development and persistence of a polyarthritis in a susceptible host. These mechanisms include the structural and functional mimicry seen in rheumatic fever, the direct toxic effects present in Lyme disease, and the superantigen-mediated immune activity evident in *M. arthritidis* arthritis. Together these observations suggest a potential way in which an infection could contribute to the development of rheumatoid arthritis.

B. Nonantimicrobial Considerations

Recent observations have suggested a number of antibiotic actions, seemingly unrelated to antimicrobial actions, that might in and of themselves exert a beneficial effect on a chronic inflammatory polyarthropathy. Most of these observations stem from the efficacious use of tetracyclines in the treatment of periodontitis and certain dermatological conditions [19]. In a manner parallel to the initial use of antibiotics in rheumatoid arthritis, antibiotic agents were first used in these conditions on the supposition that they were secondary to recurrent or persistent bacterial infection. Nonantimicrobial actions which have been described for the tetracyclines include inhibition of protein synthesis in susceptible, rapidly dividing bacteria and in certain eukaryotic cells [20] as well as perturbation of leukocyte functions, including chemotaxis [21], phagocytosis [22], and lymphocyte proliferation [22–25]. Also described are anti-inflammatory effects [26] which are probably related to antioxidant activity [27] and blockade of phospholipase A^2 [28].

Additionally, the tetracyclines have been found to inhibit the activity of host-derived collagenases and other matrix metalloproteinases [29,30]. Of particular interest is the fact that minocycline appears to inhibit collagenase in rheumatoid synovial tissue [31]. This inhibition of collagenase activity was demonstrated in vivo by treating rheumatoid arthritis patients undergoing sequential total joint arthroplasty with oral minocycline during the interval between surgeries. Comparative study of synovial tissue obtained at the first and second surgery showed a significant reduction in collagenase activity in six of seven patients following institution of minocycline. In vitro, an inhibition of collagenolytic activity by doxycycline has been shown, with the inhibitory effect apparently being reversed by the addition of calcium or zinc [32]. As metalloproteinases depend on heavy metals to maintain their structural integrity, chelation of such ions by tetracyclines offers a possible explanation for these observations of collagenase inhibition. Interestingly, tetracyclines which have been chemically modified and thereby lack antimicrobial activity seem to retain anticollagenase effects.

Nontetracycline antibiotics have not been examined as extensively as have the tetracyclines for the presence of any nonantimicrobial properties. Ampicillin, cloxacillin, and penicillin G have been found to have comparatively little anticollagenase activity [33]. However, the flouroquinolone ciprofloxacin has been shown to inhibit the in vitro production of interleukin-1β and tumor necrosis factor α by human monocytes and appears to exert a preventative effect in vivo on the development of collagen-induced arthritis in rats [34].

These nonantimicrobial actions of antibiotics, which appear to affect both the immune and inflammatory responses, provide an alternative mechanism by which antibiotic administration could exert a beneficial effect on the course of rheumatoid arthritis. Further characterization and study of the tetracyclines, nontetracyclines, and chemically modified tetracyclines should help to define whether antibiotics exhibit an antirheumatic effect as a consequence of their antimicrobial properties, their nonantimicrobial properties, or by some yet unidentified mechanism.

III. CLINICAL EXPERIENCE

Several antibiotic compounds have been shown to attenuate or prevent the development of synovitis in animal models which simulate rheumatoid arthritis and/or to exhibit immunosuppressive and anti-inflammatory effects in vitro. These observations are important and of considerable interest; however, this section will examine only those antibiotic regimens where data from human clinical studies are available.

A. Tetracyclines

Most of the presently available clinical experience with antibiotics as antirheumatic therapy involves tetracycline and its derivative minocycline. Interest in the tetracyclines can be traced to 1948 when Dienes et al. [35] reported that pleuropneumonia-like organisms were capable of producing joint inflammation. The apparent isolation of these organisms (subsequently renamed mycoplasma's) from rheumatoid synovial fluid [36] together with the demonstration that these species appeared to inhibit the migration of leukocytes from rheumatoid arthritis patients [37] led to the hypothesis that rheumatoid arthritis might be the consequence of a persistent mycoplasmal infection. The recognition that mycoplasma-induced genitourinary tract infections were responsive to tetracyclines suggested that this class of antibiotics might also be beneficial in rheumatoid arthritis. Early reports of marked improvement in rheumatoid arthritis patients treated with long-term tetracycline, written by Brown et al. [38,39] and Sanchez et al. [40], produced a continuing interest in tetracycline therapy and led to a number of clinical trials which reached different conclusions.

In 1971, Skinner et al. [41] published the results of a double-blind controlled study in which 30 patients with rheumatoid arthritis were treated for 1 year with either tetracycline 250 mg daily or placebo. Treatment was well tolerated, as 14 of the 15 patients taking tetracycline completed the study. Efficacy measures included grip strength, ring size, morning stiffness, total tender joints, total swollen joints, walking time for 50 ft, and erythrocyte sedimentation rate. Although minor improvement in ring size and the total number of swollen joints was observed in the tetracycline-treated group, the only change of statistical significance was in the duration of morning stiffness, and that change favored the placebo group. No individual patient was observed to have a remission nor substantial improvement, which led the investigators to conclude that tetracycline therapy was not beneficial.

However, the efficacious use of tetracyclines in the treatment of a number of chronic inflammatory disease processes, specifically periodontitis and a number of dermatoses, continued to suggest that this family of antibiotics might also have a beneficial effect on inflammatory arthritides. Interest focused principally on minocycline and resulted in two open studies which both suggested minocycline efficacy in rheumatoid arthritis.

Breedveld et al. [42] treated 10 patients with a maximal minocycline daily dose of 400 mg for 16 weeks in a dose-finding study. All patients had three or more swollen joints and at least two other measures of disease activity, which were defined as a Ritchie articular index score of at least 9, morning stiffness of at least 45 min, and/or a Westergren erythrocyte sedimentation rate of at least 28 mm/h. The initial dose of minocycline was 200 mg daily, which was increased to 300 mg after 8 weeks and to 400 mg after 12 weeks depending on clinical response and adverse effects. Efficacy measures included the number of swollen joints, Ritchie articular index, duration of morning stiffness, grip strength, erythrocyte sedimentation rate, and platelet count. Vestibular side effects, primarily dizziness and vertigo, limited the dose of tetracycline in 6 of the 10 patients and required one patient to withdraw after 8 weeks of treatment. All patients showed some benefit by 4 weeks of treatment, and all efficacy measures were statistically improved compared with pretreatment levels when the study concluded after 16 weeks.

Langevitz et al. [43] treated 18 patients with rheumatoid arthritis for 48 weeks with minocycline at a daily dose of 200 mg. All patients had previously failed at least two second-line agents and had active disease as defined by the presence of six or more swollen joints and at least two other measures of disease activity, including nine or more tender joints, morning stiffness of at least 45 min, and/or a Westergren erythrocyte sedimentation rate of at least 28 mm/h. Previous second-line therapy had to have been stopped for at least 1 month prior to study entry, but stable concomitant treatment with nonsteroidal anti-inflammatory agents and prednisone (not exceeding 10 mg daily) was permitted. Six patients did not complete the study. Three of these were withdrawals for lack of efficacy, two were withdrawals for adverse effects attributed to minocycline (dizziness and leukopenia), and one patient was lost to follow-up. Statistically significant improvement in patient and physician global assessment, grip strength, and erythrocyte sedimentation rate was seen in those completing the study. Three of the 12 patients who completed the study were judged to have had a complete remission, whereas the remaining 9 had either substantial (3 patients) or moderate (6 patients) improvement defined, respectively, as >50% and >25% improvement in the number of active joints and morning stiffness.

This favorable experience subsequently led to two large, randomized, placebo-controlled minocycline trials—one conducted in the Netherlands and one in the United States. Similar both in design and conclusion, these two studies have provided the most credible evidence to date of antibiotic efficacy.

Kloppenburg et al. [44] studied 80 patients with active rheumatoid arthritis equally randomized to either minocycline 200 mg daily or placebo for a 26-week treatment period. All patients had previously been treated with at least one second-line agent and 58 of the 80 study participants (69%) continued second-line therapy during the study. Other allowable background therapy during the trial included nonsteroidal anti-inflammatory agents and stable corticosteroid use not exceeding 10 mg daily. All patients satisfied commonly accepted criteria of active inflammatory disease at study enrollment. Seropositivity and erosive disease were present in 89 and 95% of patients, respectively. Determination of efficacy measures, which included pain on active movement and at rest, fatigue, duration of morning stiffness, grip strength, functional capacity, Ritchie articular index, and number of swollen joints, was performed at study weeks 0, 4, 12, and 26 as well as 4 weeks after discontinuation of the study medication. Five of the 40 patients (12.5%) randomized to minocycline treatment were withdrawn for medication-related adverse effects, primarily gastrointestinal intolerance and dizziness, whereas one patient was withdrawn for an intercurrent illness. Statistically significant improvement for the minocycline-treated group was seen in morning stiffness ($P = .006$), functional capacity ($P = .002$), Ritchie articular index ($P = .002$), and the number of swollen joints ($P = .008$). The improvement in these clinical parameters was corroborated by more pronounced changes in laboratory measures, including the erythrocyte sedimentation rate, hemoglobin, platelet count, and C-reactive protein (all P values $< .001$). No improvement in any clinical or laboratory parameter for the placebo-treated group was seen.

A second double-blind, placebo-controlled trial [45], frequently referred to by the acronym MIRA (Minocycline In Rheumatoid Arthritis), used the same dose of minocycline (200 mg/day) as the Kloppenburg trial but employed a larger study population and a longer study duration. Utilizing six clinical centers, 219 patients with rheumatoid arthritis were enrolled according to selection criteria that permitted a previous therapeutic trial of only one second-line agent other than hydroxychloroquine. To facilitate study recruitment but prevent enrollment of patients who potentially had unresponsive disease, a patient who had received more than one second-line agent was eligible for study entry only if the reason for discontinuation of any additional second-line therapy had been toxicity and the duration of treatment had been for a subtherapeutic length of time. No use of a second-line therapy within 4 weeks of study enrollment was allowed, which contrasted with the Kloppenburg study in which concurrent use of second-line agents was permitted. All patients had active inflammatory disease defined as at least six swollen joints and at least nine tender joints. Randomization between treatment and placebo arms yielded comparable patient populations, however, the frequency of seropositivity (56%) and erosive disease (68%) was much lower than the study population of Kloppenburg, perhaps indicating that the MIRA study population had milder disease. Efficacy evaluation included the number of tender joints, number of swollen joints, grip strength, morning stiffness, functional capacity, and physician and patient global assessments. The primary outcome measures were improvement in joint swelling and joint tenderness, with a patient considered to have improved if at least 50% of affected joints were less swollen or less tender at study completion compared with baseline. Despite a larger than expected placebo response, improvement in both joint swelling and joint tenderness by the minocycline group did achieve statistical significance ($P = .023$ and $P = .021$, respectively). Similar to the Kloppenburg study, significant improvement of several laboratory parameters in the minocycline group was also observed. Compared with placebo, minocycline was associated with statistically significant improvement in the erythrocyte sedimentation rate, hematocrit, and platelet count (all P values $< .001$), whereas no significant change was observed in grip strength, patient and physician global assessment, functional capacity, and morning stiffness. There were six patient withdrawals from minocycline (6%) for toxicity; contrasting with the higher withdrawal rate seen in other studies. This may be attributable to the fact that the medication dose could be adjusted during the study if an adverse event occurred.

In addition to the study of systemic tetracycline as antirheumatic therapy, a preliminary report using intrabursal tetracycline as sclerotherapy in rheumatoid arthritis patients with olecranon bursitis has been published [48]. In this small open study, resolution of the bursitis was seen in three of seven patients following a single instillation of tetracycline 250 mg, whereas an additional three patients experienced resolution after as many as five tetracycline injections at monthly intervals. A seventh patient was not responsive. The only adverse effect observed was occasional bursal pain immediately following injection. Although tetracycline has been used successfully as sclerotherapy for such processes as pleural and pericardial effusions, further controlled study is needed to establish the efficacy of such treatment for rheumatoid bursitis.

In summary, apparent minocycline efficacy and acceptable patient tolerance in the treatment of rheumatoid arthritis patients has now been demonstrated by both open and controlled clinical trials. These data notwithstanding, acceptance of minocycline as a standard antirheumatic therapy is not at present universal among rheumatologists and further study is needed.

B. Rifampin

Rifampin is a complex macrocyclic antibiotic frequently used as first-line therapy for tuberculosis as well as for a variety of other intracellular and extracellular infections. It has a wide variety of antibacterial properties, including inhibition of bacterial cell wall protein synthesis [47], as well as putative immunosuppressive effects [48]. Unlike other studies of antibiotics in the treatment of rheumatoid arthritis, clinical investigations of rifampin have utilized both intra-articular and systemic administration.

In 1982, Caruso et al. [49] reported a double-blind study of 30 rheumatoid arthritis patients with persistent knee effusions who received weekly intra-articular treatment with either placebo or the rifampin derivative, rifamycin SV, in a dose of 500 mg for a maximum of 12 weeks. Synovial fluid was drained completely prior to each injection and treatment was discontinued as soon as no reaccumulation of the effusion was evident. After a 5-year follow-up period consisting of evaluations at 3-month intervals, only one treated patient had experienced a recurrence of effusion in contrast to patients treated with placebo who were reported to have had no significant change. In a subsequent study, Caruso et al. [50] reported further on the efficacy of intra-articular injections with rifamycin SV. Forty patients with rheumatoid arthritis were randomized to weekly injections of rifamycin SV or perfloxacin, a flouroquinolone antibiotic. Improvement was seen in clinical measures as well as in the erythrocyte sedimentation rate and C-reactive protein for the rifamycin group.

McConkey et al. [51], having observed significant joint improvement in a rheumatoid arthritis patient with tuberculosis following rifampin therapy, studied 20 patients treated with rifampin 600 mg daily alone (10 patients) and in combination with isoniazid 300 mg daily (10 patients). Eighteen patients (90%) completed 3 months of treatment in this pilot study. Improvement was seen in six of the seven patients, who had a duration of rheumatoid arthritis that was less than 3 years. In contrast, the 11 patients with longer standing disease were unimproved. The presence of isoniazid appeared to have neither a beneficial nor a deleterious effect on efficacy or tolerance. A second pilot study [52] involved eight patients with active, seropositive rheumatoid arthritis and a mean disease duration of approximately 13 years. All patients were treated with oral rifampin at a daily dose of 600–1200 mg for 6 months. No significant benefit in any clinical or laboratory measure of disease activity was seen.

Subsequently, Borg et al. [53] studied 16 patients with a disease duration of less than 12 months. Randomization resulted in nine patients being treated with rifampin 600 mg daily and seven patients with hydroxychloroquine 400 mg daily. No significant improvement in clinical or laboratory measures of disease activity was seen at either 6 or 12 months of rifampin treatment. Similarly, Cox et al. [54] reported no significant improvement in 21 patients with disease duration of less than 3 years who were treated with rifampin 600 mg and isoniazid 300 mg daily for 6 months. The 15 patients with a disease duration of less than 18 months did have a significant decrease in erythrocyte sedimentation rate and C-reactive protein; however, no corresponding clinical improvement of significance was detected.

In summary, preliminary observations suggesting that oral rifampin might be beneficial in the treatment of patients with early rheumatoid arthritis have not been confirmed in subsequent and more rigorous evaluations. The reports of benefit from intra-articular rifampin are preliminary and require confirmation.

C. Dapsone

Dapsone is a sulfone antibiotic presently used as the primary treatment of dermatitis herpetiformis and for the treatment of leprosy. It has been shown to be bacteriocidal against *Mycobacterium leprae*, but its mechanism of action in dermatitis herpetiformis is unknown. A possible immunosuppressive effect has been postulated [55,56]. In open studies, McConkey et al. [57,58] reported both clinical and laboratory improvement in dapsone-treated rheumatoid arthritis patients. Swinson et al. [59] subsequently conducted a 14-week double-blind trial in which 22 patients received dapsone and 19 patients received placebo. Dapsone-treated patients received 50 mg daily for the first week and 100 mg daily thereafter. Improvement which was judged to be significant was observed for both clinical (five of seven measures) and laboratory (erythrocyte sedimentation rate and C-reactive protein) parameters in patients taking dapsone. Adverse reactions were not uncommon in the dapsone-treated group and resulted in three patient withdrawals (14%); one each for rash, nausea, and leukopenia. An anecdotal report by Roger et al. [60] has associated the resolution of skin (subcorneal pustular dermatosis) and joint disease in a rheumatoid arthritis patient after 4 months of dapsone treatment. More recently, Haar et al. [61] reported on 80 patients with active rheumatoid arthritis who were randomized to treatment for 24 weeks with dapsone, hydroxychloroquine, or a combination of both. Sixty-three patients (79%) completed the trial, with most withdrawals being from the combination group for hemolytic anemia. No hemolytic anemia, however, was seen in the group treated with dapsone alone. There was no significant improvement in clinical or laboratory measures of disease activity among the three treatment groups, although the clinical response appeared slightly more pronounced in patients receiving hydroxychloroquine and dapsone together.

The available data suggest that dapsone may have a beneficial clinical effect on rheumatoid arthritis but likely has considerable toxicity. Additional study will be needed to determine its efficacy and define its safety.

D. Ceftriaxone

Efficacious use of the third-generation cephalosporin ceftriaxone in the treatment of Lyme disease led Caperton et al. [62] to study its use in a number of patients with chronic inflammatory arthritides. A total of 60 patients with an inflammatory arthritis and antibody titers to *Borrelia burgdorferi* were randomized to treatment with either intravenous ceftriaxone 2 g daily for 2 weeks or placebo. After 1 month of double-blind evaluation, placebo-treated patients were identified and given the option of being treated with ceftriaxone. Clinical measures were obtained periodically for 6 months following treatment and consisted of both patient and physician assessment of disease activity. Patients were considered responders if they demonstrated improvement in clinical measures which persisted for 2 consecutive months, with the quality of the response being categorized as none, fair, good, excellent, or cure. Of the 58 patients treated with a full course of ceftriaxone, 12 had seropositive rheumatoid arthritis. Five of these 12 patients were considered responders, and the response was characterized as being excellent for two, good for two, and fair for one. The duration of the response varied from 2 to 7 months. Diarrhea was common, occurring in 48% of patients. The magnitude of the *Borrelia* antibody titer was not predictive of response. Ceftriaxone is not presently known to have anti-inflammatory or immunosuppressive actions.

E. Griseofulvin

Based on the premise that polymorphonuclear leukocytes are likely important in the development of inflammation in rheumatoid arthritis, the antimycotic griseofulvin, which is known to inhibit leukocyte chemotaxis in vitro, has been considered as a possible treatment [63]. During a 1-year study period, 20 patients with mild to moderate rheumatoid arthritis received griseofulvin and were compared with 19 placebo-treated patients. No significant clinical or laboratory benefit from griseofulvin was seen. Moveover, the observation that the placebo group showed more improvement has led to speculation that impairment of leukocyte chemotaxis might retard tissue repair and, thereby, have a deleterious effect.

IV. MONITORING AND ADVERSE REACTIONS

The spectrum of adverse reactions and need for monitoring will depend on the particular antibiotic regimen under consideration. Hypersensitivity to the antibiotic or an agent which is chemically similar would represent an obvious contraindication as would pregnancy for regimens presently under discussion. Potential drug interactions, such as antacids and anticoagulants with tetracyclines, also need to be carefully considered.

Regular laboratory screening for bone marrow, hepatic, and renal toxicity would seem prudent. In the MIRA trial, laboratory studies were obtained initially at 4-week intervals and subsequently at 6-week intervals; however, the actual monitoring frequency needed to optimize cost/risk considerations is presently unknown.

A concern common to all antibiotic regimens is the occurrence of serious opportunistic or resistant infections. In the 48-week MIRA experience, upper respiratory tract infections were actually less frequent in the minocycline group (11% compared with 16%) but vaginitis was more frequent (9% compared with 3%). No life-threatening infections were observed.

V. RECOMMENDATIONS

Mincoycline is the only antibiotic therapy in rheumatoid arthritis for which data from clinical trials of adequate size and duration are available; therefore, all other antibiotic regimens should at present be considered experimental and be confined to study in the setting of a clinical trial. Even minocycline presently lacks U.S. Food and Drug Administration (FDA) approval as an antirheumatic therapy. Importantly, the routine use of any treatment regimen in clinical practice can only be justified when well-designed and properly controlled studies have unequivocally demonstrated both efficacy and safety.

The precise place of minocycline in the array of therapies for rheumatoid arthritis is uncertain and can only be determined by head-to-head studies with other antirheumatic agents. It is of note that minocycline efficacy was shown predominantly in patients with relatively mild inflammatory disease.

The present data do support the continued investigation of antibiotics in the treatment of rheumatoid arthritis which, it is hoped, will contribute to the development of safer and more efficacious therapy in the future. Particularly, the study and characterization of antibiotics with differing antimicrobial and nonantimicrobial properties may define a mechanism of antirheumatic action and, in so doing, further elucidate the etiopathogenesis of rheumatoid arthritis.

REFERENCES

1. Forestier, J. Rheumatoid arthritis and its treatment by gold salts. J Lab Clin Med 1935; :827.
2. Watson D. Chloroquine protection against virus induced cell damage without inhibition of virus growth. J Gen Virol 1972; 14:100.
3. Pullar T, Hunter J, Capell H. Which component of sulphasalazine is active in rheumatoid arthritis? Br Med J 1985; 290:1535–1538.
4. Bisno A. Group A streptococcal infections and acute rheumatic fever. N Engl J Med 1991; 325:783–793.
5. Zabriskie J, Lavenchy D, Williams R. Rheumatic fever associated B cell alloantigens as identified by monoclonal antibodies. Arthritis Rheum 1985; 28:1047–1051.
6. Baird R, Bronze M, Kraus W, et al. Epitopes of group A streptococcal M protein shared with antigens of articular cartilage and synovium. J Immunol 1991; 146:3132.
7. Steere A, ED, Winchester R. Association of chronic Lyme arthritis with HLA-DR4 and HLA-DR2 alleles. N Engl J Med 1990; 323:219–223.
8. Nocton J, Dressler F, Rutledge B, et al. Detection of Borrelia burgdorferi DNA by poly-

merase chain reaction in synovial fluid from patients with Lyme arthritis. N Engl J Med 1994; 330:229–234.
9. Aberer E, Brunner C, Suchanek G. Molecular mimicry and Lyme borreliosis: a shared antigenic determinant between Borrelia burgdorferi and human tissue. Ann Neurol 1989; 26:732–737.
10. Schentag J, Ballow C. Tissue-directed pharmacokinetics. Am J Med 1991; 91:3A-5S–3A-11S.
11. Steere A, Green J, Schoen R. Successful parenteral antibiotic therapy of established Lyme arthritis. N Engl J Med 1985; 312:869–874.
12. Dattwyler R, Volkman D, Halperin J, Luft B. Treatment of late Lyme borreliosis—randomized comparison of ceftriaxone and penicillin. Lancet 1988; 1:1191–1194.
13. Cole BC, Washburn LR, Taylor-Robinson D. Mycoplasma induced arthritis. In: Razin S, Bairle MF, eds. The Mycoplasmas. Vol. 4. New York: Academic Press, 1985:107–160.
14. Cole BC, Sawitzke AD. Mycoplasmas, superantigens and autoimmune arthritis. In: Henderson B, Pettifer R, eds. Mechanisms and Models in Rheumatoid Arthritis. London: Academic Press, 1994: 47–66.
15. Cole B, Kartchner D, Wells D. Stimulation of mouse lymphocytes by a mitogen derived from Mycoplasma arthritidis (MAM). VIII. Selective activation of T-cells expressing distinct Vβ T cell receptors (TCR) from various strains of mice by the "super-antigen" MAM. J Immunol 1990; 144:425–431.
16. Kundsin R, Praznik J. Pharyngeal carriage of mycoplasma species in healthy young adults. J Epidemiol 1967; 86:579–583.
17. Taylor-Robinson D, Furr P, Webster A. Ureaplasma urealyticum in the immunocompromised host. Pediatr Infect Dis 1986; 5(Suppl):236–238.
18. Biberfield G. Infection sequelae and autoimmune reactions in mycoplasma pneumoniae infection. In: Razin S, Barile M, eds. The Mycoplasmas. Vol. 1. Orlando, FL: Academic Press, 1985:293–311.
19. Golub L, Lee H, Lehrer G. Minocycline reduces gingival collagenolytic activity during diabetes: preliminary observations and a proposed new mechanism of action. J Periodont Res 1983; 18:516–524.
20. Riesbeck K, Bredberg A, Forsgren A. Ciprofloxin does not inhibit mitochondrial functions but other antibiotics do. Antimicrob Agents Chemother 1990; 34:167–169.
21. Martin R, Warr G, Couch R, Yeager HVK. Effects of tetracycline on leukotaxis. J Infect Dis 1974; 129:110–116.
22. Forsgren A, Schmeling D, Quie P. Effect of tetracycline on the phagocytic function of human leukocytes. J Infect Dis 1974; 130:412–415.
23. Thong Y, Ferrante A. Inhibition of mitogen-induced human lymphocyte proliferative responses by tetracycline analogues. Clin Exp Immunol 1979; 35:443–446.
24. Ingham E, Turnbill L, Kearney J. The effects of minocycline and tetracycline on the mitotic response of human peripheral blood lymphocytes. J Antimicrob Chemother 1991; 27:609–617.
25. MacDonald T, Carter P. Requirement for bacterial flora before mice generate cells capable of mediating the delayed hypersensitivity reaction to sheep red blood cells. J Immunol 1979; 122:2624–2630.
26. Plewig F, Schopf E. Anti-inflammatory effects of antimicrobial agents, an in vivo study. J Invest Dermatol 1975; 65:532–536.
27. Van Barr H, Van De Kerkhof P, Mier P, Happle R. Tetracyclines are potent scavengers of the superoxide radical. Br J Rheum 1987; 117:131–132.
28. Pruzanski W, Greenwald R, Street I, et al. Inhibition of enzymatic activity of phospholipase A2 by minocycline and doxycycline. Biochem Pharmacol 1992; 44:1165–1170.
29. Golub L, Ramamurthy N, McNamara T, et al. Tetracyclines inhibit tissue collagenase activity. J Periodont Res 1984; 19:651–655.

30. Golub L, Wolff M, Lee H. Further evidence that tetracyclines inhibit collagenase activity in human crevicular fluid and from other mammalian sources. J Peridontal Res 1985; 20:12–13.
31. Greenwald R, Golub L, Lavietes B. Tetracyclines inhibit human synovial collagenase in vivo and in vitro. J Rheumatol 1987; 14:28–32.
32. Yu LP, Smith GN, Hasty KA Brandt KD. Doxycycline inhibits type XI collagenolytic activity of extracts from human osteoarthritic cartilage and of gelatinase. J Rheumatol 1991; 18:1450–1452.
33. Milwidsky A, Finci-Yeheskel Z, Mayer M. Direct inhibition of proteases and cervical plasminogen activator by antibiotics. Am J Obstet Gyncol 1992; 166:606–612.
34. Breban M, Fournier C, Gougerot-Pocidalo M-A, et al. Protective effects of ciprofloxacin against type II collagen induced arthritis in rats. J Rheumatol 1992; 19:216–222.
35. Dienes L, Ropes M, WES. The role of pleuropneumonia-like organisms in genitourinary and joint diseases. N Engl J Med 1948; 238:509–515, 563–567.
36. Bartholomew L. Isolation and characterization of mycoplasma (PPLO) from patients with rheumatoid arthritis, systemic lupus erythematosus and Reiter's syndrome. Arthritis Rheum 1965; 8:376–388.
37. Williams M, Brostoff I, Roitt IM. Positive role of Mycoplasma fermentans in pathogenesis of rheumatoid arthritis. Lancet 1970; 2:277–280.
38. Brown T, Bush S, Felts W. PPLO and their possible relation to articular disease. In: American Rheumatism Association Rheumatic Diseases. Philadelphia, Saunders, 1952:401.
39. Brown TM, Bush S, Felts W. Rheumatoid diseases and gout, long-term illnesses: management of the chronically ill patient. In: Wohl M, eds. Long-term Illnesses: Management of the Chronically Ill Patient. Philadelphia: Saunders 1959:93–125.
40. Sanchez I. Tetracycline treatment in rheumatoid arthritis and other rheumatic diseases. Braz Med 1968; 82:22–31.
41. Skinner M, Cathcart E, Mills J, Pinals R. Tetracycline in the treatment of rheumatoid arthritis: a double-blind controlled study. Arthritis Rheum 1971; 14:727–732.
42. Breedveld F, Trentham D. Suppression of collagen and adjuvant arthritis by a tetracycline. Arthritis Rheum 1988; 31:R3.
43. Langevitz P, Bank I, Zemer D, et al. Treatment of resistant rheumatoid arthritis with minocycline: an open study. J Rheumatol 1992; 19:1502–1504.
44. Kloppenburg M, Ferdinand C, Terwiel J, et al. Minocycline in active rheumatoid arthritis. Arthritis Rheum 1994; 37:629–636.
45. Tilley BC, Alarcon GS, Heyse SP, et al. Minocycline in rheumatoid arthritis: 48-Week, double-blind, placebo-controlled trial. Ann Intern Med 1995; 122:81–89.
46. Hassell A, Fowler P, Dawes P. Intra-bursal tetracycline in the treatment of olecranon bursitis in patients with rheumatoid arthritis. Br J Med 1994; 33:859–860.
47. Hartmann G, Honikel KO, Knusel F, Nuesch J. The specific inhibition of DNA-directed RNA synthesis by rifamycin. Biochim Biophys Acta 1967: 145:843–4.
48. Nessi R, Pallanza R, Fowst G. Rifampicin and immunosuppression. Arzneimittelforschung 1974; 24:832–6.
49. Caruso I, Montrone F, Fumagalli M, et al. Rheumatoid knee synovitis successfully treated with intra-articular rifamycin SV. Ann Rheum Dis 1982; 41:232–236.
50. Caruso I, Boccassini L, Cazzola M, et al. Multiple intra-articular treatment of rheumatoid arthritis: a randomized prospective study comparing rifamycin SV with pefloxacin. J Int Med Res 1992; 20:27–39.
51. McConkey B, Situnayake RD. Effects of rifampicin with and without isoniazid in rheumatoid arthritis. J Rheumatol 1988; 15:46–50.
52. Gabriel SE, Conn, DL, Luthra H. Rifampin therapy in rheumatoid arthritis. J Rheumatol 1990; 17:163–166.

53. Borg A, Davis M, Fowler P, et al. Rifampicin in early rheumatoid arthritis. Scand J Rheumatol 1993; 22:39–42.
54. Cox N, Prowse M, MCM, Maddison P. Treatment of early rheumatoid arthritis with rifampicin. Ann Rheum Dis 1992; 51:32–34.
55. Barranco CP. Inhibitions of lysosomal enzymes by dapsone. Arch Dermatol 1974; 110:563–566.
56. Barnetson RS, Barnetson C, Pearson JMH, Rees RJW. Evidence for prevention of borderline leprosy reactions by dapsone. Lancet 1976; 2:1171–1172.
57. McConkey B, Davies P, Crockson RA, et al. Dapsone in rheumatoid arthritis. Rheumatol Rehabil 1976; 15:230–234.
58. McConkey B, Davies P, Crockson RA, et al. Effects of gold, dapsone, and prednisone on serum C-reactive protein and haptoglobin and the erythrocyte sedimentation rate in rheumatoid arthritis. Ann Rheum Dis 1979; 38:141–144.
59. Swinson D, Zlosnich JLJ. Double-blind trial of dapsone against placebo in the treatment of rheumatoid arthritis. Ann Rheum Dis 1981; 40:235–239.
60. Roger H, Thevenet JP, Stouteyrand P, Sauvezie B. Subcorneal pustular dermatosis associated with rheumatoid arthritis and raised IgA: simultaneous remission of skin and joints involvements with dapsone treatment. Ann Rheum Dis 1990; 49:190–191.
61. Harr D, Solvkjaer M, Unger B, et al. A double-blind comparative study of hydroxychloroquine and dapsone, alone and in combination, in rheumatoid arthritis. Scand J Rheumatol 1993; 22:113–118.
62. Caperton E, Heim-Duthoy K, Matzke G, et al. Ceftriaxone therapy of chronic inflammatory arthritis: a double-blind placebo controlled trial. Arch Intern Med 1990; 150:1677–1682.
63. Nilsson F, Norberg B, Frederiksen B, Eriksson S. The role of the MA-sensitive leukocyte chemotaxis in rheumatoid arthritis. a randomized double-blind clinical trial of griseofulvin treatment. Scand J Rheumatol 1983; 12:113–118.

21

Management of Spondylarthropathy

Maxime Dougados and Michel Revel
Hôpital Cochin, Paris, France

Muhammad Asim Khan*
Case Western Reserve University, Cleveland, Ohio

1. CONCEPT OF SPONDYLARTHROPATHY

A. Definition

The group of diseases collectively labeled spondylarthropathies consists of several disorders: reactive arthritis, psoriatic arthritis, arthritis related to inflammatory bowel disease, a subgroup of juvenile chronic arthritis, and ankylosing spondylitis, with the last mentioned being the prototype of this group of interrelated disorders [1,2]. It can be difficult to differentiate these disorders, because they may occur simultaneously or sequentially; in addition, some of the clinical characteristics of these diseases, such as enthesiopathy and eye involvement, are similar whatever the diagnosis.

The monitoring and, to a lesser degree, the diagnosis and treatment of these diseases are related more to their clinical presentation than to the precise diagnosis (Table 1) [3]. The rheumatic manifestations include spinal symptoms but also extraspinal joint disease and enthesiopathic lesions may be seen. The extra-articular manifestations of the disease may be similar whatever the subgroup of spondylarthropathy (e.g., acute anterior uveitis) or may be specific to a subgroup of spondylarthropathy such as the skin lesion in psoriatic arthritis, the gut involvement in inflammatory bowel disease, and the oculourethrosynovial triangle in Reiter's syndrome.

B. Interest

Recognition of this concept of spondylarthropathy is of great importance in daily practice and has at least a threefold effect: (a) it permits earlier diagnosis, (b) it facilitates patient education, and (c) it permits establishment of a prognosis.

**Current affiliation*: MetroHealth Medical Center, Cleveland, Ohio

Table 1 Clinical Presentation of Spondylarthropathy

Spondylarthropathy	
Disease subgroups	Clinical features
Ankylosing spondylitis	Rheumatological manifestations
Psoriatic arthritis	Axial involvement
Reactive arthritis	Peripheral arthritis
IBD related arthritis	Enthesiopathy
Undifferentiated spondyloarthropathy	Extraarticular features
	Acute anterior uveitis
	Endocarditis
	Genetic background
	Family history
	HLA-B27 antigen
	Specific manifestations
	psoriasis
	inflammatory bowel disease etc.

1. Early Diagnosis

The cornerstones of treatment of all rheumatic diseases are early accurate diagnosis and effective patient education. Early diagnosis enables treatment before permanent rigidity and deformity have taken place. It also allows detection of the early changes in spinal position and therefore prevention of the abnormal postures associated with these diseases. The criteria for ankylosing spondylitis may be helpful in establishing standard diagnostic levels for similar groups of patients, but they are not of much use in everyday clinical practice for diagnosis in an individual patient [4]. This is due to two major factors: Detection of radiographic evidence of sacroiliitis may sometimes take 3–7 years after disease onset and extraspinal and/or extra-articular involvement are common features of ankylosing spondylitis. The use of sets of spondylarthropathy criteria (the Amor criteria [5] and/or the European Spondylarthropathy Study Group criteria [6]; Table 2) may be more helpful. For example, the Amor criteria permit establishment of the diagnosis of spondylarthropathy whatever the target symptom; for example, enthesiopathy or uveitis. Both criteria permit determination the diagnosis of spondylarthropathy even in the absence of radiographic sacroiliitis.

2. Patient Education

Patient education is crucial for the successful management of patients with spondylarthropathy [4a,4b]. As soon as the diagnosis is made, the patient must be given a clear description of the nature of the disease, including three main points: (a) explanation of the various potential clinical presentations, (b) explanation of the possible progression of the target symptom, and (c) explanation of the possible occurrence of other clinical symptoms of spondylarthropathy.

To clarify this approach, we will take the example of a young patient presenting with inflammatory low back pain:

1. The patient has to be informed clearly about the differences between back pain due to spondylarthropathy and back pain due to a mechanical problem. The physician must keep in mind that the patient has previously received or will

Table 2 Classification Criteria for Spondylarthropathy

Amor criteria	
Parameters	Scoring
A. Clinical systems or past history of	
1. Lumbar or dorsal pain at night or morning stiffness of lumbar or dorsal pain	1
2. Asymmetrical oligoarthritis	2
3. Buttock pain	1
or	
if alternate buttock pain	2
4. Sausage-like toe or digit	2
5. Heel pain or other well-defined enthesiopathy	2
6. Iritis	2
7. Nongonococcal uretritis or cervicitis within 1 month before the onset of arthritis	1
8. Acute diarrhea within 1 month before the onset of arthritis	1
9. Psoriasis, balanitis, or inflammatory bowel disease (IBD) (ulcerative colitis or Crohn's disease)	2
B. Radiological findings	
10. Sacroiliitis (bilateral grade 2 or unilateral grade 3)	2
C. Genetic background	
11. Presence of HLA-B27 and/or family history of ankylosing spondylitis, reactive arthritis, uveitis, psoriasis, or IBD	2
D. Response to treatment	
12. Clear-cut improvement within 48 h after NSAID intake or rapid relapse of the pain after their discontinuation	2

A patient is considered as suffering from a spondylarthropathy if the sum is ≥ 6.

ESSG Criteria for Spondylarthropathy		
Inflammatory spinal pain	or	Synovitis asymmetrical or predominantly in the lower limbs

and

One or more of the following:
- Alternate buttock pain
- Sacroiliitis
- Enthesiopathy
- Positive family history
- Psoriasis
- Inflammatory bowel disease
- Uretritis or cervicitis or acute diarrhea occurring within 1 month before arthritis

get various information concerning back pain from different sources (such as friends or newspapers). The most frequent mistaken notions are that (a) nonsteroidal anti-inflammatory drugs (NSAIDs) are more toxic than efficient and (b) physiotherapy has no effect on the long-term outcome of back pain.

2. Information concerning the possible occurrence of spinal ankylosis in abnormal postures will lead to better compliance with proposed treatments, such as NSAIDs, and physiotherapy and will give the patient a better understanding of the benefits of a routine annual visit.
3. The patient must be informed about the possibility of the occurrence of other clinical symptoms of spondylarthropathy. For example, in this patient, the risk of the occurrence of acute anterior uveitis has to be clearly explained together with the need for an emergency visit to an ophthalmologist in such a case.

3. *Prognosis*

Most clinicians feel that the severity (in terms of risk of the occurrence of spinal ankylosis) of the disease is decreasing [7]. However, this notion has not been clearly demonstrated. Whatever the case, we must keep in mind that a large proportion of patients seen at an early stage of the disease will never develop spinal ankylosis, whereas some of them will.

To determine the predictive factors of long-term outcome in patients with spondylarthropathy, Amor has conducted a study in a cohort of 151 patients monitored by a single investigator over a period of at least 10 years [8]. The presence of the following factors during the first 2 years of the study was correlated with poor outcome: hip arthritis, first hour erythrocyte sedimentation rate (ESR) over 30 mm, poor efficacy of NSAID, limitation of lumbar axis, oligoarthritis, and onset before the age of 16 years. It should be emphasized that information on these factors was collected by questioning of the patient. Definitions were as follows:

1. Hip arthritis was defined by the presence of pain localized in the groin together with lameness.
2. ESR was considered increased when observed on at least two examinations.
3. Efficacy of NSAID was defined by a clear-cut improvement of rheumatic complaints within 24 to 48 h or a relapse within 24 to 48 h of NSAID discontinuation.
4. Limitation of lumbar axis was defined as difficulty in bending lumbar spine and/or moving the neck.
5. Dactylitis was defined as the presence of sausage-like fingers or toes.
6. Oligoarthritis was defined as peripheral joint pain.
7. Age at onset was defined by the date of the first symptoms related to spondylarthropathy.

These factors are predictive of severity, but more interestingly, their absence during the first 2 years of evolution (i.e., often before diagnosis) seems highly predictive of mild disease. It might therefore be possible to give patients not only the bad news of having an ankylosing spondylitis or another spondylarthropathy but also the good news: mild disease with a benign long-term outcome and practically no risk of chronic disability, the need for symptomatic but efficient treatment, and no limitation of professional or sports activities.

II. AXIAL INVOLVEMENT

A. Objectives

The objectives of treatment of the axial involvement of spondylarthropathy are to reduce and/or prevent the deleterious clinical effects of the three main clinical characteristics of the disease; that is, inflammation, ankylosis, and abnormal postures.

Inflammation is not only responsible for the subjective clinical symptoms of inflammatory pain and morning stiffness but also for objective clinical measurements such as reduction in spinal mobility.

Ankylosis is responsible for reduction in spinal and thoracic mobility. Reduction in spinal mobility can hamper daily activities, and reduced chest expansion can lower respiratory capacities.

Abnormal postures result from both inflammation and ankylosis. Because of inflammation, the most analgesic posture (but also usually the most abnormal one) is unconsciously chosen by the patient; after a certain time, this reversible abnormal posture becomes permanent because of ankylosis. For example, because of the maximum occurrence of inflammation during the night, the patient usually sleeps in a fetal position. If ankylosis of the spine occurs, kyphosis will be observed.

It is important to keep in mind these three main characteristics of the disease for optimal patient management. Moreover, although a rare phenomenon, it appears that ankylosis can occur even in the absence of clinical symptoms of inflammation.

B. Monitoring

1. Available Assessment Criteria

Pain. Spontaneous pain is usually assessed using a 100 mm length visual analogue scale [9]. Other semiquantitative scales such as the Licker scale may be also useful.

Pain can also be recorded at physical examination. We have proposed an articular index in order to detect pain and/or tenderness at physical examination on 10 articular sites [10]. Results are obtained using a semiquantitative scale, ranging from 0 = no pain to 3 = very severe pain. The range of the total score is 0–30.

Inflammation. Two subjective clinical symptoms suggestive of the inflammatory aspect of pain, pain at night and morning stiffness, can be of interest to monitor patients:

Pain at night is responsible for nocturnal awakenings. This parameter can be used as either a quantitative variable by asking the patient how many times he or she awakes during the night because of pain (number of nocturnal awakenings) or a dichotomous variable by asking the patient if he or she awakens during the night because of pain (nocturnal awakening: yes/no).

Morning stiffness is of great interest to evaluate the degree of inflammation of spondylarthropathy. This parameter is usually calculated as a quantitative or semiquantitative variable evaluating the time required for resolution of early morning stiffness.

Biological parameters are not of great interest in the monitoring of the axial involvement of spondylarthropathy [11]. There is a poor correlation between the change in the biological parameters of inflammation; for example, C-reactive protein, erythrocyte sedimentation rate, and IgA and the changes in the clinical condition of patients after several months of time. These laboratory variables are not abnormal in every patient with active disease and appear to be primarily associated with peripheral arthritis and extra-articular features.

Mobility. Physical therapy and spinal orthosis are prescribed according to appropriate clinical parameters to assess the stiffness of dorsolumbar, cervical, costovertebral, and peripheral joints, to assess the changes in pelvic lumbar posture, dorsolumbar curves and cervicocephalic posture, and to assess ventilatory function, fitness level, and disability. The measurements must be reproducible, rapid, and simple enough to be collected on routine examination at each follow-up in addition to the assessment of the grade of progression of the disease. The decision to initiate and to conduct some of the physical treatments is inferred from the evolution of these various parameters.

1. Assessment of the stiffness of dorsolumbar joints: Numerous techniques have been described to measure spinal mobility in the sagittal plane [12–15]. Skin distraction methods are sensitive, simple, and rapidly performed. More popular are the Schöber test and the modified Schöber test, but they assess only mobility in flexion of the lower lumbar region [16]. The modified Schöber test extended to the whole spine allows evaluation all the segments and to direct the exercises to the site of earlier decreased mobility.

With the patient standing erect, the lumbosacral junction is defined by the spinal intersection of a line joining the dimples of Venus. Using a tape measure, a first mark is made 5 cm below, a second mark 10 cm above, and every 10 cm up to the upper dorsal spine. The patient then bends forward as far as possible, keeping the knees fully extended, and the distances between the marks are remeasured. The skin distraction between the marks from the lower to the upper segment is, respectively, about 4–6 cm, 3–4 cm, 2–3 cm. and 1–2 cm (Figs. 1 and 2). It is possible but not necessary to measure spinal extension. The fingertip to floor distance gives additional information on subpelvic mobility, especially hip mobility and tightness of the posterior leg muscles and ligaments. The subject standing erect with shoes removed and feet together bends forward as far as possible with fingers reaching toward the floor while maintaining the knees in extension. The distance between the tip of the right middle finger and the floor

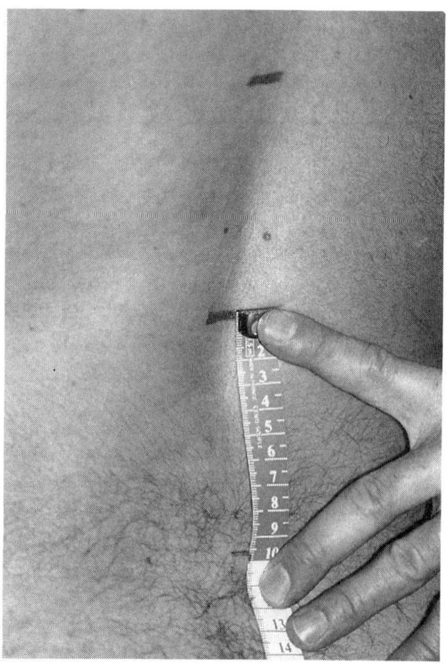

Figure 1 Marks, patient standing erect.

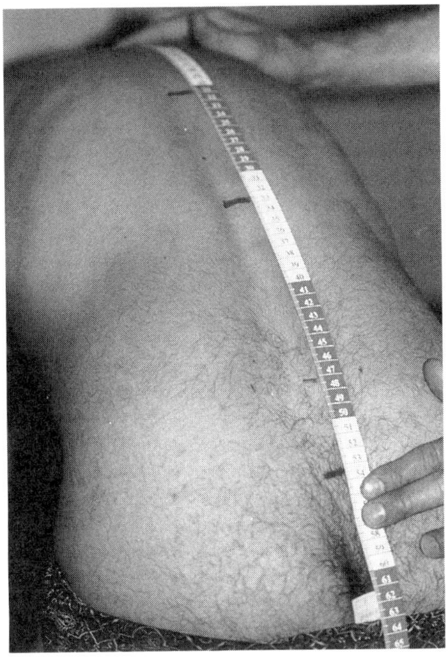

Figure 2 Same marks, patient bending forward as far as possible.

is measured in centimeters with a tape measure (Fig. 3). The fingertip to malleoleus distance gives information on mobility in the coronal plane but does not lead to specific exercises.

2. Assessment of the stiffness of cervical joints: The overall range of cervical mobility can be easily obtained by linear measurements using a tape measure. Flexion and extension are evaluated by the chin to sternum distances (jaws closed) and rotations by the chin to acromion distances expressed in centimeters (Figs. 4 and 5). Even using a reference position (shoulders in lower position, hands clasped behind the back), rotation measurements are less reproducible than the measurements of flexion and extension.

3. Assessment of the stiffness of costovertebral and peripheral joints: Chest expansion is measured with a tape measure placed circumferentially around the chest wall with the patient in standing position. The difference between the thoracic circumference in maximal inspiration and in maximal expiration represents chest expansion expressed in centimeters and mainly indicates costovertebral mobility. The measurements should be taken both at the fourth intercostal space and at the level of the xyphoid process to direct the exercises toward either the upper or the lower ribs (Fig. 6).

In peripheral joint assessment, special attention is paid to hip mobility even without defined arthritis, because mobility can be restricted by tightness of muscles and ligaments. The use of a goniometer is not necessary for measurement of the range of mobility. Flexion and extension are the motions first involved. They should be evaluated with the knees flexed and extended to take into account the respective role of joint stiffness and muscle tightness (rectus femoris in hip extension and hamstring group in hip flexion) (Fig. 7).

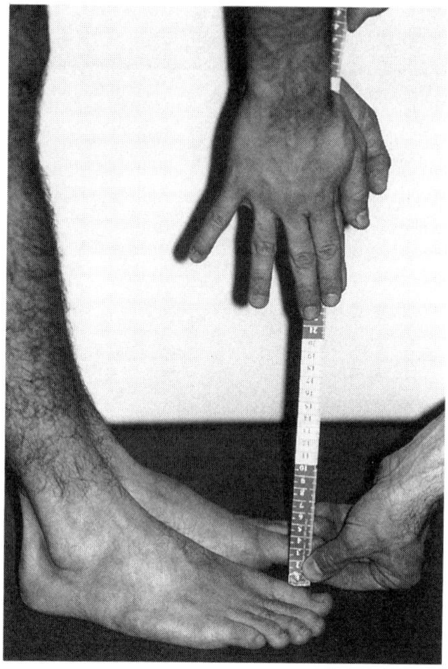

Figure 3 Fingertip to floor distance.

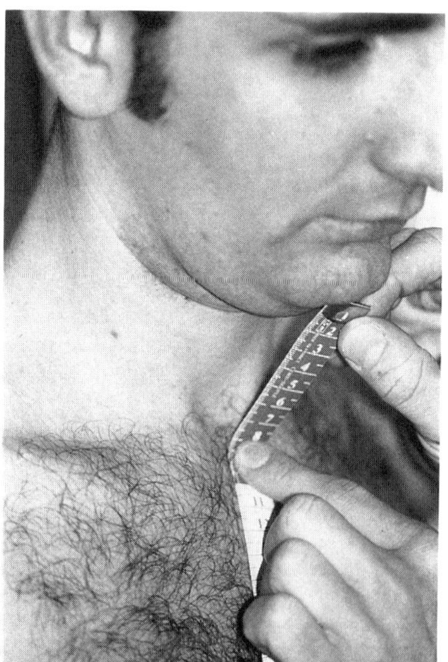

Figure 4 Chin to sternum distance.

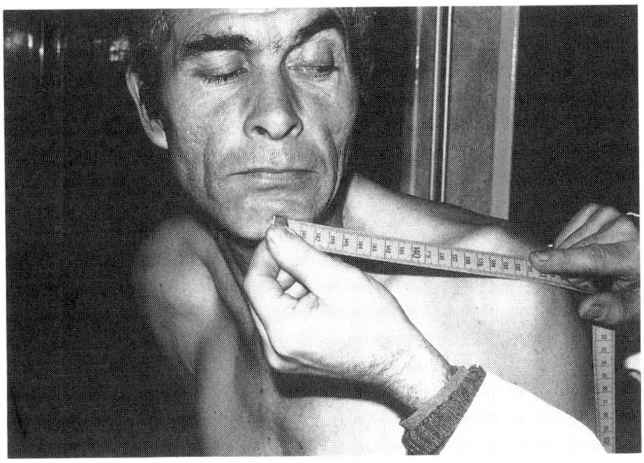

Figure 5 Chin to acromion distance.

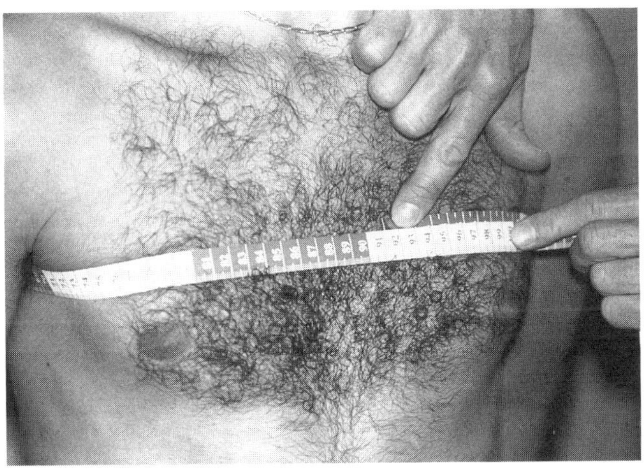

Figure 6 Thoracic circumference measured at the fourth intercostal space.

Abnormal Postures. Clinical assessment of changes in posture and spinal curves requires only a tape measure, a scale, a plumb line and/or a wall, and a measuring apparatus. Reduction in full height is a simple overall evaluation of an increase in spinal curves.

Dorsal and lumbar curves: The patient in standing position, the plumb line is placed in contact with the spine, hanging down in the buttocks pleat. The site of contact indicates the top of the dorsal curve. The distance of the plumb line to the spinous process of C7 (first spinous process easily perceived) represents the measurement of dorsal kyphosis expressed in centimeters (normally about 3–5 cm). The distance of the plumb line to the L3 spinous process represents the measurement of the lumbar curve (normally about 3–4 cm) (Figs. 8 and 9).

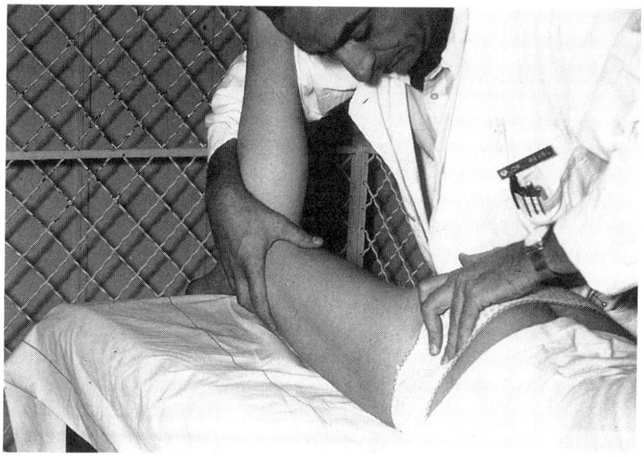

Figure 7 Assessment of rectus femoris tightness.

Gradual increase in the dorsal curve can be esthetically unpleasant, but in the case of major kyphosis, it can also lead to severe disability by restricting the vertical field of vision. The loss of lumbar curve associated with pelvic retroversion generally precedes dorsal kyphosis. The result is a gradual shift forward of the center of gravity, which facilitates the spread of dorsal kyphosis. Changes in pelvic lumbar posture should therefore be evaluated early to institute appropriate exercises and orthosis.

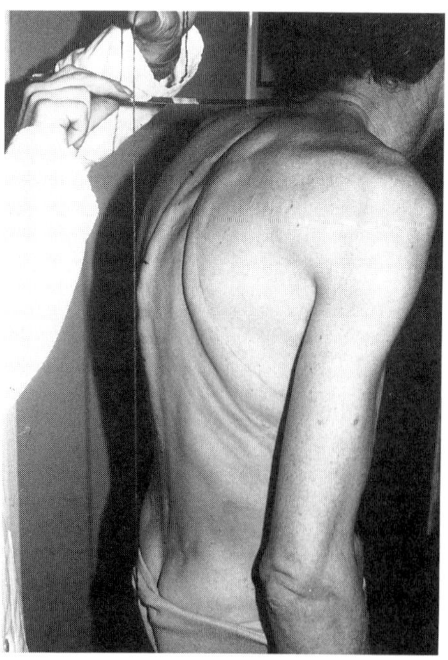

Figure 8 Distance plumbline to spinous process of C7 (dorsal kyphosis).

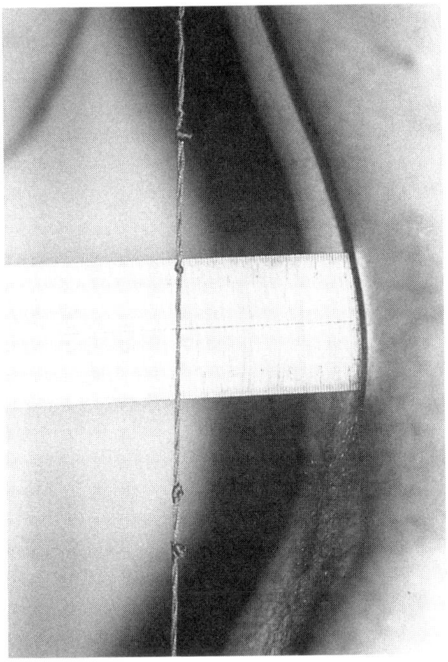

Figure 9 Distance plumbline to spinous process of L3 (lumbar curve).

Cervicocephalic posture: The abnormal posture of the neck tends to a forward transfer of the head as a result of increased lower cervical spine flexion and upper cervical spine extension to maintain the gaze in a horizontal plane. This posture can be assessed by two measurements.

1. The patient standing erect, feet together, back and heels against a wall, tries to reach the wall with the occiput. A cervical spine that is mobile and without deformity allows occiput-wall contact. The distance occiput to wall, measured with a tape measure, represents the grade of forward position of the head (Fig. 10).
2. The distance of the nape of the neck (C4) to the wall represents the grade of flexed position of the lower cervical spine but is less reproducible than the occiput to the wall.

Assessment of Ventilatory Parameters, Fitness Level, and Disability.

Although it has been demonstrated that regular exercise has a significant effect on both vital capacity and exercise tolerance as measured by the subject's maximum oxygen capacity (Vo_2 max) [17,18], pulmonary function tests, including dynamic and static spirometry tests, are not necessary to prescribe and conduct physical therapy. Therefore, unless there are coexistent cardiovascular and respiratory diseases, only chest expansion measurements are of interest on routine examination [19].

The assessment of physical fitness by fatigue tests and Vo_2 max and disability by various indices is necessary in clinical trials evaluating physical therapy but too heavy in routine management of ankylosing spondylitis (AS). These

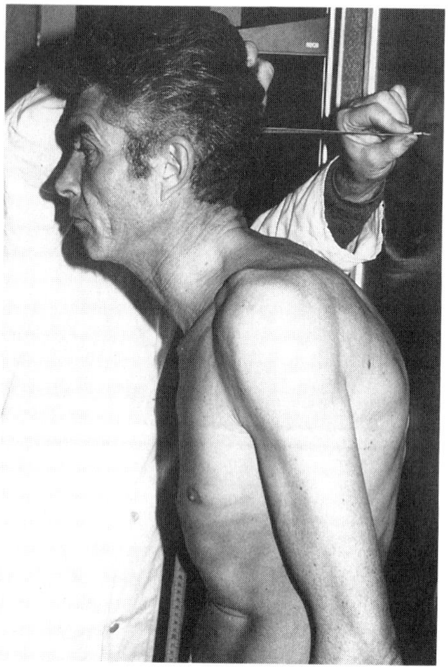

Figure 10 Assessment of the forward position of the head by the distance occiput to wall.

parameters can be indirectly evaluated by the patient, rating subjectively his or her fitness level and disability in daily life activities on a 100-mm VAS (visual analogue scale). More interesting is assessment of the ability to perform assiduously the exercise program : impossible, 0; possible with difficulties, 1; possible without difficulties, 2. Scores 0 and 1 require an adjustment of the exercises and/or drug therapy but infrequently a temporary interruption of physical therapy.

Physical treatments should be established and directed according to these various parameters and particularly to their changes between two visits.

2. Physical Treatments

The aims of physical treatments, including physical therapy, regular exercises, and spinal orthosis, are to improve mobility, strength, and fitness and to prevent or reduce spinal curve abnormalities [39–43]. Physical treatments are an integral part of the management of ankylosing spondylitis, in addition to and not instead of anti-inflammatory drugs. Indeed, most of the techniques and methods are inoperative and even impossible until inflammation and pain are under medical control. On the other hand, drugs alone cannot prevent stiffness and deformities. Physical treatments are based on the techniques of physical therapy and include regular exercises and spinal orthosis.

Physical Therapy. The prescription of physical therapy should follow three questions: Who should benefit from physical therapy? At what stage of the disease? And which techniques for which objectives? Every patient, once spondylarthropathy is diagnosed, should be informed as to the importance of physical therapy in the treatment of the disease.

1. At the early stage, when stiffness is not yet pronounced and no abnormal posture is observed, a short series of six to eight sessions conducted by a physiotherapist once a week is enough to teach an individualized exercise and posture program [41,42]. The exercises are directed to the spine, mainly the lumbar and the dorsal columns, the costovertebral joints, and the hips with the aim of maintaining mobility and strength of the back muscles. The patient is encouraged to perform assiduously at home for the program taught by the physiotherapist 10–20 min daily. Compliance and ability to perform the program is assessed by the physician at each visit. Examples of key exercises and postures (and shown in Figs. 11–14).

2. At an advanced stage of the disease, as soon as stiffness and abnormal postures are observed from comparison of the measurements at two visits, a serie of 15–20 sessions of physical therapy directed against the observed changes should be prescribed.

If the modified Schöber test shows that stiffness predominates on the lower dorsal column, limbering up exercises will be directed toward this part of the spine (Fig. 15).

If the stiffness involves the cervical spine, the exercises will be mainly directed toward strengthening the muscles acting against the limited motion; that is, in most cases, the extensors of the neck. This group of muscles is strengthened in isometric contraction from its maximal elongation (neck flexed, to its maximal shortened position (neck extended) (Fig. 16).

If the range of movement of one hip is limited compared with the opposite side, whatever the mechanism and provided drugs are active against pain, exercises should try to recover a range of movement as close as possible to functional hip mobility [44]. In the case of limitation of extension and mainly in the case of *flexion contracture*, the key exercise is the stretching of flexor

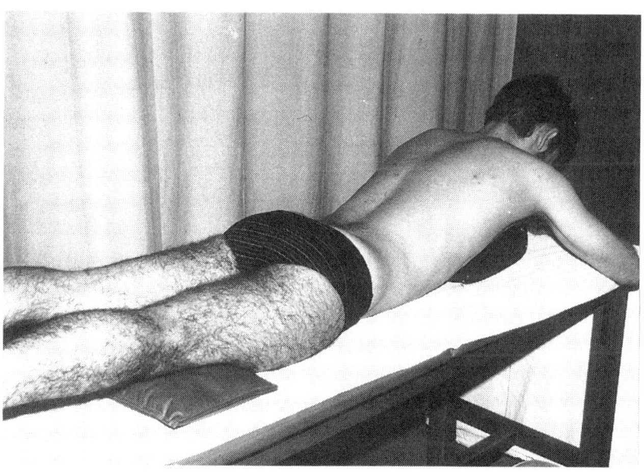

Figure 11 Example of posture to prevent the loss of hip extension and lumbar curve.

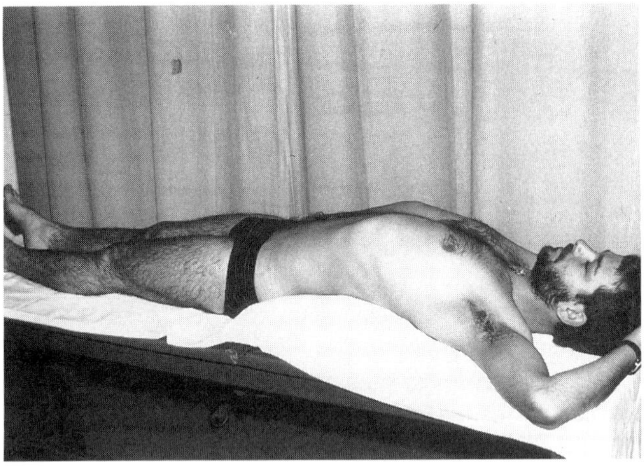

Figure 12 Exemple of posture to prevent dorsal kyphosis.

muscles and anterior soft tissues. The procedure comprises a "contract-relax" technique followed by a passive stretch. The stretching position is gradually shifted from flexion to extension.

If the chest expansion measurements suggest stiffness involving mainly the upper costovertebral joints, the thoracic opening exercises will be directed toward mobility of the upper ribs (Fig. 17).

If comparison of the plumb line to spine distances indicates the beginning of loss of lumbar curve or of dorsal kyphosis, the physical therapy program should include passive extension of the spine either at the lumbar or the dorsal level and exercises to strengthen the back muscles in extended position (Fig. 18).

The program conducted by the physiotherapist should be complemented by information and demonstration of correct postures while lying, sitting, and

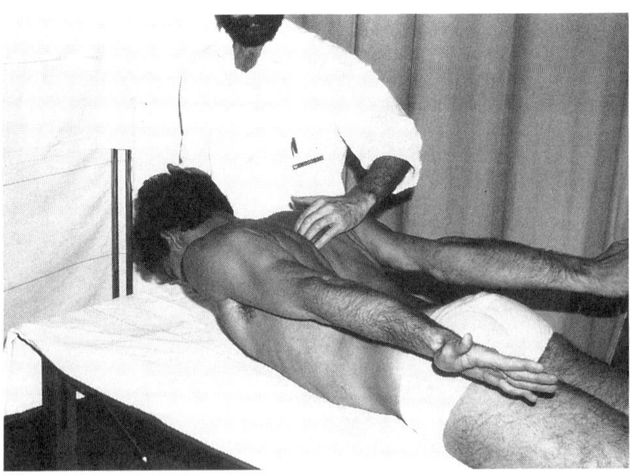

Figure 13 Strengthening of back muscles.

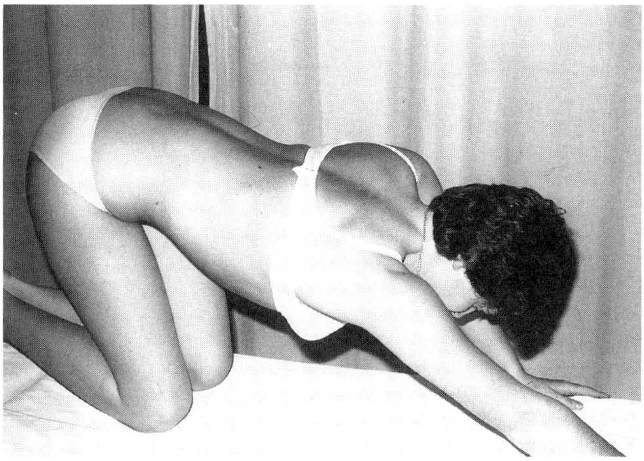

Figure 14 Limbering up exercice for the whole spine.

standing. In addition, the patient should be prompted to have regular physical activities (if necessary with adjustment of the NSAIDs) and mainly to perform regularly the self-administered daily exercise program to pursue the objectives of the physical therapy sessions. Compliance to the program and the clinical outcome should be assessed by the physician at each visit.

3. At the stage of severe ankylosis: In the case of ankylosis of the whole spine as assessed by nil skin distraction all along the spine in the Schöber test and mainly by extended ossification of the interspinous processes and facet joint spaces on frontal radiographs and of the anterior longitudinal ligament on lateral view, passive mobilization and posture are ineffective and even dangerous. At this stage of the disease, only isometric strengthening of back muscles, diaphram, and large abdominal muscles is useful and safe. Strenuous passive stretching of the back can induce syndesmophite

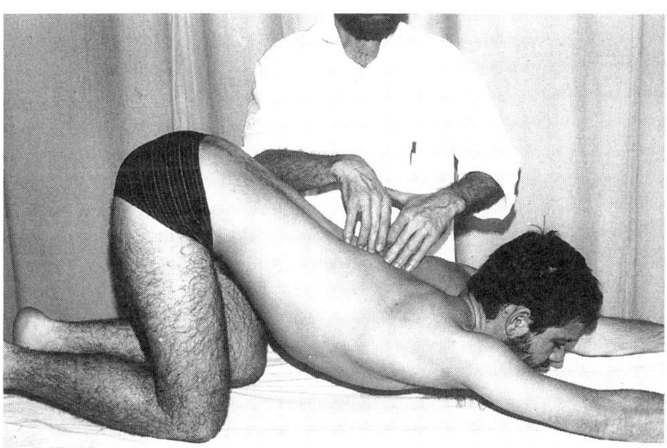

Figure 15 Limbering up exercice directed to the lower dorsal column.

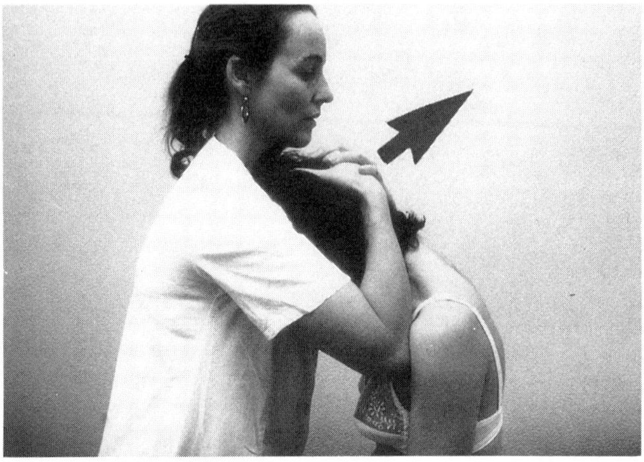

Figure 16 Isometric strengthening of neck muscles.

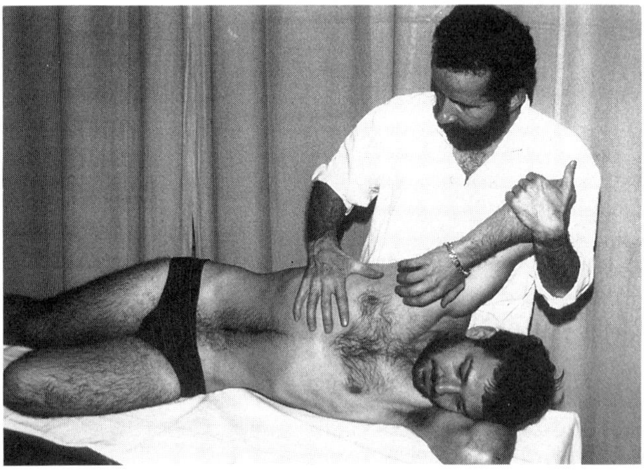

Figure 17 Exercise directed toward mobility of the upper ribs.

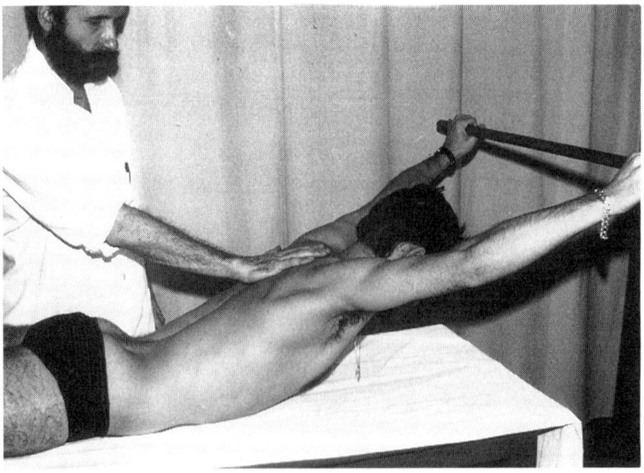

Figure 18 Exercises for back muscles.

fractures. Ankylosis of the cervical spine generally involves the segments under C3 level. Therefore, repetitive motions of the head lead to overuse of occiput-C1 and C1-C2 levels with an increase of mechanical pain as a result.

2. Spinal Orthosis

When physical therapy and regular home exercises fail to improve an abnormal posture of the spine within 5 to 6 months or when a deformity progresses rapidly, for example, an increase of the distance of the occiput to the wall of 3–4 cm, an increase of the distance of the plumb line to C7 of 3–4 cm or a decrease of the distance of the plumb line to L3 of 1–2 cm within a few months, exercise alone has little or no chance of succeeding. If clinical and radiographic examination do not reveal ankylosis, the deformity can be reduced using proper orthosis, the principle of which is permanent active self-correction.

1. Cochin lumbar curve orthosis (Fig. 19): The principle of this custom-molded three-point thoracolumbar brace is similar to that of the Jewett brace with two anterior points and one posterior point of force [45]. The differences are that this orthosis should be custom-fitted, adapted to each morphology, and light enough to be worn for several months. In addition, as with the Jewett brace, the two anterior supports cross the sternum and the pelvic symphysis but the posterior support crosses the middle of the lumbar spine to obtain lumbar extension. The tension of the strap between the lumbar pad and the two anterior pads should be adjusted so as to exert a continuous forward thrust on the lumbar spine without, however, inducing pain.

The gradual loss of lumbar curve is likely to be the result of an unconscious analgesic posture to relieve the strain on tender facet joints. This abnormal posture is very difficult to reduce with exercises alone even before the stage of ankylosis. Therefore,

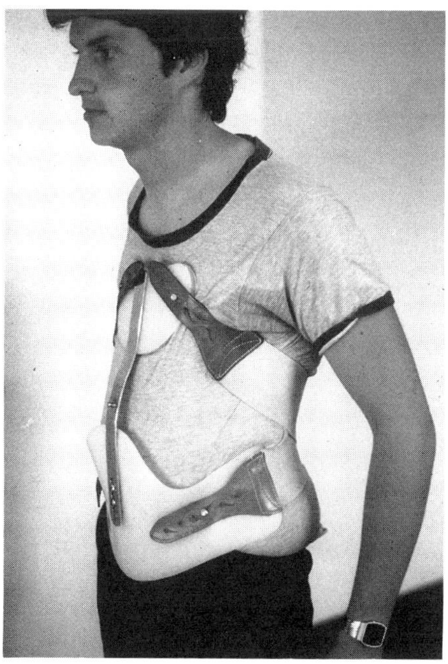

Figure 19 Three-point light brace to prevent the loss of lumbar curve.

a lumbar curve orthosis should be prescribed as soon as a loss of curve is established from repeated measurements. It should be worn full time except during exercises and possibly during sleep. A period of 12–18 months is generally necessary to obtain a gain of lumbar curve. At the stage of true ankylosis, it is too late to prescribe a corrective orthosis.

2. The corset of Swaim (Fig. 20): The corset of Swaim functions according to a principle of active correction that is close to that of the Milwaukee brace for dorsal kyphosis [46]. The orthosis is a jacket, custom fitted and molded in the upright position with the dorsal curve as corrected as possible. The lower part is applied to the pelvic girdle and extended to the trochanters. The upper part extends to the manubrium anteriorly and just under the apex of the dorsal kyphosis posteriorly. The anterior support should be in contact with the skin to give a reference point away from which the patient may actively move. As the patient progressively rectifies his back, the anterior contact is maintained by inserting felt pads between the support and the chest. When the space becomes too large, the brace is made again.

Owing to the situation of the posterior support, the correction is located at the apex of the dorsal curve. The patient continually pulls away from the anterior support, employing the back muscles to be less constrained and to allow free chest expansion during inspiration. If the anterior support is extended to the throat just under the chin, the imposed motion is a backward transfer of the head. The orthosis is then similar to the Milwaukee brace.

The corset of Swaim with sternal support is used to correct dorsal kyphosis, and the orthosis with a throat-chin support is used to correct flexion of the neck associated with a forward transfer of the head. Contrary to the loss of lumbar curve, these deformities of the upper spine can be rectified by a sustained program of physical therapy

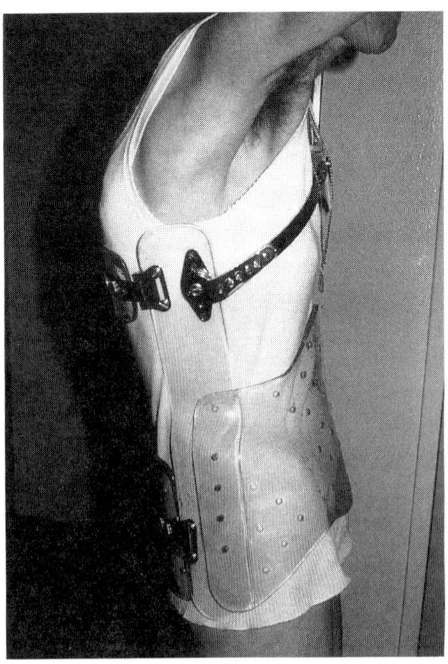

Figure 20 Example of brace with the principle of the corset of Swaim.

and home exercises in addition to an adjustment of NSAIDs. Therefore, when an increase of the occiput to the wall and/or the plumb line to C7 distance is established from repeated measurements, the first step is to intensify physical therapy. If no result is observed after 3–6 months, the orthosis should be prescribed. As with the lumbar curve, orthosis is useless at the stage of definite ankylosis. If some spinal and costovertebral mobility is still present, correction can be obtained within a 1- to 3-month period, but stable effects require 12–18 months. The plaster orthosis should be worn full time during the first period, then the plastic can be replaced by a lighter material like resin, and the corset can be removed during exercises and possibly during sleep. In all cases, the patient is taught to make efforts of pulling away from the anterior supports.

3. *Radiotherapy*

Several forms of radiation have been used therapeutically in ankylosing spondylitis. Refractory symptomatic axial involvement has been treated by either rœntgen therapy and/or thorium X.

Use of rœntgen therapy in the treatment of axial involvement of ankylosing spondylitis was quite frequent in the 1940s. Rœntgen therapy was finally abandoned because of serious long-term side effects, particularly an increased risk of malignancies [47–52].

Thorium X (^{224}radium) is a disintegration product of thorium. Its half-life is 3.85 days and the emitted radiation is largely made up of alpha particles (92%), with the remainder being beta and gamma rays [53]. This treatment is administered intravenously. Such treatment was widely used in Germany several decades ago and seemed to have a long-term beneficial effect [54]. However, long-term follow-up of patients indicated a higher risk of developing cataract [55]. It appears that its use has been abandoned.

4. *Surgical Therapy*

Surgical management may be needed in some patients [4a,4b]; for example, those with severe advanced hip joint disease have dramatically benefited from total hip arthroplasty with marked functional improvement. Loosening of the bone-cement interface may occur after many years and may require revision surgery. Noncemented hip arthroplasty is now preferred in more active and younger patients. Some patients with extreme spinal kyphosis have benefited from wedge osteotomy with relative straightening of the spine, but the surgery carries a high degree of the risk of neurological damage that can even cause paraplegia. Cardiac conduction defects may require a pacemaker, and those with severe aortic incompetence resulting from dilatation of the aortic root and adjacent ascending aorta may require valve replacement surgery. The ankylosed osteoporotic spine is very vulnerable to fracture even after a relatively minor trauma. Overlooking spinal fracture may have disastrous consequences, since the fracture usually occurs in the lower cervical spine and is usually unstable [4a,4b]. A fracture dislocation at this level may result in quadriplegia, which is the most dreaded complication with a high mortality. Magnetic resonance imaging is most sensitive in detecting fracture and visualizing any cord compression or soft tissue swelling and hematoma. Controversy regarding surgical versus conservative management of spinal fracture continues to persist. Rigid spine and limited chest expansion produce technical difficulties for anesthesiologists. Undiagnosed or untreated fractures may result in spondylodiscitis (discovertebral erosion and destruction), pseudoarthrosis, or marked spinal deformity. Patients with spondylodiscitis and back pain may require immobilization of the affected segment with a rigid orthosis to allow fusion to occur, but surgical fusion may be needed in some patients. These complications of ankylosing spondylitis usually persue a benign clinical course, but they can cause spinal cord compression requiring appropriate surgical management. Isolated or multiple vertebral compression fractures may also occur as a result of severe osteoporosis, and sometimes without any trauma.

Spontaneous atlantoaxial subluxation can occur in ankylosing spondylitis and related spondyloarthropathies but is less commonly observed than in rheumatoid arthritis. The occurrence of neurological signs and severe referred occipital pain may require surgical spinal in some patient.

A slowly progressing cauda equina syndrome is a rare but significant complication of long-standing ankylosing spondylitis. There is unfortunately no specific treatment, and current data suggest that surgical treatment should be resisted, because it may worsen the problem. Only palliative treatment can be offered, including the standard management of urinary and fecal incontinence in the advanced stage of the syndrome.

5. Drug Therapies

Analgesics. Simple analgesics are usually considered to have a limited role in treating inflammatory rheumatic diseases. The dramatically significant beneficial effect of NSAIDs in spondylarthropathy results in little use of analgesics. However, in some particular patients, this treatment may have a sparring effect on NSAID intake.

Nonsteroid Anti-inflammatory Drugs. NSAIDs are considered the cornerstone of drug therapy of spondylarthropathy. The NSAID response to inflammatory back pain is so strong that this criterion (symptomatic effect of NSAIDs) is considered as one of the 12 items in the Amor criteria. In the multicenter cross-sectional study conducted in more than 2000 patients to evaluate the different sets of criteria of spondylarthropathy, 741 patients (69 ankylosing spondylitis and 672 controls) complained of back pain [24]. In the subgroup of ankylosing spondylitis, 53 (77%) considered that NSAID treatment was very efficient; this was the case in only 102 (15%) of controls. This prospective, cross-sectional study conducted during 1 week in all consultants permitted to calculate the positive and the negative predictive value of this factor. The probability of suffering from ankylosing spondylitis in case of NSAID efficacy was 34% (positive predictive value) and the negative predictive value was 97%. Thus, in this population, in the case of NSAID inefficacy, the probability of ankylosing spondylitis was very low (3%).

Axial involvement is probably the clinical presentation which responds the most dramatically to NSAIDs. Numerous studies have been conducted with various NSAIDs in order to evaluate the rapid, symptomatic effect of these drugs [25–28]. Most of these trials clearly show a substantial, quick relief of symptoms. The problem is that we do not know whether this symptomatic effect obtained in the short term will correlate with an improvement in the long-term prognosis. One of the recent emerging questions is whether spondylarthropathies, and especially ankylosing spondylitis, have become less severe since the introduction and the long-term use of NSAIDs. Members of the French Society of Rheumatology tried to answer this question [29]. Despite numerous possible biases (absence of control group, requirement of long-term follow-up), it appeared that the disease is less severe than it was several decades ago and that this better prognosis might be at least in part due to the long-term use of NSAIDs. To our knowledge, only one study has compared the radiographic progression of the disease (in terms of spinal ossification) in patients treated with high or low doses of phenylbutazone [30]. This study, presented only as an abstract in a congress in 1985, suggests that a delay in spinal ossification can be obtained by using daily high doses of phenylbutazone.

In summary, the use of NSAIDs in active spondylarthropathy is beneficial. NSAIDs intake must be restricted to painful periods of the disease. When treating a patient without pain who is receiving NSAIDs, the problem is to differentiate between a clinical spontaneous remission of the disease and a NSAID-induced clinical remission. The first hypothesis suggests stopping NSAIDs therapy, whereas the second suggests continuing it. The simple, pragmatic method to resolve this problem is to propose treatment discontinuation to the patient and to reintroduce the drug in case of flare of the disease.

Several NSAIDs are available for use in spondylarthropathies. Phenylbutazone is probably the most effective but potentially the most toxic. Phenylbutazone, the first NSAID available, was immediately recognized as being very effective in the treatment of ankylosing spondylitis, and it became the drug of choice. Subsequently, the problem of potential toxicity appeared with the publication of several observations of agranulocytosis associated with this treatment. In some countries, phenylbutazone is now no longer available, but we still feel that the risk-benefit ratio of this compound permits the following approach: in ankylosing spondylitis, NSAIDs other than phenylbutazone have to be used as first-line drugs; however, before classifying a patient as being refractory to NSAIDs, phenylbutazone has to be tried at up to a 400- to 600-mg daily dosage with proper patient management, and any unwanted effect is looked for.

Introduced in 1963, indomethacin soon challenged phenylbutazone as the drug of choice for ankylosing spondylitis. Indomethacin is now probably the most widely used NSAID in ankylosing spondylitis. However, numerous clinical trials have been conducted with other NSAIDs, and they clearly show a similar beneficial effect in ankylosing spondylitis. For a given patient, it is impossible to predict which NSAID will be both efficient and well tolerated. Therefore, successive trials of the use of different NSAIDs might be helpful in making this choice.

Whatever the selected NSAID, treatment should be based on both the schedule of clinical symptoms (mostly pain) and the pharmacokinetic properties of the drug. For example, in the case of a patient who awakes at 4 a.m. because of inflammatory lumbar pain, a short half-life NSAID taken the day before during the evening meal might be absolutely ineffective. It would instead seem logical to propose that the patient should take an NSAID with a long duration of action during the evening (just before bedtime) and a quick-acting NSAID during the morning (on awaking). To enhance patient compliance, NSAIDs that need to be taken once or twice daily may be preferable to those that need to be taken more often.

Another important point to consider concerns the daily dosage of the NSAID. It must be kept in mind that most of the available NSAIDs have been developed to correspond to the lowest efficient dosage in inflammatory rheumatic diseases, usually in rheumatoid arthritis. Moreover, the toxicity of NSAIDs in inflammatory rheumatic diseases has also been mostly evaluated in rheumatoid arthritis. Spondylarthropathy is very different from rheumatoid arthritis, and one could argue that the tolerability of NSAIDs is better in the latter; perhaps because of younger patient age and the absence of concomitant therapies. Therefore, we fell that the first logical step when dealing with ankylosing spondylitis is to propose the official recommended dosage of the NSAID. In the case of efficacy, the minimum efficient dosage can be determined by successive lowering of this dosage. In the case of inefficacy, we feel that the next logical step is therefore to increase the daily intake of NSAID. Examples of proposed daily dosages: naproxen 1500–2000 mg; diclofenac 200 mg; ketoprofen 400–450 mg.

Corticotherapy. Corticosteroids can be administered locally or systemically.

Local Corticotherapy. Localized articular involvement (sacroiliac, interapophysal, costovertebral, manubriosternal, sternoclavicular) represents the best indication of intra-articular corticotherapy.

The problem here is to recognize the anatomical structure which is responsible for the clinical symptoms of the patient. This information is usually easy to obtain for the manubriosternal and sternocostal joints. However, in some cases, it may be difficult to recognize the anatomical origin of the pain. In such situations, one may need to give a local injection of lidocaine (Xylocaïne) 1% and perform a complete, detailed clinical examination just before and 30 min after the injection. The injected site is considered to be responsible for the patient's clinical symptoms if there is at least a 75% improvement within the 30 min following the injection [31]. Radiographic imaging may be required to ascertain localization of the injection at the desired site. Injection for anterior chest wall pain can usually be performed without radiographic control.

Some of these localized axial involvements may respond well to the local injection of corticosteroids, but controlled studies are lacking to document their efficacy.

To our knowledge, there has been only one prospective double-blind study evaluating the effects of the intrasacroiliac injection of corticosteroids in patients with ankylosing spondylitis [32]. Although involving a very small number of patients (10 patients, 13 evaluated joints), this study demonstrated a statistically significant improvement in pain (evaluated on a visual analogue scale) and the patient's overall assessment in the group of 7 patients who had received an intra-articular injection of 3.75 mg cortivazol compared with the group of 6 patients who had received placebo.

Systemic Corticotherapy. Corticosteroids given orally are of little if any use in the treatment of ankylosing spondylitis; they do not halt the progression of the disease process and their chronic use causes unwanted side effects.

In a few cases, NSAIDs may remain ineffective even at high doses. In these cases, pulse therapy using methylprednisolone 15 mg/kg during 3 consecutive days may promptly and temporarily control painful and disabling acute attacks. Such a beneficial effect has been reported in a double-blind controlled trial comparing high-dose (1000 mg) to low-dose (375 mg) methylprednisolone pulse therapy administered intravenously in patients with active ankylosing spondylitis [33].

Second-line Drugs. The presentation of the studies conducted to evaluate the effects of second-line drugs in ankylosing spondylitis frequently does not allow drug evaluation to be feasible. Most of the studies indicate that the recruited patients fulfilled the diagnostic criteria for ankylosing spondylitis without giving any information concerning clinical presentation at study entry (axial and/or peripheral articular involvement). Often even when this information is given, no correlation is made with the efficacy of the study drug. For example, the description of patient characteristics, states that 60% of them had peripheral arthritis at entry, and the results section states that the study drug was effective in 40% of the patients, but there is no mention as to whether the efficacy was observed or not only in the subgroup of patients with peripheral articular involvement. In any case, it is clear that these second-line drugs are commonly prescribed in patients with refractory and persisting peripheral articular involvement. Therefore, we will describe in more detail the data obtained with such drugs in the section of this chapter related to the treatment of peripheral articular involvement.

However, there is still the question as to whether there is a place for second-line drugs in the treatment of the axial involvement of spondylarthropathy. Two drugs, sulfasalazine and methotrexate, have been sufficiently studied to try to answer this question.

Sulfasalazine is the most investigated second-line drug in the field of spondylarthropathy. Four studies clearly mentioned the efficacy of the drug with regard to the clinical presentation of the recruited patients [34–37]. When analyzing the results obtained in studies including patients with and without peripheral articular involvement and when analyzing the results using a dichotomous variable (response to treatment: yes/no), all these studies conclude in favor of sulfasalazine in patients with axial involvement. When analyzing the results obtained in the outcome measurements specifically intended to assess axial involvement (spinal pain, spinal mobility), most of the placebo-controlled studies favor sulfasalazine with an acceptable safety profile. Its action seems to begin after 4–8 weeks of treatment and the plateau of efficacy is obtained only after 12–16 weeks. Therefore, in daily practice, sulfasalazine can be proposed to patients with symptomatic refractory axial involvement with the following guidelines:

The patient has to be informed that sulfasalazine is a slow-acting drug.
Sulfasalazine has to be given in combination with an appropriate NSAID (at least during the first few weeks of treatment).
Sulfasalazine has to be given at least 16 weeks before considering it to be ineffective.

At variance, there are still no data suggesting a disease-modifying effect (i.e., clinical spinal ankylosis and/or radiographic spinal ossification) of sulfasalazine. Therefore, there is no reason systematically to propose such a treatment for a long-term period in patients with axial involvement.

Methotrexate has been investigated in a small number of patients in open controlled studies and has showed clinical improvement in pain and/or spinal mobility [38]. These preliminary results have to be confirmed in other studies including a larger number of patients and a longer duration of follow up.

III. PERIPHERAL ARTICULAR INVOLVEMENT

A. Objective

The objectives of treating potential articular involvement are similar to those of treating axial involvement (e.g., to reduce and/or to prevent the deleterious effects of the three main clinical characteristics of the disease: inflammation, cartilage breakdown, and abnormal postures.

1. Inflammation is not only responsible for the subjective clinical symptoms of inflammatory pain and morning stiffness but also for the objective clinical measurement, synovitis.
2. Cartilage breakdown is the local consequence of synovitis but is not a sys-

tematic phenomenon. Intact cartilage can be observed even after several years of persisting synovitis.

3. Abnormal posture and joint contractures may result from both inflammation and cartilage breakdown.

B. Monitoring

1. Inflammation

Pain. The evaluation of pain due to peripheral articular involvement is similar to that of axial involvement except for pain recorded at physical examination. For this purpose, indexes used to assess rheumatoid arthritis can be of great interest [56].

Inflammation. The evaluation of inflammation due to peripheral articular involvement is similar to that of rheumatoid arthritis (Chapter 19). Several outcome parameters can be of interest for this purpose:

Nocturnal awakening due to pain.
Duration of morning stiffness.
Number of swollen joints.
Nonspecific laboratory markers of inflammation, i.e., erythrocyte sedimentation rate [ESR] and C-reactive protein [CRP].
Several studies suggest that immunoglobulin A serum levels might be of particular interest in the monitoring of spondylarthropathy.

Cartilage Breakdown. Apart from the variables of pain and functional impairment, cartilage breakdown is beast evaluated by radiographic analysis. There is no specific radiographic scale of the cartilage breakdown observed in spondylarthropathy. However, the different radiographic scoring systems used in rheumatoid arthritis might be of interest in spondylarthropathy [57].

Abnormal Posture. Abnormal posture and joint contractures must be detected early; they can develop during a relatively early phase of the disease. This is the case of retracted toe in inflammatory arthritis of the feet and/or hip flexion contracture in the case of hip arthritis.

C. Treatment

Indication of the different therapeutic modalities is based on both the extent of the articular involvement (local therapies are devoted to monoarticular and/or pauciarticular involvement and systemic therapies to polyarticular involvement) and the duration of symptoms (second-line drugs are used for the persisting [at least 3 months] clinical symptoms).

1. Local Therapies

Several different treatments have been proposed and some beneficial effects have been reported in open, uncontrolled studies for each. In increasing order of activity (which in daily practice means in chronological order of administration), the following treatments can be proposed: intra-articular injection of corticosteroids, arthroscopic synovectomy and intra-articular injection of osmic acid, and/or radioactive products. Two particular localizations should be mentioned:

The first localization to consider is hip involvement. Because of the frequency and severity of hip involvement in ankylosing spondylitis, systematic radiographic evaluation of the pelvis has been recommended to be performed every 2 years. However, we must keep in mind that the aim of an early diagnosis of hip involvement is to provide the possibility of administering local therapy in order to prevent chondrolysis due to synovial inflammation. Two arguments are not in favor of such routine radiographic evaluation: (a) there are no data clearly showing that local treatment can be prevent chondrolysis, and (b) it does not seem logical to treat patients without pain. At variance, any unexplained pain in this area requires radiographic evaluation, since it might be difficult to differentiate between hip involvement and pelvic enthesiopathy.

The second localization to consider are the toes. Toes are frequently involved by the disease, especially during reactive arthritis episodes. Retraction of the affected toes is a frequent complication which can occur very quickly. The inflammation due to the disease process usually disappears spontaneously but, the retraction is frequently a disabling sequala. Therefore, toe involvement, even if moderate in terms of inflammation, has to be considered as a therapeutic emergency necessitating local anti-inflammatory treatment (intra-articular injection of corticosteroids) together with physical therapy.

2. *Systemic Therapies*

Quick-acting Drugs. These drugs are similar to those used in the treatment of axial involvement of spondylarthropathy, but there are two differences :

1. The first difference is related to the efficacy of NSAIDs, which are also effective in this indication but to a lesser degree.
2. The second difference, which is at variance, is related to the efficacy of systemic low-dose prednisone (between 5 and 10 mg per day) and might be of interest.

Slow-acting Drugs.

Sulfasalazine. Sulfasalazine was developed and manufactured to cure rheumatoid arthritis by eliminating the then suspected putative cause—group B streptococcal intestinal infection. It has long been accepted as the drug of choice in the treatment of inflammatory bowel disease [58]. After temporary disfavor, sulfasalazine has regained a position as a second-line antirheumatic, disease-modifying drug, mainly through the work of McConkey et al. [59]. Although the stimulus for using sulfasalazine in the treatment of spondylarthropathy did not derive directly from its use in patients with rheumatoid arthritis, there are several arguments for considering it: (a) the common association between inflammatory bowel disease and spondylarthropathy [60]; (b) the description of inflammatory lesions in the ileum of patients with spondylarthropathy [61,62]; and (c) the reported association between a disturbance in bowel flora and ankylosing spondylitis [63]. Much of the rationale postdated the early clinical studies [64]. Since 1984 a number of workers have shown that sulfasalazine may be effective in the treatment of spondylarthropathies. Meta-analysis carried out on five randomized controlled trials [34–36,65,66) suggests that sulfasalazine is a safe and effective drug in the short-term treatment (3–6 months) of ankylosing spondylitis [67].

The mechanism of action of sulfasalazine in ankylosing spondylitis is still unresolved. For example, it is still unclear which of its constituents is the active moiety in spondylarthropathy. Most of an oral dose of sulfasalazine is delivered intact to the distal ileum, where bacterial enzymes reduce the azobound, releasing 5-aminosalicylic acid and sulfapyridine [68]. Most of the sulfapyridine is absorbed, whereas more than 95% of the 5-aminosalicylic acid remains in the lumen and is delivered to the colon. A 24-week controlled study comparing the effects of sulfasalazine 2 g daily, sulfapyridine 1.25 g daily, and 800 mg daily was conducted in 90 patients with active disease [69]. This study supports the conclusion that sulfapyridine is the active moiety of sulfasalazine in spondylarthropathy. In this study, there was also a trend suggesting a better outcome in the sulfasalazine group when compared with sulfapyridine alone. On the other hand, a recently reported open study suggests that olsazaline, a dimer of 5-aminosalicylic acid, might be effective in ankylosing spondylitis [70].

Most of these studies clearly emphasize the fact that the most impressive effects are observed in patients with peripheral articular involvement [37]. However, there are at least three reasons not to prescribe this drug routinely in all patients with peripheral articular involvement: (a) most episodes of articular involvement spontaneously resolve within a few weeks of evolution; (b) most episodes of articular involvement affect only a few joints, and this monoarticular and/or oligoarticular involvement generally responds to local treatment; and (c) the long-term evolution of peripheral articular involvement in spondylarthropathy. One practical problem is management of patients who are in clinical remission after several months of sulfasalazine treatment. In rheumatoid arthritis, it is clear that discontinuation of the drug, in this situation, is usually responsible for a flare of the disease several weeks later. In spondylarthropathy, this is far from the rule. Such a lack of recurrence reflects the heterogeneous evolution and raises the question of the usefulness of continuing the drug in a spondylarthropathy patient who is in clinical remission. In our practice, after a 2-year period of remission, we discontinue the drug and clinically and biologically monitor the patients each month and reinstate sulfasalazine in the case of a flare of the disease.

Antibiotics. Antibiotic treatment is currently being evaluated in patients with reactive arthritis. Microbial material, triggered by Chlamydia, Salmonella, Shigella, or Yersinia, has been demonstrated in the synovium and the synovial fluid of patients with reactive arthritis [71–75]. Intracellular and extracellular particles highly suggestive of Chlamydia have also been found in the joints of some patients with sexually acquired reactive arthritis. Some chlamydial infections can be clinically inapparent and not detectable by standard culture or antibody-based screening methods but can be detected by polymerase chain reactions (PCRs) designed to amplify a conserved region of the major outer membrane protein (MOMP) gene of Chlamydia trachomatis or defied by a molecular hybridization screening system directed toward chlamydial ribosomal RNA. These findings suggest that, at least under some circumstances, potentially viable chlamydiae are present in patients with reactive arthritis/Reiter's syndrome even when they are not detectable by the conventional laboratory screening methods. Such inapparent joint infection with Chlamydia may be critical during the initial development of reactive arthritis, and reactivation of such infection may account in large part for the recurrent episodes of arthritis activity seen in many patients with Reiter's syndrome.

Antibiotic treatment of the triggering infection is recommended if the presence of infection can still be identified after the onset of arthritis. For example, in Yersinia infections, the aim of such antibiotic therapy is to minimize the spread of infection within the patient's family or among close associates. Several studies have demonstrated that short-term antibiotic treatment does not influence the course of postenteric reactive arthritis. It is obvious that once the trigger has been pulled, the chain of events pursues its path. Some studies indicate that long-term antibiotic treatment of Chlamydia-triggered acute reactive arthritis may lead to more rapid recovery and less chronicity [76]. The lack of therapeutic efficacy of antibiotics in postenteric reactive arthritis suggests that a different pathogenetic mechanism may be involved in this form of reactive arthritis or that such antibiotic therapy does not effectively eradicate the enteric pathogens in the gut that trigger reactive arthritis. Antibiotic treatment in order to prevent recurrence is probably of value in Chlamydia-induced reactive arthritis.

Recently, a study of Greenland Eskimos demonstrated that vigorous antibiotic treatment of Chlamydia reinfections significantly reduced relapses of Chlamydia-induced reactive arthritis [77]. The value of antibiotic treatment in chronic forms of reactive arthritis is not yet settled. There are findings suggesting that some benefit is obtained [78]. However, more research with sufficient numbers of patients is still needed.

Other Second-line Drugs. In some spondylarthropathy patients with mainly active peripheral arthritis of chronic duration, second-line drugs currently used in rheumatoid arthritis have been prescribed.

1. Methotrexate. This appears to be the most frequent drug used in this indication, probably owing to its beneficial effect on psoriasis and psoriatic arthritis and its place of choice in the treatment of rheumatoid arthritis. Some anecdotal observations have reported efficacy of this drug on the axial involvement of spondylarthropathy [3,79–81].
2. Gold. No placebo-controlled studies with intramuscular gold salts in spondylarthropathy are available. Some open studies and/or anecdotal observations suggest that in a dosage very similar to that recommended in rheumatoid arthritis, intramuscular gold might produce a significant long-term beneficial effect in only 20% of patients, with a resulting decreased need for general or local corticosteroid treatment, reduction of NSAIDs consumption, and normalization of erythrocyte sedimentation rate. The oral gold compound auranofin was studied in a double-blind placebo-controlled trial of 6 months' duration. No difference in clinical and laboratory variables could be found between treatment with auranofin or placebo [82].
3. Thiol compounds (D-penicillamine, tiopronine). Conflicting reports have been published concerning the efficacy of D-penicillamine in spondylarthropathy. Some anecdotal observations suggest a certain degree of efficacy [83–85]. However, the only placebo-controlled study (of 6 months' duration in 17 patients) failed to demonstrate a significant favorable effect of D-penicillamine [86].
4. Antimalarial Compounds. No controlled studies with antimalarial drugs are available in spondylarthropathy. Several anecdotal observations suggest that antimalarial drugs are of little if any use in the treatment of the articular involvement of spondylarthropathy.

IV. ENTHESIOPATHY

A. Definition

The enthesis is the anatomical site of insertion of a tendon, ligament, or articular capsule into bone. Widespread enthesitis leads to many of the articular and nonarticular manifestations of spondylarthropathy. This preliminary definition is important not only to improve our knowledge of the physiopathology of the disease but also to help us in the daily monitoring of a spondylarthropathy patient. Local and/or region pain occurring in a spondylarthropathy patient reflects enthesiopathy. Moreover, considering this definition, most of the clinical presentations of spondylarthropathy (axial involvement, peripheral articular involvement) might be related to enthesiopathy. In this chapter, we will focus on the monitoring of the most frequent and distinct enthesiopathy; that is, heel pain

B. Objectives

Enthesiopathy is responsible for local inflammation and local bone remodeling.

Inflammation is responsible for the subjective clinical symptoms (i.e., pain).
Bone remodeling is responsible for stiffness and decreased mobility when enthesis is located in particular areas such as the spine. When enthesis is located in other areas such as the heel, whether the clinical symptoms are related to bone remodeling is questionable.

C. Treatment

We will focus on heel pain, keeping in mind that this therapeutic approach can be applied to other localizations of enthesiopathy.

Heel pain due to Achilles enthesiopathy, Achilles bursitis, or plantar fasciitis is the most frequent extravertebral symptom of spondylarthropathy (in our experience, 171 of 441 patients, 38% [87]).

Inferior heel pain is the most frequent (148 of the 171 patients 85%), but it can be associated with posterior heel pain (77 of the 171 patients, 45%). The presence of heel pain is important in considering the diagnosis of spondylarthropathy. However, it requires a specific treatment in only one subgroup of patients (72 of the 171 patients 42%). In these cases, several treatments can be proposed: heel pads, NSAIDs, or local injections of steroids. In our experience, NSAIDs were sufficient to control heel pain in 40 of the 64 patients in whom we used such treatment, and local injection of corticosteroids was considered to be effective in 45 of the 53 patients given such therapy. Even in the case of ineffective therapy, heel pain spontaneously disappeared after a mean duration of 16 $\pm$ 14 months (0.5–60.0 months). Because of this natural benign course, we consider only heel pain persisting after a period of 2 years to be refractory. This was the case in only 11 patients (6%) in our experience: Sulfasalazine was specifically prescribed in 5 patients with a good result in 4. In the patient who failed on sulfasalazine and in four others who complained of chronic and disabling heel pain, local anti-inflammatory radiotherapy was performed with good and definitive results in three and no effect in one patient. Similar good outcome and minimal short-term side effects have also been reported by others [88]. Surgery was proposed to four patients, including the patient who failed on sulfasalazine and who had only transitory benefit from radiotherapy. It was finally not performed, however, because the clinical symptoms completely resolved while surgery was being planned. Good results were obtained from surgery in only one of the three remaining patients.

REFERENCES

1. Arnett FC. Seronegative spondylarthropathies. Bull Rheum Dis 1987; 37:1–12.
2. Moll JMH, Haslock I, MacRae IF, Wright V. Associations between ankylosing spondylitis, psoriatic arthritis. Reiter's disease, the intestinal arthropathies, and Behcet's syndrome. Medicine (Baltimore) 1974; 53:343–364.
3. Dougados M. Diagnosis and monitoring of spondylarthropathy. Compr Ther 1990; 16:52–56.
4. van der Linden S, Valkenburg HA, Cats A. Evaluation of diagnostic criteria for ankylosing spondylitis; a proposal for modification of the New York criteria. Arthritis Rheum 1984; 27:361–368.
4a. Khan MA. Medical and surgical treatment of seronegative spondylarthropathy. Curr Opin Rheumatol 1990; 2:582–599.
4b. Toivanen A, Khan MA. Therapeutic dilemnas in ankylosing spondylitis and related spondylarthropathies. Rheumatol Rev 1994; 3:21–27.
5. Amor B, Dougados M, Mijiyawa M. Critères de classification des spondylarthropathies. Rev Rhum 1990; 57:85–89.
6. Dougados M, van der Linden S, Juhlin R, et al. The European Spondylarthropathy Study Group preliminary criteria for the classification of spondylarthropathy. Artritis Rheum 1991; 34:1218–1227.
7. Calin A. The material history and prognosis of ankylosing spondylitis. J Rheumatol 1985; 15:1054–1055.
8. Amor B, Silva-Santos R, Nahal R, et al. Predictive factors of the long term outcome of spondylarthropathies. J Rheumatol 1994; 21:1883–1887.
9. Rosenbloom D, Brooks P, Bellamy N, Buchanan W. Clinical Trials in the Rheumatic Diseases : A Selected Critical Review. Vol. 1. New York: Praeger, New York, 1985; 262–279.
10. Dougados M, Gueguen A, Nakache JP, et al. Evaluation of a functional index and an in articular index. J Rheumatol 1990; 17:1254–1255.
11. Dougados M, Gaudouen Y, Blan M, et al. Vitesse de sédimentation globulaire et immunoglobulines sériques au cours de la pelvi-spondylite rhumatismale. Rev Rhum Mal Ostéoartic 1987; 54:273–278.
12. Schöber P. The lumbar vertebral column and backache. MMW 1937; 84:336–338.
13. MacRae IF, Wright V. Measurement of back movement. Ann Rheum Dis 1969; 28:584–589.
14. Sturrock R, Wojtulewski JA, Hart FD. Spondylometry in a normal population and in ankylosing spondylitis. Rheumatol Rehabil 1973; 12:135–142.
15. Reynolds PMJ. Three methods of measuring spinal mobility. Rheumatol Rehabil 1975; 14:180–185.
16. Miller MH, Lee P, Smythe A, Goldsmith CH. Measurement of spinal mobility in the sagittal plane: new skin contraction technique compared with established methods. J Rheumatol 1984; 11:507–511.
17. Fisher LR, Cawley MID, Holgate ST. Relation between chest expansion pulmonary function, and exercise tolerance in patients with ankylosing spondylitis. Ann Rheum Dis 1990; 49:921–925.
18. Feltelius N, Hedenstrom H, Hillerdal G, Hallgren R, Pulmonary involvement in ankylosing spondylitis. Ann Rheum Dis 1986; 45:736–740.
19. Revel M, Rondier J, Amor B. Critères de surveillance de la pelvispondylite rhumatismale à moyen et à long terme. in: "La spondylarthrite ankylosante : actualités nosologiques et thérapeutiques" sous la direction de L Simon et C Hérisson. Paris: Masson, 1988:43–48.
20. Taylor HG, Wardle T, Beswick EJ, Dawes PT. The relationship of clinical and laboratory measurements to radiological change in ankylosing spondylitis. Br J Rheumatol 1991; 30:330–335.

21. Dougados M. Les critères d'évolutivité et de sruveillance à court terme de la spondylarthrite ankylosante. In: La Spondylarthrite ankylosante, actualités nosologiques et thérpaeeutiques. Simon L, Herisson C, eds. Paris: Masson, 1988:35–42.
22. Dougados M, Nguyen M, Listrat V, Amor B. Score d'quivalence des anti-inflammatoires non stéroïdiens (AINS). Rev Rhum Mal Osteoartic 1989; 56:276(abstr. H34).
23. Creemers MCW, van't Hof MA, Franssen MJAM, et al. Disease activity in ankylosing spondylitis: selection of a core set of variables and a first step in the development of a disease activity score. In: Clinical and Methodological Studies in Ankylosing Spondyltis, 1995. (in press).
24. Amor B, Dougados M, Listrat V et al. Evaluation des critères de spondylarthropathies d'Amor et de l'European Spondylarthropathy Study Group (ESSG). Une étude transversale de 2228 patients. Ann Med Interne (Paris) 1991; 142:85–89.
25. Dougados M, Nguyen M, Nakache JP, Amor B. Spondylarthrite ankylosante et antiinflammatoires. Concours Médical 1987; 109:2780–2786.
26. Dougados M, Caporal R, Doury P, et al. A double blind cross over placebo controlled trial of ximoprofen in A.S. J Rheumatol 1989; 16, 1167–1169.
27. Dougados M, Nguyen M, Caporal R, et al. Ximoprofen in ankylosing spondylitis: a double blind placebo controlled dose ranging study. Scand J Rheumatol 1994; 23:243–248.
28. Calin A, Grahame R. Double blind crossover trial of flurboprofen and phenylbutazone in ankylosing spondylitis. Br Med J 1974; 4:496–499.
29. Vincent G, David-Chaussee J, Dufour R, Galand F. Enquêtes sur le traitementet le devenir socioprofessionnel des spondylarthropathiques. Rev Rhum Mal Osteoartic 1987; 54:319–324.
30. Boersma JW. Retardation of ossification of the lumbar vertebral column in ankylosing spondylitis by means of phenylbutazone. Scand J Rheumatol 1976; 5:60–64.
31. Revel M, Listrat V, Chevalier X, et al. Facet joint block for low back pain: identifying predictors of a good response. Arch Phys Med Rehabil 1992; 73:824–828.
32. Maugars Y, Mathis C, Horreard F et al. Etude en double aveugle contre placebo de la corticothérapie intra-sacroïliaque: efficacité dans les sacroïliites rhumatismales. Rev Rhum 1992; 59:607.
33. Peters ND, Ejstrup L. Intravenous methylprednisolone pulse therapy in ankylosing spondylitis. Scand J Rheumatol 1992; 21:134–138.
34. Dougados M, Boumier P, Amor B. Sulphasalazine in ankylosing spondylitis: A double blind controlled study in 60 patients. Br Med H 1986; 293:911–914.
35. Feltelius N, Hallgren R. Sulphasalazine in ankylosing spondylitis. Ann Rheum Dis 1986; 45:396–399.
36. Nissila M, Lehtinen K, Leirisalo-Repo M et al. Sulphasalazine in the treatment of ankylosing spondylitis. Arthritis Rheum 1988; 31:1111–1116.
37. Dougados M, van der Linden S, Leirisalo-Repo M, et al. Sulfasalazine: a randomized multicentre, double-blind, placebo-controlled study. Arthritis Rheum 1995 (in press).
38. Bosi Ferraz M, Carrica da Silva H, Atra E. Low dose methotrexate with leucovorin rescue in ankylosing spondylitis. J Rheumatol 1991; 18:146–147.
39. Kraag G, Stokes B, Groh J, et al. The effects of comprehensive home physiotherapy and supervision on patients with ankylosing spondylitis. A randomized controlled trial. J Rheumatol 1990; 17:228–233.
40. Roberts WN, Larson MG, Liang MH, et al. Clarke AK. Sensitivity of anthropometric techniques for clinical trials in ankylosing spondylitis. Br J Rheumatol 1989; 28:40–45.
41. Hidding A, van der Linden S, de Witte L. Therapeutic effects of individual physical therapy in ankylosing spondylitis related to duration of disease. Clin Rheumatol 1993; 12:334–340.
42. Hidding A, van der Linden S, Boers M, et al. Is group physical therapy superior to individualized therapy in ankylosing spondylitis? A randomized controlled trial. Arthritis Care Res 1993; 6:117–125.

43. Vitanen JV, Suni J, Kautiainen H, et al. Effect of physiotherapy on spinal mobility in ankylosing spondylitis. Scand J Rheumatol 1992; 21:38–41.
44. Bulstrode SJ, Barefoot J, Harrison RA, Clarke AK. The role of passive stretching in the treatment of ankylosing spondylitis. Br J Rheumatol 1987; 26:40–42.
45. White AA, Panjabi MM. Spinal braces: functional analysis and clinical applications. In: Clinical Biomechanics of the Spine. 2nd ed. Philadelphia: JB Lippincott, 1990:475–509.
46. Revel M, Rondier J, Amor B. Intérêt d'une orthèse de courbure lombaire dans le traitement de la pelvispondylite rhumatismale. In: La spondylarthrite ankylosante: actualitiés nosologiques et thérapeutiques sous la direction de L Simon et C Hérisson. Paris: Masson, 1988:155–159.
47. Court Brown WM, Abbatt JD. The incidence of leukæmia in ankylosing spondylitis treated with X-rays. A preliminary report. Lancet, 1955; 1:1283–1285.
48. Graham DC. Leukemia following x-ray therapy for ankylosing spondylitis. Arch Intern Med 1960; 105:51–59.
49. Desmarais MHL. Radiotherapy in arthritis. Ann Rheum Dis 1953; 12:25–28.
50. Sharp J, Easson EC. Deep x-ray therapy in spondylitis. Br Med J 1954; 13:619–623.
51. Wilkinson M, Bywaters EGL. Clinical features and course of ankylosing spondylitis. Ann Rheum Dis 1958; 17:209–228.
52. Kaprove RE, Little AH, Graham DC. Ankylosing spondylitis. Survival in men with and without radiotherapy. Arthritis Rheum 1980; 23:57–61.
53. Delikan O. Preparation of ^{224}Ra for therapy of ankylosing spondylitis. Health Phys 1978; 35:21–24.
54. Koch W, Reske W. Die Ergebnisse der intravenösen Thorium X-Behandlung bei der Spondylarthritis ankylopoetica (M. Bechterew). Strahlentherpiie 1952; 82:439–457.
55. Chmelevsky D, Hays CW, Spiess H, et al. An epidemiological assessment of lens opacifications that improved vision in patients injected with radium 224. Radiat Res 1988; 115:238–257.
56. Smolen JS, Breedveld FC, Eberl G, et al. Validity and reliability of the twenty-eight joint counts: development and validation in a prospective longitudinal study of patients with rheumatoid arthritis. Arthritis Rheum 1994; 38:44–48.
57. van der Heidje DM, van Riel PL, Nuver-Zwart IH, et al. Effects of hydroxychloroquine and sulphasalazine on progression of joint damage in rheumatoid arthritis. Lancet 1989; 1:1036–1038.
58. Peppercorn MA. Sulphasalazine : Pharmacology, clinical use, toxicity and related new drug development. Ann Intern Med 1984; 3:377–386.
59. McConkey B, Amos RS, Durham S, et al. Sulphasalazine in rheumatoid arthritis. Br Med J 1980; 280:442–444.
60. Moll JMH. Pathogenic mechanism of B27 related seronegative polyarthritis: interplay between genetic and environmental factors. Clin Exp Rheum 1987; 5(Suppl 1):7–14.
61. Mielants R, Veys EM. Inflammation of the ileum in patients with B27 positive reactive arthritis. Lancet 1984; 1:288.
62. Dougados M, Alemanni M, Tulliez M, et al. Ileocolonoscopie systématique au cours des spondylo-arthropathies séronégatives. Rev Rhum Mal Osteoartic 1987; 54:279–283.
63. Ebringer RW, Cawdwell DR, Cowling P, Ebringer A. Sequential studies in anlylosing spondylitis. Association of Klebsellia pneumoniæ with active disease. Ann Rhum Dis 1979; 37:145–151.
64. Amor B, Kahan A, Dougados M, Delrieu F. Sulphasalazine in ankylosing spondylitis. Ann Intern Med 1984; 101:878.
65. Prieur AM, Listrat V, Dougados M, Amor B. Critères de classification des spondylarthropathies chez les enfants. Arch Fr Pediatr 1993; 50:379–385.
66. Corkill MM, Jabanputra P, Gilbson T, MacFarlane DG. A controlled trial of sulphasalazine

treatment of chronic ankylosing spondylitis: failure to demonstrate a clinical effect. Br J Rheumatol 1990; 9:41–45.
67. Ferraz MB, Tugwell P, Goldsmith CH, Atra E. Metanalysis of sulphasalazine in ankylosing spondylitis. J Rheumatol 1990; 17:1481–1488.
68. Dougados M. Sulphasalazine in rheumatic disease. Agents Actions 1993; 44(Suppl):197–201.
69. Taggart AJ, Gardiner PV, McEvoy FM. et al. Which is the active moiety of sulphasalazine in ankylosing spondylitis? Arthritis Rheum 1994; 37:S354(abstr. 1159).
70. Chapman CM, Zwillich SH. Olsalazine in ankylosing spondylitis: a pilot study. J Rheumatol 1994; 21:1699–1701.
71. Granfors K, Jalkanen S, von Essen R, et al. Yersinia antigens in synovial-fluid cells from patients with reactive arthritis. N Engl J Med 1989; 320:216–221.
72. Granfors K, Jalkanen S, Lindberg AA, et al. Salmonella lipopolysaccharide in synovial cells from patients with reactive arthritis. Lancet 1990; 335:685–688.
73. Keat A. Thomas B. Dixey HJ, et al. Chlamydia trachomatis and reactive arthritis—the missing link. Lancet 1987; 1:72–74.
74. Hammer M, Zeidler H, Klimsa S, et al. Yersinia enterocolitica in the synovial membrane of patients with Yersiniainduced arthritis. Arthritis Rheum 1990; 33:1795–1800.
75. Granfors K, Jalkanen S, Toivanen P, et al. Bacterial lipopolysaccharide in synovial fluid cells in shigella triggered reactive arthritis. J Rheumatol 1992; 19:500.
76. Lauhio A, Leirisalo-Repo M, Lähdevirta J, et al. Double-blind, placebo-controlled study of three-month treatment with lymecycline in reactive arthritis, with special reference to Chlamydia arthritis. Arthritis Rheum 1991; 34:6–14.
77. Bardin T, Enel C, Cornelis F, et al. Antibiotic treatment of venereal disease and Reiter's syndrome in a Greenland population. Arthritis Rheum 1992; 35:190–194.
78. Toivanen A, Yli-Kerttula T, Luukkainen R, et al. Effect of antimicrobial treatment on chronic reactive arthritis. Clin Exp Rheumatol 1993; 11:301–307.
79. Handler RP. Favorable results using methotrexate in treatment of patients with ankylosing spondylitis. Arthritis Rheum 1989; 32:234.
80. Yamane K, Saito C, Natsuda H, et al. Ankylosing spondylitis successfully treated with methotrexate. Intern Med 1993; 32:53–56.
81. Sampaios-Barros PD, Costallat LTL, Fernandes SRM, et al. The use of methotrexate in the treatment of ankylosing spondylitis: pilot study. Rev Esp Reumatol 1993; 20 (Suppl 1):485.
82. Grasedyck K, Schattenkirchner M, Bandilla K. Zur Behandlung der Spondylitis ankylosans mit Auranofin (Ridaura). Z Rheumatol 1990; 49:98–99.
83. Scharf Y, Nahir M. Penicillamine in ankylosing spondylitis. Arthritis Rheum 1976; 19:122.
84. Bird HA, Dixon ASJ. Failure of d-penicillamine to affect peripheral joint involvement in ankylosing spondylitis or HLA-B27-associated arthropathy. Ann Rheum Dis 1977; 36:289.
85. Jaffe IA. Penicillamine in seronegative polyarthritis. Ann Rheum Dis 1977; 36:593–594.
86. Steven MM, Morrison M, Sturrock RD. Penicillamine in ankylosing spondylitis: a double blind placebo controlled trial. J Rheumatol 1985; 12:735–737.
87. Ebringer RW, Cawdwell DR, Cowling P, Ebringer A. Sequential studies in ankylosing spondylitis. Association of Klebsellia pneumoniæ with active disease. Ann Rhum Dis 1979; 37:145–151.
88. Dougados M, Contreras L, Maetzel A, Amor B. Les talalgies des spondylarthropathies: présentation clinique et traitement. Rev Rhum Mal Osteoartic 1992; 59:611(abstr. A12).

22
Therapy of Systemic Rheumatic Disorders in Children

Anne-Marie Prieur
Hôpital des Enfants-Malades, Paris, France

I. INTRODUCTION

There are several reasons why it can be more difficult to use a given drug in children with rheumatic conditions than in adults with these conditions. Some drugs have not been granted a license for pediatric use, and many formulations are unsuitable for very small children. Also, certain drugs have specific side effects in children. Finally, the pharamacokinetics of a product can differ in very young children. However, all drug classes used in rheumatology can be given to children as long are the risks are borne in mind and treatment is closely monitored.

After reviewing the different products used in pediatrics, we will describe their indications according to the various rheumatic diseases, focusing on the three forms of juvenile arthritis chronic (JCA), spondylarthropathies, systemic lupus erythematosus (SLE), polydermatomyositis, and vasculitides.

II. THE DIFFERENT DRUGS

A. Nonsteroidal Anti-inflammatory Drugs

Acetylsalicyclic acid has been the first licensed product for children of all ages. Other nonsteroidal anti-inflammatory drugs (NSAIDs), such as diclofenac, naproxen, and ibuprofen, can be used in most countries. But legal recommendations are not uniform, and some drugs can be available in some countries for pediatric use and not in others.

1. Acetylsalicyclic Acid

Acetylsalicyclic acid (ASA) is available in many different formulations, meaning that the unit dose per kilogram is easy to prepare (Table 1).

Recommended Doses. These vary according to the indication. They are generally 60–80 mg/kg daily for nonfebrile conditions and 100–120 mg/kg daily for highly febrile

Table 1 Nonsteroidal Anti-inflammatory Drugs (NSAIDs)

Drug	Dose
Acetyl salicylic acid	50–100 mg/kg/d (max 4 g)
Naproxen	15–20 mg/kg/d (max 1.5 g)
Ibuprofen	40–60 mg/kg/d (max 2.4 g)
Kétoprofen	3–5 mg/kg/d (max 300 mg)
Fenoprofen	40–50 mg/kg/d (max 3.2 g)
Flurbiprofen	3–4 mg/kg/d (max 300 mg)
Diclofenac	2–3 mg/kg/d (max 200 mg)
Sulindac	4–6 mg/kg/d (max 400 mg)
Meclofenamate	4–7 mg/kg/d (max 300 mg)
Piroxicam	0.3 mg/kg/d
Indometacin	1–3 mg/kg/d (max 200 mg)
Tolmetin	20–30 mg/kg/d (max 1.8 mg)

systemic forms. The daily dose is divided into three or four fractions for nonfebrile forms but is given every 4 h (even during the night) for systemic forms.

Blood salicylate levels must not exceed 150–200 mg/L 2 h after ASA intake, as there is otherwise a risk of salicylate intoxication. Various factors can influence blood salicylate concentrations. The plateau is reached after about 10 days. At high doses, even a minor change in dose can considerably modify the blood salicylate level. An increase in urinary pH increases ASA clearance; this occurs, for example, with aluminum- and magnesium hydroxide–containing antacids. Urinary excretion increases 10-fold when the pH rises from 5.5 to 8.0 [1]. Absorption is slowed when ASA is taken with a meal. The hypoalbuminemia associated with inflammatory diseases increases the volume of distribution. Combination with steroids cuts blood salicylate levels by one-third [2]. Serum levels, however, only reflect the overall extracellular concentration of salicylate, not the bound fraction (especially that diffusing through the tissues). As a result, a low blood salicylate value does not necessarily reflect low tissue concentrations. It is thus possible to obtain a satisfactory clinical effect despite an apparently inadequate blood salicylate level. In contrast, a blood salicylate level approaching 200–250 mg/L may point to overdose and a risk of intoxication.

Side Effects. The practitioner must be on the lookout for adverse effects during long-term and high-dose ASA therapy. Parents must also be informed of the clinical signs of intolerance.

Certain side effects are dose dependent, such as hearing loss and tinnitus, behavioral changes (irritability), polypnea (not to be confused with polypnea due to pericarditis), nausea, and vomiting.

Most of these side effects are independent of the dose.

Allergic reactions are rare, and usually consist of a urticarial rash or exceptionally anaphylactic shock.

A bleeding tendency can arise because of the bruise inhibition of platelet aggregation; children in whom this is present will, for example, bruise easily while playing. Epistaxis and occasionally severe gastrointestinal bleeding can also occur.

Gastrointestinal manifestations appear to be less frequent in children than in adults. Gastric irritation is relatively mild and can occur at the beginning of treatment, generally resolving after a few days. Occult bleeding is probably fairly frequent. Iron supplementation has been shown to increase low hemoglobin levels during ASA therapy of JCA [3]. Certain ASA preparations, especially enteric-coated forms and salicylates, reduce the risk of side effects. Antacids reduce blood loss but also diminish blood salicylate levels by increasing urinary pH. Cimetidine is exempt from these problems. Marked bleeding is rare, and it is due to local lesions and the anticoagulant effect of aspirin.

Renal toxicity is very rare, and consists of papillary and tubular necrosis [4].

Hepatotoxicity must be watched for closely during ASA therapy in children with JCA. Liver damage can be reflected by a simple increase in transaminase activity, which is fairly frequent. A concomitant fall in the prothrombin time requires ASA to be withdrawn [5] to avoid the danger of complex manifestations with a hemorrhagic syndrome reminiscent of intravascular coagulation, together with hepatic and neurological signs; some specialists consider that these manifestations correspond to Reye's syndrome. In fact, the syndrome resembles certain rare familial syndromes affecting the monocyte lineage, such as the Chédiak-Higashi syndrome in the accelerated phase and familial lymphohistiocytosis. Owing to these similarities, this syndrome in JCA should be named "macrophage activation syndrome" (MAS). These complications, which are not always associated with elevated blood salicylate levels, were recently reviewed [5,7].

B. Other NSAIDs

Table 1 shows the NSAID doses in pediatric indications. In general, their action is similar to that of aspirin, and their tolerability is often better. In addition, their mode of administration (two to three daily doses) improves compliance with treatment. The few available pharmacokinetic studies in older children have shown only minor differences with adults; the half-life in synovial fluid is longer than in plasma [8]. In contrast, noteworthy differences have been found in infants [9]. NSAIDs are usually rapidly effective, but some investigators have found that they only act after several weeks [10].

The most frequent side effects are gastrointestinal (mainly abdominal pain), cutaneous (urticaria, rash, and hypersensitivity [11]), and hematological (anemia). Rare cases of renal damage and central nervous system disorders (headache and dizziness) have been reported. Allergic reactions can also occur. The main side effects of NSAIDs in children are summarized in Table 2, which is based on 427 therapeutic sequences [12].

C. Slow-acting Antirheumatic Drugs

In pediatric rheumatic diseases, the most used slow-acting antirheumatic drugs (SAARDs) are gold salts and D-penicillamine. Other thiole derivatives can be used, such as tioponine and sulfasalazine. Synthetic antimalarials are occasionally used to treat children, at least in France. These treatments all take several weeks to act and carry a risk of side effects that are now well documented in adults. Their use in children must take account of age and the clinical form. An improvement is usually observed during the first 6 months, and there is no point in continuing treatment if no result is obtained after this period.

Table 3 summarizes the main preparations and their doses and side effects.

Table 2 Side Effects Observed with NSAIDs in 427 Therapeutic Sequences

	Increased transaminases 100%	Anemia 100%	Blood in hematuria 100%	Stools 100%	Proteinuria 100%
Aspirin	25	-	1.4	-	-
Tolmétin	-	2.2	-	1.1	-
Naproxen	5.7	3.8	1.1	-	-
Fenoprofen	-	6.5	6.5	6.4	4.3
Ibuprofen	-	3.0	3.0	-	-
Others	-	4.3	7.1	-	2.4

Source: After ref. 12.

Several prospective studies have been carried out in the pediatric setting. D-penicillamine has been the subject of three comparative trials, which yielded somewhat contradictory results. A French study comparing D-penicillamine with a placebo showed that the active drug had a degree of efficacy [13], whereas an American-Russian study comparing D-penicillamine, hydroxychloroquine, and a placebo showed no difference in efficacy or tolerability among the three groups [14]. The frequency of side effects in these two studies was acceptable, whereas a Norwegian team reported side effects

Table 3 Slow-acting Antirheumatic Drugs (SAARDs) in Pediatric Rheumatic Diseases

Drug	Dose	Side effects
Gold salts (intramuscular)	Weekly: 1/2 mg, then 1 mg/kg Monthly: 1 mg/kg	Rash Cytopenia Bone marrow aplasia MAS at the second injection in the systemic forms
Auranofin (oral)	0.5 mg/kg/d (max 9 mg)	Diarrhea Same as above but weaker
D-penicillamine (oral)	5, then 10, then 15 mg/kg/day	Rash Cytopenia Proteinuria Pneumopathy Autoimmunity: myasthenia, lupus
Tiopronine (oral)	10, then 20 mg/kg/day	Same as D-penicillamine
Sulfasalazine (oral)	20–30 mg/kg/day	Rash Cytopenia Increased transaminases Neurological complications in systemics
Hydroxychloroquine (oral)	5–7 mg/kg/day (max 200 mg)	Retinopathy Cutaneous symptoms Neuropathies Cytopenia

MAS, macrophage-activation syndrome.

in 25% of patients on D-penicillamine in a comparative study with gold salts [15]. Certain studies indicate that gold salts given by the oral route are more beneficial than a placebo [16], an effect that persists beyond 5 years [17].

Among the thiol derivatives, tiopronine had similar efficacy and tolerability to D-penicillamine in a personal study. Several pediatric trials of sulfasalazine have been done. Sulfasalazine appears to be beneficial in certain forms, especially spondylarthropathies [18], but it is poorly effective in systemic JCA [19], in which very serious side effects can be observed [20].

Published results on SAARDs are mediocre (Table 4). A meta-analysis of 6-month efficacy on disease activity confirmed the lack of spectacular improvements (Giannini). In addition, most of these studies did not distinguish between the different forms of JCA. There is no evidence that combinations of SAARDs are effective in children.

D. Intraveneous Immunoglobulins

The efficacy of IV immunoglobulin in certain autoimmune manifestations, especially those of idiopathic thrombocytopenic purpura and Kawasaki's disease [21], together with their effect on various autoimmune diseases [22], has led to trials in systemic JCA [23,24]. Their tolerability is excellent, but the very high cost of this treatment (generally used at 1 g/kg/injection) and the lack of concrete proof of efficacy mean that the results of placebo-controlled trials should be awaited before extending the indications.

E. Steroids

Steroids a very powerful tool but often have unacceptable side effects in children. They can be given systemically or locally.

1. Systemic Steroids

Systemic steroids can be used at a daily dose of up to 2 mg/kg/day prednisone, or at a low dose of <0.5 mg/kg/day, or as an alternate-day therapy, or as an intravenous bolus of 30 mg/kg methylprednisolone. Table 5 shows the different forms of systemic steroids and their equivalence. Forms not inducing marked sodium retention are preferred for children.

The side effects of systemic steroids are still the main problem in pediatric use. Rapid weight gain can only be avoided by a strict diet, which must be not only sodium free but also poor in slow resorption carbohydrates. The most troublesome cutaneous side effects are indelible striae, but these appear to be rare when weight gain is controlled by dieting. Arterial hypertension and diabetes can develop. Osteoporosis can lead to very painful vertebral collapse which necessitates immobilization in a corset. The use of deflazacort, available in some countries, apparently lessens the impact of steroids on bone metabolism [25]. Aseptic joint necrosis, especially of the hips, is far from rare and complicates underlying diseases that can also involve the joints. The onset of steroid-induced cataracts must be watched for closely. Finally, above all in children, daily steroid therapy arrests growth. This is overcome by alternate-day dosing when possible [26].

2. Local Steroid Therapy

Local steroid therapy can be applied to the joints and eyes.

Table 4 Results of SAARDs in Juvenile Chronic Arthritis

Drugs	No. of patients	Type of study	Results VG/G 100%	M 100%	N 100%	W 100%	Side effects[a] 100%	Ref.
D-penicillamine 10–30 mg/kg/day	235	Open retrospective	49	28	23	-	12	65
D-penicillamine 15–30 mg/kg/day	26	Open comparative	69	-	-	8	21	
Gold salts	24	(1st choice)	62	-	-	20	17	66
D-penicillamine 10 mg/kg/day	24	Open	33	16	16	10	25	
Gold salts 0.7 mg/kg/wk	23	Open comparative	40	31	16	0	13	67
Hydroxychloroquine 5 mg/kg/day	25		40	31	25	4	0	
D-penicillamine 10 mg/kg/day	54		26	-	28	16	18	
Hydroxychloroquine 6 mg/kg/day	57	Double-blind comparative	72	-	26	2	27	14
Placebo	51		53	-	41	6	18	
D-penicillamine 10 mg/kg/day	38	Double-blind comparative	60	5	7	3	5	13
Placebo	36		40	3	12	11	0	
Auranofin 0.5–0.20 mg/kg/day	231	Double-blind comparative	69	-	-	-	30	7
Placebo			60	-	-	-	15	

VG, very good; G, good; M, mild; N; Nil; W, worse.
[a]Side effects leading to withdrawal.

Table 5 Various Steroid Preparations

	Anti-inflammatory effect	Dose (mg) (equivalent)	Sodium-retaining potency	Half-life (h)
Cortisone	0.8	25	++	8–12
Hydrocotrisone	1	20	++	8–12
Deflazacort	4	6	+	1.5
Prednisone	4	5	+	12–36
Prednisolone	4	5	+	12–36
Methylprednisolone	5	4	0	12–36
Triamcinolone	5	4	0	12–36
Dexamethasone	20–30	0.75	0	36–54
Betamethasone	20–30	0.6	0	36–54

Intra-articular steroid injections have totally modified the prognosis of oligoarticular forms of JCA. Among the many available products, only triamcinolone hexacetonide gives satisfactory results. It is fairly caustic and must thus be used with care to avoid local complications (mainly cutaneous atrophy at the injection site).

These products are simple to apply to large joints such as the knee, but general anesthesia may be necessary before treating small and/or tight joints, especially in the very young child. There is no lower age limit for this type of treatment, as long as the precautions for use are respected; this also means that an experienced practitioner must treat the joints of small children. In general, the volume injected must be adapted to the volume of the joint, and the product must not be injected "under pressure." The joint must be rested with a splint for 3 days. Complications are rare and mainly consist of cutaneous atrophy at the injection site or untroublesome intra-articular calcifications. Needless to say that the important causticity of this preparation contraindicates it for injection of tendon sheaths where only hydrosoluble steroids can be used.

In regard to the eyes, uveitis, a very frequent complication of oligoarticular forms of JCA with antinuclear antibodies, is treated with steroid-based eye drops and mydriatic agents.

F. "Immunomodulatory" Treatments

Immunomodulatory treatments may be of value in severe forms of JCA. However, their efficacy is often difficult to appreciate objectively because of the small number of sound, prospective, multicenter trials. Too many specialists continue to use a given treatment in "selected cases," meaning that the results are uninterpretable. Ideally, as in oncology, multicenter protocols should be established to accelerate the assessment of the efficacy and tolerability of experimental treatments.

1. Methotrexate

Methotrexate (MTX) is one of the most widely used immunomodulatory treatments. The use of MTX in children with rheumatic diseases was proposed when its efficacy and acceptable tolerability were established in adults [27]. The recommended dose is 10 mg/m^2/week [28], but certain investigators use higher doses for particularly resistant forms [29].

The tolerability of MTX in children is acceptable [30,31]. Combination with NSAIDs can increase MTX blood levels [32]. A few cases of severe liver damage have been reported [33]. Side effects, which are generally mild, must be sought for every month or two. Most patients (almost 30%) show an increase in transaminase levels. Values usually return to normal when the dose is reduced or treatment is suspended. Nausea is fairly frequent immediately after MTX intake after a few months of treatment, and these patients may benefit from a switch to the intramuscular route. Oral aphthae, cytopenia, and pulmonary manifestations are rarely observed.

MTX seems to have clear efficacy in some cases, especially certain forms of JCA. Systemic forms appear to be less sensitive than polyarticular forms with antinuclear antibodies (ANAs) [34,35]. A European multicenter double-blind trial is underway to confirm this notion. MTX is classically indicated for dermatomyositis [36].

2. Azathioprine

Azathioprine (AZ), 2.0–2.5 mg/kg/day is used by certain specialists in the treatment of JCA. Its tolerability is acceptable. The long-term risk of cancer must, however, be borne in mind, and this means that the product should only be used in severe cases [37]. In JCA, AZ appears to be a little more effective than a placebo [38]. Certain investigators consider it to be effective in lupus-associated kidney involvement [39].

3. Alkylating Agents

Alkylating agents can be used when "classic" treatments fail to control disease progression in JCA and in the case of life-threatening visceral involvement.

Chlorambucil. The use of chlorambucil at a maximum dose of 0.2 mg/kg/day leads to a very significant reduction in disease activity. However, a personal series of 40 children revealed a very high mutagenic risk [40], and we thus only recommend this treatment for life-threatening complications such as secondary amylosis in JCA [41,42].

Cyclophosphamide. This is mainly used at a dose of 500–1000 mg/m^2 as an intravenous bolus every 3–6 weeks rather than as a daily oral dose. This form of administration, which must only be used in the hospital setting with forced diuresis, has fewer side effects, especially alopecia and hemorrhagic cystitis. Few trials have so far been published. A study of systemic forms of JCA requires confirmation [43]. The value of cyclophosphamide for lupus-associated kidney involvement has been confirmed in children [44], but efficacy appears to tail off after a few years [45]. Cyclophosphamide is indicated for diffuse forms of polyarteritis nodosa with visceral involvement, which is rare in children [46].

4. Cyclosporine A

Cyclosporine A is effective in adult rheumatoid arthritis at doses below 5 mg/kg/day [27]. Studies involving JCA patients have failed to show marked improvements [47], but further trials are required. In contrast, cyclosporine may be of value in macrophage-activation syndromes [7]. Some specialists consider it to be more effective than MTX in dermatomyositis [48], and this is borne out by our experience.

The pediatric side effects of cyclosporine A are identical to those observed in adults.

5. Plasma Exchanges and Lymphocyte Depletion

Plasma exchanges and lymphocyte depletion are both technically complex and costly in children, whereas the long-term benefit is often disappointing [49]. These approaches should be reserved as emergency treatments for neurological or renal manifestations of SLE [50].

III. THERAPEUTIC INDICATIONS IN THE MAIN CHILDHOOD INFLAMMATORY AND AUTOIMMUNE DISEASES

A. Juvenile Chronic Arthritis

Juvenile chronic arthritis can have three types of onset: systemic (20%), polyarticular (30%), and oligoarticular (50%) [54]. JCA covers a wide range of pathophysiological conditions that differ in terms of their response to various treatments, and also in the side effects with which they are associated. The main therapeutic indications are summarized in Table 6.

1. Systemic Forms

Systemic forms of JCA are highly febrile, affect very young children, and can spare the joints at the onset. They are characterized by a certain difficulty in controlling clinical manifestations (with the exception of steroid therapy) and by a high risk of therapeutic side effects. In France, where very few NSAIDs have been licensed for use in children with low body weights, our therapeutic approach is as follows.

NSAID Therapy Starting in the Hospital. The most commonly used NSAID in this setting is acetylsalicyclic acid (ASA) at a high dose of 100 mg/kg/day in six fractions (even at night). Doses of 110–120 mg/kg can be reached gradually as long as tolerability is satisfactory. The total daily dose must not exceed 4 g. The effect on pain is often rapid, whereas fever abates more slowly. There are no noteworthy effects on laboratory parameters [2]. This treatment can be continued for several months at home if it is effective and well tolerated. It is very important for the parents to be warned of potential side effects, and they must be able to call a physician immediately if problems arise.

In our experience, 50% of children under 5 years of age initially respond to this treatment. Other NSAIDs can be used to treat older children. Although not used in France until the age of 15 years, indomethacin is effective and shows acceptable tolerability in the older child. There have been anecdotal reports of efficacy with other NSAIDs in systemic forms of JCA [51,52]. In principle, two NSAIDs should not be combined given the increased risk of a macrophage-activation syndrome [53]. However, in cases of morning stiffness on aspirin only, indomethacin at a dose of 1–2 mg/kg/day, taken in the evening, can improve the patient's comfort.

Steroid Therapy. At a dose of 2 mg/kg/day, prednisone or equivalent orally is indicated if NSAIDs are totally ineffective after appropriate treatment (at least 1 month) or if intolerance or pericarditis arises. Once started, steroids are continued for several months, as all attempts to reduce the dose rapidly or to switch to alternate-day dosing are doomed to fail. An NSAID can be added to the steroid regimen. It should be remembered that blood salicylate levels are cut by one-third during steroid therapy. Steroids have a spectacular effect on all clinical and biological manifestations, but this benefit is only obtained at high doses, which also carry a risk of severe adverse effects. Their effect is purely suspensive and in no way appears to prevent progression to severe arthritis. Some specialists have proposed using bolus methylprednisolone [54].

Table 6 Main Therapeutic Indications in Juvenile Systemic Rheumatic Diseases

	ASA	NSAIDs	Corticosteroids		Gold salts	THIO. DER.	SLZ	Antimalarial
			General	Local				
Systemic-JCA	+++	+	+++	-	-	-	-	-
RF^+ polyarthritis	+	+++	+	++	+++	+++	+	++
RF^- polyarthritis	+	+++	+	++	+	+	-	+
Oligoarthritis	+	+	-	+++	-	-	-	-
Spondytoarihritis	+	+++	-	+++	+	+	+++	+
SLE	-	-	+++	-	-	-	-	++
Polydermatomyositis	-	-	+++	-	-	-	-	-
Kawasaki's disease	+	-	-	-	-	-	-	-
Cutaneous PAN	+	+	+++	-	-	-	-	-
Periarteritis nodosa	+	+	+++	-	-	-	-	-

ASA, acetylsalicylic acid; NSAIDs, nonsteroidal anti-inflammatory drugs; MTX, methotrexate; CYA, cyclosporine A; CHX, cyclophosphamide; JCA, juvenile chronic arthritis; RF^+, rheumatoid factor positive; RF^-, rheumatoid factor negative; SLE, systemic lupus erythematosus.

SAARDs. These are rarely active in systemic forms of JCA [55], and they may even be dangerous (especially gold salts) [53,56]. Serious adverse effects have been reported with levamisole [57] and sulfasalazine [20].

Intravenous Immunoglobulins. These are less active than in Kawasaki's disease [21]. Certain specialists suggests that they reduce steroid requirements in the systemics [24], but this requires confirmation in prospective, double-blind studies.

Immunomodulators. The effect of methotrexate is controversial in this setting, but is probably less marked than in some other forms of JCA [35]. There is no formal evidence that heavy immunosuppressive treatments are effective in the systemic forms, but multicenter trials are warranted in severe systemic forms despite the risk of side effects. An anecdotal report reflects the difficulty in controlling this disease. High-dose chemotherapy was administered for a year to a child with a misdiagnosis of malignant histiocytosis. When the correct diagnosis—systemic JCA—was finally made and therapy was switched to more "classic" means, the multiple-drug regimen failed to halt progression of the basic disease [58].

2. Polyarticular Forms

Polyarticular forms of JCA no doubt comprise several entities. Forms with rheumatoid factor (RF^+) (10% of all polyarticular forms) are generally distinguished from other forms (RF^-).

NSAIDs. These are the first-line treatment of choice; there is a fairly wide choice, as these forms mainly affect older children.

SAARDs. These are rapidly indicated in RF^+ forms given their rapid progression. The indications in these forms are similar to those in adults. As regards RF^- forms, the response varies according to the degree of clinical and biological inflammation. It appears that a subcategory of "dry" juvenile arthritis is particularly resistant to all available drugs [59].

Systemic Steroid Therapy. This is rarely indicated in these forms. However, steroids at daily doses of less than 5 mg/day or alternate-day therapy may improve these patients' comfort. Intra-articular injections can improve the function of a severely affected joint.

Immunomodulators. Among the immunomodulators, only methotrexate is indicated, mainly for RF^+ forms.

3. Oligoarticular Forms

NSAIDs. These are prescribed routinely, but they have more of an analgesic than an anti-inflammatory effect. As these forms of JCA are generally associated with little pain, we usually discontinue NSAIDs if the parents observe no effect.

Local Treatments. These have totally modified the prognosis of these forms of JCA. As soon as a joint remains inflamed for 6–8 weeks, we inject triamcinolone hexacetonide (THX). It is important to treat the inflamed knee of very small children early to avoid the risk of flexion contracture with posterior subluxation of the tibia, which can occur abruptly. Treatment must be given to young children under general anesthesia and be accompanied by physical therapy (traction), which can only be administered in pediatric orthopedic units with experience with these diseases. Local treatments give very good results on larger joints, but are less effective on tighter and more complex joints such as those of the feet and hands. The injected dose should be adapted to the volume of the joint.

Ophthalmologic Involvment. This is closely associated with circulating ANAs. The presence of ANAs calls for routine ophthalmological examination for iridocyclitis every 3–4 months for several years. Iridocyclitis occurs in about 30 and 50% of cases after 5 and 10 years, respectively, even in the absence of articular progression [60]. Ocular involvement is tenacious and thus calls for local eye-drop treatment, steroids, and mydriatic agents for several months or years. The lack of appropriate treatment can lead to cataracts and band keratopathy. Alternate-day systemic steroids can be used in some cases if local treatment fails to control ocular inflammation.

SAARDs. These are not indicated for these forms of JCA, as they are poorly active. Methotrexate appears to be active in forms with oligoarticular onset with spreading to multiple persisting joint involvement [21].

4. Spondylarthropathies

Undifferentiated forms of spondylarthropathy account for 80% of pediatric cases according to the ESSG and Amor criteria [61].

NSAIDs. These are very often very active on pain, as stressed by Amor, who included this characteristic of the spondylarthropathies in his criteria. Many NSAIDs can be used, as this condition generally affects older children. We virtually never use phenylbutazone.

SAARDs. Sulfasalasine appears to be the most active drug in the treatment of the spondylarthropathies [18].

Local (Intra-articular) Treatments. These are indicated when the arthritis is persistent and problematic. Treatment of enthesiopathies is difficult, and is based eventually on local infiltrations and physical or orthopedic approaches.

B. Systemic Lupus Erythematosus

SLE is a serious disease in childhood. Despite progress in its treatment, the mortality rate is still about 10% 10 years after diagnosis. Death is due to infections related to the disease and its treatment, renal involvement, or the frequent lack of compliance with therapy in adolescents.

1. Systemic Steroid Therapy

Systemic steroid therapy remains the cornerstone of treatment of SLE, at doses of 1–2 mg/kg/day prednisone or equivalent. Bolus methylprednisolone an be helpful in the case of severe organ involvement. It is strongly recommended to avoid alternate-day regimen despite the risk of arresting growth.

2. Immunomudulatory Treatments

Immunomodulatory treatments are used in the case of serious organ involvement (especially renal) after an initial renal biopsy. The usual treatment consists of bolus cyclophosphamide (500–1000 mg/m^2) every 3–4 weeks [44]. Certain investigators have obtained satisfactory results with azathioprine in lupus-associated renal damage [39]. Plasma exchanges have been used for severe forms.

3. Duration of Treatment

The overall duration of treatment of SLE is often several years. Treatment is essentially monitored by assaying complement and complement fraction levels together with anti-DNA antibody titers. Some specialists combine synthetic antimalarials (hydroxychloroquine 5–7 mg/kg/day) for uncomplicated lupus without visceral involvement in order to facilitate steroid withdrawal. There have been no objective pediatric studies of this approach.

C. Polydermatomyositis

Among the various categories of dermatomyositis, one group is observed mainly in children and involves inflammation of the muscles and skin. There is a major risk of muscular and subcutaneous calcinosis (about 30%).

1. Systemic Steroid Therapy

Systemic steroid therapy generally consists of prednisone 2 mg/kg/day or equivalent. Bolus methylprednisolone can be necessary in some particularly serious cases. Certain investigators start alternate-day steroid therapy soon after diagnosis. In our experience, there is a high risk of relapse in such cases, and we prefer daily doses for longer periods. Apart from a minority of children in whom steroid therapy can be administered for 1–2 years, treatment is generally necessary for several years. Efficacy is assessed solely on the basis of muscle strength.

2. Immunomodulatory Treatments

Immunomudulatory treatments are indicated in the case of relapse requiring an increase in the steroid dose. Methotrexate provides reasonable disease control in the opinion of certain specialists [36]. Cyclosporine A is valuable in our experience and that of other investigators [48]. As regards intravenous immunoglobulin, plasma exchanges, and leukopheresis [61], they have no proven value in the pediatric setting.

3. Preventive or Curative Treatments

There are no preventive or curative treatments for calcinosis.

D. Vasculitides

1. Kawasaki's Disease

Kawasaki's disease is mainly observed in children under 3 years of age. When the diagnosis is based on recommended criteria [63], intravenous immunoglobulin must be given at a dose of 1–2 g/kg. Efficacy is particularly marked when treatment is started within 10 days of onset, with a significant reduction in the risk of aneurysms [21]. The value of adding aspirin is generally agreed on, although the dose (low for an antiplatelet effect, high for an anti-inflammatory effect) remains controversial. The same is true of concomitant steroid therapy.

2. Cutaneous Forms of Polyarteritis Nodosa

The cutaneous forms of polyarteritis nodosa, which are particularly frequent in children in our experience, consists of cutaneous and muscle involvement, arthritis in many cases, and laboratory signs of a major inflammatory syndrome, and they often respond well to high-dose steroids (2–3 mg/kg/day prednisone) [64]. The steroids must be tapered slowly; often over a period of about 2 years. The frequent increase in antistreptolysins points to a possible role of streptococcal infections and suggests that relapse might be prevented by penicillin.

3. *Forms with Organ Involvement*

Forms of the vasculitides with organ involvement (especially cerebral or renal) warrant the adjunction of bolus cyclophosphamide to steroid therapy.

E. Conclusion

The treatment of children with inflammatory and autoimmune disorders must be adapted to the clinical manifestations (which may differ from those in adults), and also according to the risk of side effects, which can be severe in this age range. Rare diseases, the management of which remains to be standardized, call for prospective multicenter trials in order to group together individual experience and provide rapid answers to the many outstanding questions.

IV. SUMMARY

The drugs used in the management of the rheumatic disorders in children are similar to those used in adults. In juvenile chronic arthritis, NSAIDs must be administered first, with the systemic type requiring the maximum allowed dose. In case of failure, particulary in the systemic forms, the use of corticosteroids is can be necessary. However, growth retardation is a major problem when daily corticosteroids are given. Slow-acting antirheumatic drugs are mainly indicated in the polyarticular forms. In the systemics forms, they have little effect if any. The risk of a macrophage-activation syndrome is particularly high in systemic forms treated with gold and sulfasalazine. Methotrexate is a treatment of choice in some forms. Oligoarticular forms must be treated as such as possible with intra-articular triamcinolone hexatonide. The occurrence of chronic iridocyclitis requires a specific therapeutic approach by the ophthalmologists.

Systemic lupus erythematosus is a serious disease in childhood. Despite progress in its treatment with corticosteroids and immunosuppressive drugs, the mortality rate is still about 10% 10 years after the diagnosis. In juvenile polydermatomyositis, corticosteroids remain the best therapeutic approach. Cyclosporine A seems to be a valuable treatment in corticodependent cases. The use of intravenous immunoglobulin has transformed the prognosis of Kawasaki's disease.

ACKNOWLEDGMENT

Most of the data presented in this chapter were previously published in Prieur A-M. Rhumatismes inflammatoires des enfants. In: Thérapeutique Rhumatologique Bardin T, Kuntz D, eds. With the permission of the Médecine-Sciences, Flammarion, 1995.

REFERENCES

1. Dromgoole SH, Furst DE, Paulus HE. Rational approaches to the use of salicylate in the treatment of rheumatoid arthritis. Semin Arthritis Rheum, 1981; 11:57.
2. Prieur AM, Journo G. Résultats et tolérance du traitement par l'aspirine à dose élevée au cours des poussées systémiques d'arthrite chronique juvénile. In: Meyer P, Albin H, Jaillon

P, Worse F, eds. Actualités de pharmacologie clinique, Hôpital Necker-Enfants Malades, Flammarion Médecine-Sciences, 1984:134.
3. Koerper MA, Sempel DA, Dallman JR. Anemia in patients with juvenile rheumatoid arthritis. J Pediatr 1978; 92:930.
4. Murray T, Goldberg MM. Analgesic abuse and renal disease. Ann Rev Med 1975; 26:537.
5. Athreya BH, Moser G, Cecil HS, Myers AR. Aspirin induced hepatotoxicity in juvenile rheumatoid arthritis. A prospective study. Arthritis Rheum 1975; 18:347–352.
6. Prieur AM, Stephan JL. Macrophage activation syndrome in pediatric rheumatic diseases. Rev Rhum (Engl Ed) 1994; 6:385–388.
7. Stephan JL, Zeller J, Hubert P, et al. Macrophage activation syndrome and rheumatic disease in childhood. A report of four new cases. Clin Exp Rheumatol 1993; 11:451–456.
8. Halle F, Marfil F, Sioufi A, et al. Pharmacokinetics of pirprofen, in children, with juvenile chronic arthritis. Eur J Drug Metab Pharmacokinet, 1991; 9:16:29–34.
9. Pariente-Khayat A, Dubois MC, Vauzelle-Kervroaedan F, et al. Pharmacokinetics of tiaprotenic acid in infants after a single oral dose. Int J Clin Pharmacol Ther 1996; 34:342–344.
10. Lovell DJ, Giannini EH, Brewer EJ Jr. Time course of response to non steroidal antiinflammatory drugs in juvenile rheumatoid arthritis. Arthritis Rheum 1984; 27:1433–1437.
11. Levy ML, Barron KS, Eichenfield A, Honig PJ. Naproxene induced pseudoporphyria: a distinctive photodermatitis. J Pediatr 1990; 177:660–664.
12. Barron KS, Person DA, Brewer EJ. The toxicity of steroidal antiinflammatory drugs in juvenile rheumatoid art. J Rheumatol 1982; 9:149–155.
13. Prieur AM, Piussan CH, Manigne P, et al. Evaluation of D-penicillamine in juvenile chronic arthritis. A double-blind multicentre study. Arthritis Rheum 1985; 28:376–382.
14. Brewer EJ, Giannini EH, Kuzmina N, Alekseev L. Penicillamine and hydroxychloroquine in the treatment of juvenile rheumatoid arthritis; results of the USA-USSR double blind placebo controlled trial. N Engl J Med 1986; 314:1269–1270.
15. Kvien TK, Hoyeraal HH, Sandstad B. Gold sodium thiomalate and D-penicillamine. A controlled, comparative study in patients with pauciarticular and polyarticular juvenile rheumatoid arthritis. Scand J Rheumatol 1985; 14:346–354.
16. Giannini EH, Brewer EJ Jr, Kuzmina N, et al. Auranofin in the treatment of juvenile rheumatoid arthritis. Results of the USA-USSR double-blind, placebo controlled trial. Arthritis Rheum 1990; 33:466–476.
17. Giannini EH, Barron KS, Spencer CH, et al. Auranofin therapy in juvenile rheumatoid arthritis: results of the five-year open label extension trial. J Rheumatol 1991; 18:1240–1242.
18. Job-Deslandre C, Menkes CJ. Sulphalazine in the treatment of juvenile spondylarthropathy. Arthritis Rheum 1991; 34:S153.
19. Ansell BM, Hall MA, Woo P, et al. A multicentre pilot study of sulphasalazine in juveniles chronic arthritis. Clin Exp Rheumatol 1991; 10:201–203.
20. Herzberger-Ten Cate R, Cats A. Toxicity of sulphasalazine in juvenile chronic arthritis. Clin Exp Rheumatol, 1991; 9:85–88.
21. Newburger JW, Takahashi M, Burns JC, et al. The treatment of Kawasaki syndrome with intravenous gammaglobuin. N Engl J Med 1986; 315:341–347.
22. Kaveri SV, Dietrich G, Hurez V, Kazatchkine MD. Intravenous immunoglobulines (IV Ig) in the treatment of autoimmune diseases. Clin Exp Rheumatol 1991; 86:192–198.
23. Prieur AM, Adleff A, Debré M, et al. High dose immunoglobulin therapy in severe juvenile chronic arthritis : long term follow-up in 16 patients. Clin Exp Rheumatol 1990; 8:603–609.
24. Silvermann E, Uziel J, Schneider R, Laxer R. Intravenous immunoglobulin in systemic juvenile rheumatoid arthritis. Clin Exp Rheumatol 1993; 11(Suppl S9):abstr 70.
25. Loftus JK, Reeve J, Hesp R, et al. Deflazacort in JCA. J Rheumatol 1993; 20(suppl 37):40–42.

26. Prieur AM. The place of corticosteroid therapy in juvenile chronic arthritis in 1992. J Rheumatol 1993; 30(Suppl 37):32–34.
27. Dougados M, Awada H, Amor B. Cyclosporin in rheumatoid arthritis; double-blind, placebo controlled study in 52 patients. Ann Rheum Dis 1988; 47:127–133.
28. Giannini FH, Brewer EJ, Kuzmina N, et al. Methotrexate in resistant juvenile rheumatoid arthritis. N Engl J Med 1992; 326:1043–1049.
29. Wallace C, Sherry D, Salmonson K. Treatment of juvenile rheumatoid arthritis with higher dose methotrexate. Arthritis Rheum 1991; 34:S152.
30. Graham LD, Myones, BL, Rivas-Chalon RF, Pachman LM. Morbidity associated with long-term methotrexate therapy in juvenile rheumatoid arthritis. J Pediatr 1992; 120:468–473.
31. Truckenbrodt H, Hafner R. Methotrexate therapy in juvenile rheumatoid arthritis: a retrospective study. Arthritis Rheum 1986; 29:801–807.
32. Dupuis LC, Koren G, Shore A, et al. Methotrexate-non steroidal antiinflammatory drug interaction in children with arthritis. J Rheumatol 1990; 17:1469–1473.
33. Keim D, Ragadale C, Heidelberger K, Sullivan D. Hepatic fibrosis with the use of methotrexate for juvenile arthritis. J Rheumatol 1990; 17:846–848.
34. Halle F, Prieur AM. Evaluation of methotrexate in the treatment of juvenile chronic arthritis according to the subtype. Clin Exp Rheumatol 1991; 9:297–302.
35. Speckmaier M, Findeisen J, Woo P, et al. Low dose methotrexate in systemic onset juvenile chronic arthritis. Clin Exp Rheumatol 1989; 67:647–650.
36. Miller LC, Sisson SA, Tucker LB, et al. Methotrexate treatment of recalcitrant childhood dermatomyositis. Arthritis Rheum 1992; 35:1143–1148.
37. Silman AJ, Petrie J, Hazleman B, et al. Lymphoproliferative cancer and other malignancy in patients with rheumatoid arthritis treated with azathioprine. A 20 year follow-up study. Ann Rheum Dis 1988; 47:988-992.
38. Kvien TK, Hoyeraal HM, Sandstad B. Azathioprine versus placebo in patients with rheumatoid arthritis: a single center double-blind comparative study. J Rheumatol 1986; 13:118–123.
39. Felson DT, Anderson J. Evidence for the superiority of immunosuppressive drugs and prednisone over prednisone alone in lupus nephritis. Results of a pooled analysis. N Engl J Med 1984; 311:1528–1533.
40. Prieur AM, Balafrej M, Griscelli C, Mozziconacci P. Résultats et risques à long terme des traitements immunosuppresseurs dans l'arthrite chronique juvénile. Rev Rhum 1979; 46:85–90.
41. Deschennes G, Prieur AM, Hayem F, et al. Renal amyloidosis in juvenile chronic arthritis. Evolution after chlorambucil treatment. Pediatr Nephrol 1990; 4:463–469.
42. Woo P. Complications in juvenile arthritis. An Overview including amyloidosis. In: Woo P, White PH, Ansell BM, eds. Pediatric Rheumatology Update. Oxford, Oxford University Press, 1990:38–46.
43. Shaikov AV, Maximov AA, Speransky A, et al. Repetitive use of pulse therapy with methylprednisolone and cyclophosphamide in addition to oral methotrexate in children with systemic juvenile rheumatoid arthritis. Preliminary results of a long term study. J Rheumatol 1992; 19:612–616.
44. Lehman TJA, Sherry DD, Wagner-Reine I, et al. Intermittent intravenous cyclophosphamide therapy for lupus nephritis. J Pediatr 1989; 114:1055–1060.
45. Wagner-Weiner L, Emery H, Spencer C, et al. Intravenous pulse cyclophosphamide therapy (IVCT), variable renal outcome at 3 to 7 year follow-up. Arthritis Rheum 1991; 34:S58.
46. Fort JG, Abruzzo JL. Reversal of progressive vasculitis with intravenous pulse cyclophosphamide and methylprednisolone. Arthritis Rheum 1988; 31:1194–1198.
47. Ostensen M, Hoyeraal HM, Kass E. Tolerance of cyclosporin A in children with refractory rheumatoid arthritis. J Rheumatol 1988; 15:1536–1538.

48. Heckmatt J, Saunders C, Peters AM, et al. Cyclosporin in juvenile dermatomyositis. Lancet 1989: 1:1063–1067.
49. Nickleson RW, Brewer EJ, Rossen RD, et al. Plasma exchange in selected patients with juvenile rheumatoid arthritis. J Pediatr 1981; 98:194–200.
50. Lewis EJ, Hunsicker LG, Lan SP et al. A controlled trial of plasmapheresis therapy in severe lupus nephritis. N Engl J Med 1992; 326:1373–1379.
51. Brewer EJ. Non steroidal antiinflammatory agents. Arthritis Rheum 1977; 20(Suppl):513–525.
52. Gewanter HL, Baum J. The use of tolmetin sodium in systemic onset juvenile rheumatoid arthritis. Arthritis Rheum 1981; 24:1316–1319.
53. Hadchouel M, Prieur AM, Griscelli C. Acute hemorragic, hepatic and neurologic manifestations in juvenile rheumatoid arthritis; possible relationship to drug or infection. J Pediatr 1985; 106:561–566.
54. Prieur AM. Arthrite chronique juvénile. EMC, Paris, Pédiatrie, 4048 K10, 1992:1–8.
55. Manners PJ, Ansell BM. Slow acting antirheumatic drug use in systemic onset juvenile chronic arthritis. Pediatrics 1986; 77:99–103.
56. Jacobs JC, Gorin LJ, Hanissian AS, Simon JL. Consumption coagulopathy after gold therapy for JRA. J Pediatr 1984; 105:674–675.
57. Prieur AM, Buriot D, Lefur JM. Possible toxicity of levamisole in children with rheumatoid arthritis. J Pediatr 1978; 93:304–305.
58. Heaton DC, Muller PW. Still's disease associated with Coxsackie infection and hemophagocytic syndrome. Ann Rheum Dis 1985; 44:341–344.
59. Jean S, Leiva I, Prieur AM. Les formes à début polyarticulaire d'arthrite chronique juvénile (ACT) : une entité très hétérogène. Rev Rhum 1992; 59:668 (abstr G06).
60. Peralta JL, Prieur AM. Arthrite chronique juvénile avec présence d'anticorps antinucléaires sériques. Arch Fr Pédiatr 1990; 47:497–502.
61. Prieur AM, Listrat V, Dougados M, Amor B. Critères de classification des spondylarthropathies chez les enfants. Arch Fr Pédiatr 50:379–385.
62. Miller FW, Leitman SF, Cronin ME, et al. Controlled trial of plasma exchange and leukapheresis in polymyositis and dermatomyositis. N Engl J Med 1992; 326:1380–1384.
63. Sekiguchi M, Takao A, Endo M, et al. On the mucocutaneuos lymph nodes syndrome or Kawasaki disease. In: Yu PN, Goodwin JF, eds. Progress in Cardiology 13. Philadelphia: Lea & Febriger, 1985:97.
64. Halle F, Guillard J, Gire R, et al. Cutaneous poyarthritis nodosa (PAN) in childhood. Scand J Rheumatol 1991; (Suppl 89),5 (abstr 54).
65. Schairer H, Stoeber E. Long-term follow-up of 235 cases of juvenile rheumatoid arthritis treated with D-penicillamine. In: Munthe. Penicillamine Research in Rheumatoid Disease (Penicillamine Symposium). Oslo: Fabritius, 1977:279–281.
66. Ansell BM, Hall MA. Penicillamine in chronic arthritis in childhood. J Rheumatol 1981; 8(Suppl 7):112–115.
67. Kvien TK, Hoyeraal HM, Sandstad B. Slow acting antirheumatic drugs in patients with juvenile rheumatoid arthritis-evaluated in a randomized, parallel 50 week clinical trial. J Rheumatol 1985; 12:533–539.

23

Palindromic Rheumatism and Recurrent Arthritis

Pierre-André Guerne
University Hospital of Geneva, Geneva, Switzerland

I. PALINDROMIC RHEUMATISM AND RECURRENT ARTHRITIDES

Palindromic rheumatism (PR), originally described in 1944 by Hench and Rosenberg [1], is characterized by recurrent attacks of mostly oligoarticular arthritis with periarticular and paraarticular tissue inflammation that leave no residual clinical and radiographic changes. This condition was separated from rheumatoid arthritis because of totally distinct clinical features, but it soon became evident that a substantial part of the cases evolve into rheumatoid arthritis (RA) [2–4], which led to consider PR a variant or a mode of presentation of RA.

However, 60–70% of the patients do not evolve toward RA, including 50% who remain with palindromic rheumatism, 15% who go into remission, and some who develop another disease, such as systemic lupus erythematosus, Wegener's granulomatosis, or seronegative spondarthropathies. Therefore, the palindromic syndrome appears to be a heterogeneous entity, encompassing a few inflammatory conditions at the early stages of their evolution, but also including an entity whose relationship with RA is evident but still unclear and should be called PR; evolution of up to 30–40% of these patients into otherwise typical rheumatoid arthritis (RA), commonly accompanied by the conversion to rheumatoid factor seropositivity, the frequent occurrence of nodules, and the observed familial aggregation of the two conditions indicate that PR is part of the spectrum of RA. However, the fact that close to 50% of the cases will remain palindromic even after many years of evolution, with well-defined and recognizable clinical manifestations, including a different pattern of distribution of the arthritis, the frequent distinctive periarticular manifestations, a general absence of significant constitutional symptoms, the lack of progression, chronicity and/or radiographic changes, and the absence of female preponderance justify the recognition of PR as a distinct identity and the necessity of a specific therapeutic approach [5-7].

As seen in Table 1, diagnostic criteria have been proposed for PR, but require the exclusion of other arthritides in order to be met.

Table 1 Proposed Diagnostic Criteria for Palindromic Rheumatism

1.	A 6-months history of brief sudden-onset and recurrent episodes of mono- or rarely polyarthritis or of soft tissue inflammation
2.	Direct observation of one attack by a physician
3.	Three or more joints involved in different attacks
4.	Absence of erosions on radiographs
5.	Exclusion of other arthritides

Source: Adapted from refs. 5 and 6.

Several other well-defined conditions whose joint manifestations generally (or frequently) present as intermittent arthritis similar to PR (Table 2) have been progressively recognized. Since some of them require very specific treatments, the first and crucial issue is to establish the diagnosis as accurately as possible when considering the treatment of an intermittent or recurrent arthritis.

In addition, in view of the recent interest in initiating the treatment of RA early, in particular with medications directed against the T lymphocytes [8], pre-RA forms of PR might represent suitable opportunities for such interventions. However, parameters reliably predicting evolution toward RA and/or the future severity of the disease would be necessary.

A. Diagnosis

1. Clinical Manifestations

Very sudden attacks of monoarticular (rarely oligoarticular) arthritis, usually without any obvious inciting event, remain the most distinctive feature of PR [1,6]. The disease can strike almost any joint, although the spine and the hips are rarely affected. When the spine is involved, it is usually at the cervical level. The joints most frequently involved are the wrists and the small joints of the hands, followed by the knees, shoulders, ankles, and feet. Morning stiffness and pain in several joints at once [9] are more common among the patients who ultimately develop RA. The pain is generally described as very severe or excruciating, often confining the patient to bed [1,6,10]. In addition, extra-articular tissue inflammation is observed in about 30% of the patients [1,6]; usually characterized by prominent swelling and redness, it can be a tendinitis, but frequently swelling involves undefined para-articular structures, often remote enough from a joint to allow clear distinction from articular involvement. The size of these para-articular swellings vary from 2 cm to much larger areas.

The PR attacks last less than 2 days in most cases, and sometimes as short as 2 h [1], but they can rarely extend to more than 2 weeks [1,10]; their frequency is highly variable, from a few to more than 250 per year [1,5,10]. Patients who experience frequent attacks (more than one per month) may be more likely to develop frank RA [11]. Only a few patients display constitutional reactions such as fever or weight loss, and they appear to be more frequently rheumatoid factor (RF) positive and prone to later progression into erosive RA.

A peculiar feature of PR is the occasional occurrence of transient nodules, which are usually the size of a pea and frequently overlying the tendons of the hands. Their appearance parallels the arthritis attacks and generally last at most a week, but they can be more sustained [1,3,4,10].

Table 2 Differential Diagnosis of Recurrent Arthritis

Affection	Attack length	Articular involvement	Distinctive features
Palindromic rheumatism	Hours-days (<2–3 week)	Mono- or oligoarthritis (mainly hands, knees, and shoulders)	Para-articular involvement; nodules or rheumatoid factor frequently present
Mediterranean fever	Days	Arthralgias, mono- or oligoarthritis (large > small joints, lower > upper limbs)	Onset usually in childhood Fever and serositis[a]
Intermittent hydrarthrosis	Days (usually 2–4)	Mono- or oligoarthritis (mainly knees)	Absence of inflammatory signs Generally painless
Microcrystalline arthritis	Days	Mono- > oligo- > poly-arthritis	Crystals present in synovial fluid; typical radiographic signs frequently present
Behçet's disease	Days–weeks	Mono- or oligoarthritis	Painful orogenital ulcers Posterior or panuveitis
Chronic sarcoidosis	2–3 weeks	Oligo- or polyarthritis Symmetrical, additive	Lung parenchymal disease ± hilar adenopathies Frequent destructive bone lesions
Eosinophilic-allergic synovitis	1–2 weeks	Oligo- or polyarthritis	History of allergy or parasitic infection Elevated IgE in blood Eosinophilia in synovial fluid (usually >10%)
Hereditary angioedema	Hours–days	Nonarticular swelling Rare oligoarthritis	Painless and nonpruritic swelling
Types II and IV hyperlipidemia	Days–2 weeks	Mono- or oligoarthritis (peripheral large joints)	Hyperlipidemia, xanthomas
Whipple's disease	Days–weeks	Oligo- or polyarthritis Large > small joints	Diarrhea-abdominal pain-malabsorption[a] Frequent lymphadenopathy
Lyme arthritis	Weeks–months	Mono- or oligoarthritis (mainly knees and ankles)	History of tick bite and/or erythema migrans Positive serology
Reactive arthritis	Weeks–months	Mono- or oligoarthritis Asymmetrical	Frequent history of diarrhea or urethritis Frequent ocular or mucocutaneous manifestations

[a]Can be absent at the beginning of the disease.

The mean age of onset of PR is about 45 years, with cases reported from the early twenties to the eighties. The prevalence of this disease is difficult to establish but is estimated to be one-eighth [6] to one-twentieth [5] that of RA. Despite the absence of female preponderance, pregnancy can induce remission as well as in RA [12]. In one-third to one-half of PR patients, the interval before the conversion to chronic disease varies from a few months to more than 20 years.

2. Laboratory Features

Laboratory blood abnormalities are rare in PR and are not specific. The erythrocyte sedimentation rate (ESR) is frequently increased during or just after the attacks but rarely between them [1,3,10]; elevation might indicate subsequent development into RA [1]. The percentage of rheumatoid factor seropositive patients is clearly increased in PR. The patients who remain palindromic appear to be more frequently positive than the normal population [6]. Among the cases of PR that have evolved into a chronic arthritis, the percentage of seropositivity is not different than in RA [6,10,11], and about one-third of the patients turn from negative to positive, usually shortly before evolution to chronic arthritis. In addition, patients with PR and positive RF seem more susceptible to develop RA [6]. Antinuclear antibody (ANA) studies, on the other hand, are usually negative in PR cases [11,13].

Radiographic studies are always normal in PR patients [1,3,10,11] as long as they do not evolve into a chronic arthritis. Absence of radiographic signs is thus among the six diagnostic criteria proposed by Pasero and Barbieri [5].

Analysis of the synovial fluid does not appear to be of much help. The rare studies that have been reported [14] show variable leukocyte counts (150-12700/mm^3) and differentials (2–66% polymorphonuclear cells) that do not correlate with the severity of the symptoms or attacks.

HLA antigen status in PR, in view of its debated autonomy from RA, and the potential prognostic value of the HLA-DR1 and DR4 "shared epitope" in RA, assumes some importance. Data on a possible association of HLA-DR1 or HLA-DR4 with PR are scarce and generally show an absence of a clear association of PR with HLA-DR4 [11,15–17], which might contribute to an alternate expression of the disease. In one study, it was shown that the PR patients who developed RA during follow-up carry more frequently the HLA-DR4 [16].

B. Treatment

A number of different treatments of PR have been evaluated with various and sometimes inconsistent results, but none of the interventions has been submitted to rigorous controlled studies. Inconsistencies are likely due to the relative rarity of the condition and possible heterogeneities both within and between the case series. However, multiple testimonials for the beneficial effects of several treatments, including nonsteroidal anti-inflammatory drugs (NSAIDs), antimalarials, and gold justify their use in PR, which can be seriously disabling.

1. NSAIDs and Analgesics

NSAIDs appear to be effective for at least partial relief of joint pain in some patients, and they can even induce long-lasting remissions in rare cases. Success, however, is variable and its rate differs considerably in different series: in a questionnaire-based study, Grattan et al. reported that in 68% of 38 patients, NSAIDs or analgesics were said to be effective [9], whereas in another series, only 2 cases of 60 cases had a satisfactory response to NSAIDs and did not require remission-inducing antirheumatic drugs [6]. In a more recent survey, 10 of 30 patients did not respond at all to NSAIDs, but in 20 patients, these drugs terminated or alleviated attacks [18]. On the other hand, it was noted in several studies that analgesics are inefficient during PR attacks [18,19].

2. *Antimalarials*

Because of the relatively mild severity of PR, and its observed relationship with RA, antimalarials were evaluated in several series. The response rate varies from 15% [11] to almost 80% in more recent series [20,21]. In a large and recent survey, 51 patients received antimalarials [21]. Forty-one of the 51 patients experienced marked improvement (77.5% reduction in frequency and 63% reduction in duration of the attacks). However, this type of drug did not prevent evolution toward RA in 12 of 51 patients (23%). Interestingly, in one series, effectiveness was much lower in the group of patients who remained palindromic than in the ones who developed chronic arthritis [6].

3. *Gold*

Chrysotherapy has also been widely used in the treatment of PR with frequent although highly variable testimonials for favorable results. In one survey, the disease was stopped after gold treatment in only 20% of the patients, which was not better than the spontaneous outcome, with remissions having occurred in 3 of 7 untreated patients (42%) in this series [11]. In three other series, however, good responses were observed in 50–70% of the patients treated with injectable gold [3,6,18]; the injections appeared to stop the acute attacks, or at least decrease their frequency and the intensity of pain, often within a few weeks, and usually by the time 200–500 mg had been reached. Of note is an unusually high percentage of cutaneous side effects reported in one series [3].

4. *Other DMARDs and Immunosuppressors*

Sulfasalazine has also been shown to induce favorable responses in about half the patients who used it [6,22], and it should be considered for the treatment of PR, especially in cases of intolerance or inefficiency of gold or antimalarials.

In one small series, D-penicillamine was reported to be very effective, with complete remission in four of five patients [23]. The four patients who experienced remissions were RF negative, whereas the one who did not was mildly seropositive. Good responses, however, were much rarer in two other series [6,11], and the benefits of D-penicillamine in PR are questionable in view of its frequent side effects.

Other drugs, such as chlorambucil and dapsone, have been employed more rarely in the treatment of PR, but they reportedly induced prolonged remissions in a few patients [11,24]. On the other hand, information on newer treatments such as methotrexate or cyclosporine is not available

5. *Colchicine*

Probably because of the similarity between PR and familial Mediterranean fever, colchicine has been evaluated at prophylactic doses and has been recommended on the basis of remission or good response in all subjects of a small series of five patients [25]. On the other hand, in a more recent survey, of eight patients treated with colchicine, only one reported a relief manifested as a decrease in the frequency of attacks; this medication therefore appeared to be useful only in a minority of patients.

6. *Conclusions and Treatment Guidelines*

The variable evolution of PR and its frequent spontaneous remissions together with the absence of well-defined criteria for diagnosis and treatment outcome all contribute to the difficulty of evaluating any drug intervention. The diversity of the drugs employed is an indication of the sometimes disabling nature of PR and a less than satisfactory therapeutic experience with nonspecific treatments. However, many PR patients remain free of progressive or severe disease. Therefore, once another specific entity has been reasonably ruled out (see Section II), it is quite judicious to begin by reassuring these patients of the likely possibility of a favorable outcome. Control of the attacks should first be attempted with NSAIDs. If still disabled, patients should be prescribed disease-modifying antirheumatic drugs (DMARDs) such as antimalarials or gold, which have to be considered earlier if markers indicative of potential unfavorable outcome are present (more than one attack per month, pain in several joints at once, morning stiffness, fever or weight loss, high ESR, rheumatoid factor positivity, or RA-associated HLA-DR alleles, particularly if present at double dose). Not enough information is available yet, however, to advise the early use of more progressive regimens, including T-cell–directed drugs, such as cyclosporine A, routinely in the presence of these severity markers. Such approaches will hopefully be the subject of clinical trials in reference centers.

II. DIFFERENTIAL DIAGNOSIS

Many inflammatory rheumatic diseases, including systemic lupus erythematosus, Wegener's granulomatosis, or psoriatic arthritis, to name a few, can begin by intermittent or recurrent episodes of arthritis. Conditions which more specifically present as recurrent arthritis and can remain so for prolonged periods of time are listed in Table 2. The diagnosis and treatments of familial Mediterranean fever, intermittent hydrarthrosis, sarcoidosis, Behçet's disease, Whipple's disease, hyperlipidemic arthropathy, and hereditary angioedema are described in more detail in the following sections.

III. MEDITERRANEAN FEVER

Familial Mediterranean fever (FMF) is a chronic inherited disorder of unknown etiology. It occurs mainly among Northern Africa Jews, Armenians, and Arabs, but sporadic cases are widely spread. Recessive inheritance is likely, but dominant forms have been described. Establishing the correct diagnosis is crucial because of the specific need for colchicine treatment.

A. Diagnosis

1. *Clinical Features*

The diagnosis of FMF is very easy in typical cases, being characterized by the unique association of attacks of peritonitis, arthritis, and pleuritis, usually in young children [26]. The mean age of onset is 4.9 (>50% of the cases before age 10 and 95% before age 30).

Arthritis is present in 75% of cases of FMF and constitutes the presenting sign in 26% [27]. Three types of arthritis have been described (acute, chronic, and abortive), but acute attacks, representing 95% of the cases, are by far the most characteristic. Attacks of synovitis are usually monoarticular or oligoarticular, with an abrupt onset and severe pain, and affect mainly large joints of the lower limbs. Large effusions are observed, but redness or heat are usually not prominent. Attacks usually last less than a week and their frequency is variable, generally from 0.5 to 4.0 per week. Free intervals, which sometimes extend up to a year, are totally asymptomatic. In 5% of the cases, arthritis attacks are long-standing or protracted (chronic type), with an average duration of 6 months; articular sequelae are generally absent but can occur, particularly in the hip. On the other hand, in a few cases, joint symptoms are limited to arthralgias (abortive type).

Fever, the hallmark of the disease, is essential for the diagnosis, but might be absent during some acute episodes. It generally constitutes the first manifestation of an attack, may rise up to 40°C, and can be associated with chills. Fever generally lasts less than 3 days but can extend up to 2 weeks.

Abdominal pain, representing acute peritonitis, is the next most common manifestation after fever and occurs in 94–100% of the cases. It varies in severity, but generally progresses during an episode to affect the entire abdomen, sometimes associated with nausea, vomiting, diarrhea, or constipation. Pleuritis is less common, occurring in approximately 60% of the crisis and less frequently in children.

A rarer but distincting feature of FMF is the occasional occurrence (~15% of cases) of erysipela's-like erythema. These hot and painful skin lesions cover small or large areas, generally around the ankles or extensor surfaces of the legs, and usually parallel the attacks.

2. *Radiography*

In the acute type, the most frequent radiographic findings include soft tissue swelling and transient osteoporosis [28]. In more chronic forms, delay in closure of epiphysis, enlargement of femoral condyles, together with marked and extended regional osteoporosis can be observed; coarse trabecular osteoporosis with pseudocysts reflects long-term immobilization. With chronicity, lytic intra-articular lesions and degenerative changes can develop; these changes, characterized by joint space narrowing and proliferative marginal bony changes, are most prominent in the hips and knees, and they are partly reversible [29].

3. *Laboratory Features*

No specific laboratory test for FMF has been discovered yet. ESR and acute phase proteins are significantly to markedly elevated (ESR > 60 mm) in most patients during acute episodes [26], but they are usually normal between attacks. The white blood cell count is elevated in a minority of patients. In synovial fluid, white cell counts are generally markedly elevated; exceeding $100000/mm^3$.

4. *Amyloidosis*

AA amyloidosis, due, at least in part, to the excessive release of the acute phase protein SAA, determines the prognosis of the disease [26]. Its incidence varies markedly (from 0–2% in Armenian-Americans to 30–60% in Israeli and Turkish individuals), and can develop early (before age 20 in ~30% of the cases). Nephropathy and splenomegaly are the most common manifestations of FMF amyloidosis, whereas gastrointestinal, cardiac, adrenal, and hepatic dysfunctions are rare. However, rectal biopsy remains the procedure of choice for diagnosis.

B. Treatment

Before the era of colchicine, many treatments for FMF were evaluated, including psychotherapy, antibiotics, steroids, and NSAIDs. None proved really effective neither to significantly reduce the frequency, severity, and length of the attacks, nor to prevent the development of amyloidosis, whose natural history is to progress to end-stage renal failure within 2–13 years after the appearance of proteinuria [30].

1. Colchicine

The outcome of FMF completely changed when colchicine was introduced in 1972 by Goldfinger, who first demonstrated that this drug prevents febrile attacks of FMF [31]. This was confirmed by several controlled studies, and colchicine has become the mainstay of FMF treatment since 1973 [32].

Colchicine for Prevention of FMF Attacks and Amyloidosis. Complete remission of febrile attacks of FMF were shown to be achieved in 64% of 350 children and partial remission in 31%, whereas protracted attacks of arthritis virtually disappeared [33]. The benefits of colchicine were further demonstrated for the prevention of amyloidosis in FMF. The appearance of proteinuria is prevented in virtually all colchicine-treated patients with doses between 1 and 2 mg/day [33,34]. Dosages currently used are between 0.02 and 0.033 mg/kg/day up to a maximum of 2 mg/day [26] given in one or two divided doses. The treatment can be initiated at half doses and increased progressively, which might decrease gastrointestinal side effects. Colchicine, which should be taken throughout life, appears to be safe and side effects are minimal. Reported side effects include nausea, vomiting, diarrhea, bone marrow suppression, malabsorption, myopathy, neuropathy, alopecia, azoospermia, and chromosomal abnormalities, but these hardly represent a major issue. Side effects of long-term colchicine treatment in children with FMF were recently evaluated: growth, development, and subsequent fertility were normal, and colchicine did not produce major side effects [33]. Life-threatening events are very rare. Only one case of reversible thrombocytopenia was described in a series of 101 children, and colchicine could be reinstituted after 3 months without side effects [26]. Teratogenic effects appear to be extremely rare as well: no abnormalities occurred in a series of 16 infants born to mothers having taken colchicine [35]. Currently, it is advised not to discontinue this treatment before and during pregnancy. Thus, the efficacy and safety of long-term colchicine in children with FMF make this treatment lifesaving, and early diagnosis of prime importance.

Colchicine for the Treatment of Overt FMF Amyloidosis. Colchicine treatment can resolve proteinuria ($\sim$6% of the cases) or stabilize its progression ($\sim$80%) in patients who have proteinuria but not nephrotic syndrome [36]. When nephrotic syndrome is present, regression is more difficult; a favorable response, however, can occur, but it appears to require doses $\geq$1.5 mg/day. In a recent study, factors affecting the outcome of colchicine treatment in AA amyloidosis of familial Mediterranean fever were evaluated [37]. In this retrospective study, among 68 FMF patients presenting with proteinuria ($>$0.5 g/24 h) but with creatinine values $<$2.5 mg/dL, 31 were observed to worsen. Deterioration was related to initial serum creatinine ($\geq$1.5 mg/dL) and to mean colchicine dosage, confirming that therapeutic dosage for amyloidosis in FMF is >1.5 mg/day in adults.

2. *Other Treatment Modalities*

In most cases, colchicine is sufficient to allow a perfectly adequate management. However, in the rare occurrences of colchicine failure, or when treatment has been undertaken too late, other therapeutic modalities can be required, in particular to control chronic synovitis or manage irreversible damages related to synovitis or amyloidosis.

NSAIDs. The place of NSAIDs is very limited in FMF, since they are not helpful for the prevention of the attacks or amyloidosis. However, they can be beneficial during the acute attack, in particular because colchicine, although very effective in decreasing the frequency and intensity of the attacks, is not as good to abort them once they have started.

Synovectomy and Joint Replacement. In the case of protracted or chronic synovitis, which in rare cases can show resistance to colchicine and NSAIDs, synovectomy has been reported to significantly reduce joint symptoms [27]. Given the propensity of the chronic arthritis of FMF to lead toward joint damage, and the recognized effects of synovectomy in other diseases such as rheumatoid arthritis, this approach might be useful in selected cases. In cases of advanced articular destruction, in particular of the hip, joint replacement can be necessary. In such cases, implantation of cementless prostheses following meticulous synovectomy is recommended [38].

Renal Transplantation. In patients with end-stage renal failure due to amyloidosis, renal transplantation has been shown to be a valuable procedure [36,39]. After transplantation, the graft can be efficiently protected from amyloidosis by preventive treatment with colchicine provided the dose is sufficient (≥1.5 mg/day) [36].

IV. INTERMITTENT HYDRARTHROSIS

Intermittent hydrarthoris, or periodic hydrarthosis, is defined as the recurrence of joint effusions, usually of the knees, without signs of local or systemic inflammation [40]. Although most rheumatologists can recall a few such cases, reports are very rare in the literature, and the clinical description can be variable.

A. Diagnosis

1. *Symptoms*

Reported cases of intermittent hydarthosis usually begin early in life, but can present at any age. Women are more frequently affected than men in some but not in all reports, and episodes are sometimes reported to be associated with the menses. A single joint, usually the knee, is affected in most cases, but the disease can rarely be bilateral, and involve elbows, hips, or ankles. The average interval between attacks is 1–4 weeks. The effusion is relatively painless, without other sign of inflammation such as warmth, redness, or tenderness. Total resolution of the effusion usually occurs after 2–4 days.

2. *Laboratory Features*

In synovial fluid of patients with intermittent hydarthrosis, leukocyte counts are very low, rarely reaching a few thousand. Hemogram, ESR, and acute phase proteins typically remain normal during and between attacks, and autoantibodies, including rheumatoid factor and antinuclear antibodies, remain negative. The diagnosis of hydrarthrosis demands such an absence of biological abnormalities, as well as normal radiographic tests except for soft tissue swelling.

B. Treatment

A number of therapeutic interventions in intermittent hydrarthrosis have been based on the presumed etiology of the disorder. The etiology is still enigmatic, but it is very likely that a few different heterogeneous entities have been reported under this appellation. Because some patients have a strong allergic history and/or develop giant urticaria, urticarial or allergic synovitis has been suggested [41]. Joint laxity, primary or acquired, is also known to produce intermittent hydrarthrosis [42,43] and probably accounts for some cases.

No treatment significantly changes the course of intermittent hydrarthrosis, which is spontaneously benign [40]. Because of the observed relation with allergic manifestations, antiallergic medications, including antihistamines, were tested but did not appear to be efficient. Numerous anecdotal observations have been reported on the beneficial effect of different anti-inflammatory therapies, including injection of steroids, which might reduce the severity and frequency of attacks. However, because of the benignity of intermittent hydrarthrosis, its variable evolution, the constant possibility of spontaneous resolution, and the rarity of the condition, evaluation of any therapeutic modality is virtually impossible. In most cases, any treatment is likely to be potentially more harmful then beneficial. Accordingly, many patients fail to consult physicians, particularly once they have learned more about the favorable course of their condition and how little can or need be done.

Consideration, however, should be given to the possibility of a primary condition requiring a specific approach. In case of joint hyperlaxity, treatment first consists in emphasizing appropriate exercise to develop protective reflex reactions and strengthen surrounding musculature, especially in weight-bearing or very mobile joints. In selected (serious) cases, surgical procedure designed to improve joint stability can be advocated [42,43].

V. HYPERLIPIDEMIA

A transient recurrent or migratory polyarthritis associated with hyperlipidemia is frequently reported, but appears to be rare, Nevertheless, since these manifestations can antedate the diagnosis of hyperlipidemia, their recognition can be very important by contributing to early diagnosis and appropriate treatment.

A. Diagnosis

1. Epidemiology and Clinical Features

Recurrent polyarthritis was first described in a series of patients with homozygous hypercholesterolemia (type II hyperlipidemia) [44]. Ten of 18 patients (56%) experienced rheumatic manifestations which were recurrent in 4. Large joints were involved more frequently. Attacks lasted from 2 days to a month and pain varied from mild to incapacitating. Joint swelling with warmth and tenderness was consistently observed and fever sometimes occurred during the attacks. Xanthomata were not consistently associated with rheumatic manifestations. Several case reports confirmed these findings [45]. In heterozygous patients, subsequent studies reported similar manifestations in up to 32% of the patients [46], but others questioned the association between an arthropathy and hyperlipidemia, and the reported manifestations appeared somewhat variable. Recurrent oligoarthritis involving large and small joints and lasting days to weeks has also been described in type IV hyperlipidemia [45,47]. A recent controlled study confirmed an association between rheumatic manifestations and hyperlipidemia [48]. Most frequent manifestations, however, were Achilles tendinitis and oligoarthritis, whereas recurrent or migratory polyarthritis appeared to be less frequent and to be limited to cases of adult familial hypercholesterolemia.

2. Laboratory Features

No specific laboratory abnormalities are reported in hyperlipidemia except for elevated lipid levels. Cholesterol, in particular, has been shown to be significantly higher in hyperlipidemic patients with rheumatic manifestations than in those without them [45]. In homozygous hypercholesterolemia, ESR were noted to be elevated during but also between attacks [44], whereas in heterozygous patients, ESRs were reported normal even during attacks [46]. In most cases, synovial fluids are not inflammatory, with only one report of elevated cell count [45]. Cholesterol or lipid crystals are found only in a minority of fluids.

B. Treatment

In most cases, attacks of arthritis in type II hyperlipidemia resolve spontaneously [45]. NSAIDs can be used, but evidence for shortening of the duration of the acute episode is lacking [46]. Since a relationship between the onset of joint symptoms and undue exercise has been observed [46], adapted physical activities can be advised.

In fact, the most important issue is to prescribe an adequate lipid-lowering treatment. In addition to decreasing the development of atherosclerosis and the occurrence of ischemic complications, such treatments appear to reduce the frequency and severity of the attacks of arthritis in many patients. In a small series of 10 patients on cholestyramine or colestipol therapy, 6 continued to experience recurrent episodes of arthritis [46], but the lipid status during arthritis was not reported. A case report suggested that the decrease in the frequency of the attacks might be related to the correction of the hyperlipidemia [49]. In a recent survey, among 30 patients able to state whether their rheumatic symptoms had been modified by lipid-lowering treatment, 19 (63%) had improved (reduction in frequency or severity of the attacks), whereas 11 (37%) had not noted any difference.

In type IV hyperlipidemia, articular symptoms also appear to be correlated with the correction of the lipid levels: in one series, 30% of patients experienced an improvement of their attacks of arthritis, correlating with a decrease in the triglyceride levels [47].

Fibrates remain the treatment of choice in moderate hypercholesterolemia (<7.8 mmol/L), mixed hyperlipidemias, and hypertriglycyceridemias, but inhibitors of cholesterol synthesis (HMG CoA reductase inhibitors) should be used in severe hypercholesterolemias whether or not associated with hypertriglycyceridemia [50]. In resistant cases, ion exchange resins, but not fibrates, can be associated to HMG CoA reductase inhibitors. Ideally, such treatments should be supervised by a specialist.

VI. SARCOIDOSIS

Sarcoidosis is a granulomatous disorder of unknown etiology that may affect many organs including the musculoskeletal system. Two types of disease, with profoundly different outcomes and therapeutic needs, are classically distinguished as acute and chronic. Acute sarcoidosis, which is frequently associated with acute arthritis and erythema nodosum, has a benign prognosis; chronic sarcoidosis, often but not always preceded by the acute form, is frequently associated with a chronic polyarthritis that may subside and recur. Other rheumatic features include muscular and osseous sarcoidosis.

A. Diagnosis

1. Epidemiology and Clinical Features

Sarcoidosis is a frequently occurring disorder with a prevalence ranging from less than 1 per 100,000 in Spain to 64 per 100,000 in Sweden. Involvement of the lungs is the most common feature and source of morbidity and mortality. Acute disease frequently presents with arthritis, erythema nodosum, and stage 1 pulmonary involvement (see Chest radiographs below); respiratory symptoms, including cough, dyspnea, and retrosternal discomfort, are frequent but can be lacking. Chronic disease generally manifests as progressive respiratory manifestations, including nonproductive cough, dyspnea, nonspecific chest pain, and stage II (25% of patients at presentation) or stage III pulmonary disease (15% of patients at presentation), associated with chronic recurrent arthritis in 25 to 50% of the patients.

Other manifestations of sarcoidosis include fever, fatigue, hepatic and splenic enlargement, and symptoms of hypercalcemia. Less common manifestations include lupus pernio, anterior and posterior uveitis, cardiac conducting defects and left ventricular wall abnormalities, upper respiratory tract stuffiness, neurosarcoidosis (cranial nerve abnormalities, meningitis, space-occupying lesions), muscular and osseous sarcoidosis, and endocrine dysfunctions.

2. Diagnostic Procedures and Laboratory Features

A number of tests and procedures can help in the diagnosis of sarcoidosis, but they differ in sensitivity and specificity, depending on the presentation, stage, and duration of the disease [51].

Chest Radiographs. Chest radiographs are abnormal in about 90% of patients and provide the basis for the staging of the disease: hilar (bilateral in 90–95% of patients) or mediastinal lymphadenopathies in stage I, hilar lymphadenopathies with parenchymal disease in stage II, diffuse parenchymal infiltrates without adenopathy in state III, widespread cystic destruction and fibrosis in stage IV.

The triads consisting of acute arthritis, erythema nodosum, and hilar adenopathies or uveitis, erythema nodosum, and hilar adenopathies are sufficiently specific to allow diagnosis without histological confirmation. Isolated hilar adenopathies in asymptomatic patients have long been considered sufficiently specific too, but it is now recognized that other conditions such as lymphoma can present like this; if histological confirmation is not obtained in this setting, a very close follow-up is mandatory. In most cases, however, radiographic findings are too unspecific and biopsy should be performed.

Biopsy and Histology. Diagnosis of sarcoidosis is generally made by the demonstration of noncaseating granulomas in an appropriate clinical setting; however, a number of disorders able to produce similar histological changes must imperatively be excluded; these include infectious conditions (mycobacteria, leprosy, histoplasmosis, coccidioidomycosis), autoimmune disorders (Crohn's disease, Wegener's granulomatosis, primary biliary cirrhosis), neoplasms (lymphoma, carcinoma), reactions to chemicals (beryllium, talc), and hypersensitivity reactions.

Palpable lymphnodes or skin nodules (except erythema nodosum) should be biopsied if present. Scalene node biopsy or transbronchial biopsy are other means to obtain tissues; the former should be preferred in stage I and the latter in stage II or III disease [51]. Broncholalveolar lavage, on the other hand, is too unspecific to be suitable for routine diagnostic use. Mediastinoscopy has a very high sensitivity but is rarely necessary.

It is now advocated to perform polymerase chain reaction (PCR) for *Tropheryma whippelii* in biopsy samples, because of the possible sarcoid presentation of Whipple's disease [52].

Pulmonary Functions. Pulmonary function testing is very unspecific but vital capacity and carbon monoxyde diffusing capacity (DLCO) are very helpful to determine an eventual need for aggressive treatment, to monitor response to treatment, and to detect exacerbation and changes.

Blood Tests. Angiotensin-converting enzyme levels are elevated in up to 60% of cases, more commonly in the presence of pulmonary infiltrates, but they can be abnormal in many granulomatous conditions mimicking sarcoidosis and is not recommended for diagnosis. This test, however, can be helpful to monitor the body granulomatous mass.

Other findings that can suggest the diagnosis but are unsensitive and unspecific include hypercalciuria (10% of patients) and increased plasma levels of 1,25-dihydroxycholecalciferol (calcitriol, 5% of patients).

HLA-B8 and HLA-DR3, which appear to be associated with acute sarcoid arthritis but not with the chronic type, are of limited diagnostic value.

B. Treatment

Treatment of sarcoidosis depends on the manifestations and stage of the disease. It must be kept in mind that spontaneous resolution is common and occurs in 65–90% of patients with stage I disease, 50% with stage II, and 20% with stage III. These data indicate how difficult it can be to differentiate therapeutic benefits from the natural course of the disease, and that many patients should not be exposed to the potentially severe side effects of aggressive drugs. On the other hand, severe manifestations, including progressive lung disease (which can lead to pulmonary fibrosis, cor pulmonale, and respiratory failure) and heart and central nervous system involvement require drastic treatments.

1. Sarcoid Arthritis, Myositis, and Osteitis

Acute Sarcoid Arthritis. Acute sarcoid arthritis involves the ankles, knees, wrists, and proximal interphalangeal joints in decreasing frequency, and it is frequently accompanied by tenosynovitis and periarticular swelling [53]. The course of the disease is usually benign and joint destructions are unusual.

Acute sarcoid arthritis and erythema nodosum respond well to NSAIDs in most patients, and resolution occurs in 92% of these patients [54]. In rare cases, symptoms are more troublesome or resistant to NSAIDs, and a short course of oral prednisolone or prednisone (≤0.5 mg/kg/day) generally leads to rapid improvement. In most cases, pulmonary involvement is benign, but the lungs and other major organs must always be watched closely and appropriate treatment eventually administered.

Chronic Sarcoid Arthritis. Chronic sarcoid arthritis involves the same joints, but may subside and recur for months to years. Irreversible destructive lesions can take place.

The treatment of chronic disease is dictated in most cases by the major systemic manifestations and includes medications that control the arthritis as well (see below). Occasionally, a disabling chronic arthritis can occur without major organ involvement. When resistant to NSAIDs or acceptable courses of oral prednisolone or prednisone (initial doses of ≤40 mg/day and maintenance doses ≤7.5-12 mg/day), such cases can generally be controlled with weekly low doses of methotrexate [55]. Beneficial effects were observed within 8–12 weeks with methotrexate doses ranging from 7.5 to 15.0 mg, which allowed a reduction of approximately 60% of the corticosteroid posology without significant toxicity. It appears that the effects of methotrexate are dose dependent and that in some patients, better and quicker improvement can be obtained with treatments ranging between 15 and 25 or even 35 mg/week. Hydorxycholoroquine or cyclosporine can be useful alternatives.

Muscular and Osseous Sarcoidosis. Muscle involvement, as evidenced by granulomas on biopsy, occurs in 75–100% of patients with acute sarcoid arthritis but is usually asymptomatic. Three types of symptomatic muscle involvement can be seen: an acute type of myositis, producing myalgia and muscular tenderness can occur in the early stage of the disease; a chronic myopathy has similar features, but frequently leads to atrophies; finally, a nodular type, which can manifest as cramping, is very rare but can be a presenting manifestation.

Osseous lesions occur in 1–13% of patients and most commonly involve the hands and the feet, generally under the form of localized punched out lytic lesions, trabecular alterations, or pathological fractures. Osseous involvement is frequently asymptomatic but can be painful.

Sarcoid myositis and osteitis should be treated as chronic arthritis. It can be mentioned that muscular nodules have been successfully treated with intralesional injections of triamcinolone hexacetonide. Magnetic resonance imaging can be very useful in the diagnosis and follow-up of myositis and osteitis, which can improve without radiographic modification.

2. Mild Pulmonary Disease

Because of the potential side effects of most treatments and their good prognosis (up to 90% spontaneous remissions at 2 years), patients with mild acute pulmonary disease do not require treatment [56]. Definition of such mild cases is somewhat varying, but it is generally agreed that patients with an abnormal radiograph (any stage) with mild or no symptoms and little or no impairment of pulmonary functions (FEV_1, vital capacity, total lung capacity, and DLCO) do not require active treatment [56,57]. Observation, however, is mandatory, with further radiographs and pulmonary functions every 2–3 months. Since extensive radiographic changes can occur with little or no functional impairment, it is considered that radiographs should not be used as a guide to therapy.

3. Severe or Progressive Pulmonary Disease

Severe or progressive pulmonary disease requires more aggressive treatment, including corticosteroids. Opinions vary concerning their indication and use, but marked symptoms or progressive disease, usually defined by recent deterioration of pulmonary functions during follow-up, even in the absence of symptoms, generally require corticosteroids [57]. It is less clear whether treatment is required for an asymptomatic patient who has impaired lung function at diagnosis; in any case, if not treated, such patients should at least be followed up very closely.

Corticosteroids. Corticosteroids are extremely efficient in most serious manifestations of sarcoidosis and are generally considered the mainstay of its treatment. Opinions also vary concerning the optimal dose and the duration of the treatment. For patients with moderate function deterioration, a single daily dose of 30–40 mg prednisone is generally advocated. Higher doses may be required but usually not exceeding 1 mg/kg/day. Symptomatic improvement is generally observed within a few weeks. Initial prednisone doses should be maintained for a couple of months. Doses can then be tapered progressively, but treatment should be continued at a maintenance dose of 10–15 mg/day for 6–12 months or even longer in some cases. In most patients, the process stabilizes and eventually burns out. Relapses occurred in only 5 of 37 patients treated with daily doses of 1 mg/kg/day prednisolone for 6 weeks and reducing to 0.25 mg/kg for 1 year [56]. Alternate-day therapy is not recommended as initial therapy, but it can be adequate early in patients with only mild symptoms and impairment of lung functions. Such regimen, which can minimize side effects, necessitates close follow-up to rule out progression of the disease. In some patients with disease confined to the lungs, high doses of inhaled corticosteroids (e.g., budesonide 1.6 mg/day) have been advocated as an alternative [58] and a recent double-blind placebo-controlled study demonstrated the potential of such regimen to reduce deterioration and postpone the need for systemic corticosteroids [59].

Cytotoxic and Immunosuppressive Agents. Several cytotoxic and immunosuppressive drugs have been evaluated for the treatment of patients who do not respond adequately to steroids or who require prolonged treatments with unacceptably high doses. These agents are lacking controlled trials to date, but many reports and open studies indicate therapeutic benefits for several of them.

Methotrexate at weekly low doses (7.5–25.0 mg/weeks) has been shown to be a useful alternative therapy and an effective corticosteroid-sparing agent for refractory lung manifestations of sarcoidosis [55,60,61]. A recent study suggests that the prolonged use of methotrexate allows significant improvement in pulmonary disease (vital capacity), skin lesions, and central nervous system involvement (evidenced by magnetic resonance imaging), as well as a decrease or discontinuation of corticosteroids [62]. Supplementation with folic acid should be considered in patients with relatively high doses, macrocytosis, or mucocutaneous side effects; although there are no data showing it, such a supplementation is not likely to decrease the effects of methotrexate in sarcoidosis, as in rheumatoid arthritis.

Cyclosporine initially proved disappointing as an isolated treatment in pulmonary sarcoidosis [63]. More recent studies, however, showed beneficial effects of this drug in patients with neurosarcoidosis [64] and severe pulmonary sarcoidosis [65]. Several cases of pulmonary sarcoidosis were documented to show objective clinical improvement, falls in bronchoalveolar lavage counts, or regression of ground-glass lesions on computed tomographic (CT) scanning. In two cases, regression of life-threatening endobronchial lesions were observed to regress only with cyclosporine. It appears that responsiveness of pulmonary sarcoidosis to cyclosporine is probably dependent on relatively high doses (150–500 ng/mL). It may prove, however, possible to use lower doses to maintain remissions. Cyclosporine may thus be a valuable alternative in patients with refractory disease. Azathioprine, cyclophosphamide, and chlorambucil have also been used with testimonials for favorable results but lack controlled trials to date.

Organ Transplantation. In a few patients, sarcoidosis progresses with the development of advanced lung fibrosis despite vigorous treatment with corticosteroids and immunosuppressive agents. In these patients, lung or heart-lung transplantation is an option, but recurrence of the primary disease appears terribly high: two out of two patients who were grafted for sarcoidosis were described to have recurrence in a recent report, which also illustrates the possible resistance of this disease to massive immunosuppression [66].

4. Other Manifestations

Benign Hepatosplenic, Cutaneous, and Ocular Manifestations. Asymptomatic liver and spleen disease are common and generally benign and do not require specific intervention. Treatment, however, may be required in cases of liver function deterioration, hypersplenism, or portal hypertension, and splenectomy can be helpful in selected cases [67]. Mild skin and ocular disease can sometimes be controlled by topical corticosteroids; chloroquine [68] and thalidomide [69] have also ben suggested to be valuable in cutaneous sarcoidosis. More serious disease, however, requires systemic therapy, including corticosteroids and, in most severe cases, immunosuppressive agents.

Serious Extrapulmonary Manifestations. The most serious extrapulmonary disease involve the central nervous system (CNS) and the heart. CNS manifestations, which usually develop within 2 years of onset of systemic sarcoidosis, are generally expressed as cranial neuropathy, facial palsy, aseptic meningitis, hydrocephalus, mass lesions, seizures or diffuse encephalopathies [64]. Cardiac involvement generally presents as arrhythmias, heart block, or cardiomyopathy, sometimes associated with sudden death. Severe extrapulmonary manifestations are sometimes asymptomatic and should be routinely sought by careful examination, electrocardiogram, and, in any case of suspicion, brain CT scan or magnetic resonance imaging. It is generally agreed that patients with objective evidence of serious extrapulmonary disease must be treated with high doses of corticosteroids (1–2 mg/kg/day initially in divided doses for the most severe cases). Methotrexate at weekly low doses (7.5–25.0 mg/weeks) has been shown to be a useful adjunctive therapy and an effective corticosteroid-sparing agent for neurological cutaneous, ocular, and hepatic manifestations as well as for refractory lung sarcoidosis [55,60,61]. Cyclosporine has also been shown to be beneficial in patients with neurosarcoidosis [64]. A recent retrospective study indicates that immunosuppressive agents are beneficial in neurosarcoidosis refractory to corticosteroids [64]. In this study, cyclosporine was suggested to be the best choice with azathioprine: The former is proposed to be better in the presence of liver or hematological disease and the latter in the presence of high blood pressure or renal disease; methotrexate, cyclophosphamide, chlorambucil, and radiation therapy were shown to be alternatives. A few patients, however, have progressive disease and die despite the addition of immunosuppressive agents to high doses of corticosteroids.

5. *Conclusions and Considerations on Antibiotic Treatments*

The occurrence of spontaneous remission in many patients is an indication for conservative treatment in mild cases. On the other hand, the possibility of a fatal issue justifies the use of aggressive interventions in more severe cases. Treatment has therefore to be closely adapted to the disease type, severity, and activity. Although rare cases proved to be resistant to all therapeutic interventions, immunosuppressive agents appear to be efficient in most severe cases, and most patients can eventually be offered an adequate control of their disease.

A few reports recently suggested an association between mycobacterial infection and sarcoidosis [70]. This may obviously arouse temptations for antimycobacterial drugs, especially for patients with resistant disease. Despite the similarities between sarcoidosis and tuberculosis, no studies could convincingly demonstrate any benefits of the classic antimycobacterial drugs, but other trials with newer drugs will undoubtedly be undertaken. In the meantime, it is certainly not justified to use antibiotics in the treatment of sarcoidosis, at least in patients responding to conventional therapies.

VII. WHIPPLE'S DISEASE

Whipple's disease is a multisystemic disorder, caused by the bacillus *Tropheryma Whippelii*, in which recurrent arthralgias or arthritis are the commonest nonintestinal complaint [71,72]. In many cases, rheumatic manifestations appear years (up to 35) before any other symptoms, including gastrointestinal ones. Since irreversible lesions, particularly in the CNS can occur, early diagnosis is of prime importance.

A. Diagnosis

1. *Epidemiology and Clinical Features*

Whipple's disease is rare, and it usually presents in middle-aged men. In most cases, rheumatic manifestations appear as an acute symmetrical migrating polyarthralgia or polyarthritis lasting, in the beginning, from a few days to a few weeks [71]. As the disease progresses, symptom-free intervals may fade and disappear. The joints most commonly involved are (in decreasing frequency) the knees, ankles, hips, finger joints, wrists, elbows, and spine. Objective signs of synovitis are absent in most cases, but swelling, warmth, and decreased range of motion can occur. The arthritis is generally nondestructive. Spondylitis has been described in 4–8% of patients and is often accompanied by a unilateral or bilateral sacroiliitis.

Besides arthralgia, the commonest clinical presentations are gastrointestinal complaints, which include weight loss, diarrhea, abdominal pains, and less frequently nausea, vomiting, and constipation. Malabsorption of fat, proteins, and carbohydrates is common. Eighty percent of patients have occult blood in their feces, but macroscopic bleeding is rare. Enlargement of the spleen and lympadenopathies, particularly mesenteric, are frequent. The heart is frequently involved with pericarditis, endocarditis, and myocarditis occurring in up to 80, 50, and 10%, respectively. CNS involvement can occur with varied symptoms and signs which include dementia, supranuclear ophthalmoplegia, truncal ataxia, hypothalamic syndrome (impotence and sleeping and eating disorders), and uveitis. Other clinical manifestations include skin changes (hyperpigmentation of light-exposed areas), pleuritis and cough, sarcoid-like illness, wasting syndrome, and fever.

2. Laboratory Features and Diagnostic Procedures

Joint fluid only shows a variable leukocytosis and is very unspecific, as well as blood findings such as anemia (90% of the patients), low serum iron and folates (30%), and hypoalbuminaemia (90%) [71]. Profound leukocytosis or leukopenia is mainly seen in seriously ill patients. Increased fecal fat is present in more than 90% of cases but is very unspecific. Shilling's test and xylose absorption are more specific of malabsorption and are positive in 15 and 78% of patients, respectively.

Once Whipple's disease is suspected, the procedure of choice is duodenal biopsy [52], which shows very specific foamy macrophages with inclusions intensely stained by periodic acid-Schiff (PAS). Diagnosis is more difficult in the rare cases with absent intestinal involvement, because periodic acid–Schiff is either unsensitive or unspecific in other tissues [52]. Demonstration of the bacilli by electron microscopy is highly specific but not always feasible. PCR has recently proved to be a very useful and sensitive technique and should be used in case of normal duodenal biopsy. PCR demonstrates the presence of bacterial RNA in different tissue samples, including lymphnodes, pleural cells, vitrectomy material, histologically normal duodenal biopsy, and even peripheral blood mononuclear cells [52,73].

B. Treatment

1. General Considerations

If left untreated, Whipple's disease is uniformly progressive and fatal, whereas treatment with antibiotics results in a dramatic improvement and, in most cases, complete recovery. The goals of the antibiotic treatment are to treat the disease manifestations but also to prevent relapses. Since relapses occurred in up to 35% of cases in a large study, there is a consensus for long-term (1 or 2 years) treatment. However, because of the rareness of the disease, recommendations on the duration of the treatment remain empirical and anecdotal. In addition, since *T. whippelii* cannot be cultured, its pattern of resistance is still unknown and antibiotic choices are largely historical or based on experience [71]. The first report of Ruffin and coworkers, who used chloramphenicol, streptomycin, penicillin, or tetracycline and achieved complete remission in 10 patients [74], has been particularly influential, and some textbooks still recommend the use of penicillin followed by long-term tetracycline. From several studies, however, it emerges that tetracycline and penicillin treatments are associated with a significant rate of relapses.

2. Antibiotic Regimens

An important study of Whipple's disease, based on a review of the literature and questionnaires sent to gastroenterological centers, reports relapses in 31 or 88 patients, with 13 of them affecting the CNS [75]. Most of the patients who relapsed had been treated with tetracycline alone (21 of 49, involving the CNS in 9). Frequent relapses also occurred with penicillin alone (three of eight, two in the CNS), and penicillin plus streptomycin (two of five, none in the CNS). Only two relapses occurred in 15 patients treated with a combination of penicillin, streptomycin, and tetracycline (none in the CNS) and none in three patients treated with trimetoprim-sulfamethoxazole. Non-CNS relapses responded well to a second treatment, but among 11 patients with CNS relapses, 6 died and 3 responded poorly. These data, as others, indicate that antibiotics such as tetracycline and penicillin, which penetrate poorly the blood-brain barrier unless the meninges are inflamed, are less efficient in preventing relapses, particularly in the CNS. They also highlight the poor prognosis of these CNS relapses and the importance of their prevention. On this basis, several investigators have recommended parenteral treatment with penicillin (1.2 MIE daily) and streptomycin (1 g daily) for 14 days followed (because of the low penetrance of these two antibiotics through the blood-brain barrier) by a treatment with sulfamethoxazole (800 mg) and trimethoprim (160 mg) twice daily for a year [76,77].

Treatment with sulfamethoxazole and trimethoprim alone (800 and 160 mg, respectively, three times daily for a fortnight and then twice daily), whose good penetration through the blood-brain barrier is well documented, has been advocated, more recently. This regimen has been found to be definitely superior to tetracyclines, allowing complete clinical remission in 12 of 13 patients [78]. In several cases, however, this treatment did not prevent cerebral involvement, sometimes severe and irreversible, despite remission of other manifestations [78,79]. It was therefore concluded that trimethoprim-sulfamethoxazole is no safeguard treatment against severe cerebral recurrence, maybe owing to the absence of bactericidal and opsonic activity of the cerebral fluid. Third-generation cephalosporins, on the other hand, have been shown to induce remission of cerebral disease in a few case reports even after sulfamethoxazole-trimethoprim failure [79,80].

On this basis, it can be concluded that a treatment course of 3 weeks with a highly active bactericidal compound that readily crosses the blood brain-barrier must be used initially. Parenteral third-generation cephalosporins such as ceftriaxone are certainly the best choice at the present time. This initial treatment should be followed by long-term treatment (1–2 years) with sulfamethoxazole-trimetroprim or oral third-generation cephalosporin.

3. *Assessment of the Response and Treatment Duration*

Evaluation of the treatment of Whipple's disease should be based on clinical as well as laboratory parameters. Apart from spondylitis, rheumatic and most other manifestations respond well to the antibiotic treatment within days to weeks, but the presence of CNS involvement indicates a poor prognosis, with little response to treatment, and death frequently occurring within months to a few years. Blood abnormalities (increased ESR and C-reactive protein [CRP]) may take several months to normalize. Small bowel biopsy may remain abnormal, with PAS-positive macrophages in up to 50% of patients for years despite an optimal response to treatment and life-long remission. On the other hand, the reappearance of typical Whipple's bacilli in the lamina propria may announce an imminent relapse even in asymptomatic patients. In addition, relapses may extend to other organs, sometimes exclusively extraintestinal, not involved during the primary attack. The duration of the treatment necessary for clinical and bioptical cure is highly individual, with a mean duration of 16 months [78]. The effective treatment is generally not shorter than 6 months.

4. *Conclusions and Treatment Guidelines*

Because of the absence of sensitivity testing of *Tropheryma whippelii*, treatment of Whipple's disease is still experimental. From available studies, however, it can be concluded that the best choice at the present time is 1–2 years of treatment with sulfamethoxazole and trimethoprim (800 and 160 mg, respectively, three times daily for 3 weeks and then twice daily) preceded, particularly if cerebral involvement in suspected, by a 2-weeks treatment course with parenteral ceftriaxone (1 g daily). When clinical manifestations persist after 1 month, compliance and antibiotic choice should be reevaluated. In case of allergy or intolerance, ceftriaxone can be substituted by penicillin plus streptomycin or possibly a quinolone. Sulfamethoxazole-trimetroprim can be substituted by oral third-generation cephalosporin or, but less favorably, tetracycline or penicillin. Small bowel biopsies should be performed at 3- to 6-month interval. Treatment should be continued until disappearance of symptoms and eradication of intracellular and extracellular bacteria. After 2 years, the persistence of single PAS positive macrophages should, per se, not be an indication for continuation of antibiotic treatment [78], but patients should be carefully followed clinically, biologically, and bioptically.

VIII. BEHÇET'S DISEASE

Behçet's disease is a multisystemic disorder of unknown etiology. In addition to the classic triad (uveitis and oral and genital ulcerations), practically any organ system can be affected, including the joints. Disease severity is variable, but morbidity and even mortality are fairly high, especially in young males, justifying the use of aggressive treatments.

A. Diagnosis

1. Epidemiology and Clinical Features

Distribution and Prevalence. Behçet's disease is generally considered rare except in Mediterranean countries, the Middle East, and Japan where its prevalence reaches 1:10000. The disease, however, may not be that uncommon in other countries, as suggested by a recent study in Olmstedt County, Minnesota, showing a prevalence of 1:15000 [81].

Diagnostic Criteria. Although combinations of characteristic features (Table 3 make the diagnosis of Behçet's disease easy in many patients, the decision may be more difficult in others because of its heterogeneous onset, variable organ involvement, lack of specificity of many features of the disease, and the absence of universally accepted diagnostic test. To help overcome this difficulty, a number of diagnostic or classification criteria have been put forward, including a set recently proposed by an international study group (Table 4), which is now being adopted for use in clinical and epidemiological studies [82].

2. Laboratory Features and Diagnostic Procedures

No laboratory tests are specific for Behçet's disease. Many abnormalities can be encountered, including decreased hemoglobin or increased ESR and CRP, but these parameters frequently remain normal despite active disease [82].

In Japan and the Middle East, HLA-B5, and more specifically the HLA-B51 rather than the HLA-B52 subtype, appear more frequent in patients with Behçet's disease (50–69%). More recent studies indicate that HLA-B51 may be associated only with more

Table 3 Frequency and Specificity of Clinical Features in Behçet's Disease

Feature	Frequency (%)	Specificity (%)
Oral ulcers	97–99	Very low
Folliculitis and/or erythema nodosum	81	75
Genital ulcers	77	95
Uveitis or retinal vasculitis	60	93
Pathergy phenomenon	58	90
Arthralgia	56	38
Arthritis	38	38
Family history	20	73
Subcutaneous thrombophlebitis	16	95
Deep vein thrombosis	13	96
CNS involvement (pyramidal, cerebellar, and sensory signs, meningeal irritation)	10	89
Epididymitis	8	100
Gastrointestinal problems (colicky abdominal pain and diarrhea	9 (30 in Japan)	82
Aneurysms and/or arterial occlusions	3	98

Source: Adapted from refs. 117 and 118.

severe disease; determination of HLA-B5 may thus contribute to predict severity in addition to help determine the diagnosis in some early cases with partial expression of the disease.

Specialized ophthalmological procedures, including slit-lamp examination performed by an ophthalmologist, are indicated even in the absence of symptoms in order to detect and stage ocular lesions early.

Although CT appears to be very unsensitive, magnetic resonance imaging (MRI) and single photon emission CT (SPECT) can be useful in identifying lesions in patients with CNS involvement [83,84]. However, signal changes have also been found in neurologically asymptomatic patients. The significance of these clinically silent lesions remains unresolved, and the role of MRI in monitoring disease activity is still uncertain [83].

Table 4 Criteria or the Diagnosis of Behçet's Syndrome (International Study Group)

In the absence of other clinical explanations, patients must have

1. Recurrent oral ulceration (aphtous or herpetiform) observed by the physician or patient, recurring at least three times in one 12-month period and at least two of the following
2. Recurrent genital ulceration
3. Eye lesions: anterior uveitis, posterior uveitis, cells in the vitreous or retinal vasculitis observed by slit-lamp examination by an ophthalmologist
4. Skin lesions: erythema nodosum, pseudofolliculitis, papulopustular lesions, or acneiform nodules in postadolescent patients not on corticosteroids
5. Pathergy, read by a physician at 24–48 h

Source: Adapted from refs. 117 and 118.

3. *Disease Severity and Activity*

Because of the variable outcome of the disease and the severe side effects of many of its treatments, the availability of reliable measures of disease activity is of prime importance in monitoring the management of Behçet's disease. Separating new disease activity from established damage and predicting disease severity are especially important [82].

In the absence of adequate laboratory markers, assessment of disease severity has to be based largely on history and clinical features. Complete Behçet's disease, multiple organ involvement, especially neurological, ocular, and vascular, male sex, Mediterranean or Far Eastern origin, and HLA-B51 are recognized markers of disease severity.

As to disease activity, no laboratory tests, including hemoglobin, ESR, and CRP, consistently reflect the activity of the disease; it has been noted, however, that ESR and CRP, although frequently normal despite active disease, can be useful when raised in clinically inactive patients and should prompt further investigation. Aiming at providing better evaluation of disease activity, several instruments have been developed, including the recent "European Behçet's Disease Current Activity Form," which is presently undergoing evaluation but can already be used to help monitor activity in routine clinical management [82].

B. Treatment

1. *General Considerations*

Many drugs have been used in the treatment of Behçet's disease. It is widely considered that treatment is largely determined by the type and severity of organ involvement, but few interventions have been evaluated in controlled trials. The aim of the treatment is to suppress inflammation early and prevent progression of irreversible lesions, particularly in the eyes and in the brain. In general, treatment must be more aggressive in patients with markers of disease severity (see above). Patients with recent-onset disease must be followed up very closely, and any major organ involvement treated early. It has even been proposed to consider prophylactic immunosuppressive treatment with azathioprine in patients with a high risk of developing aggressive disease [85].

Eye involvement is the most common serious manifestation of Behçet's disease; it has been the object of most clinical studies and its treatment generally governs the management of seriously affected patients.

2. *Treatment of Ocular Manifestations*

Ocular involvement is a serious manifestation in that legal blindness usually ensues within 4 years unless the patients is treated with immunosuppressive drugs. It is a sign of disease severity, and up to 30% of these patients (at least in Northern Europe and the United States where the prevalence is higher) have an associated neuro-Behçet's.

It is generally considered that treatment must be initiated early in order to be effective. The goals are to suppress inflammation, particularly any involvement of the retina, and to reduce the frequency and severity of the recurrences. Immunosuppessive agents are the mainstay of the treatment in most patients, but the choice of the medication is determined by the severity of the disease. In addition to general signs of severity (see above), multiple recurrences of uveitis and retinal and bilateral involvement are indications for more aggressive treatment. In addition to local treatments, the most commonly used systemic treatments are corticosteroids, immunosuppressive agents, and colchicine.

Local treatment. Local mydriatics should be used in the acute inflammatory stage to prevent the formation of synechiae. The role of topical steroid is less clear: drops, with or without periocular injections, are generally adequate to control inflammation limited to the anterior segment; in some cases of posterior segment inflammation, corticosteroid drops can be useful and allow the use of lower doses of systemic corticosteroids.

Systemic Corticosteroids. Systemic corticosteroids have a rapid and potent anti-inflammatory effect in all phases of Behçet's disease, including ocular manifestations. They are particularly effective in the acute phases of the disease but fail to prevent visual deterioration and the eventual development of blindness [86]. Corticosteroids are therefore very useful in acute phases or exacerbation of the disease, but must be associated with other agents. Systemic corticosteroids are always required to control inflammation of the posterior segment. They are generally used at initial doses ranging between 1.0 and 1.5 mg/kg/day. In severe cases, doses can be divided (up to four) or preceded by methylprednisolone pulses (0.5–1.0 g/day) for a few days (generally 3 consecutive days). Corticosteroids are usually introduced in association with a cytotoxic agent or cyclosporine. Once this latter treatment becomes affective, usually after 3–6 weeks, the corticosteroids are tapered gradually. Since there is no formal evidence that long-term systemic corticosteroids are effective, toxicity should be a concern: Ideally, maintenance doses in chronic cases should not exceed 7.5–12.5 mg/day.

Immunosuppressive Agents. Azathioprine, cyclosporine, and chlorambucil can be used alone or in combination in the treatment of Behçet's disease.

Chlorambucil. Chlorambucil, the first cytotoxic drug evaluated in Behçet's disease, is still widely used in many centers. The effects of this alkylating agent are similar to those of cyclophosphamide. It allows substantial corticosteroid-sparing and long remissions, and it was reported to achieve total control of blinding ocular manifestations in 70% of patients in an American series [87]. Chlorambucil is currently strongly recommended by some experts [87,88].

A favorable response is generally obtained within 1–3 months with initial doses of 0.2 mg/kg/day. The dosage can then be reduced and maintained for 1–2 years. In refractory cases, dosages of up to 22 mg/day have been advocated [87]. However, because of its high risk/benefit ratio (especially myelotoxic and oncogenic), other immunosuppressants are now frequently preferred over chlorambucil.

Cyclophosphamide. Cyclophosphamide has also been shown to be better than corticosteroids in controlling uveitis and can be used at a maximum dose of 2 mg/kg/day with close monitoring of the blood cell counts. As in other diseases, monthly intravenous pulses are probably less toxic than oral administration, although they are not as efficient in severe cases. Several studies have reported the efficacy of intravenous pulses in Behçet's disease, and cyclophosphamide has even been used successfully in cases of uveitis refractory to chlorambucil [87].

Azathioprine. Azathioprine has been the object of a careful double-blind study. At 2.5 mg/kg/day, it was found to be more effective than placebo in maintaining visual acuity and preventing the emergence of new eye disease [89]. This therapy, however, was not shown to improve compromised vision. More recently, the same group reported a study indicating that long-term results are better when azathioprine is introduced early in the course of the disease. Others found the effects of azathioprine to be less spectacular, but its relative safety makes it a very useful drug in the management of Behçet's disease. Azathioprine might also be beneficial when associated with cyclosporine in severe and unresponsive cases (personal observation).

Cyclosporine. Cyclosporine has been the object of numerous studies. In a double-blinded controlled study, cyclosporine at 10 mg/kg/day proved to be better than colchicine in decreasing the frequency and severity of ocular attacks [90]. The side effects, however, were higher with cyclosporine at this dosage. For long-term treatment, doses had to be decreased to 3–5 mg/kg/day, but the drug appeared to retain its effects. At 5 mg/kg/day, cyclosporine was shown, in a single masked trial, to be better than monthly pulse intravenous cyclophosphamide at 6 months, although it appeared equivalent at 2 years [91]. Other groups confirmed the efficacy of cyclosporine even in cases poorly controlled by other immunosuppressive agents [92–95]. In some series, on the other hand, low doses were ineffective in up to 30% of the patients, particularly in the presence of retinal vasculitis [95]. In addition, the effects can decrease over time. The effects of cyclosporine, however, are improved when corticosteroids are associated [94]. In cases of resistance, the addition of another agent, such as azathioprine, can allow to gain or regain control of the disease. Because of frequent side effects, cyclosporine should not be used at doses higher than 5 mg/kg/day, at least in the long term. The proposed guidelines for the use of cyclosporine in rheumatoid arthritis should be adequate to monitor the treatment properly [96]. It is important to maintain efficient doses (2.5–5.0 mg/kg/day) for a prolonged period of time (24 months) after resolution of the activity, even when complete, otherwise the disease can reactivate and become difficult to control. Because of its relative safety at low doses and efficiency in most patients, cyclosporine is certainly a very useful drug for the management of Behçet's disease.

Colchicine. The anti-inflammatory effects of colchicine are only mild and not sufficient to prevent the development of irreversible ocular lesions in most cases. Several studies, however, indicate that when colchicine is added to immunosuppressive agents, it can allow patients to decrease their dosage [87]. Initial doses are usually of 1.0–1.5 mg/day and can be decreased to 0.5 mg/day once the symptoms have stabilized.

Alternative Treatments. Interferon-α has been reported to allow tapering of corticosteroids in a patient with severe ocular manifestations resistant to corticosteroids, colchicine, cyclosporine, and cyclophosphamide [97], and this warrants further studies.

FK506, a very powerful immunosuppressive agent analogous to cyclosporine has recently been evaluated in a phase II open study. It was found to be beneficial in most patients [98]; side effects (mainly renal and neurological) appeared to be acceptable in this study but are still poorly appreciated in the long-term treatment of immunoinflammatory diseases. FK506 also warrants further studies, but it might already be helpful in the management of selected cases, even serious, in the absence of satisfying response to other treatments.

Surgery. Surgery may be indicated in selected patients with Behçet's disease to correct structural changes. It has to be kept in mind, however, that the trauma associated with surgery can (re)activate inflammation, presumably because the pathergy phenomenon may occur at sites other than the skin.

3. Treatment of CNS Manifestations

CNS manifestations of Behçet's disease are one of the major causes of fatalities, especially in Northern Europe and the United States where the prevalence reaches 10–25%

of the patients. No controlled studies have been performed on the treatment of CNS manifestations to date. These manifestations are therefore usually treated as severe ocular disease, with high doses of corticosteroids and immunosuppressive agents. It has been suggested, however, that cyclosporine might be less effective for the treatment of CNS involvement [99].

Headaches are frequent but have to be considered clinically important only when associated with other neurological manifestations [100]; otherwise, symptomatic treatment is adequate. On the other hand, headaches associated with intracranial hypertension require corticosteroids, which are highly effective; prednisone at doses between 1.0 and 1.5 mg/day with gradual tapering is usually satisfactory.

Psychiatric disturbances are frequently encountered. They might represent either an organic manifestation of the disease, a reaction toward the disease, or a side effect of the treatment (steroid induced psychoses). Depending on the setting, attempting a treatment with corticosteroids or, on the other hand, tapering high doses of corticosteroids can be informative and useful.

4. *Treatment of Mucocutaneous Manifestations*

Mucocutaneous manifestations of Behçet's disease are generally less severe but affect virtually all patients. In most cases, they consist only of minor aphtous ulcers. General measures of oral hygiene are required, including the avoidance of certain foods when these are felt to precipitate the symptoms. Topical preparations, adhering to the mucosa, of anesthetics (2% lidocaine gel), steroids, or steroids combined with antibiotics can alleviate symptoms of oral and genital ulcers; topical steroids might even shorten the duration of ulcerations and be more effective when given early, if possible, during the prodromal manifestations (tenderness, red papule) [85]. Colchicine (1.5 mg/day) has been shown to be effective particularly in erythema nodosum.

Very rarely, mucocutaneous manifestations can be very severe and disabling and require systemic corticosteroids or immunosuppressive treatments even in the absence of major organ manifestations. Both azathioprine [85] and cyclosporine [90] have been shown to be effective and can be used in such settings. Thalidomide (200–400 mg/day) has also been used with success, but its use is limited by the lack of studies and its high teratogenicity [85].

Interferon-α has more recently been reported to be effective by several independent groups: it controlled skin manifestations such as oral and genital ulcers as well as pustular vasculitis in a noncontrolled study on 14 patients [101] and in a self-controlled study on 20 patients [102]. Interferon-α might therefore be useful in severe as well as in more benign mucocutaneous manifestations. On the other hand, the antiviral agent acyclovir gave negative results.

5. *Treatment of Articular and Muscular Manifestations*

Not infrequently, articular manifestations reveal Behçet's disease and can precede other manifestations by many months or years. Joint involvement typically takes the form of recurrent, nondestructive peripheral oligoarthritis (less than five joints), generally affecting large joints (knees, ankles, hips, elbows, and wrists), but it may rarely involve small joints of the hands and feet. Episodes usually last from a few days to a few weeks, but chronic arthritis can occasionally be seen. Back pain is uncommon and the frequency of sacroiliitis is not increased.

Rest, simple analgesics, and NSAIDs are adequate to control symptoms in most patients, although the efficacy of NSAIDs, or at least some of them, has been questioned [85,103]. Colchicine has also been shown to decrease joint manifestations. Intra-articular corticosteroids can be helpful in cases of resistant single-joint inflammation. In more severe cases, methotrexate or interferon-α [97] can be considered.

Muscular involvement can be seen, generally as local myositis, but generalized forms with elevated enzymes can also occur. A case of generalized myositis resistant to steroids and azathioprine has reportedly been treated successfully with cyclosporine [104].

6. Vascular Manifestations

Thrombophlebitis. Thrombophlebitis usually affects peripheral veins, especially from the calf, but the thrombus is usually firmly attached to the endothelial wall, and the occurrence of pulmonary embolism is rare in Behçet's disease. In such cases, antiplatelet agents, such as low-dose aspirin, are usually recommended [85]. Severe cases, however, can involve the superior and inferior venae cavae and eventually lead to the development of the Budd-Chiarri syndrome. Involvement of the veins of the central nervous system can also occur and be life threatening. Early diagnosis and treatment are essential for the management of such cases. Recent advances in the diagnosis of vasculo-Behçet's disease have been brought about by the use of radionuclide venography [105,106]. In severe cases, anticoagulants are indicated and fibrinolytic agents can be beneficial [105,106].

Arteritis and Aneurysms. Arteritis can involve any arterial tree, including the aorta and pulmonary vessels. Both occlusions and aneurysms can be life threatening. In some cases, pulmonary arteritis can be difficult to differentiate from pulmonary embolism (although rare) in patients with the coexistence of arteritis and deep vein thrombosis (Hughes-Stovin syndrome). Advances in the diagnosis of arteritis have recently been achieved with the use of computed tomography and ultrasonography.

Operative therapy is often recommended for the management of arterial aneurysm, with their rupture being one of the leading causes of death in Behçet's disease. The disease activity, however, should be controlled as much as possible before and after the intervention with adjuvant immunotherapy because of the propensity of surgery to (re)activate inflammatory lesions [107]. Severe vasculitis is treated as other major organ manifestations with high doses of corticosteroids and immunosuppressive agents. Cyclophosphamide, either orally or by intravenous pulses, is generally recommended [108]. Plasma exchange might also be beneficial in serious cases, such as severe cutaneous necrotizing vasculitis [109].

7. Gastrointestinal Manifestations

Inflammatory bowel disease is seen particularly in Japanese patients and can affect any segment of the gastrointestinal tract. Sulfasalazine (2-4 g/day) has been reported to be beneficial, although no controlled study supports its effects. In some cases, resection surgery may be required because of the propensity of gastrointestinal ulcers to perforation. It is probably wise to avoid NSAIDs in the presence of such manifestations.

8. Conclusions and General Guidelines

In many patients, Behçet's disease is mild and symptomatic treatment is sufficient. Regular evaluation is required, however, to detect involvement of major organs early, especially in patients with more severe prognosis (see above). Such manifestations must be treated aggressively with corticosteroids and immunosuppressive agents (Table 5). The choice of the immunosuppressor is governed by its specificities, including potential side effects, as well as by the physician's experience. In some cases, immunosuppressors can be combined, which sometimes allows a decrease in dosages and results in a decrease side effects. The natural tendency of the disease for exacerbations and remissions and the usual improvement over time indicate that treatment must be regularly reevaluated. When remission occurs, treatment must be maintained and tapered only very progressively. It is considered, however, that after 2 years of complete resolution, in particular of ocular manifestations, further treatment is not required.

IX. HERIDITARY ANGIOEDEMA

Hereditary angioedema, defined biochemically by a deficiency in the functional activity of C1 esterase inhibitor (C1INH), is frequently mentioned in the differential diagnosis of recurrent arthritis. It rarely presents with true synovitis, but the attacks of edema can localize about a joint and mimic synovitis. Hereditary angioedema, though, can also present with recurrent episodes of synovitis in some patients [110]. In addition, hereditary angioedema is frequently associated with immunoinflammatory disorders involving the joints, such as Sjögren's syndrome or rheumatoid arthritis [111,112].

Because of the severity of the conditions, which can be fatal, and the need for specific treatment, diagnosis must be made rapidly [113].

A. Diagnosis

1. Epidemiology and Clinical Features

Hereditary angioedema is rare, with its estimated prevalence ranging between 1 in 10,000 and 1 in 50,000. In mot cases, the condition results from an autosomal dominant genetic defect, but it can also result from spontaneous mutations; symptoms generally appear during early childhood, but they may emerge well into adulthood. An acquired form, generally associated with lymphoproliferative disorders, is well described.

Hereditary angioedema is characterized by episodic bouts of subcutaneous nonpitting, circumscribed swelling without erythema that primarily involves the extremities, the face, the larynx, and the abdomen. Episodes last from 1 to 4 days. Swelling of the extremities is painless, but nausea, vomiting, diarrhea, and severe abdominal pain can occur, resulting from swelling of the gastrointestinal mucosa. Involvement of the upper airways leads to severe and life-threatening dyspnea. CNS symptoms, including severe headaches, aphasia, and hemiplegia, can also occur.

2. Blood Tests

On immunological measurement, 85% of patients with hereditary angioedema have decreased levels of C1INH (type 1 disease) whereas the remaining have normal or increased levels (type 2 disease). On the other hand, almost all patients have low plasma levels of C4. In the few patients with normal C4, diagnosis can be established by measuring functional C1INH [114]. In the acquired form, C1 is distinctly decreased in addition to the decrease in C1INH and C4.

Table 5 Summary of the Medications used in Behçet's Disease

Type of manifestations	Medication	Dosage
Ocular		
Mild anterior uveitis	Topical corticosteroids	
	Colchicine	1.5 mg/day
	Azathioprine?	1.0–2.5 mg/kg/day
Severe involvement	Oral corticosteroids	0.1–2.0 mg/kg/day[a]
	or IV methylprednisolone boluses	0.5–1.0 g for 3 consecutive or alternate days before oral
	and immunosuppressives	
	azathioprine	2.5 mg/kg/day
	cyclosporine	3–5 mg/kg/day
	chlorambucil	0.2 mg/kg/day
	cyclophosphamide	oral: 1.5–2.0 mg/kg/day
		IV pulses: 1.0–1.5 g/month
	Colchicine (with immunosuppressives)	1.5 mg/day (optional)
CNS (not isolated headaches)	Corticosteroids and immunosuppressives	Compare severe ocular manifestations

Mucocutaneous		
Genital and oral ulcers	Topical anesthetics, topical corticosteroids ± topical antibiotics	
	Colchicine?	1.5 mg/day
Severe involvement	Thalidomide?	200–400 mg/j
	Azathioprine or cyclosporine	Compare severe ocular manifestations
	Interferon-α (see text)	
Erythema nodosum	Colchicine	1.5 mg/day
Articular and muscular	Analgesics or NSAIDs	
	Colchicine	1.5 mg/day
	Methotrexate (severe cases)	7.5–25.0 mg/week
	Cyclosporine (diffuse myositis)	3-5 mg/kg/day
Vascular		
Peripheral thrombophlebitis	Antiplatelet agents	
Arteritis and life-threatening thrombophlebitis	Steroid + immunosuppressives (cyclophosphamide preferred) and anticoagulants ± fibrinolytics (see text)	See severe ocular manifestations

[a]Equivalent prednisone.

B. Treatment

1. *Treatment of the Attacks*

Before adequate treatment and prophylaxis, the mortality of hereditary angioedema, essentially due to attacks involving the upper airways, exceeded 25%. Treatment has been considerably improved by the availability of purified concentrates which produce their effect within minutes. A recent double-blind controlled study showed that vapor-heated C1INH concentrate (25 plasma units/kg) markedly and significantly reduces the severity and length of the episodes without evidence of toxicity [115]. C1INH concentrate is now certainly the treatment of choice for acute laryngeal obstruction or severe abdominal pain. Yet, indications for treatment with C1INH concentrate are not unrestricted. Although heat treatment reduces the transmission of hepatitis C, and no transmission of human immunodeficiency virus has been reported, safety is nevertheless a concern and patients must be followed carefully. For this reason, and because of its cost, the use of C1INH concentrate for benign, harmless, subcutaneous edema is more controversial, and it is probably inappropriate so far [113]. No other drug, including antihistamines, corticosteroids, adrenergics, and androgens, proved to be really effective for the treatment of the attack, but analgesics, including narcotics, may be required for abdominal pains.

2. *Prophylaxis*

Attenuated androgens are very effective in preventing attacks of hereditary angioedema, and stanozolol (0.5–2.0 mg/day) and danazol (50–400 mg/day) are now widely used [116]. At optimal dosage, which must be determined for each patient, they achieve their effect after approximately 5 days. Androgens, however, are transiently and poorly effective in the acquired form. In addition, attenuated androgens are contraindicated in prepubertal patients except for short courses of 5 days before elective surgical or dental procedures. Before such elective procedures, it is recommended to give two to three times the usual dose.

Prophylactic infusions of heated C1 inhibitor concentrate (25 plasma units/kg every third day) was also shown to decrease significantly the frequency and the severity of the attacks but not to prevent them completely [115]. Because of safety and cost concerns, and because of the effectiveness of androgens, it is still probably inappropriate to use concentrate for long-term prophylactic use [113] except in patients who are resistant or cannot tolerate the attenuated androgens.

REFERENCES

1. Hench PS, Rosenberg EF. Palindromic rheumatism. A "new" oft recurring disease of joints (arthritis, periarthritis, para-arthritis) apparently producing no articular residues. Report of thirty-four cases: its relation to "angio-neural arthrosis", "allergic rheumatism" and rheumatoid arthritis. Arch Intern Med 1944; 73:293–321.
2. Ansell BM, Bywaters EGL. Palindromic rheumatism. Ann Rheum Dis 1959; 18:331–3332.
3. Mattingly S: Palindromic rheumatism. Ann Rheum Dis 1966; 25:307–317.
4. Williams MH, Sheldon PJ, Torrigiani G, et al. Palindromic rheumatism. Clinical and immunological studies. Ann Rheum Dis 1971; 30:375–380.
5. Pasero G, Barbieri P. Palindromic rheumatism: you just have to think about it. Clin Exp Rheumatol 1986; 4:197–199.

6. Hannonen P, Möttönen T, Oka M. Palindromic rheumatism. A clinical survey of sixty patients. Scand J Rheumatol 1987; 16:413–420.
7. Guerne P-A, Weisman MH. Palindromic rheumatism: Part of or apart from the spectrum of rheumatoid arthritis. Am J Med 1992; 93:451–460.
8. Pincus T. Is control of rheumatoid arthritis using available therapies a realistic goal? Rheumatology 1994; 8:3–4.
9. Grattan CE, Kennedy TD, Yates DB. Prognostic factors in palindromic rheumatism. Bristol Med Chir J 1984; 99:51–54.
10. Wajed MA, Brown DL, Currey HL. Palindromic rheumatism. Clinical and serum complement study. Ann Rheum Dis 1977; 36:56–61.
11. Bregeon C, Dajon JL, Renier L, et al. [Palindromic rheumatism]. Rev Rhum Mal Osteoartic 1986; 53:441–449.
12. Verwilghen J, Panayi GS. Influence of pregnancy of disease activity in a patient with palindromic rheumatism. J Rheumatol 1992; 19:292–293.
13. Barbieri P, Benedettini G, Ciompi ML, Campa M. Failure to detect a lymphocyte imbalance during acute attacks of palindromic rheumatism (letter). Clin Rheumatol 1987; 6:102–103.
14. Schumacher HR. Palindromic onset of rheumatoid arthritis. Clinical, synovial fluid, and biopsy studies. Arthritis Rheum 1982; 25:361–369.
15. Fisher LR, Kirk A, Awad J, et al. HLA antigens in palindromic rheumatism and palindromic onset rheumatoid arthritis. Br J Rheumatol 1986; 25:345–348.
16. Gran JT, Husby G, Thorsby E. HLA antigens in palindromic rheumatism, nonerosive rheumatoid arthritis and classical rheumatoid arthritis. J Rheumatol 1984; 11:136–140.
17. Barbieri P, Ciompi ML, Menicucci A, Pasero G. HLA antigens in palindromic rheumatism. An Italian study. Clin Rhemuatol 1988; 7:470–473.
18. Eliakim A, Neumann L, Horowitz, J, et al. Palindromic rheumatism in Israel—a disease entity? A survey of 34 patients. Clin Rheumatol 1989; 8:507–511.
19. Hardo HG. Palindromic rheumatism: a review. J R Soc Med 1981; 74:521–524.
20. Hannonen P, Möttönen T, Oka M. Treatment of palindromic rheumatism with cholorquine (letter). Br Med J (Clin Res) 1987; 294:1289.
21. Youssef W, Yan A, Russell AS. Palindromic rheumatism: A response to cholorquine. J Rheumatol 1991; 18:35–37.
22. Golding DN. Sulphasalazine for palindromic rheumatism (letter). Br J Rheumatol 1988; 27:79.
23. Huskisson EC. Treatment of palindromic rheumatism with D-penicillamine. Br Med J 1976; 2:979.
24. Meyer O, Ryckewaert A. [Palindromic rheumatism: efficacy of dapsone (letter)]. Rev Rhum Mal Osteoartic 1985; 52:596–597.
25. Schwartzberg M. Prophylactic colchicine therapy in palindromic rheumatism (letter). J Rheumatol 1982; 9:341–343.
26. Gedalia A, Adar A, Gorodischer R. Familial Mediterranean fever in children. J Rheumatol 1992; 35(Suppl):1–9.
27. Garcia-Gonzalez A, Weisman MH. The arthritis of familial Mediterranean fever. Semin Arthritis Rheum 1992; 22:139–150.
28. Hernes D, Makin M. Articular damage in familial mediterranean fever. J Bone Joint Surg (Am) 1975; 57:265–267.
29. Sneh E, Pras M, Michaeli D, et al. Protracted arthritis in familial Mediterranean fever. Rheumatol Rehabil 1977; 16:102–106.
30. Sohar E, Gafni J, Pras M, Heller H. Familial mediterranean fever: a survey of 470 cases and review of the litterature. Am J Med 1967; 43:227–253.
31. Goldfinger SE. Colchicine for familial mediterranean fever. N Engl J Med 1972; 298:1302.

32. Dinarello CA, Wolff SM, Goldfinger SE, et al. Colchicine therapy for familial mediterranean fever. A double-blind trial. N Engl J Med 1974; 291:934–937.
33. Zemer D, Livneh A, Danon Y, et al. Long-term colchicine treatment in children with familial mediterranean fever. Arthritis Rheum 1991; 34:973–981.
34. Zemer D, Pras M, Sohar E, et al. Colchicine in the prevention and treatment of the amyloidosis of familial mediterranean fever. N Engl J Med 1986; 314:1001–1005.
35. Ehrenfeld M, Brzezinski A, Levy M, Eliakim M. Fertility and obstetric history in patients with familial Mediterranean fever on long-term colchicine therapy. Br J Obstet Gynaecol 1987; 94:1186–1191.
36. Livneh A, Zemer D, Langevitz P, et al. Colchicine in the treatment of AA and AL amyloidosis. Semin Arthritis Rheum 1993; 23:206–214.
37. Livneh A, Zemer D, Langevitz P, et al. Colchicine treatment of AA amyloidosis of familial mediterranean fever. An analysis of factors affecting outcome. Arthritis Rheum 1995; 37:1804–1811.
38. Salai M, Langevitz P, Blankstein A, et al. Total hip replacement in familial Mediterranean fever. Bull Hosp Jt Dis 1993; 53:25–28.
39. Kiliccturgay S, Haberal M. Transplantation for renal amyloidosis. Ren Fail 1993; 15:629–633.
40. Lightfoot RW. Intermittent and periodic arthritic syndromes. In: Arthritis and Allied Conditions McCarty DJ, Koopman WJ, eds. Philadelphia: Lea & Febiger, 1993:1121–1137.
41. Malone DG, Wilder RL. Participation of synovial mast cells in intermittent hydrarthrosis (letter). Arthritis Rheum 1989; 32:357–358.
42. Witvoet J. [Chronic instability of the knee]. Rev Prat 1989; 39:2507–2518.
43. Finsterbush A, Pogrund H. The hypermobility syndrome. Clin Orthop Rel Res 1982; 168:124–127.
44. Khachadurian AK. Migratory polyarthritis in familial hypercholesterolemia (type II hyperlipoproteinemia). Arthritis Rheum 1968; 11:385–393.
45. Careless DJ, Cohen MG. Rheumatic manifestations of hyperlipidemia and antihyperlipidemia drug therapy. Semin Arthritis Rheum 1993; 23:90–98.
46. Rooney PJ, Third J, Madkour MM, et al. Transient polyarthritis associated with familial hyperbetalipoproteinaemia. Q J Med 1978; 47:249–259.
47. Buckingham RB, Bole GG, Bassett DR. Polyarthritis associated with type IV hyperlipidemia. Arch Intern Med 1975; 135:286–290.
48. Klemp P, Halland AM, Majoos FL, Steyn K. Musculoskeletal manifestations in hyperlipidaemia: a controlled study. Ann Rheum Dis 1993; 52:44–48.
49. Carroll GJ, Bayliss CE. Treatment of the arthropathy of familial hypercholesterolaemia. Ann Rheum Dis 1983; 42:206–209.
50. Mol MJM, Stalenhoef AFH. HMG CoA reductase inhibitors. Curr Opin Lipidol 1994; 4:41–48.
51. Poe RH, Levy PC. Diagnosis and treatment of Sarcoidosis. Compr Ther 1993; 19:209–213.
52. Dobbins WO. The diagnosis of Whipple's disease. N Engl J Med 1995; 332:390–392.
53. Fink SD, Kremer JM. Cutaneous and musculoskeletal features, diagnostic modalities, and immunopathology in sarcoidosis. Curr Opin Rheumatol 1994; 6:78–81.
54. Gran JT, Bøhmer E. Acute sarcoid arthritis: a favourable outcome? Scand J Rheumatol 1996; 25:70–73.
55. Kaye O, Palazzo E, Grossin M, et al. Low-dose methotrexate: an effective corticosteroid-sparing agent in the musculoskeletal manifestations of sarcoidosis. Br J Rheumatol 1995; 34:642–644.
56. Hunninghake GW, Gilbert S, Pueringer R, et al. Outcome of the treatment for sarcoidosis [see comments]. Am J Respir Crit Care Med 1994; 149:893–898.

57. Honda M, Yammamoto S, Cheng M, et al. Human soluble IL-6 receptor. Its detection and enhanced released by HIV infection. J Immunol 1992; 148:2175–2180.
58. Spiteri MA. Inhaled corticosteroids in pulmonary sarcoidosis. Postgrad Med 1991; 67:327–329.
59. Alberts C, van dert Mark TW, Jansen HM. Inhaled budesonide in pulmonary sarcoidosis: a double-blind, placebo- controlled study. Dutch Study Group on Pulmonary Sarcoidosis (see comments). Eur Respir J 1995; 8:682–688.
60. Lower EE, Baughman RP. The use of low-dose methotrexate in refractory sarcoidosis. Am J Med Sci 1990; 229:153–157.
61. Soriano FG, Caramelli P, Nitini R, Rocha AS. Neurosarcoidosis: therapeutic success with methotrexate. Postgrad Med 1990; 66:142–143.
62. Lower EE, Baughman RP. Prolonged use of methotrexate for sarcoidosis. Arch Intern Med 1995; 155:846–851.
63. Tanaka Y, Otsuka T, Hotokebuchi T, et al. Effect of IL-10 on collagen-induced arthritis in mice. Inflamm Res 1996; 45:283–288.
64. Agbogu BN, Stern BJ, Sewell C, Yang G. Therapeutic considerations in patients with refractory neurosarcoidosis. Arch Neurol 1995; 52:875–879.
65. O'Callaghan CA, Wells AU, Lalvani A, et al. Effective use of cyclosporin in sarcoidosis: a treatment strategy based on computed tomography scanning. Eur Respir J 1994; 7:2255–2256.
66. Kazerooni EA, Jackson C, Cascade PN. Sarcoidosis: recurrence of primary disease in transplanted lungs. Radiology 1994; 192:461–464.
67. Kruithoff KL, Gyetko MR, Scheiman JM. Giant splenomegaly and refractory hypercalcemia due to extrapulmonary sarcoidosis. Successful treatment by splenectomy. Arch Intern Med 1993; 153:2793–2796.
68. Zic JA, Horowitz DH, Arzubiaga C, King LE Jr. Treatment of cutaneous sarcoidosis with chloroquine. Review of the literature. Arch Dermatol 1991; 127:1034–1040.
69. Carlesimo M, Giustini S, Rossi A, et al. Treatment of cutaneous and pulmonary sarcoidosis with thalidomide. J Am Acad Dermatol 1995; 32:866–869.
70. Mitchell DN. Mycobacteria and sarcoidosis. Lancet 1996; 348:768–769.
71. Gaist D, Ladefoged K. Whipple's disease. Scand J Gastroenterol 1994; 29:97–101.
72. Berthelot JM, Dao T, Bregeon C, et al. Palindromic rheumatism as the first manifestation of Whipple's disease. Rev Rhum 1994; 61:39–43.
73. Rickman LS, Freeman WR, Green WR. Uveitis caused b tropheryma whippelii (Whipple's bacillus). N Engl J Med 1995; 332:363–366.
74. Ruffin JM, Kurtz SM, Roufail WM. Intestinal lipodystrophy (Whipple's disease)-the immediate and prolonged effect of antibiotic therapy. JAMA 1966; 195:182–184.
75. Keinath RD, Merell DE, Viestra R, Dobbins WL III. Antibiotic treatment and relapse in Whipple's disease. Gastroenterology 1985; 88:1867–1873.
76. Dobbins WO III. Whipple's disease. In: Principles and Practice of Gastroenterology and Hepatology. Gitnick G, ed. New York: Elsevier, 1988:426–438.
77. Flemming JL, Wiesener RH, Shorter RG. Whipple's disease: clinical, biochemical and histopathologic features and assessment of teatment in 29 patients. Mayo Clin Proc 1988; 63:539–551.
78. Feurle GE, Marth T. An evaluation of antimicrobial treatment for Whipple's Disease. Tetracycline versus trimethoprim-sulfamethoxazole. Dig Dis Sci 1994; 39:1642–1648.
79. Cooper GS, Blades EW, Remler BF, et al. Central nervous system Whipple's disease: relapse during therapy with trimethoprim-sulfamethoxazole and remission with cefixime. Gastroenterology 1994; 106:782–786.
80. Lowe GN, Fu YH, McDougall S, et al. Effects of prostaglandins on deoxyribonucleic acid

and aggrecan synthesis in the RCJ 3.1C5.18 chondrocyte cell line: Role of second messengers. Endocrinology 1996; 137:2208-2216.
81. O'Duffy JD. Behcet's disease. Curr Opin Rheumatol 1994; 6:39–43.
82. Rigby AS, Chamberlain MA, Bhakta B. Behçet's disease. Baillieres Clin Rheumatol 1994; 9:375–395.
83. Morrissey SP, Miller DH, Hemaszeski R, et al. Magnetic resonance imaging of the central nervous system in Behçet's disease. Eur Neurol 1993; 33:287–293.
84. Mizukami K, Shiraishi H, Tanaka Y, et al. CNS changes in neuro-Behçet's disease: CT, MR, and SPECT findings. Comput Med Imaging Graph 1992; 16:401–406.
85. Yazici H, Barnes CG. Practical treatment recommendations for pharmacotherapy of Behçet's syndrome. Drugs 1991; 42:796–804.
86. Faris BM, Foster S. Behçet's disease. In: Principles and Practice of Ophtalmology. Albert DM, Jakobiec FA, eds. Philadelphia: Saunders, 1996:1018–1027.
87. Baer JC, Raizman MB, Foster CS. Ocular Behçet's disease in the United States: clinical presentation and visual outcome in 29 patients. In: Proceedings of the 5th International Symposium on the Immunology and Immunopathology of the Eye. Masahiko U, Shigeaki O, Koki A, eds. Tokyo, March 13–15 1990. New York: Elsevier, 1990:383–393.
88. O'Duffy JD. Behçet's syndrome. N Engl J Med 1990; 322:326–328.
89. Yazici H, Pazarli H, Barnes CG, et al. A controlled trial of azathioprine in Behçet's syndrome. N Engl J Med 1990; 332:281–285.
90. Masuda K, Urayama A, Kogure M, et al. Double-masked trial of cyclosporin versus colchicine and long-term open study of cyclosporin in Behçet's disease. Lancet 1989; 1:1093–1096.
91. Ozyazgan Y, Yurdakul S, Yazici H, et al. Low dose Cyclosporin A versus pulsed cyclophosphamide in Behçet's syndrome: a single masked trial. Br J Ophtalmol 1992; 76:241–243.
92. Pacor ML, Biasi D, Lunardi C, et al. Cyclosporin in Behçet's disease: results in 16 patients after 24 months of therapy. Clin Rheumatol 1994; 13:224–227.
93. Kotake S, Ichiishi A, Kosaka S, et al. Low dose cyclosporin treatment for ocular lesions of Behçet's disease. Nippon. Ganka. Gakkai, Zasshi. 1992: 96:1290–1294.
94. Whitcup SM, Salvo EC, Nussenblatt RB. Combined cyclosporine and corticosteroid therapy for sight-threatening uveitis in Behçet's disease. Am J Ophthalmol 1994; 118:39–45.
95. Atmaca LS, Batioglu F. The efficacy of cyclosporin-a in the treatment of Behçet's disease. Opthalmic Surg 1994; 25:321–327.
96. Panayi GS, Tugwell P. The use of cyclosporin A in rheumatoid arthritis: conclusions of an international review. Br J Rheumatol 1994; 33:967–969.
97. Durand JM, Kaplanski G, Telle H, et al. Beneficial effects of interferon-a2b in Behçet's disease. Arthritis Rheum 1993; 36:1025–1026.
98. Sakane T, Mochizuki M, Inaba G, Masuda K. A phase II study of FK506 (tacrolimus) on refractory uveitis associated with Behçet's disease and allied conditions. Ryumachi 1995; 35:802–813.
99. Mizushima Y: Recent research into Behçet's disease in Japan. !!!BADKEY -- Journal Name Lost 1988; 1282:-7711.
100. Serdaroglu P, Yazici H, Ozdemir C. Neurological involvement in Behçet's syndrome: a prospective study. Arch Neurol 1989; 46:265–269.
101. Alpsoy E, Yilmaz E, Bacsaran E. Interferon therapy for Behçet's disease. J Am Acad Dermatol 1994; 31:617–619.
102. Hamuryudan V, Moral F, Yurdakul S, et al. Systemic interferon a2b treatment in Behçet's syndrome. J Rheumatol 1994; 21:1098–1100.
103. Moral F, Hamuryudan V, Yurdakul S, Yazici H. Inefficacy of azapropazone in the acute arthritis of Behccet's syndrome: a randomized, double blind, placebo controlled study. Clin Exp Rheumatol 1995; 13:493–495.

104. Lingenfelser T, Duerk H, Stevens A, et al. Generalized myositis in Behçet's disease: treatment with cyclosporine. Ann Intern Med 1992; 116:2651-653.
105. Hashimoto T, Haraoka H. [Vasculo-Behccet's disease]. Nippon Rinsho 1994; 52:138-2142.
106. Sulimovic H, Flaisler F, Teissier JM, et al. [Cerebral thrombophlebitis disclosing Behccet disease. Value of high resolution MRI]. Rev Rhum Ed Fr 1993; 60:69–73.
107. Tuzun H, Sayin A, Karaozbek Y, et al. Peripheral aneurysms in Behçet's disease. Cardiovasc Surg 1993; 1:220–224.
108. Hamuryudan V, Yurdakul S, Moral F, et al. Pulmonary arterial aneurysms in Behccet's syndrome: a report of 24 cases. Br J Rheumatol 1994; 33:48–51.
109. Cornelis F, Sigal-Nahum M, Gaulier A, et al. Behçet's disease with severe cutaneous necrotizing vasculitis: response to plasma exchange-Report of a case. J Am Acad Dermatol 1989; 21:576–579.
110. Ley SJ, Williams RC Jr. A family with hereditary angioedema and multiple immunologic disorders. Am J Med 1987, 92:1046–1051.
111. Brickman CM, Tsokos GC, Balow JE, et al. Immunoregulatory disorders associated with hereditary angioedema. I. Clinical manifestations of autoimmune disease. J Allergy Clin Immunol 1986; 77:749–757.
112. Duncan IJ, Tymms KE, Carney G. Rheumatoid arthritis and hereditary angioedema. J Rheumatol 1988; 15:700–702.
113. Cicardi M, Agostoni A. Hereditary angioedema (editorial; comment). N Engl J Med 1996; 334:1666–1667.
114. Gigli I, Rosen F. Angioedema associated with complement abnormalities. In: Dermatology in General Medicine. Fitzpatrick TB, Eisen AZ, Wolff K, et al., eds. New York: McGraw-Hill, 1993:1494–1497.
115. Waytes AT, Rosen FS, Frank MM. Treatment of hereditary angioedema with a vapor-heated C1 inhibitor concentrate (see comments). N Engl J Med 1996; 334:1630–1634.
116. Cicardi M. Longterm treatment of hereditary angioedema with attenuated androgens: a survey of a 13 -year experience. J Allergy Clin Immunol 1991; 87:768–776.
117. International Study Group for Behçet's disease. Evaluation of diagnostic (classification) criteria for Behçet's disease-towards internationally agreed criteria. Br J Rheumatol 1992; 31:299–308.
118. Yazici H. Behçet's syndrome. In: Rheumatology. Klippel JH, Dieppe PA, eds. London: Mosby, 1994:1–6.

24
Adult Still's Disease

Pierre-André Guerne
University Hospital of Geneva, Geneva, Switzerland

I. INTRODUCTION

Rheumatologists can be faced with cases of adult-onset Still's disease (AOSD) as well as with cases of juvenile onset disease (JOSD) persisting into adulthood, since approximately 50% of these patients will have chronic disease, usually with progression of the arthritis.

AOSD, as well as JOSD, is a disorder of unknown etiology, primarily characterized by spiking fever, rash, and arthritis. Adult- and juvenile-onset diseases are very similar as to presentation, treatment, and prognosis [1,2]. Disease severity is variable, but disability can be severe in some cases and fatal issues can occur, which eventually justifies the use of aggressive treatments. In the absence of pathognomonic symptoms or laboratory markers, diagnosis can be difficult and other entities, especially infectious, must be carefully eliminated.

II. DIAGNOSIS

A. Epidemiology and Clinical Features

AOSD is rarer than its juvenile counterpart and primarily affects young adults between the ages of 16 and 30, with a prevalence decreasing as a function of age. It is found worldwide, and it is equally distributed among men and women.

Fever, characteristically spiking once a day over 39°C, is present in >90% of the patients [3,4]. A salmon pink macular or maculopapular rash is present in about 90% of the patients but can be difficult to visualize because of its evanescent character. It generally parallels the fever, can be precipitated by mechanical irritation, and is most commonly found on the trunk, proximal extremities and the face, where it can be limited.

Arthralgias are always present, whereas frank arthritis occurs in only 75–95% of the patients. Arthritis affects mainly the knees and the wrists, but most joints, including the distal interphalangeals, can be involved.

In addition to fever, rash, and arthritis-arthralgia, multiple organ manifestations can occur, including myalgia (80% of the patients), lymphadenopathy and splenomegaly (60%), abdominal pain (50%), hepatomegaly (40%), pleuritis and pericarditis (30%), and pneumonitis (25%). Sore throat is common (90%), probably due to cricoarythenoid arthritis in most patients.

Severe and life-threatening complications include acute hepatic necrosis, disseminated intravascular coagulation (DIC), frequently associated with hemophagocytosis, acute respiratory distress syndrome, and myocarditis.

B. Investigations

1. Blood Tests

Many biological abnormalities can occur in associations with Still's disease, but none is specific of the disease. The most universally encountered reflect the marked acute phase reaction and include elevated erythrocyte sedimentation rate (ESR), and C-reactive protein (CRP), thrombocytosis, and hypoalbunimemia. Very high serum ferritin levels, compared with other inflammatory disorders, have been proposed to be a diagnostic marker of Still's disease [5,6]. Comparable levels, however, are also found in other conditions, such as infections or neoplasias, which may be difficult to differentiate clinically from Still's disease. Isoferritins might be better tools for the diagnosis of active adult Still's disease [6], but they need further evaluation. Leukocytosis (over 15000 in more than 75% of the patients) is also a characteristic but unspecific feature of Still's disease. Anemia, elevation of liver function tests and complement C3 and C4 are also frequently encountered. On the other hand, autoantibodies such as rheumatoid factor and antinuclear antibodies should be absent [7], but can be detected transiently.

2. Radiography

Radiographs of affected joints may eventually show a characteristic pattern of pericapitate and intercarpal, nonerosive, joint space narrowing in the wrist, evolving toward bony ankylosis. Radiographic findings also include distinctive joint changes of interphalangeal joints that result in Heberden-like nodes, and nonspecific soft tissue swelling, periarticular osteopenia, and occasional erosions or joint space narrowing, especially about the ankles, knees, and hips.

C. Diagnostic Criteria and Differential Diagnosis

Confronted with frequent difficulties in establishing diagnosis and with the absence of specific clinical or laboratory features, a number of diagnostic or classification criteria have been put forward. The most widely used are those proposed by Cush et al. [7] (Table 1). Although helpful, these criteria are not satisfied by many patients, particularly early in the course of the disease, whereas a number of patients with other diseases do satisfy them. Therefore, a major challenge in treating patients with suspected Still's disease remains excluding other entities, especially those requiring a specific treatment. Diseases that can mimic Still's disease are listed in Table 2.

III. DISEASE COURSE: MARKERS OF SEVERITY AND ACTIVITY

A. Disease Course

AOSD has a highly variable course. Some patients enter prolonged remissions, some have intermittent exacerbations, and some develop a chronic and severe disorder [8].

Table 1 Criteria for the Diagnosis of Adult Still's Disease

Diagnosis of adult Still's disease requires the presence of *all* of the following:
Fever ≥39°C
Arthralgia and/or arthritis
Rheumatoid factor <1/80
Antinuclear antibodies < 1/100
In addition to *any 2* of the following
White blood cell count ≥15000/mm^3
Evanescent macular or maculopapular rash
Pleuritis or pericarditis
Hepatomegaly
Splenomegaly
Generalized lymphadenopathy

Source: Adapted from ref. 7.

Three main types of disease course have been described: monocyclic systemic (single episode of illness, 25–30% of patients), polycyclic systemic (25–30%), chronic articular (30–50%) [7,9,10]. In most patients, the disease is benign, and after 5 years, approximately 50% of them do not require medication [8]. On average, patients have low levels of pain, physical disability, and psychological disability compared with patients with other rheumatic diseases. In half of the patients, however, the articular prognosis is poor, with severe joint destruction [8,11]. Secondary amyloidosis occurs not infrequently in AOSD [1,11]. These data indicate how important is a personalized therapeutic approach adapted to disease severity and activity.

B. Predictors of Disease Severity

Among the clinical parameters, the type of arthritis at onset appears to be the best predictor of arthritis progression: early polyarthritis (within 6 months of onset) and involvement of proximal limb joints have been found to be significantly associated with chronic articular disease in many studies [7,10,12,13]; corticosteroid requirement for over 2

Table 2 Differential Diagnosis of Adult Still's Disease

Infections	Viral: rubella, parvovirus, HIV, Coxsackie, Epstein-Barr, cytomegalovirus Bacterial: subacute bacterial endocarditis, meningococcemia, tuberculosis, leprosy, Lyme disease, rheumatic fever, Whipple's disease
Malignancies	Leukemia, lymphoma, atrial myxoma
Granulomatous and inflammatory disorders	Sarcoidosis, Crohn's disease, ulcerative colitis, idiopathic granulomatous hepatitis, familial Mediterranean fever, crystal-induced arthropathies (gout, chondrocalcinosis)
Connective tissue diseases	Systemic lupus erythematosus, mixed connective tissue disease
Vasculitis	Periarteritis nodosa, serum sickness, Wegener's granulomatosis, Takayasu's arteritis

years has been associated with poorer long-term function [7]. On the other hand, isolated arthralgia was predictive of monocyclic or polycyclic systemic disease [10], and the absence of a rash reported to denote a better outcome [13].

The transient presence of rheumatoid factors and/or antinuclear antibodies might reflect a more severe inflammatory state and be associated with more prolonged active disease [13]. On the other hand, no HLA-DR allele was reproducibly shown to be associated with disease severity.

C. Markers of Disease Activity

Elevations of ESR and CRP levels and peripheral blood leukocytes are very useful to monitor disease activity and treatment. Serum ferritin has also been proposed to be a marker of disease activity [5,6]. High levels, however, can be found during secondary infections, whereas normal levels can be encountered in active disease. Isoferritins might be better tools for the assessment of disease activity [6], but their place in clinical practice needs further evaluation.

IV. TREATMENT

A number of different treatment regimens have been evaluated, but few of them have been submitted to rigorous controlled studies. Treatment recommendations are based in part on experience with rheumatoid arthritis and juvenile Still's disease.

Treatment has to be directed at the systemic features, as well as at the arthritis, whose managements are not identical. Systemic features usually predominate during the acute early phase, whereas arthritis is a major feature of chronic disease. In addition to medications, global management (education, physical and occupational therapy) are essential in the proper management of the disease.

A. Nonpharmacological Global Management

Education, which is generally felt as insufficiently delivered by most patients, is especially important in young adults between the ages of 16 and 30, who are predominantly affected by this disease. The psychosocial impact of the perspective of a chronic incapacitating disease is indeed likely to be more devastating at a time when one attempts to make his or her own way as an independent adult. Problems of denial and poor compliance are frequent and their consequences are especially detrimental. Education has been shown to improve pain, physical disability, and psychosocial impact of the disease [14]. In addition to information about medications (purpose, duration of the treatment, posology, side effects) advice should be given about rest, nutrition, appropriate use of joints in daily life, exercise programs, sport, and professional choices when applicable.

Appropriate programs of physical therapy and rehabilitation are important as well and should be especially directed at preservation of joint and muscle integrity and function. A good collaboration between all health professionals, sometimes including psychologists, is essential as well as contact with, and support from, family members, teachers, or employers.

B. Drug Therapy of Systemic Features

1. Nonsteroid Anti-inflammatory Drugs

Nonsteroidal anti-inflammatory drugs (NSAIDs) are still generally considered to be the first-line therapy of adult-onset Still's disease. These drugs are sufficient in only a minority of cases and can be (rarely) associated with severe side effects, but they are certainly useful in many patients. Because alternatives are not without flaws, an initial trial with NSAIDs is certainly appropriate.

Because of the wide experience gathered with salicylates and the fact that their levels are easily measured in serum, enteric-coated aspirin is still advocated by many specialists. Optimal levels range between 150 and 250 mg/L, and the doses required to reach adequate control of the manifestations are frequently much higher than for other diseases. Aspirin, however, appears to be less efficient than other NSAIDs [10,15] and has been specifically associated with severe side effects.

Other NSAIDs that can be used and are beneficial, even in patients whose disease is inadequately controlled by aspirin, include indomethacin and naproxen [10, 12,15]. Required doses are often larger than in other diseases (indomethacin up to 250 mg/day and naproxen up to 1500 mg/day). Although reported cases of toxicities are not as frequent with other NSAIDs than with aspirin [4], severe side effects can occur as well.

The most severe side effects linked with aspirin and other NSAIDs appear to be hepatic necrosis and intravascular coagulation, which are frequently associated. In most cases of acute hepatic necrosis reported in adults, NSAIDs were incriminated and the situation shown to be reversible after the cessation of the treatment [4]. At least one case of acute hepatic necrosis has been shown to develop with aspirin and regress after a switch to indomethacin [4]. Aspirin toxicity seems to be promoted by hypoalbuminemia, which is frequent in Still's disease and increases free salicylates; frequent hepatic controls and albuminemias are therefore required in patients treated with aspirin or other NSAIDs. Intravascular coagulation, sometimes in association with hemophagocytic syndrome, has also been reported to be triggered by NSAIDs in JOSD and AOSD, but the fact that these manifestations can occur in the absence of NSAIDs casts doubt on the reality of a causal link. In any event, frequent monitoring of clotting tests is mandatory while the disease remains active.

It is generally considered that NSAIDs should be continued at least three months after disease manifestations have remitted. Despite their efficacy, NSAIDs ensure a satisfactory control of the disease in only 10–25% of the patients [10,13]. In cases of failure, corticosteroids and/or disease-modifying antirheumatic drugs (DMARDs) are required.

2. Corticosteroids

The proportion of patients treated with corticosteroids has tended to increase over the recent years, as reflected by three large series [10,12,13]: Forty-seven percent of the patients were prescribed steroid in the 1986 series, 66% in the 1991 series, and 88% in the 1995 series. This tendency probably reflects higher expectations on quality of life and outcome from patients and physicians. When prescribed, corticosteroids should always be associated with measures directed at the prevention of osteoporosis.

Initial doses usually required to provide control of the acute manifestations range between 0.5 and 1.0 mg/kg/day. With such doses, symptoms generally disappear in

48 h. Initial high doses can be advantageously replaced by methylprednisolone boluses: In a retrospective French study, boluses (1 g/day for 3 consecutive days) induced a rapid and frank improvement in all cases, and allowed long-term remission in half of the patients, without the disadvantages of high daily oral doses [16].

The additional use of NSAIDs may be beneficial in some patients and in rare cases, indomethacin appeared to be more effective than large doses of corticosteroids, which underlines the fact that corticosteroids should not be the first-choice medication for non-life-threatening acute manifestations.

Absolute indications for corticosteroids include intravascular coagulation, hemophagocytosis, rising liver function tests, in particular while receiving NSAIDs, acute respiratory distress syndrome, myocarditis, pericardial tamponade, and meningoencephalitis. In the presence of such manifestations, methylprednisolone intravenous boluses (1 g/day) for a few days (generally 3 consecutive days) can be beneficial before the introduction of oral treatment at high doses (1.0–1.5 mg/day). Megadose pulse methylprednisolone proved effective in a patient with fulminant multiple organ involvement unresponsive to oral therapy [17].

Tapering must be initiated slowly once the disease manifestations are controlled (generally after 2–4 weeks), but this must be done very carefully, since disease exacerbations are frequent. Alternate-day therapy, which theoretically leads to fewer side effects, is generally inadequate but has been used successfully in a few cases [15]. Very low doses should be continued for several months after remission in order to prevent and minimize relapses. On the other hand, large doses (>7.0–12.5 mg/day) should not, as a rule, be used for more than 6 months. If disease manifestations cannot be controlled with reasonable corticosteroid regimens, introduction of slow-acting antirheumatic or immunosuppressive drugs is required.

3. *Slow-acting Antirheumatic and Immunosuppressive Agents*

Cyclosporine, methotrexate, and cyclophosphamide can be helpful in the management of systemic manifestations of AOSD, whereas agents such as gold, D-penicillamine, salazopyrine, hydroxycholorquine, or azathioprine have mainly been shown to be beneficial in chronic articular manifestations. Cyclosporine, methotrexate, and cyclophosphamide lack controlled trials in AOSD, but case reports and the growing experience gathered in JOSD and adult rheumatoid arthritis all indicate that these drugs can be beneficial without excessive side effects.

Methotrexate. Methotrexate at low doses (7.5–25.0 mg/week) is mainly used for chronic disease but has also been reported to control systemic manifestations [18,19]. Considering its now well-recognized tolerability and its potential additional benefits on articular manifestations, methotrexate can be considered early in patients with severe systemic manifestations and/or poor response to more conventional regimens.

Cyclosporine. Cyclosporine can be used both as a corticosteroid sparing agent or as an adjunct for the management of cases resistant to steroids. It has been observed to be efficient in JOSD, causing disappearance of fever, improvement of joint manifestations, and reduction of corticosteroids [20]. Cyclosporine has also been used with success in cases of AOSD [21]; in particular for treating severe manifestations such as disseminated intravascular coagulation resistant to pulse methylprednisolone [22]. As in rheumatoid arthritis, treatment should be initiated at low doses (2.5 mg/kg/day), increased progressively, and not exceed 5 mg/kg/day [23]. There appears to be no correlation between blood levels and clinical efficacy and/or side effects [20]. In case of remission, the treatment should not be stopped before a gradual tapering over several months, since untimely withdrawal or tapering almost invariably induces a relapse (personal observation).

Cyclophosphamide. Although generally avoided in children with Still's disease because of possible long-term side effects, cyclophosphamide has been proved beneficial in severe cases: repetitive pulses (every 3 months), in association with pulses of methylprednisolone and oral methotrexate resulted in a rapid suppression of all articular and systemic manifestations in all children of a group of 18. Such regimens have also been shown (in case reports) to be efficient and useful in AOSD [24]. Cyclophosphamide, however, should be reserved for selected patients with particularly severe disease.

4. *Intravenous Immunoglobulins*

A few case series suggest that intravenous immunoglobulins (IVIgs) can be helpful in AOSD [1], but controlled trials are lacking; IVIg therapy has been extensively evaluated in the juvenile form of the disease. Three studies from a same center indicated that monthly IVIg infusions at a dosage of 1 g/kg/day for 2 consecutive days can be beneficial in most patients with JOSD [25–27]. The investigators concluded that IVIg should be used in patients with severe AOSD with prolonged unresponsiveness to standard therapy. Disappointing results, however, were obtained by other groups [28]. Although considered relatively safe [29], IVIgs can occasionally lead to complications [28,29]; in addition to being very expensive. In the absence of more convincing data on their effectiveness, IVIgs should therefore not be considered a first-line therapy in AOSD but can be attempted when other regimens fail.

C. Management of Relapses

After complete remission and cessation of all medications, relapses occur in about 50% of cases. Relapses, however, tend to be milder and shorter than the initial episode. Early relapses are probably an indication that treatment has been tapered or discontinued prematurely. Relapses usually respond similarly to the therapeutic regimens used for the initial episode.

D. Drug Therapy of Chronic Articular Disease

Chronic disease is generally defined as persistent activity 12 months after diagnosis. Most commonly, chronic polyarthritis or oligoarthritis uncontrolled by NSAIDs and/or acceptable doses of prednisone for long-term treatment (<7.5–12.5 mg/day, depending on the sex and size of the patient) predominates. Other chronic manifestations include fever, rash, serositis, lymphadenopathies, and hepatosplenomegaly, but are less frequent, at least in white individuals. It is now indicated to introduce second-line drugs in the case of chronic disease, and even before 12 months when symptoms are severe: Given the potential of AOSD for severe articular destruction, an approach similar to that now proposed in rheumatoid arthritis (earlier use of aggressive treatments in cases with poor prognosis) can be advocated (see predictors of disease severity). Several second-line agents have been used to control articular symptoms, but they lack controlled study.

1. Methotrexate

Methotrexate has recently been reported by several investigators to be effective in AOSD [10,19,30,31]. Its use was associated with the concomitant evolution toward complete remission in up to 50% of the patients [19]. In addition, methotrexate has a steroid-sparing effect in almost all cases [10,19], even those unresponsive to other medications such as sulfasalazine, azathioprine, and/or cyclophosphamide. It also controlled severe manifestations such as disseminated intravascular coagulopathy (DIC) [30]. It has to be mentioned that the use of methotrexate has been associated with episodes of fever, arthralgias, and/or rash occurring after the injections [10,19]. Nevertheless, its efficacy and usual tolerability make methotrexate one of the first-choice second-line therapy in chronic articular AOSD.

2. Gold

Intramuscular gold has been used often in Still's disease, and up to 40% of patients may improve coincidentally with its introduction according to uncontrolled studies. In the juvenile form of the disease, gold injections have been associated with death, generally occurring after the second injection [32,33], and very strong advise against its use in this disease has been formulated [33]. Death is generally due to DIC, sometimes combined with acute hepatolysis and hemophagocytosis. This syndrome, which can also occur in the absence of treatment, occurs in the adult-onset form as well [30,34]. Caution is indicated when using intramuscular gold in AOSD, and other therapeutic options, in particular methotrexate, should be considered first. Oral gold, whose toxicity profile is very different, is probably safer than the intramuscular preparations; oral gold has been used successfully in AOSD [35] but is probably not as efficient.

3. Other Second-line Drugs

Sulfasalazine, D-penicillamine, azathioprine, and hydroxychloroquine have all been used with testimonials for some degree of benefits in the control of articular symptoms, but experience with these treatments is restricted [10,13]. The frequent switches from one treatment to another though, is an indication of the limited effectiveness of these compounds.

The use of immunoglobulins for the control of articular manifestations is rarely reported [1]. Their effectiveness for this indication is difficult to evaluate but appears lower, in altering the course of chronic arthritis than in improving the acute systemic manifestations in JOSD [27].

Cyclosporine, on the other hand, appears to be effective in the treatment of the chronic articular manifestations of AOSD even in patients failing to improve after multiple other second-line treatments [21]. This drug has been shown to decrease the progression of erosions in RA, but the doses required to control AOSD, at least in some patients, seem high and may not be acceptable in the long-term.

4. Combination Therapy

Given the severity and poor prognosis of some cases, a more aggressive approach is warranted in selected patients. Some combinations of second-line agents, which have recently been the object of several studies in RA and proved to decrease significantly disease activity [36], are certainly applicable to patients with Still's disease. Association of methotrexate ≤15 mg/week) with cyclosporine (2.5–5.0 mg/day), which is likely to be one of the most powerful of these combinations, although acceptable in terms of toxicity [37], has been shown to control all disease manifestations in patients with intractable disease necessitating prolonged and very high doses of corticosteroids (personal observation). Such therapies, which must be restricted to severe cases and be the object of very careful monitoring, might minimize joint destruction in addition to dramatically improving quality of life in some patients [36].

E. Treatment of Secondary Amyloidosis

Secondary amyloidosis and associated mortality, might be more frequent in AOSD (up to 35% in a French series) than in its juvenile-onset counterpart [1]. Once present, amyloidosis has a very poor prognosis if not treated aggressively and specifically, but it appears to have a potential to respond to alkylating agents and enter into remission as well as rheumatoid arthritis [38,39]. A decrease in the number of deaths from sec-

Table 3 Proposed Therapy in AOSD Disease

Main manifestations	Medication	Usual dosages
Acute-systemic		
Mild	NSAIDs	High
Moderate or unresponsive to NSAIDs	Oral corticosteroids ± NSAIDs	0.5–1.0 mg/kg/day initially*
Severe (life threatening) or unresponsive to initial therapy	Oral corticosteroids or IV methylprednisolone boluses ± NSAIDs	1–2 mg/kg/day initially* 1.0 g/day for 2–3 consecutive days before oral corticosteroids
Unresponsive to steroids or requiring unacceptable doses of steroids for ≥6months	Add second-line agents: methotrexate, or cyclosporine or IVIG	 7.5–25.0 mg/week 3–5 mg/kg/day 1 g/kg/day for 2 consecutive days monthly
Life threatening and uncontrolled by other agents	Cyclophosphamide (with high doses corticosteroids)	oral: 1.5–2.0 mg/kg/day or IV pulses: 1–1.5 g/month
Chronic-articular		
Mild	NSAIDs and/or corticosteroids	 ≤7.5–12.5 mg/day*
Severe or uncontrolled by initial therapy	Add second-line agents methotrexate or cyclosporine	 7.5–25.0 mg/week 3–5 mg/kg/day
(less efficient, recommended or documented)	(hydroxychloroquine or sulfasalazine or D-penicillamine or gold or azathioprine)	
Uncontrolled by single second-line agents	Combination therapy for ex. cyclosporine + methotrexate	 2.5–5 mg/kg/day 7.5–15 mg/kg/week
Amyloidosis	Steroids + alkylating agent chlorambucil or cyclophosphamide	See text

*Equivalent predinisone.

ondary amyloidosis in JOSD has recently been shown to be explained by an increased use of cytotoxic drug treatments [40]. Symptoms or signs of amyloidosis (proteinuria/renal insufficiency, diarrhea/obstipation/malabsorption, goiter, neuropathy, or hepatomegaly) should therefore rapidly prompt a rectal, abdominal fat, or kidney biopsy [41].

Alkylating agents, such as, cyclophosphamide and chlorambucil have both been shown to be effective, although chlorambucil is preferred by some investigators [39]. Alkylating treatment is indicated in case of proteinuria or decreased glomerular filtration and when amyloidosis is proved by biopsy (preferably renal). It is then generally advised to use chlorambucil in association with high doses of prednisone (0.5–1.0 mg/kg/day) to bring the number of leukocytes down to less than 1.0×10^9 and achieve a complete remission (quasinormalization of SAA amyloid and/or CRP). When remission is obtained, prednisone can be reduced progressively to ≤7.5 mg/day, but chlorambucil should be continued for about 6 months at a dose allowing maintenance of the remission [39].

F. Conclusions and Treatment Guidelines

On one hand, the occurrence of spontaneous remission in many patients and the absence of controlled trials are indications for conservative treatment in mild cases of Still's disease. On the other hand, the possibility of fatal issues and frequent evolution toward severe and destructive articular disease justify the use of aggressive interventions for acute-systemic or chronic-articular manifestations in more severe cases. Treatment has therefore to be adapted to disease type, severity, and activity (Table 3).

When remissions occur, very progressive tapering is indicated. Second-line agents, when used, are proposed by some investigators to be maintained indefinitely. Relapses, however, are usually milder and respond to the rapid reintroduction of the treatment. In any event, second-line agents should not be stopped before at least 1–2 years. Switch to a safer agent may be an alternative. Introduction of hydroxychroloroquine may in particular be indicated before attempting to stop methotrexate.

REFERENCES

1. Cabane J., Michon A., Ziza J. M., et al. Comparison of long term evolution of adult onset and juvenile onset Still's disease, both followed up for more than 10 years. Ann Rheum Dis 1990; 49:283–285.
2. Tanaka S, Matsumoto Y, Ohnishi H, et al. [Comparison of clinical features of childhood and adult onset Still's disease]. Ryumachi 1991; 31:511–518.
3. Esdaile JM. Adult Still's disease. In: Rheumatology. Klippel JH, Dieppe PA, eds. London: Mosby, 1994:21.1–21.7.
4. Masson C, Le Loët X, Lioté F, et al: Adult Still's disease. Part I. Manifestations and complications in sixty five cases in France. Rev Rhum Engl Ed 1995; 62:748–757.
5. Schwarz Eywill M, Heilig B, Bauer H, et al. A: Evaluation of serum ferritin as a marker for adult Still's disease activity. Ann Rheum Dis 1992; 51:683–685.
6. Van Reeth C, Le Moel G, Lasne Y, et al. Serum ferritin and isoferritins are tools for diagnosis of active adult Still's disease. J Rheumatol 1994; 21:890–895.
7. Cush JJ, Medsger TA Jr, Christy WC, et al.: Adult-onset Still's disease: clinical course and outcome. Arthritis Rheum 1987; 30:186–194.

8. Sampalis JS, Esdaile JM, Medsger TA Jr, et al. A controlled study of the long-term prognosis of adult Still's disease. Am J Med 1995; 98:384–388.
9. Wouters JMGW, Reekers P, Van de Putte LBA. Adult onset Still's disease: disease course and HLA associations. Arthritis Rheum 1986; 29:415–418.
10. Masson C, Le Loët X, Lioté F, et al. Adult Still's disease. Part II. Management, outcome and prognostic factors. Rev Rhum Engl Ed 1995; 62:758–765.
11. Cabane J, Michon A, Ziza JM et al. Comparison of long term evolution of adult onset and juvenile onset Still's disease, both followed up for more than 10 years. Ann Rheum Dis 1990; 49:283–285.
12. Wouters JMGW, Van de Putte LBA. Adult-onset Still's disease; clinical and laboratory features, treatment and progress of 45 cases. Q J Med 1986; 61:1055–1065.
13. Pouchot J, Sampalis JS, Beaudet F, et al. Adult Still's disease: manifestations, disease course, and outcome in 62 patients. Medicine 1991; 70:118–136.
14. Lorig K, Lubeck D, Kraines RG, et al.: Outcomes of self-help education for patients with arthritis. Arthritis Rheum 1985; 28:680–685.
15. Larson EB. Adult Still's disease, evolution of a clinical syndrome and dagnosis, treatment and follow-up of 17 patients. Medicine 1984; 63:82–91.
16. Bisagni Faure A, Job Deslandre C, Menkes CJ. [Treatment of Still's disease with bolus methylprednisolone. Retrospective study of 7 patients]. Rev Rhum Mal Osteoartic 1992; 59:228–232.
17. Khraishi M, Fam AG. Treatment of fulminant adult Still's disease with intravenous pulse methylprednisolone therapy (see comments). J Rheumatol 1991; 18:1088–1090.
18. Kraus A, Alarcón-Segovia D. Fever in adult onset Still's disease. Response to methotrexate. J Rheumatol 1991; 18:918–920.
19. Aydintug AO, Cruz D, Cervera R, et al.: Low dose methotrexate treatment in adult Still's disease. J Rheumatol 1992; 19:431–435.
20. Pistoia V, Buoncompagni A, Scribanis R, et al. Cyclosporin A in the treatment of juvenile chronic arthritis and childhood polymyositis-dermatomyositis. Results of a preliminary study. Clin Exp Rheumatol 1993; 11:203–208.
21. Shojania K, Chalmers A. Rangno K. Cyclosporin A in the treatment of adult Still's disease. J Rheumatol 1995; 22:1391–1392.
22. Mori T, Tanigawa M, Iwasaki E, et al. [Cyclosporine therapy of adult onset Still's disease with disseminated intravascular coagulation]. Rinsho Ketsueki 1993; 34:147–152.
23. Panayi GS, Tugwell P. The use of cyclosporin A in rheumatoid arthritis: conclusions of an international review. Br J Rheumatol 1994; 33:967–969.
24. Sato M, Takeda A, Honzu H, et al. Adult Still's disease with Sjogren's syndrome successfully treated with intravenous pulse methylprednisolone and oral cyclophosphamide. Intern Med 1993; 32:730–732.
25. Silverman ED, Cawkwell GD, Lovell DJ. Intravenous immunoglobulin in the treatment of systemic juvenile rheumatoid arthritis: A randomized placebo controlled trial. J Rheumatol 1994; 21:2353–2358.
26. Silverman ED, Laxer RM, Greenwald M, et al. Intravenous gamma globulin therapy in systemic juvenile rheumatoid arthritis. Arthritis Rheum 1990; 33:1015–1022.
27. Uziel Y, Laxer RM, Schneider R, Silverman ED. Intravenous immunoglobulin therapy in systemic onset juvenile rheumatoid arthritis: a followup study. J Rheumatol 1996; 23:910–918.
28. Prieur AM. Intravenous immunoglobulins in Still's disease: Still controversial, still unproven. J Rheumatol 1996; 23:797–799.
29. Schiff RI. Intravenous gammaglobulin. 2. Pharmacology, clinical uses and mechanisms of action. Pediatr Allergy Immunol 1994; 5:127–156.

30. Aellen P, Raccaud O, Waldburger M, et al.: [Still's disease in adults with disseminated intravascular coagulation]. Schweiz Rundsch Med Prax 1991; 80:376–378.
31. Kenouch S, Fessi H, Mery JP, et al.: Oral low-dose methotrexate (MTX) to be efficient in refractory rheumatoid arthritis and adult-onset Still's disease (letter). Am J Kidney Dis 1989; 14:76–77.
32. Silverman ED, Miller JJ, Bernstein B, Shafai T. Consumption coagulopathy associated with systemic juvenile rheumatoid arthritis. J Pediatr 1983; 103:872–876.
33. Jacobs JC. The hazards of gold injections in children with juvenile rheumatoid arthritis. Arthritis Rheum 1993; 36:1636.
34. Hisano C, Nakamura M, Mayumi T, et al. [A case of hemophagocytic syndrome manifesting adult Still's disease and acute hepatitis]. Nihon Rinsho Meneki Gakkai Kaishi 1995; 18:256–264.
35. Take H, Kubota K, Tamura K, et al.: Successful treatment with auranofin in a patients with elderly-onset Still's disease. J Med 1994; 25:393–397.
36. Furst DE. Rational disease-modifying anti-rheumatic drug (DMARD) therapy: is it possible? Br J Rheumatol 1996; 35:707–710.
37. Tugwell P, Pincus T, Yocum D, et al. Combination therapy with cyclosporine and methotrexate in severe rheumatoid arthritis. N Engl J Med 1995; 333:137–141.
38. Blanche P, Menkes CJ. [Immunosuppressive therapy of secondary amyloidosis associated with rheumatoid arthritis or Still's disease]. Rev Rhum Mal Osteoartic 1992; 59:784–789.
39. Berglund K, Thysell H, Keller C. Results, principles and pitfalls in the management of renal AA-amyloidosis; a 10-21 year followup of 16 patients with rheumatic disease treated with alkylating cytostatics. J Rheumatol 1993; 20:2051–2057.
40. Savolainen HA, Isomake HA. Decrease in the number of deaths from secondary amyloidosis in patients with juvenile rheumatoid arthritis. J Rheumatol 1993; 20:1201–1203.
41. Gertz MA, Kyle RA. Secondary systemic amyloidosis: response and survival in 64 patients. Medicine 1991; 70:246–256.

25
Systemic Lupus Erythematosus

Naomi F. Rothfield and Ann Parke
University of Connecticut Health Center, Farmington, Connecticut

I. OVERVIEW

The goals of the management of patients with systemic lupus erythematosus (SLE) is the control of the disease so that the patients may live as normal lives as possible in the present and in the future. These goals may conflict, since the long-term complications of therapy may be as severe as the immediate threat to life and well-being. The goals must be balanced for each patient, since each patient has a unique set of manifestations of the disease. Thus, treatment in SLE is individualized for each particular patient. Some general rules of management are important for every patient and are discussed below.

II. GENERAL MANAGEMENT

Patients with recently diagnosed SLE usually need significant psychological support from family and from the physician. Questions about prognosis and treatment are raised over and over again and should be handled with patience. Some patients become anxious and others become depressed. Depression is most often a reactive depression due to the fact of the diagnosis, the disfiguration from corticosteroid therapy, alopecia, and facial rash. Reassurance is essential to calm fears of further rashes and loss of hair. It is helpful to have a knowledgeable SLE patient who is on a low dose of corticosteroids but who once had cushingoid symptoms talk to the newly diagnosed patient to reassure her.

Patients must be instructed to call the physician if a fever or signs of infection occur. Pustules can grow rapidly to abscesses and otitis can become septicemia in SLE patients on high or moderate corticosteroid therapy or on immunosuppressive therapy.

Patients must be instructed to call the physician if they think the signs or symptoms of SLE are getting worse or recur so that the physician can evaluate the patient and adjust therapy if necessary.

We warn our patients against the use of hair dyes or other possible sources of allergic reactions. Patients have reported flares of disease after exposure to paint fumes, hair dyes, and other agents, although this has not been well substantiated [1]. We prefer to avoid immunizations except in postspelenectomy patients who should receive PneumoVax. Pregnancy must be discussed along with the use of contraceptive devices (see below).

Although only about 40% of patients with SLE have a sun-sensitive rash sometime during the course of the disease, we warn all patients to avoid the sun and tell them to wear long-sleeved dresses and wide brimmed hats and to use a sun screen.

A very important aspect of management is the exercise program that all patients should maintain. Exercise is important for osteoporosis prevention and for generalized well-being and muscle strengthening. We suggest walking each day, and for those who can do aerobics, low-impact aerobics should be done three times a week. Recently diagnosed patients whose disease is not yet under control should rest when they are tired, which is usually in the afternoon. Chronic fatigue is not a part of SLE, but severe fatigue does occur in untreated patients with active disease and in patients who are experiencing a flare of the disease in other systems. The treated patient has a loss of fatigue if the treatment is adequate and then should be encouraged to move around, walk, and exercise rather than sitting or lying in bed all day.

A. Use of Other Medications

Commonly used drugs containing sulfa compounds such as gantrisin, trimethopterin, and sulphasalazine [2] may lead to a flare of SLE, so we recommend patients not receive these agents. Similarly, griseofulvin has been associated with SLE flares in our patients as well as in reports in the literature [3].

III. SPECIFIC THERAPIES

A. Prednisone

The use of corticosteroids is the basis for the treatment of SLE. Whereas a small number of patients may be managed with a combination of antimalarials and aspirin, the great majority of SLE patients require some corticosteroids for complete disease control.

Patients with mild disease severity may sometimes be treated with aspirin and antimalarials, but usually a small dose (10–20 mg prednisone) is needed to relieve the fatigue, improve the arthritis/arthralgia, and alleviate the moderate anemia and leukopenia so common in SLE patients.

Patients with moderately severe disease require more prednisone (25–30 mg) to relieve their fatigue, arthritis, pericarditis, nonhemolytic anemia, leukopenia, and the cutaneous manifestations.

Patients with severe disease require at least 40 mg prednisone for the relief of fatigue, arthritis, pleurisy, pericarditis, nephritis, hemolytic anemia, leukopenia, cutaneous manifestations, vasculitis, thrombocytopenia, and central nervous system disease (acute onset of seizures of organic brain disease). Most patients can be successfully treated with oral prednisone given on an every 6-h regimen, but some individuals require intravenous corticosteroid therapy (see below).

B. Antimalarial

Antimalarial drugs have been used in the treatment of SLE since the 1950s and were previously used successfully in the treatment of discoid lupus [4,5]. All antimalarial drugs have been used including quinacrine (Atabrine), chloroquine, and hydroxychloroquine (Plaquenil). The efficacy of these drugs was first analyzed in a retrospective study of SLE patients treated with the agents from the time of diagnosis to many years later when other patients were being studied for the first time for the presence of ocular abnormalities [6]. As soon as we noted ocular abnormalities, the drug was discontinued. Patients continued to be followed as before. Thus, matched years on and off antimalarials could be compared in the same patients. The data revealed that there were fewer flares of the disease while on 500 mg chloroquine and that general manifestations such as fatigue, weight loss, and fever occurred statistically significantly less frequently during the years on the drug. In addition, there were significantly fewer episodes of skin manifestations while on the drug. We found no difference in arthritis, pleuritis, and other manifestations of SLE. More recently, a Canadian multicentered study evaluated SLE patients while on antimalarials and then after the antimalarials were discontinued according to the study protocol. The results supported the belief that antimalarials are helpful in mild to moderate SLE [5,7]. Recently, a number of studies have suggested that antimalarials lower the levels of cholesterol and triglycerides [8–10].

Hydroxychloroquine is given in a dose of 200 mg twice daily. If the patient has severe skin lesions, mucosal ulcers, or severe alopecia, it is wise to initiate therapy with 600 or 800 mg of hydroxychloroquine for a few weeks and then decrease the dose to a maintenance dose of 400 mg. The skin lesions respond rapidly to antimalarial therapy [11,12]. After the disease in general has gone into remission and the prednisone dose is lowered to 10 mg, it is wise to reduce the Plaquenil dose to 200 mg daily. Many patients can have their prednisone dose reduced further while maintained of 200 mg of hydroxycholorquine.

If the patient's skin disease does not respond to 400 mg hydroxychloroquine after 3 months of therapy, chloroquine (250 mg bid) or *quinacrine* (100 mg bid) (which may not be available) may be substituted, since it has been noted that some patients respond to one antimalarial, but not to another.

1. Side Effects

Some patients become nauseated on antimalarials and may tolerate the drug better if taken with meals. Usually, the nausea disappears after a few weeks while the patient continues to take the drug. The ocular complications may be significant [13,14]. We were the first to note asymptomatic ocular complications when the eyes of our patients who had been on antimalarials for up to 12 years were first examined. Corneal deposits of the drug were noted, and in some of these patients, night driving was difficult because of halos seen around street lights. These deposits disappear gradually after the drug is discontinued. Patients had difficulty accommodating owing to the effects on the extraocular muscles. The most serious problem involves pigment mottling around the macula which, in some patients, led to edema of the macula "bull's eye". It should be noted that many patients had more than 5 years of ingestion of 500 mg chloroquine and their eyes had never been examined. Some of these patients lost vision 5 years after the initial macula mottling had been noted and the drug discontinued. The appearance of macular lesions is directly related to the total ingested dose of the drug and rarely is noted prior to 3 years of therapy with either 500 mg of chloroquine or 400 mg of Plaquenil. It is generally recommended that the eyes be examined twice yearly by an ophthalmologist familiar with the ocular complications of antimalarial drugs. Over the last 25 years, many fewer patients have been noted to have macular mottling, and when this is noted, the drug is discontinued. We have had no patients going on to partial blindness during the past 25 years.

Other rarer complications include pigment mottling, usually of the lower extremities, and blackish lines crossing over the nails due to quinacrine. Conduction disorders have been reported [15].

Only 3.3% of pregnancies with exposure to either chloroquine or hydroxychloroquine had congenital abnormalities [16].

C. Cyclophosphamide

Cyclophosphamide may be used in an oral daily dose or as intravenous doses given every 3–4 weeks. It is our impression that the oral daily dose appears to be more effective in patients with severe cutaneous vasculitis with ulcerations and gangrene. Intravenous pulse therapy is used in patients who are severely ill with life-threatening manifestations such as pulmonary hemorrhage, seizures unresponsive to corticosteroids, and acute severe renal disease with renal insufficiency. The data on its use in these situations are anecdotal but are most suggestive of some therapeutic help in these catastrophic situations. Monthly intravenous cyclophosphamide is now recognized as the treatment of choice for diffuse proliferative lupus nephritis and may be effective even in membranous lupus nephritis (see below) [17].

Amenorrhea is a common effect of intermittent monthly pulse cyclophosphamide treatment and is more common in patients older than 25 years and in patients treated for 15 months or longer [18]. More serious complications of therapy are hemorrhagic cystitis, bladder fibrosis, and bladder carcinoma due to the metabolite acrolein. Patients should be well hydrated and some physicians routinely give mesna (2-mercaptoethanolsulfonate), which binds the acrolein. Patients should be monitored carefully with complete blood counts and urinalysis every month for oral therapy and 10 days to 2 weeks after intravenous therapy. Unexplained hematuria should be evaluated by cytology. Patients treated for prolonged periods with cyclophosphamide should be followed indefinitely for the possibility of bladder fibrosis and cancer.

D. Plasmapheresis

Plasmapheresis, in general, has not proven to be successful in the treatment of SLE. There have been no studies showing the value of plasmapheresis in the long-term outcome of SLE [19]. It has been used alone and in conjunction with pulse intravenous cyclophosphamide. At present, we use plasmapheresis along with intravenous corticosteroids and intravenous cyclophosphamide in SLE patients with pulmonary hemorrhages. It is our impression that more patients have survived this catastrophe who have been so treated than those treated with only corticosteroids or with corticosteroids plus intravenous cyclophosphamide.

E. Sex Hormones

Sex hormones influence normal immune responses [20]. Both humoral immunity and cell-mediated immunity are different in females compared with males, as females have higher immunoglobulin levels, an increased resistance to infection, and accelerated graft rejection.

As the female/male ratio for SLE is 9:1 overall, rising to 15:1 during the child-bearing years, it is clear that sex hormones influence the expression of this disease. It has also been shown that both female and male SLE patients metabolize estrogens abnormally [21]. Animal studies have shown detrimental effects of estrogen in some autoimmune models of disease, and removal of the protective effects of androgens, by castrating NZB/NZW hybrid male mice, results in an accelerated onset of disease, producing a pattern of disease typical of that found in the female mice, with early onset of disease, devastating end-organ failure, and premature death [22]. Similarly, exogenous estrogens may stimulate flares of disease in patients with SLE [23], and a recent study suggests that postmenopausal estrogen therapy is associated with an increased risk for developing SLE [24]. Flares of disease have also been related to the menstrual cycle. A recent report described three patients whose infertility was treated with clomiphene citrate, a nonsteroidal compound which stimulates the pituitary resulting in a significant rise in levels of serum gonadotropins and estradiol. These patients developed SLE after several cycles of this ovulation-induction treatment [25]. Various hormonal manipulations have been tried. Our report of the beneficial effects of danazol (an antigonadotropic agent) in two patients who suffered severe premenstrual exacerbations of their disease [26] was supported by a subsequent paper by Agnello et al., who described benefit in seven SLE patients treated with danazol [27]. Cyproterone (another antigonadotropic agent) has also been tried. Several women with SLE were treated with cyproterone and followed for several months. The number of flares of disease was lower during the treatment period compared with a similar pretreatment period and the dosages of corticosteroids and antimalarial therapy were reduced [28].

Tamoxifen (an estrogen antagonist) has been demonstrated to be of benefit in murine models of SLE [29], but concerns about a potential for developing carcinoma of the uterus will almost certainly limit its use in young SLE patients. Initial reports of the use of 19-nortestosterone decylate (Nandrolone decanoate) in patients with SLE demonstrated a lack of improvement in the treated female patients and an exacerbation of disease in the treated male patients that was considered to be due to the nandrolone suppressing the production of free testosterone [30].

Dehydroepiandroesterone (DHEA) is a naturally occurring adrenal steroid that is subsequently metabolized into both testosterone and estrogens. A recent report describing the use of DHEA in 10 patients with SLE demonstrated that after 3–6 months of DHEA treatment, disease activity and physician overall assessment were both improved and corticosteroid therapy was reduced in these patients [31]. Multicenter national studies of DHEA in lupus patients are now underway. Hormonal manipulation has obvious potential, but this therapeutic approach is still in its infancy 15 years after the first experiments clearly documented benefits in murine models of SLE [22].

F. Methotrexate

Concerns about the toxic effects of the usual therapies used to manage SLE have resulted in a search for steroid-sparing agents. The benefits of antimalarial agents are well documented, but these agents are limited in their effects and have not been demonstrated to be of use in the management of renal or central nervous system disease. The past 15 years have clearly determined that methotrexate is a very potent and effective anti-inflammatory agent that is useful in the management of inflammatory arthritis. This agent is comparatively well tolerated, and even though drug toxicity remains the main reason for discontinuing therapy, rheumatoid patients tolerate methotrexate for longer periods of time than they do most other second-line therapies.

Methotrexate also appears to be of benefit in patients with SLE. Rothenberg et al. reported benefit in 7 of 10 steroids-resistant SLE patients [32], which supports previous reports [33,34]. These investigators note that because this drug is excreted by the kidney, it must be monitored very carefully in patients with renal disease, and they even suggest that subclinical renal disease may have been responsible for the development of toxicity in two of their patients [32]. Walz LeBlanc et al. report benefit in five SLE patients reviewed retrospectively [35]. In each of these patients, there was a decrease in their corticosteroid requirements, and in two patients, proteinuria was noted to improve, suggesting that perhaps this agent can be used in SLE patients with renal disease. Studies done here have agreed with these reports, but we have found methotrexate to be of particular benefit in the management of arthritis [36]. To date, there have been no large randomized studies of the use of methotrexate in patients with SLE but initial reports seem to be encouraging.

G. Intravenous Gamma Globulin

Intravenous gamma globulin (IVIG intravenous immunoglobulin) is useful in managing a variety of autoimmune diseases, in particular, autoimmune thrombocytopenic purpura. The precise mechanism whereby IVIG is beneficial in these diseases is not known, but it has been suggested that it may be related to an anti-idiotypic activity against a variety of autoantibodies, an enhancement of T suppressor cell function, or other mechanisms modulating macrophage–T-cell interaction. In an attempt to find less toxic therapies for patients with life-long autoimmune disease, IVIG is now being used in the management of patients with systemic lupus erythematosus. Unfortunately, the majority of these studies have been open, unrandomized studies involving only small numbers of patients.

Francioni et al. recently reported clinical and laboratory improvement in 11 of 12 patients with resistant SLE treated with monthly boluses of IVIG for periods of 6–24 months [37]. Other case reports have suggested that IVIG may be of benefit in patients with resistant SLE [38,39], but reports of acute renal failure associated with IVIG treatment [40] must give rise to concerns about its use in patients predisposed to renal damage [41]. Our results from using IVIG in patients with SLE and Sjörgen's syndrome were disappointing [42]. Intravenous gamma globulin does have a place in the management of autoimmune thrombocytopenia [43], and previous reports have demonstrated the suppression of phospholipid antibodies in patients treated with IVIG and thrombocytopenia associated with the lupus anticoagulant. This has led to a current vogue to consider the use of intravenous gamma globulin in both pregnant and nonpregnant phospholipid antibody (aPL) patients [44]. However, this treatment is very expensive and the appropriate studies necessary to conclude that IVIG is truly beneficial in these patients have not been done.

H. Aspirin and Nonsteroidal Anti-inflammatory Drugs

Some patients with mild SLE may be controlled using aspirin and nonsteroidal anti-inflammatory drugs (NSAIDs) plus antimalarial drugs. On the other hand, these agents may be very toxic in patients with SLE, since their use may lead to interstitial nephritis [45]. It is very important to monitor the serum creatinine levels in SLE patients taking NSAIDs. We have had a number of patients whose "lupus nephritis" was directly due to the ingestion of NSAIDs. Other severe side effects that we have observed include gastrointestinal perforation and two fatal silent gastrointestinal hemorrhages in patients taking 12 or more tablets of aspirin in addition to 10–20 mg of prednisone. In addition, these agents may produce liver disease in SLE patients [46].

In our experience and in those of some others [47], pleuritis or pericarditis warrants treatment with from 40 to 60 mg of prednisone rather than treatment with indomethacin.

Aseptic meningitis continues to be reported in patients with SLE treated with NSAIDs (e.g., ibuprofen and naproxen) [48]. In addition, interstitial nephropathy induced by NSAIDs [48] has been reported. Discontinuation of NSAIDs and the institution of corticosteroid therapy was followed by improvement in renal function and remission of nephrotic syndrome. Proteinuria associated with treatment with tolmetin has been reported [49].

IV. USE OF LABORATORY TESTS IN MANAGEMENT OF SLE

It is very important to measure anti-DNA antibodies and complement proteins in the diagnosis of SLE. The presence of both anti-DNA antibodies and low C3 is highly predictive of the diagnosis of SLE [50]. In most patients, the anti-DNA antibody level, if it is elevated during the acute onset of disease, will fall gradually during treatment and become normal when the disease is fully suppressed. The anti-DNA should be measured using double-stranded DNA rather than a preparation of DNA containing single-stranded regions. The use of the latter leads to a false-positive anti-DNA assay, since what is specific and clinically relevant is anti-double-stranded DNA rather than anti–single-stranded DNA. Complement levels may be low in patients with active disease and the levels go back to normal during remission [50]. Thus, these tests have been shown to reflect disease activity and are very helpful in following the disease, since the tests may become abnormal prior to the development of clinical signs or symptoms or other laboratory test abnormalities [51]. In a prospective study, Appel et al. guided immunosuppressive therapy according to changes in CH50 and anti–double-stranded DNA [52]. Their 5-year follow-up suggested that normalization resulted in a trend toward stabilized renal histology, creatinine clearance, and a lower serum creatinine at a lower final mean dose of prednisone [53].

V. SPECIAL PROBLEMS

A. Renal Disease

The National Institutes of Health (NIH) group has been studying the effects of various treatment regimens on lupus nephritis for many years [17,54–57]. Their study of the use of pulse methylprednisolone versus two regimens of pulse cyclophosphamide in severe lupus nephritis showed that the extended course (monthly for 6 months and then quarterly for 2 years) of pulse cyclophosphamide is more effective than just giving the short course (monthly for 6 months) or than the 6 months of pulse methylprednisolone. The patients treated with pulse methylprednisolone had a higher probability of doubling their serum creatinine than those treated with the extended course of cyclophosphamide, although there were no data presented regarding overall mortality [57]. In the previous report from the NIH by Steinberg and Steinberg, it was shown that the probability of progression to end-stage renal disease was less in patients treated with intravenous cyclophosphamide and oral cyclophosphamide and combined oral azathioprine and cyclophosphamide [54]. However, the changes in survival are based on very few patients followed for more than 5 years, and in the use of actuarial life tables, the small number of patients greatly magnified any error, as pointed out in a review by Danadio and Glassock [58]. These nephrologists also emphasize that the effect of therapy on patient survival did not differ in any of the treatment groups in the NIH trials [54–56] and conclude, "Although these immunosuppressive agents may have favorable effects on the overall activity of systemic lupus erythematosus, their long-term effects per se on renal disease are in question and could be attributed to lower prednisone dosage and better medical management of hypertension, hyperlipidemia, infection and other metabolic consequences of the disease." In this respect, it is important to recognize that the NIH trial protocols do not consider fluctuations in complement levels or anti-DNA antibodies as indicators for raising or lowering the doses of oral corticosteroid. We have long felt that the onset of clinical renal disease (i.e., onset of hematuria and proteinuria), can be predicted by a simultaneous fall in complement levels and a rise in anti-DNA antibodies, as first described by Schur and Sandson in 1968 [51].

The use of laboratory tests and the aggressive treatment of hypertension, hyperlipidemia, and infection may have played a major role in the current improvement in survival from severe lupus nephritis compared with that of more than 25 years ago.

The Lupus Nephritis Collaborative Study Group concluded that there was a lack of efficacy of plasmapheresis in treating severe lupus nephritis [59]. It is especially hazardous to use NSAIDs in patients with lupus nephritis, since proteinuria, nephrotic syndrome, and interstitial nephritis may result from this treatment.

B. Skin Disease

Most dermatological manifestations of SLE, including the butterfly blush, alopecia. maculopapular eruptions, and mucosal ulcers, will respond to adequate prednisone given for other moderate to severe manifestations of the disease; that is, from 25 to 60 mg daily in divided doses. In addition, patients with such manifestations should be started on antimalarial therapy; that is, hydroxychloroquine 200 mg bid [12]. It is sometimes possible to use 30 mg of prednisone in a split dose in patients with such skin manifestations who do not have significant hematological, serological (low C3 and/or high anti-DNA), central nervous system (CNS), or renal disease but may have arthritis and pericarditis/pleuritis. Maintenance on antimalarials is essential as the dose of prednisone is decreased gradually until less than 10 mg daily. It may be possible then to decrease the hydroxychloroquine to one tablet daily.

SLE patients with severe skin lesions due to vasculitis should be tried on prednisone and antimalarials, but ultimately daily oral cyclophosphamide may be needed if ulcerations do not heal.

For SLE patients with annular or papular subacute lesions who do not respond to 30 mg of prednisone or who initially respond but have a recurrence on less than 20 mg prednisone daily, other therapy should be tried. This is necessary in less than 10% of SLE patients. Such treatments as methotrexate, dapsone, thalidomide, and accutane have all been reported to be effective in "steroid- and antimalarial-resistant" cutaneous lupus [60]. Most of these agents, however, are only effective while the patient continues to take them, and the skin lesions recur promptly after the drugs are discontinued.

C. CNS Lupus

We define CNS lupus as the presence of major organic brain disease as outlined in the American Psychiatric Association's *Diagnostic and Statistical Manual*, 3rd edition, revised (DSM-III-R) [61]. The most common feature is organic brain disease, which was present in 64 patients and was present in 44 patients at the time of diagnosis of SLE studied [62].

Organic brain disease usually has a rapid onset, occurring within a week or so, while the patient realizes that "something is wrong with my head." Patients are disoriented to time and place and have an impairment of perception, memory, and the ability to calculate. Some patients, in addition to the above, hallucinate and have seizures.

The second most common manifestation of CNS lupus is seizures, which are frequently associated with the presence of organic brain disease. Seizures are also most common at the onset of disease and are associated with other manifestations of SLE. At Bellevue Hospital in New York City, 29 patients had seizures at onset, and of these, 15 had grand mal seizures. Status epilepticus may occur and has an ominous prognosis.

Unfortunately, there have been no prospective randomized studies of the various treatments for CNS lupus. Treatment of the organic psychosis at the time of diagnosis in a febrile SLE patient with multiple organ disease activity should be prednisone in a dose of 20–30 mg given every 6 h. If the patient is too severely ill to take the pills, intravenous methylprednisolone should be started at an equivalent dose and regimen. Most patients treated thus become afebrile within a few days and respond within 10 days with clearing of the sensorium along with improvement of the other manifestations of disease. This was the experience of one of us (NFR) at Bellevue Hospital during the late 1950s and 1960s when all psychotic SLE patients from throughout the city were transferred to the Bellevue psychiatric wards. Some patients responded to 120 mg/day of prednisone and become totally irrational on 100 mg/day. Tapering of the prednisone must be done carefully and also must be done slowly at doses less than 30–40 mg/day. Some of the Bellevue patients were mentally well on 10 mg but began to have hallucinations on 7.5 mg. Complete recovery is the usual result of treatment, but some patients have residual impairment of mental processes such as the ability to do calculations. Some of these patients have had to find different employment from their previous occupations.

Pulse cyclophosphamide has been used in patients with severe CNS lupus who have failed treatment with corticosteroids. A recent report described 31 patients treated with intravenous cyclophosphamide after failing to respond to various doses and regimens of corticosteroids [61]. There was substantial improvement in 61% of patients and only 10% deteriorated.

The group from the NIH reported on patients with severe neuropsychiatric lupus (defined as focal neurological deficits with/without seizures and organic brain disease with psychosis) who responded to cyclophosphamide 0.75–1.0 g/m body surface area [63]. Eight of the nine patients had complete recovery. Included were six patients who had been unresponsive to a higher dose of the drug.

Steroid psychosis must be differentiated from the organic brain disease due to SLE. Steroid psychosis is noted after patients are placed on high (60 mg/day or more) doses of prednisone and is not accompanied by other manifestations of SLE. On the other hand, a similar organic brain disease due to SLE is usually associated with other manifestations of SLE and is present at the time of diagnosis or during a severe flare of the disease. It has recently been noted that patients with mildly active SLE on no corticosteroids may have some form of cognitive impairment and this is improved by taking corticosteroids (0.5 mg/kg of prednisone for 3 weeks) [64].

D. Transverse Myelitis

Seven SLE patients treated with pulse methylprednisone followed by pulse cyclophosphamide for a mean of 6 months had an excellent outcome [65]. These patients had failed to respond to medium to high doses of oral prednisone.

E. Pregnancy

Concerns for the lupus patient who wishes to become pregnant are numerous. First, there are the effects of the physiological changes of pregnancy, which are a particular problem for the patient who has renal disease or pulmonary hypertension. Second, there are the effects of the disease on the pregnancy. Patients with SLE have no trouble becoming pregnant, but there is increased fetal wastage in these patients and an increased potential for preterm birth [66,67]. The reasons for the increase in fetal wastage in these patients are numerous, but one of the most important is control of disease activity [68]. It is absolutely vital for the patient with SLE to plan for pregnancy, and our usual instruction for these patients is to wait until the disease has been quiescent for at least 6 months before trying to become pregnant. Unfortunately, this advice is not always taken, making management of the patient and her fetus more difficult.

It is very important that the pregnant lupus patient is managed by the same rheumatologist throughout her pregnancy. Patients who are educated to their disease know which symptoms are due to their disease and which are not. As it is so vital to keep the disease under control during pregnancy, it is very useful to ask the patient if she thinks her disease is active, particularly as important laboratory markers of disease activity such as complement levels are less helpful during pregnancy as these are elevated in normal pregnancy. Buyon et al. suggest that activated components of complement are useful for determining which patients have active disease and which have toxemia of pregnancy [69]. Using Ba and Bb as measures of activation of the alternate complement pathway, Buyon has concluded that the ratio of CH50/Ba is less than 100 in patients with active lupus nephritis and greater than 100 in patients with preeclampsia [69]. As these measurements of complement activity are not routinely available, it is helpful to measure the complement levels regularly in order to be aware of any fall in them, as this would be unusual in a normal pregnancy and may signify a flare of disease. Buyon has suggested that C4 levels and CH50 levels are more useful than C3 levels [69].

The other important factors that may determine the outcome of pregnancy in SLE patients are maternal autoantibody production. Two autoantibodies in particular are associated with fetal and placental pathology and it is therefore vital to know if these autoantibodies are present.

1. Neonatal Lupus Syndrome

The neonatal lupus syndrome is known to be associated with the presence of Ro antibodies, even in patients who do not have criteria for connective tissue diseases and who may have no clinical complaints at the time of the abnormal pregnancy [70]. The features of this syndrome include a transient photosensitive rash, transient hematological disorders, and permanent primary congenital complete heart block [71]. The syndrome is considered to be a consequence of the transplacental passage of a maternal autoantibody [72,73], with primary congenital complete heart block the end result of a conducting system that has been permanently damaged by a maternal autoantibody. Ninety-eight percent of these mothers have Ro antibody, 72% have antibodies to the 52-kD Ro fraction, and 52% have antibodies to the 60 kD Ro faction [69]. Eight-six percent of mothers of infants with primary congenital complete heart block also have antibodies to La [69].

As mortality in these infants with primary congenital complete heart block can reach 30% [74], various therapeutic attempts at preventing this pathology have been tried, including plasmapheresis, in an attempt to lower levels of maternal autoantibody and high doses of dexamethasone or betamethasone, corticosteroids that cross the placenta, aimed at reducing fetal cardiac inflammation [75,76]. Close monitoring with frequent fetal echocardiography is probably one of the most beneficial prophylactic steps, as it identifies the fetus at risk.

One problem in identifying the fetus at risk for permanent cardiac damage is that there are fetal factors that determine the development of this syndrome that are yet to be identified. The same mother, with the same antibody, can produce both normal and abnormal infants even in a twin pregnancy [77]. It is therefore difficult to predict which infants are at particular risk (except for the presence of maternal autoantibodies to Ro and La), and it is even more difficult to determine the benefit of various prophylactic therapeutic regimens unless the fetus demonstrates cardiac inflammation in utero which is improved by treatment [76,78].

2. Phospholipid Antibody Syndrome

The phospholipid antibody syndrome is a prothrombotic state that is associated with the presence of antibodies to phospholipids (aPL) measured as (a) a lupus anticoagulant (LAC); (b) a biologically false-positive test for syphilis (VDRL); and (c) cardiolipin antibodies (aCL). This thrombotic states leads to recurrent clinical thrombosis, both arterial and venous, and therefore may present with a variety of complaints, including recurrent deep venous thromboses, premature dementia (a consequence of recurrent cerebral infarctions), and recurrent fetal wastage. It is considered that the recurrent fetal wastage is a direct consequence of thrombosis in the placental bed [79,80] which leads to placental insufficiency and subsequent fetal death. This is usually late fetal death.

Although there are some patients who may also experience fetal loss in the first trimester, it usually occurs after 10 weeks of gestation [81].

The association of these phospholipid antibodies with a predisposition to recurrent fetal wastage has resulted in a variety of therapeutic approaches being adopted in an effort to prevent fetal wastage. The initial reports in the early 1980s suggested that the patients should be treated with large doses of corticosteroids, in an attempt to suppress autoantibody production, as well as antithrombotic agents such as low-dose aspirin [82]. Since then it has been become apparent that this is not essential and it is sometimes not possible to suppress the level of these autoantibodies with high doses of corticosteroids. Other regimens, including subcutaneous heparin and aspirin, low-dose prednisone (20 mg/day) and baby aspirin, as well as other immunosuppressive agents such as intravenous gamma globulin have all been tried [83–85]. Unfortunately, to date, there have been no large randomized well-controlled studies which have conclusively proven the benefits of any one therapeutic regimin over others. There is, however, no question that doing something is much better than doing nothing at all, as the fetal wastage rate in these patients can be as high as 90%. Our experience has been that the fetal wastage rate falls to less than 30% using a variety of therapeutic regimens, all of which have included subcutaneous heparin and aspirin.

The presence of high-titer IgG cardiolipin antibodies and/or a lupus anticoagulant in particular are associated with the presence of recurrent fetal wastage. Patients who have these autoantibodies and have an obstetrical history which has demonstrated previous fetal loss must be considered at high risk for subsequent fetal loss. It is important, therefore, to discuss with these patients the potential for recurrent fetal wastage and the potential toxicities of any therapeutic regimens to be tried in subsequent pregnancies. There is never any guarantee that any therapeutic regimen will be successful in preventing a fetal wastage, and indeed our placental studies in these patients have demonstrated that the thrombotic diathesis continues despite subcutaneous heparin, baby aspirin, and intravenous gamma globulin [86]. The placental pathology that is found in one pregnancy appears to be repeated in subsequent pregnancies, and at best, we feel that the therapeutic interventions may delay the onset of significant placental pathology enough to enable to the fetus to attain sufficient size and maturity to be able to survive independently.

Patients who have had a previous clinical thrombotic event, especially if this was related to pregnancy or oral contraception, must be treated throughout pregnancy with subcutaneous heparin at therapeutic doses (i.e., 10,000 units bid). In patients with partial prothrombin times (PTTs) that are prolonged because of their LAC, it may be necessary to monitor plasma heparin levels in order to ascertain if the dosages of heparin are sufficient to attain therapeutic anticoagulation. Patients who have never had a previous clinical thrombotic event but do have phospholipid antibodies (particularly high-titer IgG cardiolipin and/or LAC) may need prophylactic anticoagulation with heparin at dosages of 5000 units bid. Oral anticoagulants cannot be used, as they cross the placenta and may be associated with the development of the congenital warfarin syndrome, which includes nasal and eye defects as well as deafness, seizures, hypoplasia of the extremities, and congenital heart disease, especially if they are used after 7 weeks of gestation [87]. We usually give heparin with a baby aspirin throughout pregnancy, and maintain anticoagulation for 6 weeks postpartum, changing to oral anticoagulants postpartum, as some of these patients are particularly at risk for thrombosis during pregnancy and the postpartum period [88]. We therefore do not routinely use prednisone during pregnancy just because of the presence of phospholipid antibodies. Patients with SLE and aPL who need prednisone to control their lupus and who need anticoagulation throughout pregnancy are instructed about the potential risks of combining heparin and corticosteroids, particularly the risks of osteoporosis and aseptic necrosis. Serum calcium levels need to be monitored carefully, and these patients need calcium supplementation, as some of them develop problems with muscle cramping.

Other groups continue to use prednisone during pregnancy in patients with aPL, usually combined with low-dose aspirin [83]. We have been impressed with the hypertension and toxemia of pregnancy that we have encountered in these patients and feel that prednisone just makes a bad situation worse, although we do consider using corticosteroids if the patient has demonstrated inflammatory pathology in previous pregnancies; that is, villitis, intervillousitis, and/or vasculitis [86].

The use of intravenous gamma globulin in these pregnant patients is controversial. It is extremely expensive and in our experience does not prevent placental thrombosis.

F. Thrombocytopenia

Most SLE patients with significant thrombocytopenia can be treated successfully with 60 mg of prednisone and the dose tapered slowly thereafter without a fall in platelet count. However, in some patients, the platelets fall with a concomitant prolongation of the bleeding time after the prednisone dose reaches about 20 mg daily. In some patients, repeated attempts gradually to taper the prednisone below 20 mg daily lead to a fall in the platelet count. Some of these patients have been treated with intravenous gamma globulin (see above) with good success. In other patients, the good response to intravenous gamma globulin is repeated but in others splenectomy is necessary. Other modalities that have been tried successfully in refractory thrombocytopenic include intermittent low-dose (0.25 g/m body surface area) intravenous cyclophosphamide [89]. Danazol is another choice in patients who have failed with prednisone and splenectomy [90]. However, thrombocytopenia usually recurs when danazol is discontinued. Some of the treatments used for thrombocytopenia are listed in Table 1.

G. Phospholipid Antibody Syndrome in the Nonpregnant Patient

As already stated in Section V.E.2, the phospholipid antibody syndrome is a thrombotic diathesis associated with the presence of phospholipid antibodies measured as (a) a lupus anticoagulant (LAC); (b) a biologically false-positive test for syphilis (e.g., VDRL); and (c) cardiolipin antibodies (aCL). This thrombotic diathesis may present

Table 1 Treatment of Thrombocytopenia

1.	Corticosteroids
2.	IV gamma globulins
3.	Splenectomy
4.	Danazol
5.	Low-dose IV cyclophosphamide

in a variety of ways, but it has been clearly demonstrated that these patients are predisposed to recurrent thrombotic events over time. Some patients with these phospholipid antibodies do not meet the criteria for other well-defined connective tissue diseases, and these patients are defined as having primary phospholipid antibody syndrome or a lupus-like syndrome if they have additional autoantibodies. Phospholipid antibodies are also found in patients who do meet the criteria for other connective tissue diseases such as systemic lupus erythematosus, Sjögren's syndrome, and systemic sclerosis. In some of these patients, it appears that flares of their underlying disease may precipitate recurrent thrombotic events.

In recent years, it has been identified that these phospholipid antibodies may require a cofactor. This has led to the concept that these antibodies are not just directed at phospholipids but are directed against a phospholipid protein complex. The cofactor that has been studied most aggressively is β_2-glycoprotein, which is known to have natural anticoagulant properties. As these antibodies are now known to be a family of antibodies, it is quite likely that some of them are directed against one protein phospholipid complex and others are directed against other protein phospholipid complexes. It has been suggested that a variety of proteins involved in the complement cascade may in fact be cofactors for these autoantibodies [91,92].

As the exact nature of this thrombotic diathesis remains unclear, managing these patients with a view to preventing thromboses remains difficult. In a retrospective study of 70 patients with phospholipid antibodies who had experienced at least one clinically thrombotic event, Rosove concluded that only high-dose anticoagulation (an INR >3) was efficient at preventing rethrombosis [93]. These investigators also demonstrated that patients who previously experienced an arterial thrombotic event could subsequently expect another arterial event and similarly for patients experiencing thrombosis on the venous side of the vascular system. A subsequent paper by Dercksen addressing venous thrombotic events in patients with phospholipid antibodies came to a similar conclusion that these patients need to be maintained on long-term anticoagulants [94]. These investigators demonstrated that patients receiving oral anticoagulants had a 100% probability of surviving 8 years without a recurrent thrombotic event, whereas those patients who were not treated with long-term anticoagulants had a 50% probability of a recurrent venous thrombotic event at 2 years and a 78% probability of a recurrent event at 8 year's follow-up [92]. Our studies do not concur with these previous findings [88]. First, approximately 50% of our patients who rethombosed did so on either side of the arterial tree suggesting that venous thrombosis is not necessarily followed by a venous thrombosis. We looked at 3 treatment regimens including oral anticoagulants, low-dose aspirin, and no therapy. As our patients were followed for such a long period of time, some of these patients moved from one treatment regimen to another over many months of follow-up. Using the same statistical methods as Derksen to analyze our data, we did not demonstrate any significant change in the rate of rethrombosis among these three treatment groups, however, none of the patients in our study were treated with high-dose oral anticoagulants. Out data did show, however, that there are a variety of prothrombotic triggers that precipitated clinical thrombotic events in these patients. Pregnancy, the postpartum period, and oral contraceptives appeared to be associated with recurrent thrombotic events, particularly in our patients with primary phospholipid antibody syndrome/lupus-like syndrome who did not meet the criteria for SLE. Other prothrombotic triggers included flares of disease in those patients who did meet the criteria for SLE and events known to be prothrombotic, even in normal individuals such as elective surgery. We concluded that these patients are at risk for thrombosis, and may be triggered into clinical thrombosis by a variety of events known to be prothrombotic, and we feel that these patients would be better served by identifying these prothrombotic triggers and covering the patients prophylactically throughout these known triggering events. Patients managed on long-term high-dose oral anticoagulants will eventually run into problems. Even though Rosove's initial paper was only published 5 years ago, we are already aware of several patients who have developed major bleeding problems managed with high-dose oral anticoagulation. We, therefore, do not routinely put all of our aPL patients on life-long high-dose oral anticoagulation, but we attempt to identify known prothrombotic triggers in these patients so that they may be treated prophylactically throughout these events. In the meantime, our patients are routinely managed on a low-dose aspirin, as this is considered to be comparatively harmless.

H. Aseptic Necrosis and Osteoporosis

Aseptic necrosis and osteoporosis are particular problems for SLE patients, as both the disease [95] and corticosteroid treatment predispose them to develop these complaints. Predicting SLE patients who will develop aseptic necrosis is difficult, but some studies have suggested both clinical and laboratory associations with the development of this complaint [96]. Obviously minimizing the length and amount of corticosteroid therapy is desirable, but some patients appear to tolerate long-term, high-dose corticosteroid therapy much better than others without the development of side effects.

As corticosteroids interfere with the absorption and metabolism of calcium, lupus patients on corticosteroid therapy should take supplemental calcium and vitamin D unless contraindicated. We encourage our patients to exercise regularly and to participate in osteoporosis programs but do not advise taking exogenous estrogens, as these may flare the disease [24]. Calcitonin is very effective at relieving pain but otherwise it is not particularly indicated for patients on corticosteroids. Didronel may be used in a dose of 400 mg per day for 2 weeks every 3 months, but it is not formally approved for use in these patients. The benefits of nasal calcitonin and second generation parsphosphonates (i.e., alendronate), in these patients, need further evaluation.

I. Heart Disease

Inflammation may occur in any layer of the heart in patients with SLE. Twenty-five percent of all SLE patients will develop pericarditis, whereas myocarditis is less common and is usually found in the patient with severe multisystem disease. Recent work has suggested that valvular abnormalities occur more frequently in patients with phospholipid antibodies [97], but endocardial disease per se may be found in up to 50% of SLE patients coming to autopsy. Libman-Sacks endocarditis (verrucous endocarditis) is a pathological diagnosis which may predispose patients to bacterial endocarditis. We therefore recommend that all SLE patients are covered with prophylactic antibiotics for any dental work.

Recent studies have demonstrated that patients with SLE are predisposed to develop ischemic heart disease [98,99]. It appears that as new antibiotics and antihypertensive agents have become available, the morbidity and mortality of this disease has changed, with ischemic heart disease becoming a prevalent feature found in even very young women [100]. It is probably not just a consequence of long-term corticosteroid therapy, as patients with inflammatory bowel disease and asthma do not appear to develop the same premature atherogenesis [100]. The combination of vasculitis with corticosteroid therapy appears to be a prerequisite for this pathology. This means that it is even more vital to treat hypertension appropriately and to identify and treat risk factors with lipid-lowering agents, a sensible diet, and exercise.

V. CONCLUSIONS

Over the years, the treatment of SLE has changed very little per se. Some 50 years after the discovery of corticosteroids, these potent anti-inflammatory agents are still the mainstay for treating this disease, but attempts to minimize the long-term toxicity of corticosteroids have resulted in other agents being used as steroid-sparing agents. It is hoped that a better understanding of the hormonal aberrations that are part of this disease and the influence of hormones on the immune system in general will result in the development of less toxic therapies. In the meantime, we feel the best policy for managing these patients is prevention. This means seeing the patients regularly and educating them so that they understand their disease and become aware of the signs and symptoms that signify an increase in disease activity. We also prefer that our patients do not take exogenous estrogens for any reason, and we caution our patients about exposure to exogenous chemicals. We feel that this is particularly relevant in patients with SLE, as drug-induced SLE is a well-documented phenomenon, especially in patients with abnormal drug metabolism (i.e., slow acetylators), and xenobiotic agents such as sulfonamide drugs have been shown to potentiate flares of disease even in patients with so-called idiopathic disease. Tables 2 and 3 list things that SLE patients should avoid and be alert to, respectively.

Table 2 SLE Patients Should Avoid

Sun exposure
Hair dyes
Infections
Immunizations except when necessary
Estrogens
Sulfa-containing medications
Pregnancy until disease controlled for 6 months

Table 3 SLE Patients Should Be Alert To

Infections
Rashes
Chest pain
Hair loss
Joint pain
Medications given by other physicians
Fever
Cough

REFERENCES

1. Petri M, Allbritton J. Hair product use in systemic lupus erythematosus: a case-control study. Arthritis Rheum 1992; 35:625–629.
2. Griffiths. Sulfasalazone-induced lupus syndrome in ulcerative colitis. Br Med J 1992; 2:1188–1189.
3. Almeida L, Grossman M. Widespread dermatophyte infections that mimic collagen vascular disease. J Am Acad Dermatol 1990; 23:855–857.
4. Wallace DJ. Antimalarial agents and lupus. Rhem Dis Clinics North Am 1994; 20:243–263.
5. Esdaile JM. The efficacy of antimalarials in systemic lupus erythematosus (review). Lupus 1993; 1(Suppl 2):S3–8.
6. Rudnicki RD, Gresham GE, Rothfield NF. The efficacy of antimalarials in systemic lupus erythematosus. J Rheumatol 1975; 2:323–330.
7. Anonymous. A randomized study of the effect of withdrawing hydroxychloroquine sulfate in systemic lupus erythematosus. The Canadian Hydroxychloroquine Study Group (comment). N Engl J Med 1991; 324:150–154.
8. Petri M, Lakatta C, Magder L, Goldman D. Effect of prednisone and hydroxychloroquine on coronary artery disease risk factors in systemic lupus erythematosus: a longitudinal data analysis. Am J Med 1994; 96:254–259.
9. Wallace DJ, Metzger AL, Stecher VJ, et al. Cholesterol-lowering effect of hydroxychloroquine in patients with rheumatic disease: reversal of deleterious effects of steroids on lipids. Am J Med 1990; 89:322-326.
10. Hodis HN, Quismorio FP Jr, Wickham E, Blankenhorn DH. The lipid, lipoprotein, and apolipoprotein effects of hydroxychloroquine in patients with systemic lupus erythematosus. J Rheumatol 1993; 20:661–665.
11. Lo JS, Berg RE, Tomecki KG: Treatment of discoid lupus erythematosus. Int J Dermatol 1989; 28:497–507.
12. Rothfield NF: Lupus erythematosus. In: Dermatology in General Medicine, 4th ed. Vol. II. Fitzpatrick TB, Eisen AZ, Wolff K, et al., eds. New York: McGraw-Hill, 1993:2137–2148.
13. Henkind P, Rothfield NF. Ocular abnormalities in patients treated with synthetic antimalarial drugs. N Engl J Med 1963; 269:433–439.
14. Carr RC, Henkind P, Rothfield NF, Siegel IM. The ocular toxicity of antimalarial drugs: long term follow-up. Am J Ophthalmol 1968; 66:738–742.
15. Verny C, de Gennes C, Sebastien P, et al. Heart condition disorders in long-term treatment with chloroquine. Two new cases. Presse Medi 1992; 21:800–804.
16. Levy M, Buskila D, Gladman DD, et al. Pregnancy outcome following first trimester exposure to chloroquine. Am J Perinatol 1991; 8:174–178.
17. Fessler BJ, Boumpas DT. Severe major organ involvement in systemic lupus erythematosus. Rheum Dis Clin North Am, 1995; 21:81–98.
18. Boumpas DT, Austin HA III, Vaughan EM, et al. Risk for sustained amenorrhea in patients with systemic lupus erythematosus receiving intermittent pulse cyclophosphamide therapy. Ann Intern Med 1993; 119:366–369.
19. Lewis EJ, Hunsicker LG, Lan S-P, et al. A controlled trial of plasmapheresis therapy in severe lupus nephritis. N Engl J Med 1992; 326:173–1379.
20. Ahmed SA, Penhale WJ, Talal N. Sex hormones, immune responses, and autoimmune diseases. Mechanisms of sex hormone action (review). Am J Pathol 1985; 121:531–551.
21. Lahita RG, Bradlow HL, Fishman J. Increased 16 alpha hydroxylation of estradiol in systemic lupus erythematosus. J Clin Endocrinol Metab 1981; 53:174–178.
22. Roubinian JR, Talal N, Greenspan JS, et al. Effect of castration and sex hormone treatment survival, anti-nucleic acid antibodies and glomerulonephritis in NZB x NZW F1 mice. J Exp Med 1978; 147:1568–1583.

23. Jungers P, Dougados M, Pelissier C, et al. Influence of oral contraceptive therapy on the activity of systemic lupus erythematosus. Arthritis Rheum 1982; 25:618–623.
24. Sánchez-Guerrero J, Liang MH, Karlson EW, et al. Postmenopausal estrogen therapy and the risk for developing systemic lupus erythematosus. Ann Intern Med 1995; 12:430–433.
25. Ben-Chetrit A, Ben-Chetrit E. Systemic lupus erythematosus induced by ovulation induction treatment. Arthritis Rheum 1994; 37:1614–1617.
26. Morley KD, Parke A, Hughes GRV. Systemic lupus erythematosus: two patients treated with danazol. Br Med J 1982; 284:1431–1434.
27. Agnello V, Pariser K, Gell J, et al. Preliminary observation on danazol therapy of systemic lupus: effects on DNA antibodies, thrombocytopenia and complement. J Rheumatol 1983; 10:682–687.
28. Jungers P, Kuttenn F, Liote F, et al. Hormonal modulation in systemic lupus erythematosus. Preliminary clinical and hormonal results with cyproterone acetate. Arthritis Rheum 1985; 28:1243–1250.
29. Sthoeger ZM, Bentwich Z, Zinger H, Mozes E. The beneficial effect of the estrogen antagonist, Tamoxifen, on experimental systemic lupus erythematosus. J Rheumatol 1994; 21:2231–2238.
30. Lahita RG, Cheng CY, Monder C, Bardin CW. Experience with 19-nortestosterone in the therapy of systemic lupus erythematosus: worsened disease after treatment with 19-nortestosterone in men and lack of improvement in women. J Rheumatol 1992; 19:547–555.
31. van Vollenhoven RF, Engleman EG, McGuire JL. An open study of dehydroepiandrosterone in systemic lupus erythematosus. Arthritis Rheum 1994; 37:1305–1310.
32. Rothenberg RJ, Graziano FM, Grandone JT, et al. The use of methotrexate in steroid-resistant systemic lupus erythematosus. Arthritis Rheum 1988; 31:612–615.
33. Miescher PA, Riethmuller D. Diagnosis and treatment of systemic lupus erythematosus. Semin Hemtol 1965; 2:1–28.
34. Swanson MA, Schwartz RS. Immunosuppressive therapy: the relation between clinical response and immunological competence. N Engl J Med 1967; 277:163–170.
35. Walz LeBlanc BAE, Dagenais P, Urowitz MB, Gladman DD. Methotrexate in systemic lupus erythematosus. J Rheumatol 1994; 21:836–838.
36. Wilson K, Abeles M. A 2 year, open ended trial of methotrexate in systemic lupus erythematosus. J Rheumatol 1994; 21:1674–1677.
37. Francioni C, Galeazzi M, Fioravanti A, et al. Long term IVIG treatment in systemic lupus erythematosus. Clin Exp Rheumatol 1994; 12:163–168.
38. Winder A, Molad Y, Ostefeld I, et al. Treatment of systemic lupus erythematosus by prolonged administration of high dose intravenous immunoglobulin: report of 2 cases. J Rheumatol 1993; 20:495–498.
39. Ben-Chetrit E, Putterman C, Naparstek Y. Lupus refractory pleural effusion: Transient response to intravenous immunoglobulins. J Rheumatol 1991; 18:1635–1637.
40. Pasatiempo AMG, Kroser JA, Rudnick M, Hoffman BI. Acute renal failure after intravenous immunoglobulin therapy. J Rheumatol 1994; 21:347–349.
41. Barron KS, Sher MR, Silverman ED. Intravenous gammaglobulin therapy: magic or black magic (review). J Rheumatol 1992; 33(Suppl):94–97.
42. Ballow M, Parke A. The uses of intravenous immune globulin in collagen vascular disorders. J Allergy Clin Immunol 1989; 84:608–612.
43. Borg EJ, Kallenberg CG. Treatment of severe thrombocytopenia in systemic lupus with intravenous gammaglobulin. Ann Rheum Dis 1992; 51:1149–1151.
44. Scott JR, Branch DW, Kochenour NK, Ward K. Intravenous immunoglobulin treatment of pregnant patients with recurrent pregnancy losses caused by antiphospholipid antibodies and Rh immunization. Am J Obstet Gynecol 1988; 159:1055–1056.
45. Ling BN, Bourke E, Campbell WG Jr, Delaney VB. Naproxen-induced nephropathy in systemic lupus erythematosus (review). Nephron 1990; 54:249–255.

46. Seamen WE, Ishak KG, Plotz PH: Aspirin induced hepatotoxicity in patients with systemic lupus erythematosus. Ann Intern Med 1974; 80:1–8.
47. Mills JA. Systemic lupus erythematosus. N Engl J Med 1994; 330:1871–1879.
48. Weksler BB, Lehany AM. Naproxen-induced recurrent aseptic meningitis. Drug Intel Clin Pharm 1991; 25:1183–1184.
49. Vogelgesang SA, Dennis GJ, Bauer FA. Proteinuria associated with tolmetin treatment in a patient with systemic lupus erythematosus. Arthritis Rheum 1993; 36:1181–1182.
50. Weinstein A, Bordwell B, Stone B, et al. Antibodies to native DNA and serum complement (C3) levels. Application to the diagnosis and classification of systemic lupus erythematosus. Am J Med 1983; 74:206–216.
51. Schur PH, Sandson J: Immunologic factors and clinical activity in systemic lupus erythematosus. N Engl J Med 1968; 7;278:533–538.
52. Appel AE, Sablay LB, Golden RA, et al. The effect of normalization of serum complement and anti-DNA antibody on the course of lupus nephritis: a two-year prospective study. Am J Med 1978; 64:274–283.
53. Jarrett MP, Schiffman G, Barland P, Grayzel AL: The effect of continuous normalization of serum hemolytic complement on the course of lupus nephritis. A five year prospect study. Am J Med 1981; 70:1067–1072.
54. Steinberg AD, Steinberg SC. Long-term preservation of renal function in patients with lupus nephritis receiving treatment that includes cyclophosphamide versus those treated with prednisone alone. Arthritis Rheum 1991; 34:945–950.
55. Austin HA III, Klippel JH, Balow JE, et al. Therapy of lupus nephritis: controlled trial of prednisone and cytotoxic drugs. N Engl J Md 1986; 314:614–619.
56. Balow JE, Austin HA III, Tsokos GC, et al. Lupus nephritis. Ann Intern Med 1987; 106:79–94.
57. Boumpas DT, Austin HA, Vaughan EM, et al. Controlled trial of pulse methylprednisolone versus two regimens of pulse cyclophosphamide in severel lupus nephritis. Lancet 1992; 340:741.
58. Donadio JV Jr, Glassock RJ. Immunosuppressive drug therapy in lupus nephritis. Am J Kidney Dis 1993; 21:239–250.
59. Miller ML. Treatment of systemic lupus erythematosus (review). Curr Opin Rheumatol 1992; 4:693–699.
60. Duna GF, Cash JM. Treatment of refractory cutaneous lupus erythematous. Rheum Dis Clin North Am 1995; 21:99–115.
61. Neuwelt CM, Lacks S, Kaye BR, et al. Role of intravenous cyclophosphamide in the treatment of severe neuropsychiatric systemic lupus erythematosus. Am J Med 1995; 98:32–41.
62. Rothfield NF. Clinical features of systemic lupus erythematosus. In: Kelley WN, Harris ED Jr, Ruddy S, Sledge CB, eds. Textbook of Rheumatology. Vol. II. Philadelphia: Saunders, 1981:1106–1132.
63. Boumpas DT, Yamada H, Patronas NJ, et al. Pulse cyclophosphamide for severe neuropsychiatric lupus. Q J Med 1991; 81:975.
64. Denburg SD, Carbotte RM, Denburg JA. Corticosteroids and neuropsychological functioning in patients with systemic lupus erythematosus. Arthritis Rheum 1994; 37:1311–1320.
65. Barile L, Lavalle C. Transverse myelitis in systemic lupus erythematosus—the effect of IV pulse methylprednisolone and cyclophosphamide. J Rheumatol 1992; 19:370–372.
66. Petri M. Systemic lupus erythematosus and pregnancy (review). Rheum Dis Clin North Am 1994; 20:87–118.
67. Julkunen H, Jouhidainen T, Kaaja R, et al. Fetal outcome in lupus pregnancy: a retrospective case study of 242 pregnancies in 112 patients. Lupus 1993; 2:125–131.
68. Derksen RHWM, Buinse HW, de Groot PG, Kater L. Pregnancy in systemic lupus erythematosus: a prospective study. Lupus 1994; 3:149–155.

69. Buyon JP. Systemic lupus erythematosus and pregnancy. Clin Rheumatol 1991; 1:1–8.
70. McCune AB, Weston WL, Lee LA. Maternal and fetal outcome in neonatal lupus erythematosus. Ann Intern Med 1987; 106:518–523.
71. Watson RM, Lane AT, Barnett NK, et al. Neonatal lupus erythematosus. A clinical, serological and immunogenetic study with review of the literature. Medicine 1984; 63:362–378.
72. Buyon JP, Ben-Chetrit E, Karp S, et al. Acquired congenital heart block. Pattern of maternal antibody resonse to biochemically defined antigens of the SSA/Ro-SSB/La system in neonatal lupus. J Clin Invest 1989; 84:627–634.
73. Alexander E, Buyon JP, Provost TT, Guarnieri T. Anti-Ro/SS-A antibodies in the pathophysiology of congenital heart block in neonatal lupus syndrome, an experimental model. In vitro electrophysiologic and immunocytochemical studies. Arthritis Rheum 1992; 35:176–189.
74. Waltuck J, Buyon JP. Autoantibody-associated congenital heart block: Outcome in mothers and children. Ann Intern Med 1994; 120:544–551.
75. Carreira PE, Gutierrez-Larraya F, Gomez-Reino JJ. Successful intrauterine therapy with dexamethasone for fetal myocarditis and heart block in a woman with systemic lupus erythematosus. J Rheumatol 1993; 20:1204–1207.
76. Buyon JP, Swersky SH, Fox HE, et al. Intrauterine therapy for presumptive fetal myocarditis with acquired heart block due to systemic lupus erythematosus: experience in a mother with a predominance of SS-B (La) antibodies. Arthritis Rheum 1987; 30:44–49.
77. Harley JB, Kaine JL, Fox OF, Reichlin M, Gruber B. Ro (SS-A) antibody and antigen in a patients with congenital complete heart block. Arthritis Rheum 1985; 28:1321–1325.
78. Bierman FZ, Baxi L, Jaffe I, Driscoll J. Fetal hydrops and congenital complete heart block. Response to maternal steroid. J Pediatr 1988; 108:646–648.
79. Out HJ, Koojman CD, Bruinse HW, Derksen RH. Histopathological findings in placentae from patients withintra-uterine fetal death and anti-phospholipid antibodies. Eur J Obstet Gynecol Reprod Biol 1991; 41:179–186.
80. DeWolf F, Carreras LO, Moerman P, et al. Decidual vasculopathy and extensive placental infarction in a patient with repeated thromboembolic accidents, recurrent fetal loss, and a lupus anticoagulant. Am J Obstet Gynecol 1982; 142:829–834.
81. Branch DW. Thoughts on the mechanism of pregnancy loss associated with the antiphospholipid syndrome. Lupus 1994; 3:275–280.
82. Lubbe WF, Palmer SJ, Butler WS, Liggins CG. Fetal survival after prednisone suppression of maternal lupus anticoagulant. Lancet 1983; 1:1361–1363.
83. Silver RK, MacGrego SN, Sholl JS, et al. A comparative trial of prednisone plus aspirin versus aspirin alone in the treatment of anticardiolipin antibody-positive obstetric patients. Am J Obstet Gynecol 1993; 169:1411–1417.
84. Branch DW, Silver RM, Blackwell JL, et al. Outcome of treated pregnancies in women with antiphospholipid syndrome: an update of the Utah experience. Obstet Gynecol 1992; 80:614–620.
85. Kaaja R, Julkunen H, Ämmälä P, et al. Intravenous immunoglobulin treatment of pregnant patients with recurrent pregnancy losses associated with antiphospholipid antibodies. Acta Obstet Gynecol Scand 1993; 72:63–66.
86. Parke AL, Ernst LE, Starzyk KA, Salafia CM. Placental pathology in the phospholipid antibody syndrome and systemic lupus erythematosus. Rheum Disease Clinic of North America 1994; 23:85–99.
87. Hall JG, Pauli RM, Wilson KM. Maternal and fetal sequelae of anticoagulation during pregnancy. Am J Med 1980; 68:122–140.
88. Nasr S, Parke AL. Long term oral anticoagulants are not necessary to prevent recurrent thrombotic episodes in all patients with phospholipid antibodies. New Eng U Med 1995; 333:667.

89. Roach BA, Hutchinson GJ. Treatment of refractory, systemic lupus erythematosus-associated thrombocytopenia with intermittent low-dose intravenous cyclophosphamide. Arthritis Rheum 1993; 36:682–684.
90. West SG, Johnson SC. Danazol for the treatment of refractory autoimmune thrombocytopenia in systemic lupus erythematosus. Ann Intern Med 1988; 108:703–706.
91. Bevers EM, Galli M, Barbui T, et al. Lupus anticoagulant IgG's (LA) are not directed to phospholipids only but to a complex of lipid-bound human prothrombin. Thromb Haemostas 1991; 66:629–632.
92. McNeil HP, Simpson RJ, Chesterman CN, Krilis SA. Anti-phospholipid antibodies are directed against a complex antigen that includes a lipid-binding inhibitor of coagulation: β_2-glycoprotein I (apoliproprotein H). Proc Natl Acad Sci USA 1990; 87:4120–4124.
93. Rosove MH, Brewer PMC. Antiphospholipid thrombosis: clinical course after the first thrombotic event in 70 patients. Ann Intern Med 1992; 117:303–308.
94. Derksen RHWM, de Groot G, Kater L, Nieuwenhuis HK. Patients with antiphospholipid antibodies and venous thrombosis should receive long term anticoagulant treatment. Ann Rheum Dis 1993; 52:689–692.
95. Kalla AA, Fataar AB, Jessop SJ, Bewerunge L. Loss of trabecular bone mineral density in systemic lupus erythematosus. Arthritis Rheum 1993; (12):1726–1734.
96. Migliaresi S, Picillo U, Ambrosone L, et al. A vascular osteonecrosis in patients with SLE: relation to corticosteroid therapy and anticardiolipin antibodies. Lupus 1994; 3:37–41.
97. Cervera R, Khamashta MA, Font J, et al. High prevalence of significant heart valve lesions in patients with the 'primary' antiphospholipid syndrome. Lupus 1991; 1:43–47.
98. Petri M, Perez-Gutthann S, Spence D, Hochberg MC. Risk factors for coronary artery disease in patients with systemic lupus erythematosus. Am J Med 1992; 93:513.
99. Asherson RA, Khamashta MA, Baguley E, et al. Myocardial infarction and antiphospholipid antibodies in SLE and related disorders. Q J Med 1989; 272:1103–1115.
100. Spiera H, Rothenberg RR. Myocardial infarction in four young patients with SLE. J Rheumatol 1983; 10:464–466.

26
Therapy of Systemic Sclerosis

Carol Mary Black and Christopher P. Denton
Royal Free Hospital, London, United Kingdom

I. INTRODUCTION

There is presently no cure for systemic sclerosis (scleroderma; SSc) but management strategies are possible for many aspects of the disease. In order to maximize the therapies available, it is important to understand (a) the heterogeneity of the condition, (b) the current subsetting of systemic sclerosis and staging within the subsets, (c) the organ-specific problems with the need for the earliest possible diagnosis of internal organ involvement and the use of "at-risk" markers, and (d) advances in understanding the pathogenesis of SSc and the application of this knowledge to influence treatment decisions. It is also necessary to acknowledge the lack of internationally agreed indices of disease severity and activity and the imprecise way in which this conditions is often assessed, and to be aware of the need for internationally agreed guidelines for conducting clinical trials. This chapter addresses these issues by first outlining disease heterogeneity and classification and then considering possible pathogenic mechanisms and disease assessment, The classes of drugs which have been used aiming to arrest or reverse the disease, based on its presumed mechanism of pathogenesis, will be considered together with the methods used to evaluate response to treatment. The final section addresses the problem of internal organ involvement and the management of organ-specific damage. Key points are summarized in the tables and figures within the chapter.

II. PATHOLOGICAL AND CLINICAL FEATURES OF SYSTEMIC SCLEROSIS

Systemic sclerosis forms part of the scleroderma spectrum of disorders, a group of acquired conditions characterized by skin sclerosis, vasculopathy, and immunological change, with the extent and pattern of these depending on the disease subtype. At the one end of this spectrum is localized scleroderma with its almost exclusive involvement of dermal and subdermal tissues with sclerosis and atrophy through to systemic sclerosis where vascular, sclerotic, and immunological factors intermingle and internal organ involvement is common. There are also some rare cases of visceral fibrosis and vasculopathy without skin disease, a condition known as scleroderma sine scleroderma. The extent of skin sclerosis and the accompanying pattern of internal organ involvement form the basis for one of the most used current classifications of SSc (Table 1) which divides the condition into diffuse and limited disease [1]. It is usually possible within the first year of observation to determine whether the pattern of skin sclerosis indicates diffuse disease in which sclerosis extends over the limbs and trunk or whether cutaneous involvement is restricted to the extremities and face indicating limited cutaneous SS (LcSSc). Other clinical manifestations also vary between these different forms of disease; for example, renal involvement and pulmonary fibrosis are typically seen in the more severe cases of diffuse cutaneous SSc (dcSSc), whereas vascular abnormalities and Raynaud's phenomenon are more prominent in LcSSc. The clinical course of LcSSc is generally more protracted than dcSSc, often with Raynaud's symptoms preceding other changes by many years. Some of the antibodies found in SSc are specific for different disease subsets; for example, antitopoisomerase-1 (Scl-70) and anti-RNA polymerase antibodies are typically associated with dcSSc. In contrast, anticentromere antibodies occur in LcSSc. The identification of these antibodies and the placement of

Table 1 Classification of the Systemic Sclerosis Subsets

Prescleroderma	
	Raynaud's phenomenon plus nalifold capillary changes, disease-specific circulating antinuclear autoantibodies (antotopoisomerase-1 anticentromere [ACA], or nucloelar), and digital ischemic changes.
Diffuse cutaneous SSc (dcSSc)	
	onset of skin changes (puffy or hidebound) within 1 year of onset of Raymaud's phenomenon
	trunal and acral skin involvement
	presence of tendon friction rubs
	early and significant incidence of interstitial lung disease, oliguric renal failure, diffuse gastrointestinal disease, and myocardial involvement
	nalifold capillary dilatation and dropout
	Antitopoisomerase-1 (Scl-70) antibodies (30% of patients)
Limited cutaneous SSc (LcSSc)	
	Raynaud's phenomenon for years (occasionally decades)
	skin involvement limited to hands, face, feet, and forearms (acral)
	significant (10–15%) late incidence of pulmonary hypertension with or without interstitial lung disease, skin calcification, telangiectasiaes, and gastrointestinal involvement
	high incidence of ACA (70–80%)
	Dilated nalifold capillary loops, usually without capillary dropout
Scleroderma sine scleroderma	
	Raynaud's phenomenon ±
	no skin involvement
	presentation with pulmonary fibrosis, scleroderma renal crisis, and cardiac or gastrointestinal disease
	antinuclear antibodies may be present (Scl-70, ACA, nucleolar)

a patient within a subset has both prognostic and therapeutic implications and is an important part of the management of these patients.

The two main subsets progress in different ways. During the first 5 years of diffuse disease (the early phase), the patient is fatigued and loses weight. There is rapid progression of skin disease with an increased risk of renal failure and early cardiac, pulmonary (interstitial fibrosis), and gastrointestinal disease. Arthritis, myositis, and tendon involvement can be most marked at this time. After 5 years (considered to be the late stage of diffuse disease), the constitutional symptoms have usually disappeared; the skin is stable, atrophic, or regressing; the musculoskeletal problems are not active, but have led to deformity and wasting; and there is progression of existing visceral disease, but there is a reduced risk of new organ involvement.

By contrast, in limited disease, the first 10 years is the early phase and there are few, if any, constitutional symptoms. Skin involvement is mild, often with minimal progression. Raynaud's phenomenon, pitting scars, digital ulcers, and telangiectasia can all be troublesome and esophageal symptoms are prominent. The late stage of this subset can show worsening of the vascular disease with widespread telangiectasia, digital tip ulcers, widespread calcinosis, and pulmonary vascular disease with the diagnosis of pulmonary hypertension; pulmonary interstitial disease can also occur as a late complication. The gut involvement can worsen with esophageal strictures, small bowel disease, malabsorption, pseudo-obstruction, and anal incontinence. These differences in pattern and natural history obviously influence evaluation and therapy. These different clinical patterns for the two major disease subsets are summarized in Figure 1.

The pathological hallmarks of systemic sclerosis are vascular damage, perivascular and tissue accumulation of mononuclear leukocytes, and fibrosis in the skin and internal organs [2,3]. This deposition would seem to be a response to a disruption of the normal steady state of connective tissue turnover and regulated repair. These pathological changes appear to varying degrees in both major subsets of SSc, and it is now believed that the processes are themselves related and perhaps directly linked. The current most favored explanation implicates endothelial damage/activation and mononuclear leukocyte vascular adhesion with subsequent migration into the interstitium through a leaky vascular barrier.

Mediators are released in association with these inflammatory events and a population of activated fibrogenic fibroblasts are generated [2]. Cross-talk between the major cell types or the mediators they produce is obviously central to SSc pathogenesis and these events may in the future provide avenues for therapeutic attack. There is considerable evidence that the vascular and endothelial changes precede other features of the disease. First, endothelial damage has been observed in early skin disease [4]; also, in the lung, kidney, and bowel, there is ultrastructural EC damage before abnormalities can be detected by light microscopy [5–7]. Moreover, recent studies of endothelial cell phenotype in SSc have demonstrated an increase in EC surface expression of adhesion molecules, including E-selectin, vascular cell adhesion molecule-1 (VCAM-1), and intracellular adhesion molecule-1 (ICAM-1) in clinically "yet to be involved" skin suggesting that endothelial cell (EC) activation is one of the earliest disease events [8].

Although the cellular infiltrate varies somewhat depending on the stage of disease and the organs involved, the presence of interleukin-2 (IL-2) producing T lymphocytes of the $\alpha\beta$ subset expressing typical surface antigens, including CD3, CD4, CD45, HLA-DR, and leucocyte function antigen-1 (LFA-1) is consistently noted [9]. Further clues to immune processes operating in SSc are the reported increased T-cell reactiv-

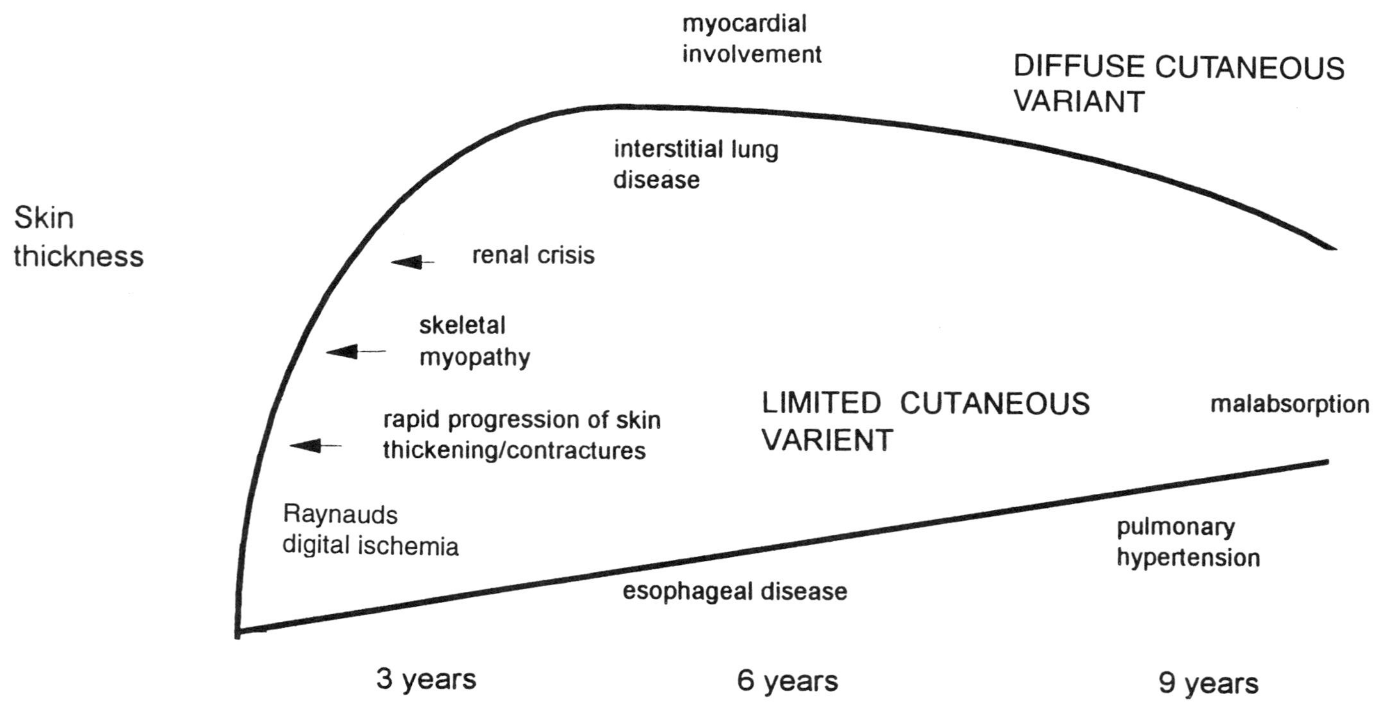

Figure 1 Typical natural history for development of visceral complicatins in dcSSc and lcSSc. (Modified from T. Medsger with permission.)

ity against collagen antigens in vitro [10] and the elevated serum levels of the immunologically active lymphocyte products IL-2 and IL-4 in some SSc patients [11]. It is, however, not yet known whether the immune activation is triggered before or after the endothelial damage [12]. In addition, intense vasospasm (Raynaud's phenomenon) often occurs in the extremities and internal organs. This could lead to structural and functional change in the endothelium which might contribute to the development of the scleroderma lesion through the local effects of endothelial cell products such as nitric oxide, superoxide anions, endothelin, or cytokines [13]. The potential role of hypoxia, physical stress, and neural mediators in the generation of SSc is also still to be fully investigated. The precise factors responsible for the generation of the scleroderma fibroblast phenotype are unknown, but a large number of cytokines of different cellular origins have been implicated as potential effectors of fibrosis. These include tumor growth factor-β (TGF-β), platelet-derived growth factor (PDGF), tumor necrosis factor-α (TNF-α), insulin-like growth factors (IGFs), basic fibroblast growth factor (BFGF) IL-1, IL-4, IL-6, IL-8, and interferon-γ (INF-γ) [14]. It is unlikely that any individual mediator can account for the complex pathology of SSc, but rather that they act in concert to establish the conditions that permit fibroblasts to develop the SSc phenotype [15]. The potential patterns of cellular interactions involved in SSc pathogenesis are summarized in Figure 2. The particular importance of any mediator may be dependent on the stage of the disease, or indeed the disease subset, but key cytokines or growth factors may be future targets for therapeutic attack.

The logical ordering of therapy in SSc must combine these three elements; that is, the vascular, the immune, and the fibrotic process to the subset and stage of the disease before the best combination of available drugs can be found for any individual patient. Different types of treatment are likely to be appropriate in different stages and subsets. For example, in early diffuse SSc, immune-directed therapies may be most successful, and in later dcSSc, antifibrotic drugs may be more effective. In LcSSc, useful treatments are likely to be primarily aimed at the vasculature.

III. CLINICAL ASSESSMENT OF SCLERODERMA

A. Staging

To stage scleroderma accurately, we need both severity and activity scores. These have proved extremely difficult to develop in SSc. After many years of collaborative work, an international group is soon to publish a suggested severity grading index [16], and an activity index also needs to be formulated. Reliable and reproducible assessment of overall SSc activity is likely to be more difficult than measuring its severity despite an increasing number of test reflecting activity within different organ systems. Some of these are sensitive, but many of them are incapable of identifying very early change or are too insensitive to monitor the slow and focal progression which so often occurs in SSc. For example, (a) an echo-Doppler examination, used for the identification of a raised pulmonary artery pressure, can only register that level once tricuspid incompetence is established—this measurement therefore misses early disease and a potential window of therapeutic opportunity; and (b) pulmonary functions tests are a rather insensitive way to document the patchy fibrosis which is usually going on in the lungs. There are fortunately an increasing number of more sophisticated techniques to help us; for example, high-resolution computed tomographic (CT) scans (HRCT) for pul-

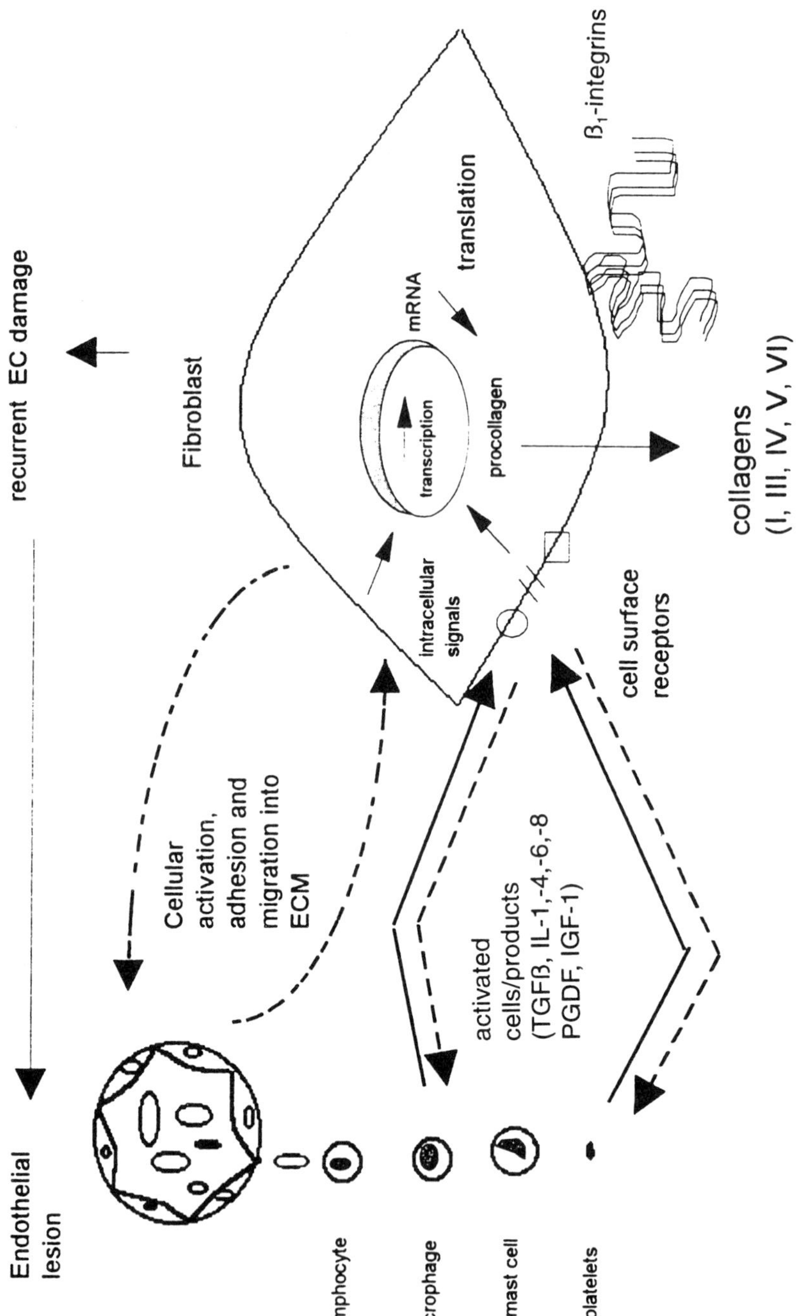

Figure 2 Interactions between endothelial cells, leukocytes, and fibroblasts in scleroderma.

monary disease (see below) and circulating markers such as soluble IL-2 receptors, IL6, IL8, soluble adhesion molecules, endothelin-1, and serum procollagen propeptides, which need to be tested in a longitudinal fashion to see whether or not they correlate with disease severity, activity, or survival in scleroderma patients.

B. Clinical Trial Methodology

It is difficult to perform a good trial in SSc. This is because the disease is rare, it is heterogeneous, the speed of progression is variable within the subsets, and the outcome measures we use are frequently too insensitive for the changes which are occurring [17]. Until recently, most trials were single center, had inadequate numbers, and were not suitably controlled with few including a placebo arm. Therefore the recent guidelines from the American College of Rheumatology's (ACR) committee on design and outcome in clinical trials in SSc is most welcome [18]. These guidelines include suggestions for patient inclusion criteria, trial design, and outcome measurements which combine clinical and laboratory parameters. Hopefully, these recommendations will be employed by the international SSc community.

IV. THERAPEUTIC STRATEGIES FOR SCLERODERMA

A. Vascular Therapy

As Reynaud's phenomenon (RP) is often the forerunner of SSc, it is appropriate to consider vascular therapy first of all. Although it is possible to improve the vasospasm, it is not yet possible to prevent or cure the more damaging proliferative structural vascular lesion which occurs in most scleroderma patients. A possible exception to this is the use of angiotensin-converting enzyme inhibitors to suppress the vascular lesion in hypertensive scleroderma renal crisis. However, based on current research, there may be newer approaches which can now be pursued (see below).

1. Principles

The treatment of RP should be a graduated process with full patient participation. RP does not always require pharmacological intervention, but all patients should stop smoking and aggravating drugs such as vasoconstricting β-blockers should be withdrawn. Keeping warm by the use of thermal underwear, body warmers, muffs, ski glove liners, fur-lined boots, and electrically heated gloves and socks can produce immediate benefit. Biofeedback techniques and physical exercise, such as the whirling of the arms, have been reported to be successful. An even ambient temperature is as important as keeping warm, because often it is not the absolute temperature but a small change in the ambient environment which precipitates an attack. Cold drafty work places should therefore be avoided.

Drug therapy is indicated for patients with prolonged frequent attacks, functional impairment, severe pain, or tissue ischemia, and the spectrum of treatment options is shown in Table 2. The treatments available provide symptomatic relief rather than cure and patient response is often idiosyncratic, so it is worth trying more than one drug with a particular class. Typically, patients with primary Raynaud's phenomenon are easier to treat than patients with secondary RP, in whom structural damage to the vessel wall is often both pronounced and fixed. Drug treatments aim to affect either the

Table 2 Treatment Options for Raynaud's Phenomenon

Treatment	Examples	Comments
Simple measures		
nondrug	Hand warmers protective clothing	Universally helpful; also useful to minimize cold exposure and ambient temperature changes in work environment.
pharmacological	Evening primrose oil	Evening primrose oil has been shown effective in controlled clinical trial.
	Fish oil capsules	
Oral vasodilators		
calcium channel blockers	Nifidipine retard Nicardipine Felodipine Amlodipine	Responses often idiosyncratic; therefore best to try several drugs in rotation to find most effective.
5-HT antagonist	Ketanserin	Only available on named-patient basis but shown effective in clinical trials.
ACE inhibitors	Captopril	In Raynaud's phenomenon; secondary to
	Enalapril	dcSSc, may protect from hypertensive renal crisis.
Topical vasodilators	GTN patches	Shown effective in short-term use but often cause headaches.
Parenteral vasodilators	Carboprostacyclin (iloprost) Prostaglandin E_1	Effective and reasonably tolerated. Given for severe frequent attacks of RP, digital ulceration, or gangrene and prior to digital surgery.
Antibiotics	Flucloxacillin Erythromycin	Important in secondary infection in RP. Prolonged oral administration may be necessary.
Surgical procedures		
lumbar sympathectomy	Chemical or operative	For severe RP of lower limbs
digital sympathectomy (radical microarteriolysis)		Useful treatment for isolated ischemia of one or two digits.
debridement amputation	Surgical or auto-amputation	Such surgery should be conservative to allow maximum possibility of spontaneous healing.

arterial wall, the blood components, the toxic products of ischemia, or the sympathetic nerves.

2. *Arterial Vasodilators*

Concern has been expressed that vasodilator drugs will divert blood through arteriovenous shunts away from areas of critical ischemia (steal syndrome). This may be a special problem in patients with Raynaud's phenomenon secondary to connective tissue disease in which proliferative, obliterative vascular lesions are prominent.

3. *Calcium Channel Blockers*

Calcium channel blockers inhibit the contraction of smooth muscle cells by reducing the cellular uptake of calcium, a process which is fundamental to contraction. Currently, the drug of choice for patients with RP is nifedipine: It reduces both the frequency and severity of the attacks and also alters platelet aggregation [19]. Adverse vasodilatory effects such as nausea, flushing, headaches, and peripheral edema are frequent. Modified-release nifedipine (e.g., nifedipine retard 20–60 mg daily) may be more acceptable, because it avoids high peak plasma concentrations.

The sublingual use of crushed nifedipine capsules (5 mg) may be helpful for the relief of an acute attack or for patients intolerant of long-term use. Other antagonists such as diltiazem (60 mg tds), nicardipine (20 mg tds), felodipine (5–20 mg daily), isradipine (2.5 mg bid), and amlodipine (5 mg od) are also effective and cause fewer side effects [19]; however, verapamil is not useful.

4. *Nitrates*

Oral glyceryl trinitrate (GTN) has no place in the treatment of RP, but topical application of a 2% ointment can be useful when the disorder affects awkward anatomical sites such as the knees and nipples. Headaches are common and often make long-term use unacceptable. Some benefits from GTN-impregnated patches have been reported [21].

5. *Alpha-Blockers*

For patients with low-grade symptoms of RP, thymoxamine, a nonselective alpha-adrenoceptor blocker may suffice. It is usually well tolerated at a dose of 40 mg three times a day with minimal side effects. Several investigators have reported favorable results with prazosin, a selective α_1-adrenoreceptor blocking agent in a dosage of 0.5–1.0 mg three times a day—the drug should be introduced cautiously at a lower dose. The α_1- and α_2-adrenoreceptors are dynamic in their functional expression, and increased numbers and/or increased sensitivity of α_2-receptors have been implicated as a causative factor in Raynaud's phenomenon [22].

6. *Angiotensin-Converting Enzyme Inhibitors*

The use of captopril (12.5–25 mg bid) and enalapril (20 mg daily) for treating RP remains controversial [23]. They have been tried when other drugs have failed, particularly in scleroderma-related Raynaud's phenomenon, but convincing evidence for their superior efficacy is still awaited. Their critical role in hypertensive renal crisis is discussed later.

7. *Serotonin Receptor Antagonists*

Serotonin receptor antagonists are of considerable interest in RP. Naftidrofuryl is an S_2-receptor blocker given orally (100–200 mg three times daily). It is well-tolerated but has not been shown to be effective in formal clinical trials. Ketanserin (40 mg tds), a selective antagonist at serotonin receptors, has proved useful for symptomatic relief of RP in several studies. It would also seem to be a well-tolerated drug [24].

8. Prostaglandins and Prostaglandin Inducers

The E and F classes of prostaglandins and prostacyclins have well-established potent vasodilatory actions [25]. The synthetic analogue of prostacyclin, iloprost (carbo-prostacyclin), also has useful rheological properties, inhibiting platelet aggregation, increasing red blood cell deformability, decreasing blood viscosity, and altering neutrophil function. It is useful in both primary and secondary RP and in critical ischemia [26]. Its use often helps to avoid the amputation of a distal part of a digit. The effects of iloprost can last for up to 16 weeks; a surprising response in view of its short duration of action [27]. The need for intravenous infusion in the hospital and their adverse effects, due to excessive vasodilatation, are considerable drawbacks to the use of prostaglandins. Day care can be utilized to reduce the hospital stay. A recent comparison of low-dose iloprost (0.5 ng/kg/min) and a standard regimen (2 ng/kg/min) showed that both were effective in decreasing severity, frequency, and duration of attacks, but that low-dose therapy caused far fewer side effects [28]. Efforts to develop an oral prostaglandin analogue which is safe and effective have been underway for several years and one such drug is soon to enter clinical trials. Fish oil (omega-3-marine triglycerides) and evening primrose oil (concentrated linoleic and gamolenic acids) which may be metabolized to prostacyclin-like or prostaglandin E_2–like materials should in theory be useful nontoxic agents, but convincing evidence of their efficacy is still awaiting [29]. These compounds are, however, popular with patients, who can purchase them without prescription.

9. Antiplatelet Drugs

Both the fibrinolytic anabolic steroid stanozolol and the thromboxane A_2-receptor antagonist dazoxiben have failed to show any clinical improvement in double-blind randomized placebo-controlled trials [30]. There is evidence for increased red cell rigidity in some patients with RP. This may explain the response to oxpentifylline (400 mg three times a day) [31] which changes the rheological properties of blood secondary to an increase in the flexibility of red cells. It may also have vasodilator properties.

10. Sympathetic Blockers

Sympathetic blocking agents such as guanethidine, reserpine, and phenoxybenzamine have no place in the treatment of RP. Their effects are short lived, and adverse effects such as apathy, depression, diarrhea, nasal stuffiness, and peptic ulcer are often unacceptable.

11. Surgery

Cervical sympathectomy usually gives only short-lived benefit and is now virtually obsolete for treating RP. However, lumbar sympathectomy still has an important place in the treatment of severe RP of the feet, since beneficial effects are often long lasting. This discrepancy between the upper and lower limbs is not understood. Recently, digital sympathectomy (radical microarteriolysis) has been shown to heal digital ulcers and relieve severe pain in patients with critical ischemia. The operation does not cure the RP, but the attacks are often less severe postoperatively. Intermediate and long-term follow-up data on this procedure are keenly awaited. An infusion of iloprost before these surgical procedures may be useful. In the most severe cases of RP, with digital gangrene, the surgeon in sometimes also called on to debride a finger, to remove an infected nail, and, in the last resort, to perform an amputation.

B. Immunomodulation

There is evidence as noted earlier than an activated immune system may play a damaging role in the earliest phase of systemic sclerosis and may be an important stimulus to both the fibrotic and vascular lesions. It is also possible that, unlike many of the other connective tissue disorders such as systemic lupus erythematosus, polymyositis, or rheumatoid arthritis, this stimulus is not a persistent or recurring one but rather is confined to early-stage disease. This hypothesis is supported by the sparsity of mononuclear cells found in the tissue except for the inflammatory infiltrate in the earliest phase of SSc. The initial immune activation could, through its cytokine and growth factor products, create autocrine loops which require no further stimulus to perpetuate the fibrotic and vascular lesions. These loops plus the nonimmune mechanisms (see Fig. 1) which may be operating could account for the relatively poor response to immune suppression seen in established SSc. All of the treatments given to date have either been generalized (e.g., corticosteroids, chlorambucil, 5-flurouracil, methotrexate, and azathioprine) or agents with intermediate specificities (e.g., cyclosporin A, antithymocyte globulin, and photophoresis). We do not as yet have sufficiently defined targets against which to design a specific attack. The immunosuppressive agents used to date and their outcome are listed in Table 3 and discussed briefly below. Many are still being evaluated, and if their usefulness is to be accurately determined, they must be employed at the earliest possible stage of diffuse disease in controlled trials of sufficient power to provide a reliable answer. The specific role of steroids and cyclophosphamide will be discussed in the context of lung disease. Recently some groups have used immunoblative treatment with cyclophosphamide combined with autologous peripheral sterocell rescue. The results of such aggresive treatment strategies are eagerly awaited.

1. *Chlorambucil and 5-Flurouracil*

Immunosuppressive drugs which have been adequately tested in the last 5 years and found not to be useful are chlorambucil and 4-flurouracil. Both had shown initial promise in open studies, but when subjected to double-blind controlled testing, neither drug showed significant clinical benefit [32].

2. *Cyclosporine A*

Cyclosporin A (CyA) is a potent suppressor of cell-mediated immunity [33] and has also been demonstrated to reduce collagen synthesis by cultured fibroblasts from SSc patients [34]. In recent years, there have been several case reports and some open studies with small numbers of patients reporting improvement of SSc with cyclosporin therapy [35–37]. The main parameter of response used in these studies was an improvement in skin score. However, the potential for cyclosporin to induce nephrotoxicity seriously limits its use in SSc. Renal parameters worsen in many patients during cyclosporin treatment, although lowering the cyclosporin dose can reduce renal insufficiency [36,38]. Renal crisis has been described in a woman treated with cyclosporin A [39], and Denton et al. [40] reported the development of hypertension and renal failure in three of eight scleroderma patients with early diffuse disease who received cyclosporin A. There are several possible explanations for this deterioration in renal function. It may be due to arteriolar hyalization and interstitial fibrosis which has been reported to occur in pa-

Table 3 Immunomodulatory Therapies for Systemic Sclerosis

Treatment	Mechanism of action	Comments	Efficacy in clinical trials
Selective immunosuppression			
cyclosporin A	Inhibits T helper cell actions by reducing IL-2 release.	Reported beneficial effects on skin sclerosis may be confounded increased incidence of renal crisis.	Yes (open study) [36]. Yes (open study) [38].
antithymocyte globulin antilympohcyte globulin	Temporary suppression of cell-mediated immunity.	Possible benefit for skin sclerosis, although controlled trial of ATG confirms considerable therapy associated morbidity.	Yes (open study) [51]. Possible benefit in placebo-controlled pilot study [52].
photophoresis	Extracorporeal photoactivated 8-methoxypsoralen inhibits activated T cells.	Benefit has been reported but good placebo-controlled clinical trial is needed.	No (open study) [47]. Yes (open study) [48]. Yes (controlled trial comparing with D-penicillamine therapy) [46]. 1992. Multicenter placebo-controlled trial currently in progress.
phasmapheresis	Removes circulating immune mediators.	Equivocal results but anecdotal benefit.	Possible benefit (open study), Jacobs et al., 1991.
pooled human gammaglobulin	Possible inhibition of lymphocyte function via regulatory idiotype cross reactivity.		Not formally evaluated.
Nonselective immunosuppression			
methotrexate	Folic acid antagonist.	Currently under formal evaluation in dcSSc.	Yes (open study) [45]. Controlled trial in progress.
cyclophosphamide chloambucil azathioprine	Alkylating agent suppressing production of immunocompetent leukocytes.	Anecdotal benefit reported open studies but controlled trial of chlorambucil failed to show superiority over placebo. Cyclophosphamide often combined with corticosteroids	Yes (cyclophosphamide in SSc lung fibrosis—open study), Akesson et al., 1994. No (chlorambucil, controlled trial, 1994).

tients treated with CyA [41]. Nonsteroidal anti-inflammatory drugs (NSAIDs), which are often prescribed for scleroderma patients, may decrease renal blood flow and therefore compound the CyA-induced damage. In addition, in vitro studies using cultured endothelial cells have demonstrated that CyA stimulates endothelial cells to synthesis endothelin [42]. Endothelin causes proliferation of smooth muscle cells and vasoconstriction and may be involved in mediating the hypertension and vasculopathy occurring with CyA therapy.

Preliminary information suggests that cyclosporin may be helpful in SSc, but if its continued use is anticipated, patients should only receive this drug as part of well-planned and closely monitored studies so that any increased risk of renal pathology can be assessed. It is also possible that newer drugs such as rapamycin may provide equal efficacy with less toxicity.

3. Methotrexate

The success of low-dose methotrexate in other rheumatological disorders has led to its use in SSc, but is tempered by the knowledge that this drug may be capable of inducing lung fibrosis. Early open studies [43,44] involved small numbers of patients at various disease stages but nevertheless suggested a beneficial effect. In addition, a recent report by Siebold et al. [45] of an open trial in early diffuse disease confirmed these findings. In this open study, 62% of patients treated with low-dose methotrexate showed more than a 25% improvement of skin score and no new visceral involvement. Confirmation of these findings in a double-blind trial is now required and such a study is currently underway.

4. Photophoresis

Photophoresis was developed as a treatment to target aberrant T lymphocytes in conditions such as T-cell lymphoma. During this therapy, patients receive the photosensitizing compound 8-methoxypsoralen and then undergo leukopheresis with exposure of the peripheral blood in an extracorporeal flow system to ultraviolet A (UVA). T lymphocytes are sensitized to UVA by 8-methoxypsoralen and UVA exposure so that they are no longer functionally competent after this treatment. Photochemotherapy therefore seemed an interesting way of eliminating activated immune cells that could mediate fibrosis and vascular damage in SSc. As yet, despite this theoretical promise, studies have yielded conflicting results: A multicenter trial reported in 1992 claimed that photophoresis was superior to D-penicillamine [46]. This study has been criticized by other investigators because of flaws in the design and analysis of results. An open study by Zacheriae et al. [47] showed no substantial clinical improvement, although Di Spaltro et al. [48] reported significant improvement of several disease parameters. It is to be hoped that the ongoing double-blind placebo-controlled trial being conducting according to ACR guidelines will finally ascertain the usefulness of photophoresis in SSc. It is likely that if photophoresis does have a role, it will be as an induction agent in the very early phase of the disease.

5. Antilymphocyte and Antithymocyte Globulin

T-cell depletion currently being pursued in some centers may have a role in the therapy of SSc. The first reports [49,50] had only two patients in each study, and therefore the positive results must be treated with great caution. The third study [51] reported nine patients with refractory autoimmune disease, three of whom had SSc. In these patients, antithymocyte globulin (ATG) was combined with other immunosuppressive agents, and therefore its true efficacy is impossible to determine. Recently, Sinclair et al. [52] reported in abstract form the results of a small placebo-controlled trial to determine over a 6-month period the effect of ATG in patients with dcSSc of less than 5 year's duration. At six months posttreatment, there was no increase in skin score or deterioration in lung function, and therefore ATG appeared to retard progression. All patients receiving ATG experienced fever with the firs dose, and one patient in each group became dialysis dependent. Again, a controlled trial with more patients is needed to assess its efficacy in the disease. It is entirely possibly that agents such as antithymocyte globulin may find their place as inducing agents and that subsequent remission will need to be maintained by other agents.

C. Antifibrotic Drugs

Once established, fibrosis is an almost impossible therapeutic problem, as there is currently no safe pharmacological means of removing the excess normal insoluble cross-linked collagen fibers without damaging the structural framework of organs and/or using highly toxic compounds. The fibrotic lesions occur both externally and internally with frightening speed in some patients—particularly those with diffuse disease. Moreover, even in LcSSc, when skin sclerosis is minimal, substantial pulmonary fibrosis may occur and perivascular adventitial collagen deposition is often present in many vascular beds. This would therefore justify starting an antifibrotic drug a soon as possible in the disease and perhaps to give it concomittantly with an immunosuppressive agent. One of the major problems is that we do not have sufficiently powerful rapidly acting antifibrotic drugs; the few therapies available all take time to act (Table 4). Our own preference in dcSSc is therefore to give both immunosuppression and antifibrotic therapy with dose escalation of the latter as rapidly as possible. In patients with LcSSc, antifibrotic drugs are not necessary for cutaneous manifestations, but a careful watch should be kept for significant visceral fibrosis.

1. D-Penicillamine

D-penicillamine (DPA), a drug capable of interfering with the intermolecular cross links of collagen [53] and possibly possessing immunosuppressive activity, has been used in the treatment of SSc since the 1970s [54–56]. The largest clinical experience with this drug comes from the Pittsburgh Group in the United States. In 1984 [57], they reported a large retrospective study of 73 patients showing a significant improvement in skin sclerosis at 2 years and an improved 5-year survival compared with similar historical controls. An updated analysis of this cohort [58] now includes 152 patients treated with DPA and 80 patients in a control group from the same period. Improvement in skin score was significantly greater in DPA patients and the 5-years survival figure was 80%, which is one of the most impressive of any survival data. Jimenez et al. [59] have also reported their 15-year uncontrolled experience in treating rapidly progressive SSc. This study was large and selected patients who had diffuse disease with a 30% increase in their skin involvement in the preceding 6 months. The results showed a 75% improvement in skin sclerosis in treated patients and an 80% 5-year cumulative survival rate. As in other studies, skin score worsens during the first 4–6 months of the study, emphasizing the necessity of a rapidly acting antifibrotic agent. There have been several other small series reported [60]. However, none of these was blinded or placebo controlled; therefore the precise effect of DPA in SSc has yet to be determined. It is hoped that the 2-year double blind multicenter study of DPA (750–1000 mg/day) versus minidose DPA (2.5 mg check dose) currently under way in the United States will resolve the controversy about this relatively safe and well-tolerated agent.

Table 4 Antifibrotic Therapies for Systemic Sclerosis

Treatment	Mechanism of action	Comments	Efficacy in clinical trials
D-penicillamine	Inhibits the formation of stable collagen cross-links by forming a complex with hydroxy-lysine aldehyde and lysine groups on collagen precursors.	Widely used as in UK, doses above 750 mg daily probably needed for any benefit. Open studies have shown beneficial effects on lung, skin, and kidney disease SSc. Placebo-controlled trial currently underway in USA.	No (controlled trial), Akesson et al., 1992. Yes (open study) [59]. Yes (open study), Saltar et al., 1990. Multicenter trial underway in USA.
Interferon-α	Inhibits collagen production by dermal SSc fibroblasts in vitro at transcriptional level. May also eliminate high collagen producing fibroblast subpopulations.	Efficacy has been confirmed in open studies and a placebo-controlled trial is currently underway in UK. Benefits must be balanced considerable morbidity of IFN administration. Recently completed UK controlled trial.	Yes (open study) [72]. No (controlled study), 1997.
Interferon-γ	As above.	Considerable support for use from open studies and in vitro properties.	Yes (open study), Bletry et al., 1993. Yes (open study) [70]. Yes (open study) [69].

2. *Interferons*

Interferons-α, -β, and -γ have been shown to inhibit collagen synthesis and dermal and synovial fibroblast proliferation in vitro [61,62]. Interferon-γ has been shown to reduce the stimulation of collagen type I gene expression by TGF-β [63] in normal fibroblasts. TGF-β is a profibrotic cytokine implicated in the pathogenesis of SSc [64]. Also, IFN-α has been shown to reduce TGF-β1 mRNA when used in the treatment of chronic liver disease [65], and the interferons have been reported to be beneficial in the therapy of various fibrotic diseases, including SSc. IFN-γ is a more potent inhibitor of collagen synthesis in vitro than IFN-α [66], but it has other effects which may be undesirable in SSc and which might actually contribute to aberrant cellular activation in the disease. Thus in vitro IFN-γ can lead to macrophage activation and class II antigen expression (DR, DP, DQ) on fibroblasts and endothelial cells; increases in IL-2 receptor expression and IgG Fc receptor expression; and upregulation of intracellular adhesion molecule-1 (ICAM-1) expression on endothelial cells [67,68]. Further in vitro experiments have also shown that interferons can stimulate the synthesis of glycosaminoglycans and fibronectin [61], two matrix proteins already increased in SSc. The choice between or interferon-α or interferon-γ must therefore balance efficacy against potential toxicity. There are several uncontrolled studies reporting the use of IFN-γ in SSc [69–71]. These studies show promise which needs to be confirmed in controlled studies, and attention should be paid to the considerable vascular side effects (including renal hypertensive crises) seen in Freudlich's study (70). IFN-α has received less attention, but an uncontrolled study of 19 patients with early diffuse disease of less than 3 year's duration indicated a favorable result with a significantly measurable reduction in type I collagen synthesis in the presclerodermatosis and involved skin fibroblasts [72]. A multicenter placebo-controlled trial has recently been undertaken in the United Kingdom; preliminary analysis does not support efficacy (personal communication). Other drugs with the potential to prevent collagen or proteoglycan deposition which have been tried unsuccessfully include colchicine [73], ketolifen [74], N-acetylcysteine [75], and cyclofenil [76]. There is an urgent need to improve our repertoire of antifibrotic agents.

V. ORGAN-SPECIFIC THERAPIES IN SYSTEMIC SCLEROSIS

Systemic sclerosis is a multisystem disease and there is often differential visceral involvement with each organ displaying to a greater or lesser extent immunological vascular and/or fibrotic damage leading ultimately to functional impairment. These abnormalities need careful investigation, and disease staging is based on the results. A patient may require either specific therapy; for example, H_2 blockage for reflux, antiarhythmics for cardiac abnormalities, or disease modifying drugs such as steroids and/or cyclophosphamide to treat complications such as pulmonary fibrosis. Increased mortality is associated with lung, renal, and cardiac disease, and these will be discussed first, which are followed by the gut, an organ involved in 95% of cases, and treatment of other relevant organs will complete this section. Tables 5 and 6 together with Figures 3 and 4 summarize our current approach to the management of the visceral complications of SSc.

Table 5 Treatment of Cardiorespiratory Disease in Systemic Sclerosis

Manifestation	Clinical features	Investigation	Treatment
Lung disease			
fibrosing alveolitis	Exertional dyspnea	Spirometry, TLCO	Prednisolone
	Bibasal crepitations	KCO, CXR	Cyclophosphamide
	Respiratory failure	HRCT scan	
	Cor pulmonale	DTPA clearance	Home oxygen
		Lung biopsy	
pulmonary hypertension	Exertional breathlessness	ECG, CXR,	Calcium channel blocker, ACE inhibitors
	Tricuspid regurgitation	Doppler echocardiogram	Warfarin
	Cor pulmonale	Right heart catheter	Prostacyclin infusion
			? Long-term oxygen
Cardiac disease			
arrhythmias	Palpitations, syncope	ECG, 24-h tape	Often no treatment required
moycardial fibrosis	Asymptomatic	MRI scan	None available
myocarditis	Variable	CK (-MB fraction)	Corticosteroids
pericarditis	Chest pain	ECG	NSAIDs, corticosteroids
	Pericardial rub		
pericardial effusion	Dyspnoea, edema	ECG, echocardiogram	Pericardiocentesis
			Pericardiotomy

Table 6 Management of Gut Involvement in Systemic Sclerosis

Site	Disorder	Symptom	Investigation	Treatment
Mouth	Tight skin	Cosmetic	None	Facial exercises
	Dental caries	Toothache	Dental radiograph	Dental treatment
	Sicca syndrome	Dry mouth	Salivary gland biopsy	Artificial saliva
Esophagus	Hypomotility	Dysphagia	Barium swallow	Cisapride
				Avoid NSAIDs and nifedipine
	Reflux esophagitis	Heartburn	Esophageal scintiscan	Omeprazole
				Bed elevation
				No late meals
				Metoclopramide
	Stricture	Dysphagia	Manometry	Dilatation
			Endoscopy	Omeprazole, Iansoprazole
Stomach	Gastric paresis	Anorexia	Scintigram	Cisapride
		Nausea		Metoclopramide
		Early satiety		
	NSAID-related ulcer	Dyspepsia	Barium meal	H_2-blockers then misoprostol
Small bowel	Hypomotility	Weight loss	Barium follow-thru	Rotational antibiotics[a]
	Stasis	Postprandial bloating	^{14C}glycocholate or	Cisapride[b]
	Bacterial overgrowth	bloating	hydrogen breath test	Metoclopramide[b]
		Malabsorption	Jejunal aspiration	Pancreatic supplements
		Steatorrhea	Fecal microscopy	Octreotide (low dose)
				Enteral and parenteral
				Nutritional support

	Pseudo-obstruction	Abdominal pain Distension	Plain abdominal radiograph	Conservative management "drip and suck"
	NSAID ulceration			
	Pneumatosis intestinalis	Diarrhea with blood benign Pneumoperitoneum	Plain abdominal radiograph	
Large bowel	Hypomotility	Alternating constipation and diarrhea	Barium enema	Dietary manipulation Cisapride may help Stool expanders (e.g., ispaghula)
	Colonic pseudodiverticula	Rare perforation	Barium enema	[resection]
	Pseudo-obstruction	Abdominal pain Distension	Plain abdominal radiograph	Conservative management "drip and suck"
Anus	Sphincter involvement	Fecal incontinance	Rectal manometry	?? Stimulation ? Surgery

[a]Useful antibiotics: ciprofloxacin, amoxycillin, metronidazole, oral vancomycin, trimethoprim.
Changing every 4 weeks with occasional "antibiotic holiday" may reduce development of resistant strains.
[b]Prokinetic drugs only useful in early neuropathic disease, not later, when smooth muscle is destroyed.

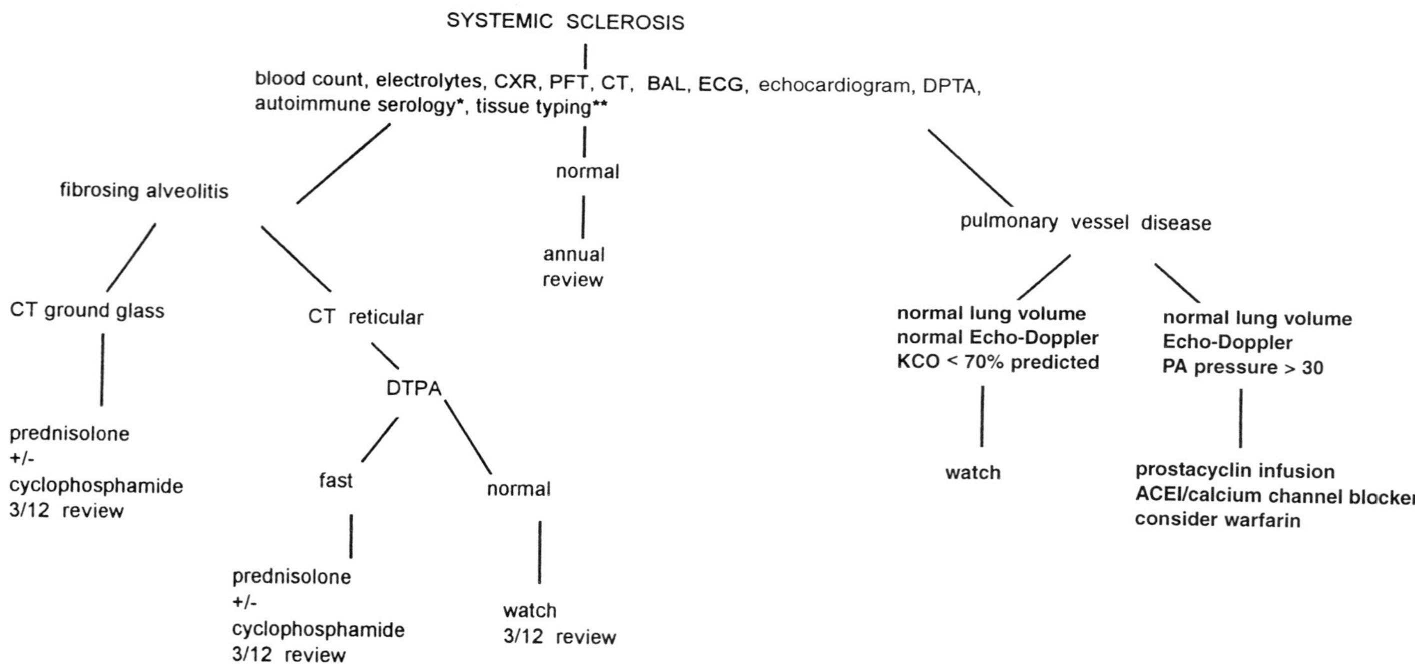

Figure 3 Algorithm for the management of lung disease in systemic sclerosis. *Anti-topoisomerase-1 is associated with pulmonary fibrosis. **HLA-DRS2A is associated with increased risk of pulmonary fibrosis in caucasoid population.

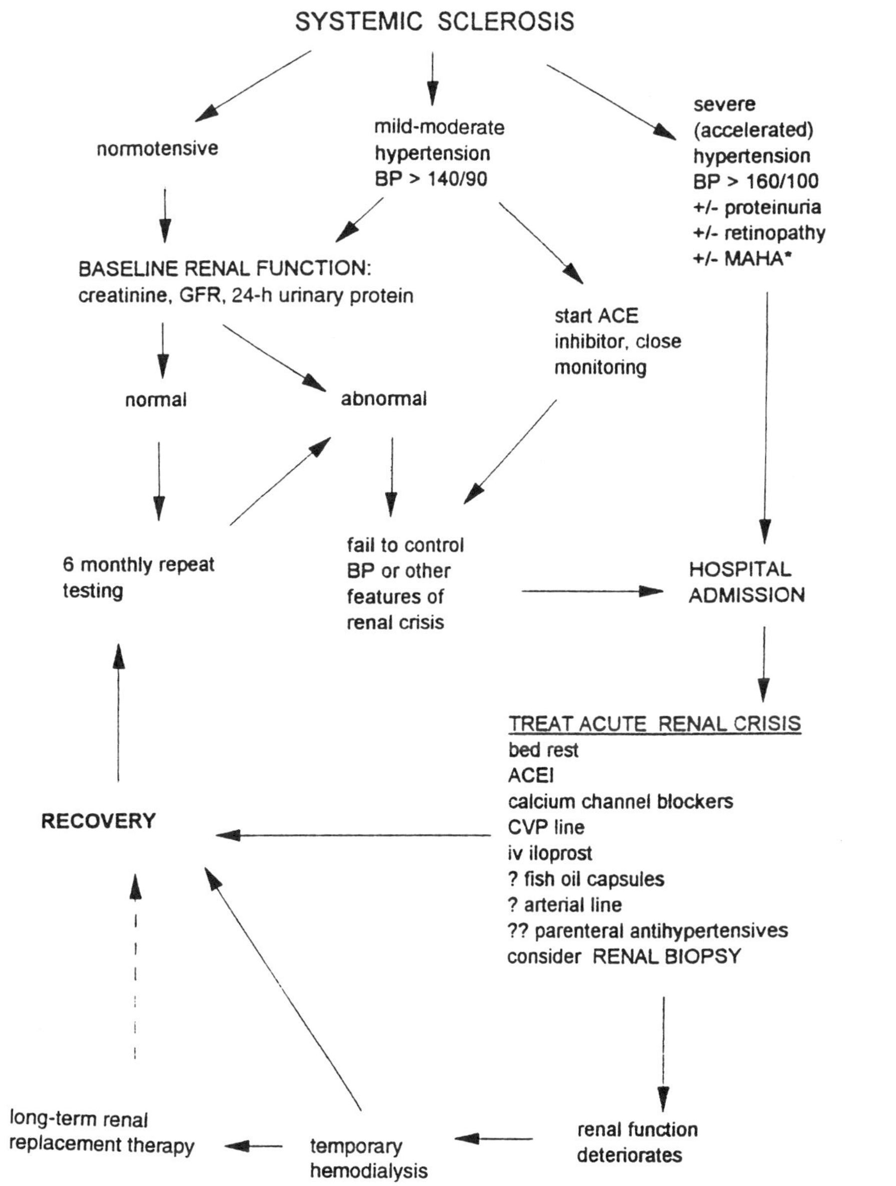

Figure 4 Algorithm for the management of scleroderma renal disease. *MAHA, microangiopathic hemolytic anaemia.

A. Pulmonary Disease

With improved survival from renal hypertensive crisis over the last 20 years, pulmonary disease (fibrosis and hypertension) is now the most frequent cause of death in SSc [77], and therefore its management is discussed in detail.

1. *Interstitial Pulmonary Fibrosis*

Initial evaluation must include a full history and examination in order to exclude factors such as previous drug history, current infection, and occupational histories which could confound the interpretation of pulmonary investigations. Chest radiography is useful as an initial screen to detect diffuse lung disease and also to check for evidence of infection or aspiration secondary to esophageal abnormalities. Lung function tests are more discriminatory. A set of normal lung function tests, particularly on exercise, can exclude the diagnosis of diffuse lung disease. Lung function tests which show normal volumes but reduced gas transfer in the face of normal imaging are suggestive of pure pulmonary vessel disease. The most common finding in patients with fibrosing alveolitis complicating SSc is a restrictive ventilatory defect indicating interstitial inflammation and fibrosis. Bronchoalveolar lavage is useful in confirming the neutrophil alveolitis associated with fibrosing alveolitis. Electrocardiography and echocardiography are performed to exclude primary SSc cardiac involvement and also to assess the effect of the lung disease on right heart function.

As yet, there is no sound evidence that any therapeutic agent used in pulmonary SSc has significantly altered its course. This may reflect an inefficacy of the drugs available or that they are not used appropriately; considering the varied nature of SSc lung disease. Alternatively, the lack of objective evidence of benefit may simply reflect the difficulties in the formal evaluation of response. Pulmonary SSc has a variable rate of progression, and pulmonary involvement has hitherto usually been identified at an established or late stage. Furthermore, treatments have been given for a variable length of time in an uncontrolled way to poorly stratified groups of patients. Most studies of treatment have been anecdotal, retrospective, or uncontrolled. A few small controlled trials have been performed, but large-scale definitive studies are essential. Many different therapies have been tried; there are at least five retrospective trials of D-penicillamine (DPA) from three centers showing some benefit with this agent over a lenthy period of treatment [78–80]. The major benefit observed was an improvement or stabilization of carbon monoxide diffusing factor (DLCO); for example, Steen et al. [78] found that long-term therapy was associated with a significant increase in DLCO: Predicted values rose from 76 to 87% among the treated group, which is significantly better than controls (from 76 to 79%). This and other studies showed no improvement in forced vital capacity (FVC). A DPA study monitoring the disease by responsiveness with bronchoalveolar lavage (BAL) showed a decline in the BAL lymphocyte count and an improvement in alveolitis. Clearly the use of DPA in lung disease needs to be clearly defined, and controlled clinical trials are currently underway. Now that there is the potential (with the use of high-resolution computer tomography (HRCT) scans, ^{99m}Tc-diethylinetriamine pentacetate (DTPA) clearance, and BAL) to recognize early inflammatory disease and predict outcome, prospective studies are urgently needed to analyze new agents and to establish the current role for those already in use. The seeming lack of efficacy of our present therapy may be due to the timing of administration and the failure to use them in early disease.

Once extensive lung damage and fibrosis are present, the best "response to treatment" that can be expected in many patients is a stabilization of disease progression; significant improvement in lung function indices will not be obtained. However, stabilization must not be regarded as failed treatment. Nowhere in scleroderma is early diagnosis and prevention more essential than in the lung.

Probably the most widely used therapeutic agents in pulmonary SSc has been the corticosteroids. An impressive literature indicates their therapeutic usefulness [83–86], but this must be balanced against a large volume of evidence suggesting a lack of efficacy [87,88]. It is possible that corticosteroids are best used in combination with cyclophosphamide [89–91]. Treatment of patients with fibrosin alveolitis in SSc with a regimen of daily oral cyclophosphamide and low-dose oral prednisolone was associated with a sustained improvement in dyspnea and an increase in FVC in 6 of 14 patients in one uncontrolled study: Changes in DLCO were not significant, although minimal improvement was noted in 5 of 13 patients at 6 months [90].

Our observational study of a group of 30 patients with biopsy evidence of SSc-associated fibrosing alveolitis (FASSc), who were all treated subsequently to the biopsy procedure (performed to "stage" the relative degrees of cellularity and fibrosis) and followed for a minimum of 1 year in the same institution, have shown that 13 of 30 patients (43%) responded to therapy. Response was defined as >15% improvement in either FVC or DLCO over pretreatment values sustained over 1 year. The treatment regimens included high-dose corticosteroids alone (60 mg/day and then taper after 1 month) and low-dose corticosteroids (20 mg on alternate days) together with cyclophosphamide. It is interesting to note that, in common with cryptogenic fibrosing alveolitis (CFA), a high percentage of neutrophils in BAL predicted a poor response to therapy [89]. The addition of plasmapheresis to an immunosuppressive regimen has shown an improvement in lung function tests [92,93] in other controlled observational studies.

The presence of alveolitis early in the disease and the ability to recognize it rapidly plus the knowledge that the greatest decline in FVC occurs in the first 2 years of the disease [58] indicate that future studies must not only be controlled and prospective but also targeted at the early active stage.

2. Pulmonary Vascular Disease

Unfortunately, there is not yet a means of detecting pulmonary hypertension at its inception; the earliest noninvasive measurement we can obtain is an estimated pulmonary arterial pressure (PAP) by Doppler echocardiography, but this reading only occurs once there is tricuspid incompetence and therefore occurs relatively late in the natural history of the process. This delay in diagnosis has inevitably resulted in disappointing responses to therapy. Pulmonary vascular disease has two major components: a reversible pulmonary vasoconstrictive element and a fixed obliterative lesion. It is the latter which probably leads to the almost universal failure of any vasodilator therapy to produce a sustained improvement, although short-term gain may be seen. Anecdotal short-term reports have advocated verapamil, hydralazine, ketanserin, and nifedipine [94–98], but evidence for long-term efficacy is still lacking, although sustained medium-term efficacy has been shown for both nifedipine and captopril. Alpert et al. [99] have reported six patients who showed an improvement in pulmonary vascular resistance following 3–6 months of oral treatment with nifedipine using the minimum dose required to achieve maximum response in a preliminary acute study. Using captopril, Alpert et al. have shown more recently both short-term and medium-term benefit (6 months) [100]. Mean pulmonary vascular resistance fell from 6.2 ± 3.6 to 4.6 ± 3.8 units) in the short-term study and improvement was maintained after 3–5 months oral therapy.

Intravenous therapy has also been tried. Prostaglandin E_1, a vasodilator, failed to alter the pulmonary artery pressure [101,102] and caused an increase in pulmonary vascular resistance presumably by increasing stroke volume. The synthetic prostacyclin analogue iloprost, which is recognized as being able to reduce pulmonary vascular resistance [103], did not improve gas transfer in one study; suggesting that the pulmonary vascular bed in SSc is not amenable to dilatation [104] Unpublished studies from our group infusing prostacyclin directly into the pulmonary artery have failed to produce significant falls in pulmonary vascular resistance, as have infusions of I-arginine, the precursor for nitric oxide (NO) (the endothelial cell–derived relaxing factor) into the pulmonary vasculature [105]. However, recent studies of continuous iloprost for primary pulmonary hypertension have been very promising and studies are ongoing in SSc. In the future, oral or inhaled iloprost formulations may be developed for use in SSc-associated PHT.

For vasodilator therapy to be of any real value, it must be effective over several years, and this has yet to be established. Furthermore, a potential complication of vasodilator therapy which must be considered is the possibility of a precipitate fall in cardiac output due to decreased systemic vascular resistance [106]. This can be life threatening, particularly in the face of fixed increases in pulmonary vascular resistance.

In primary pulmonary hypertension, warfarin therapy increases survival [107], and this is now being trialed in some centers for SSc. Oxygen therapy is a temporary help to patients with hypoxemia and pulmonary hypertension, and it has been shown to improve pulmonary vascular resistance in one controlled prospective acute study [108]. In view of the present failure to halt the disease by medical means, an increasing number of patients are being considered for transplantation. Single lung transplantation has been used to treat patients with cryptogenic fibrogenic alveolitis (CFA) and primary pulmonary hypertension. To our knowledge, only a handful of patients with SSc have received a lung transplant for either FASSc or pulmonary hypertension occurring alone, but the long-term outcome is not yet known. Clearly the presence of significant extrapulmonary disease will preclude consideration for transplantation, particularly if there is renal disease. Also, the chances of recurrence in the transplanted organs are unknown.

3. *Treatment Regimens: Our Practice*

Our own management plan of patients with pulmonary disease in systemic sclerosis is determined by the evaluation of a number of factors which are best considered as an algorithm (see Fig. 3).

Fibrosing Alveolitis. If investigations indicate that the patient has fibrosing alveolitis and if the CT pattern suggests that there is ground-glass opacification, patients are treated with low-dose prednisolone 20 mg every other day together with cyclophosphamide up to 125 mg/day for 3 months following which they are reviewed. High-dose prednisolone (greater than 20 mg/day prednisolone) is usually avoided in early diffuse disease because of the risk of precipitating renal failure.

For a female of childbearing years, however, careful counseling is needed before cyclophosphamide therapy is contemplated. More recently, we have had experience with azathioprine, and it is possible that therapy can be switched to azathioprine in a dosage of 250 mg per day (at 2.4 mg/kg) following a 3-month induction phase with cyclophosphamide.

The reason for embarking on treatment immediately with a ground-glass pattern of disease is because we know that this pattern always responds to therapy in terms of improvement of lung function and/or improvement in CT appearances and prognosis tends to be better in this group.

In the group of patients whose CT suggests a predominantly reticular pattern indicative of predominantly fibrotic disease, we use DTPA in its predictive role; if DTPA is fast, the patient is in the group whose disease is more likely to progress. If DTPA is normal, an expectant policy can be followed. In the rapid-clearance group, treatment is the same as for those in the ground-glass group. There are anecdotal data that would suggest that cyclospsorin A can be helpful, but the renal risks are high in SSc, and from the evidence, there is little to support the role for therapy such as penicillamine to treat fibrosing lung disease. This, in common with all of the treatments used to treat fibrosing alveolitis in scleroderma, needs to be the subject of a prospective controlled study which needs to be multinational and must be undertaken in the near future so that full outcome measures can be properly evaluated.

Pulmonary Vascular Disease. If first line of investigations suggest pulmonary vessel disease (normal imaging, relatively normal lung volumes, with disproportionately reduced gas transfer measurement) guidelines are less clear, because little is known about measures which can improve outcome. We know, however, that patients with gas transfers less than 50% normal have a much poorer prognosis than those whose gas transfers are above this cutoff, and certainly if gas transfer is reduced to 25% of normal, the likelihood of surviving more than 1 year is small. We therefore recommend using a cutoff of gas transfer measurement corrected for alveolar volume (KCO) of 70% as being indicative of already established vessel disease, the progression of which needs to be arrested. If KCO is less than 70% predicted and echo-Doppler suggests pulmonary hypertension (PAP > 30 mm Hg), we would recommend the introduction of a calcium channel blocker or ACE inhibitor. Nifedipine has shown to be of use in short-term studies, and there are definitive studies which show that survival has been improved. In addition, consideration needs to be given to the introduction of anticoagulants. In patients with primary pulmonary hypertension, a survival is gained by those on anticoagulants. In patients with primary pulmonary hypertension, a survival is gained by those on anticoagulants. The pattern of disease in primary pulmonary hypertension is similar to that in scleroderma, and it is possible that warfarin may benefit patients in the same way. We would recommend that they be considered in individual patients, but, again, the value and outcome measures of warfarin treatment need to be the subject of a controlled study. In similar vein, the use of prostacyclin as a vasodilator is now well established in peripheral vessel disease in scleroderma. There are good theoretical reasons why it might benefit the pulmonary vasculature, and this therapy should be considered in selected patients. Preliminary evidence supports its usefulness (ACR abstract).

4. Assessment of Response

This can be the most difficult aspect of management. Diseases which progress slowly are likely to improve slowly. Furthermore, disease which cause irreversible fibrosis and injury can often not be improved by therapy and the best that can be expected can be an arrest of decline. If that decline has been gradual, it will take a period of many months to determine with any certainty that benefit has been obtained. Clinical decision making is easier if there has been a period of observation which shows a definite decline prior to the institution of therapy, and, of course, the situation is obvious if there is significant improvement obtained in pulmonary function indices (greater than 10–15%) following therapy.

B. Renal Disease

Although renal disease has now been superceded by lung involvement as the major cause of SSc-related death [109], it remains in some ways the most important of the life-threatening complications of scleroderma, since it is amenable to treatment and because the prognosis is much better if appropriate management is instituted early. Both postmortem and antemortem studies suggest that epithelial and endothelial renal lesions occur prior to clinical evidence of renal disease in SSc [7], and they certainly precede any histological evidence of fibrosis. This supports the view that epithelial and particularly endothelial damage are important early events in disease pathogenesis [4]. Clinically, renal manifestations in scleroderma take three forms. The best characterized is the acute or subacute renal hypertensive crisis, usually occurring in dcSSc within 5 years of diagnosis and characterized by accelerated hypertension, oliguria, uremia, and evidence of microangiopathic hemolytic anemia. Histologically at renal biopsy there is typically fibrinoid necrosis, onion skin proliferative lesions of the small renal arteries, and glomerulosclerosis. Patients often present with clinical features of acute severe hypertension, including headaches, visual disturbances, hypertensive encephalopathy (especially seizures), and pulmonary edema. Occasionally, a similar pattern of renal dysfunction occurs without hypertension (normotensive renal crisis) suggesting that the pathological features are not simply the end-organ consequences of raised arterial pressure [110]. A more insidious pattern of renal involvement also occurs causing a slow reduction in glomerular filtration rate (GFR) and increased proteinuria. This is believed to reflect a more benign vascular and fibrotic process. Its relationship to the acute renal crisis is unclear [111].

Management of renal SSc must therefore involve a high index of suspicion to facilitate early diagnosis. GFR should be checked twice yearly in dcSSc for the first 5 years and annually thereafter. In LcSSc, there is less risk and less frequent monitoring is required, although an annual GFR measurement is desirable. Blood pressure should be well controlled (often antihypertensive treatments also help Raynaud's symptoms), and in dcSSc, angiotensin-converting enzyme (ACE) inhibitors are particularly appropriate since there is some anecdotal evidence that they protect from hypertensive crisis [112]. High-dose corticosteroids have now been formally demonstrated in a case-control study to increase the risk of renal crisis in dcSSc and doses above 20 mg prednisolone equivalent daily should be avoided [113].

Once diagnosed, an acute renal SSc crisis must be treated as a medical emergency. The patient should be admitted immediately and reasonable blood pressure control is a priority. Extreme caution must be taken however to avoid precipitous or excessive drops in arterial pressure and also to prevent relative or actual hypovolemia associated with vasodilatation of constricted vascular beds, both of which can further diminish renal perfusion and compound the SSc lesion with acute tubular necrosis. For this reason, powerful parenteral antihypertensives (e.g., intravenous nitroprusside or labetolol) should be avoided; an internal jugular or subclavian venous cannula should be inserted to monitor central venous filling pressure; and an indwelling arterial cannula for pressure monitoring should be considered. Hypertension should be treated using ACE inhibitors (captopril or enalapril up to a maximum dose) and calcium channel blockers (nifedipine retard initially), aiming to reduce both diastolic and systolic pressure by 20 mm Hg in the first 48 h and ultimately maintaining diastolic pressure at 80–90 mm Hg. Intravenous prostacyclin, which is believed to help the microvascular lesion without precipitating hypotension, is often administered from diagnosis. Fish oil capsules are sometimes prescribed in view of their unproven but theoretically beneficial properties outlined above (see Section V). Renal function should be closely monitored by twice weekly creatinine clearance and daily serum creatinine. Regular full blood count, clotting screen, and fibrin degradation product estimators are important to monitor the degree of microangiopathic hemolytic anemia (MAHA), which often reflects activity of the disease process. Renal biopsy is useful to confirm the diagnosis, particularly if dialysis is being contemplated to assess the extent of the renal lesion and to exclude any other coexistent pathological process such as a glomerulonephritis in the context of a SSc overlap syndrome. Short-term hemodialysis should be given if necessary and peritoneal dialysis often works well if long-term renal replacement therapy is needed. Interestingly, it has been observed in our own unit and by others that after a renal crisis, skin sclerosis and other features of SSc improve [39], particularly if a patient is undergoing maintenance dialysis. The reason for this is unknown; it may result from the removal or inactivation of circulating mediators or simply reflect the natural history of the disease. It should be remembered that there is also often considerable recovery in renal function after an acute crisis, sometimes allowing dialysis to be discontinued, and improvement can continue for up to 2 years. Therefore any decisions regarding renal transplantation should not be made before this time. A simple clinical algorithm in Figure 4 illustrates the management of scleroderma-associated renal disease.

C. Cardiac Disease

The treatment of the cardiac manifestations of SSc is primarily supportive, empirical, and of moderate value (see Table 5). There is no evidence that any of the cardiac abnormalities have been significantly altered by disease-modifying drugs.

Myocardial fibrosis does not cause infarction or angina but can cause cardiomyopathy with congestive cardiac failure. Defects in possible fibrotic areas on thallium perfusion scans at rest and reperfusion changes noted with a cold pressor test or exercise [114] suggest that repeated coronary vasospasm may contribute to fibrosis. Perfusion improved after nicardopine, dipyridamole, or captopril [114, 115, 116]. It has not as yet been shown whether such drugs used on a long-term basis would decrease or prevent the development of cardiac dysfunction as opposed to just altering perfusion.

D. Gastrointestinal Tract

After the skin, the gastrointestinal tract is the second most commonly involved organ in SSc. Studies indicate that as many as 75–90% of patients with SSc have esophageal dysmotility [117, 118], although this involvement will not always have clinical significance. Anorectal disease occurs in 50–70% of patients, small bowel hypomotility in 40% [120], and colonic involvement on barium enema in 10–50% [121]. In an excellent review, Sjogren [122] suggests an orderly series of pathological changes which cause progressive dysfunction in the gut and which permit the rational use of available therapies to try and halt the functional changes. The earliest reported gastrointestinal lesion is neural dysfunction, and there is both physiological and anatomical evidence that this may be due to arteriolar changes in the vasa nervorum [123]. The concept of initial vascular damage is central to our understanding of SSc, and it would come as no surprise to discover than the preneural lesion in the gut is a vascular one. An alternative explanation may be compression of nerve fibers by collagen deposition [124]. Neural damage, once established, produces abnormalities of function before smooth muscle contractility is impaired by connective tissue deposition. These functional changes may remain asymptomatic for lengthy periods, and treatment with prokinetic drugs at this stage is usually effective in reversing them. The next change is smooth muscle atrophy. This is the stage at which the patient usually becomes symptomatic. The muscle atrophy is superimposed on existing neural dysfunction. The muscle is capable of responding but the response is weak. The muscular dysfunction is partially reversed by prokinetic drugs. The final stage is fibrosis. The muscle cannot respond and restoration of function is not possible.

1. Esophagus

Esophageal dysmotility is the most common gastrointestinal manifestation in SSc and can lead to dyspepsia and dysphagia. Dyspepsia usually results from hypomotility and reflux and can be managed pharmacologically by suppression of gastric acid production (H_2-blockers and proton pump inhibitors) and by using prokinetic agents. Although H_2-blockers have been demonstrated to reduce gastroesophageal reflux and to improve symptoms and endoscopic appearance [125,126], it is the proton pump inhibitor omeprazole that has truely revolutionised the treatment of reflux and its sequelae. Although as yet there are few studies on the efficacy of omeprazole in SSc, it would appear that most patients with severe esophageal problems can be managed with omeprazole [127,128]. Usually 20 mg bid is required for maintenance therapy, but individual doses range as high as 80 mg/day [129]. Although the long-term safety of omeprazole has yet to be fully determined, its has been used safely in doses up to 80 mg/day for periods of up to 5 years in some individuals. Sometimes concurrent administration of cisapride helps to reduce the omeprazole requirement. Cisapride and metoclopramide are valuable prokinetic agents in SSc. These drugs work by increasing the lower esophageal sphincter pressure, by improving peristalsis, and by facilitating gastric emptying [130,131]. In addition, they seem to improve symptoms independently of their effects on motility. Should all other measures fall, antireflux surgery may be very cautiously considered; an experienced surgeon is essential, as the morbidity from these procedures is high [132,133].

2. Mid Gut

Intestinal hypomotility with its resultant symptoms (nausea, vomiting, bloating, distension, cramps, malabsorption, diarrhea, and constipation) is the hallmark of mid gut disease in SSc. The stomach and small bowel tend to function as a unit and, therefore, gastric and antroduodenal hypomotility must also be considered. Intestinal motility is dependent on the migrating myoelectric complex (MMC), which, in the fasting state, is a cyclical pattern of contractile activity with the role of clearing remnants of digestion and preventing excessive bacterial colonization in the stomach and small intestine. Patients with SSc often have an absent or dysfunctional MMC and therefore tend to develop problems such as small intestine bacterial overgrowth. Although the control of the MMC remains ill understood, hormones are probably important in its generation. Should initiation or propagation of the MMC fail, the enteric nervous system, endogenous enkephalins, and somatostatin can generate a distal MMC. Drug therapy for gastric and mid gut disorders reflects this neurohumoral control, and the long-acting somatostatin analogue octreotide, the cholinergic agonist cisapride, and the motilin agonist erythromycin have all been used. Metoclopramide and cisapride are among the most useful agents. Metoclopromide was the first effective prokinetic drug [131]. It is both a dopaminergic antagonist and a cholinergic agonist [134]. It facilitates acetylcholine release in the myenteric plexus, possibly by interaction with serotonergic receptors on nerves. Its extrapyramidal side effects do however limit its use, and, unlike cisapride, methoclopramide has little effect on the colon. Its indication is therefore restricted to the treatment of gastroparesis and small bowel stasis. Cisapride is free of antidopaminergic effects, and its primary action is to release acetylcholine in the myenteric plexus by stimulation of hydroxytryptamne (5-HT; serotonin) receptors [135]. In the stomach, it increases both fundic and antral contractions and improves antroduodenal coordination. In the small intestine, cisapride reduces transit time indices, increases propagatory contractions, and restores the MMC, and in the colon, it speeds transit time and increases contraction. The effects of cisapride seem to last longer than metoclopramide, and it has fewer side effects. Octreotide at low doses has been reported to increase intestinal peristalsis, decrease bacterial overgrowth, and relieve symptoms of nausea, bloating, vomiting, and abdominal pain in SSc [136]. It is most appropriately used for meal-related symptoms. Erythromycin has been disappointing in clinical practice. The treatment of malabsorption should be restricted to patients with significant signs and symptoms, and this includes rotational antibiotics, chosen on an empirical basis, nutritional supplements including vitamins, low-residue diets, and medium-chain triglycerides [137].

3. *Large Bowel*

Clinically significant colonic presentations are usually related to colonic pseudo-obstruction [138] and should be treated conservatively with nasogastric suction and resting of the bowel. Fecal incontinence, which is much more common, and is thought to reflect a neural defect in the myenteric plexus, is extremely difficult to treat. Surgery for colonic problems should always be viewed with great caution; however, with the help of careful manometric and radiographic localization of affected segments of stomach and small and large intestine, judicious surgical resection or venting procedures to reduce intractable symptoms may be indicated.

E. Skin Care, Telangectasia, and Calcinosis

The extent of skin sclerosis and the degree of thickening is variable and depends on the subset and the disease duration. Maintaining adequate lubrication of the skin is difficult and patients should decrease their water contact and use lubricating creams, especially the lanolin-containing ones. Intense pruritus can occur in the early stages of diffuse disease and excessive scratching and excoriation can be a major problem. There is little effective therapy, but fortunately the pruritus usually decreases with time. Telangectasia, particularly on the face, can be a cosmetic problem. These lesions can be covered with special make-up or, if particularly large, treated with laser therapy. Calcinosis occurs more frequently in LcSSc, but also troubles some patients with late-stage dcSSc. Pharmacological attempts to dissolve or prevent new lesions with probenecid, cholchicine, and warfarin [139,140] have all failed. Suitably placed lesions can be removed surgically, sometimes using a dental drill, which causes less tissue damage than conventional methods. Calcinosis may also cause chronic ulcerating lesions which can become infected and may then require antibiotics, vigorous local therapy, and possible removal. Occasionally, an acute inflammatory reaction rather like pseudo-gout occurs and should be treated with nonsteroidal anti-inflammatory drugs or colchicine.

F. Musculoskeletal System: Joints, Tendons, and Muscles

Polyarthralgias, polyarthritis, and tendon friction rubs are particular features of early dcSSc and often require significant analgesia and/or low-dose steroids to control the pain and inflammation. Early and continuous physical therapy is important in limiting contractures which result from swollen fingers, arthritis, tenosynovitis, and rapidly progressive skin sclerosis. Both active and passive exercices are necessary and adequate analgesia may be required to a permit daily regimen; the constant encouragement of the therapies and physician is also critical if function is not to be lost. Emphasis on the ultimate plateauing of the skin disease is useful. Surgery, although an exciting concept, still has an uncertain place in any therapy plan. Realignment of contracted fingers by straightening, shortening, and fusing of interphalangeal joints may improve appearance and decrease the development of digital ulcers but may not greatly improve function.

Many patients with SSc have a mild myopathy, often with little or no elevation of their serum muscle enzyme levels. Muscle biopsy typically shows occasional foci of inflammatory cells, nonspecific fiber changes, and increased perimysial and epimysial connective tissue deposition. Management is essentially physical with a program of muscle-strengthening exercises. A smaller group of patients have an inflammatory myopathy indistinguishable from polymyositis and are treated with steroids alone or in combination with methotrexate, azathioprine, or other immunosuppressive agents. The desire to give high-dose steroids must be tempered with the risk of precipitating renal failure in dcSSc and therefore 20–30 mg/daily is recommended.

VI. CONCLUSION

This chapter has reviewed the current therapies available for SSc and illustrates that although treatment remains difficult, particularly for the underlying immunological, vascular, and fibrotic disease processes, there are now specific agents of definite benefit for some visceral complications. Examples include ACE inhibitors for hypertensive renal disease in dcSSc and proton pump blockers for reflux esophagitis. It is to be hoped that the next few years will bring both a better understanding of scleroderma and its etiopathogenesis and an implementation of a generally accepted severity score which, together with the results of well-conducted placebo-controlled trials, will further improve the management of this heterogeneous disorder. Ultimate therapeutic success will probably depend on better disease stratification, using immunogenetic and serological predictors to identify those at greatest risk of specific visceral complications, and stages therapy perhaps with immunosuppressive agents given early in dcSSc followed up with antifibrotic drugs. For LcSSc, the management is likely to be directed at its vascular manifestations and toward identification of early pulmonary hypertension to allow its treatment to commence before irreversible structural changes occur in the pulmonary vasculature.

REFERENCES

1. LeRoy EC, Black CM, Fleischmajer R, et al. Scleroderma (systemic sclerosis): classification, subsets and pathogenesis. J Rheumatol 1988; 15:202–205.
2. Kahari VM. Activation of dermal connective tissue in scleroderma. Ann Med 25:511–518.
3. Uitto J, Jimenez SA. Fibrotic skin diseases: clinical presentations, aetiologic considerations and treatment options. Arch Dermatol 1990; 126:661–664.
4. Prescott RJ, Freemont AJ, Jones CJ, et al. Sequential dermal microvascular and perivascular changes in the development of scleroderma. J Pathol 1992; 166:255–263.
5. Kaye SA, Seifalian AM, Lim SG, et al. Ischaemia of the small intestine in patients with systemic sclerosis: Raynaud's phenomenon or chronic vasculopathy? Quart J Med 1994; 87:495–500.
6. Harrison NK, Myers AR, Corrin B, et al. Structural features of interstitial lung disease in systemic sclerosis. Am Rev Respir Dis 1991; 144:706–713.
7. Kovalchik MT Guggenheim SJ, Robertson JS, Steigerwald JC. The kidney in progressive systemic sclerosis: a prospective study. Ann Intern Med 1978; 89:881–887.
8. Claman HN, Giorgio RC, Seibold JR. Endothelial and fibroblastic activation in scleroderma: "the myth of uninvolved skin." Arthritis Rheum 1991; 834:1495–1501.
9. Roumm AD, Whiteside TL, Medsger TA Jr, Rodnan GP. Lymphocytes in the skin of patients with progressive systemic sclerosis, quantification, subtyping, and clinical correlations. Arthritis Rheum 1984; 27:645–653.
10. Needleman BW. Immunologic aspects of scleroderma. Curr Opin Rheum 1992; 4:862–868.
11. Needleman BW, Wigley FM, Stair RW. IL-1, IL-2, IL-4, IL-6 THFα and IFNγ levels in sera from patients with scleroderma. Arthritis Rheum 1992; 35:67–72.
12. Kahaleh MB. Vascular disease in systemic sclerosis: endothelial cell-T lymphocyte-fibroblast interactions. Rheum Dis Clinics North America 1990; 16:53–73.
13. Swerlick RA, Lawley TJ. The Role of microvascular endothelial cells in inflammation. J Invest Dermatol 1993; 100(Suppl):111S–115S.
14. Postlethwaite AE. Connective tissue metabolism including cytokines in scleroderma. Curr Opin Rheumatol 1993; 5:766–772.
15. Koch AE, Kronfield-Harrington LB, Szechnecz A, et al. In situ expression of cytokines and cellular adhesion molecules in the skin of patients with systemic sclerosis. Pathobiology 1993; 61:239–246.
16. Medsger TA Jr, Silman AJ, Steen VD. Development of a severity score for systemic sclerosis (abstr). Arthritis Rheum 1994; 37(Suppl):S260.
17. Pope JE, Bellamy N. Outcome measurements in scleroderma clinical trials. Semin Arthritis Rheum (1993); 23:22–33.
18. White B, for the American College of Rheumatology (ACR) Committee on Study Design and Response Parameters in SSc. Guidelines for clinical trials with disease modifying interventions in systemic sclerosis (SSc) (abstr). Arthritis Rheum 1993; 36(Suppl): S131.
19. Rademaker M, Meyrick TRH, Kirby JD, Kovacs IB. Effect of nifedipine on platelets and thrombolysis in systemic sclerosis. Br J Dermatol 1988; 119(Suppl 33):25–26.
20. Finch MB, Dawson J, Johnston GD. The peripheral vascular effects of nifedipine in Raynaud's syndrome associated with scleoderma: a double blind cross-over study. Clin Rheumatol 1986; 5:493–498.
21. Teh LS, Manning J, Moore T, et al. Sustained release transdermal glyceryl trinitrate patches as a treatment of primary and secondary Raynaud's phenomenon (abstr). Arthritis Rheum 1994; 37(Suppl):S262.
22. Freedman RR. Alpha-2-adrenergic function in Raynaud's disease (letter). Arch Intern Med 1992; 152:1929–1933.
23. Challenor VF, Waller DG, Hayward RA, et al. Subjective and objective assessment of enalapril in primary Raynaud's phenomenon. Br J Clin Pharmacol 1991; 31:477–480.

24. Seibold JR, Jageneau AHM. Treatment of Raynaud's phenomenon with ketanserin, a selective antagonist of the serotonin 2 (5-HT2) receptor. Arthritis Rheum 1984; 27:139–146.
25. Katoh K, Kawai T, Narita M, et al. Use of prostaglandin-E1 to treat Raynaud's phenomenon associated with connective tissue disease; Thermographic and subjective assessment. J Pharm Pharmacol 1992; 44:442–444.
26. Wigley FM, Siebold JR, Wise RA, et al. Intravenous iloprost treatment of Raynaud's phenomenon and ischaemic ulcers secondary to systemic sclerosis. J Rheumatol 1992; 19:1407–1414.
27. Tanner SB, Darton K, Watson HR, et al. Long-term follow up of iloprost therapy for secondary Raynaud's phenomenon using self report data and infra-red thermography (abstr). Arthritis Rheum 1991; 34(Suppl):S52.
28. Torley HI, Madhok R, Capell HA, et al. A double-blind, randomised, multicentre comparison of two doses of intravenous iloprost in the treatment of Raynaud's phenomenon secondary to connective tissue diseases. Ann Rheum Dis 1991; 50:800–804.
29. McCarthy GM, Kenny D. Dietary fish oil in rheumatic diseases. Semin Arthritis Rheum 1992; 21:318–375.
30. Jayson MIV, Holland CD, Keegen A, et al. A controlled study of stanazol in primary Raynaud's phenomenon and systemic sclerosis. Ann Rheum Dis 1991; 50:41–47.
31. Berman B, Duncan MR. Pentoxifylline inhibits the proliferation of human fibroblasts derived from keloid, scleroderma and morphea skin and their production of collagen, glycosaminoglycan and fibronectin. Br J Dermatol 1990; 123:339–346.
32. Furst DE, Clements PJ, Hillis S, et al. Immunosuppression with chlorambucil versus placebo for scleroderma: results of a three year, parallel, randomised, double blind study. Arthritis Rheum 1989; 32:584–593.
33. Kahane BD. Cyclosporine. N Engl J Med (1989); 321:1725–1738.
34. Frances C, Brauclet MC, Bletry O, et al. Skin changes fron scleroderma patients before and after cyclosporin A treatment. Clin Exp Dermatol 1988; 13:1–31.
35. Appelboon T, Itzkowitch D. Cyclosporin is successful control of rapidly progressive scleroderma. JAMA 1986; 82:886–887.
36. Zachariae M, Halkier-Sorensen I, Heickendorf L, et al. Cyclosporin A treatment of systemic sclerosis. Br J Dermatol 1990; 122:677–681.
37. Vayssairat M, Baudot N, Boitard C, et al. Cyclosporine therapy for severe systemic sclerosis associated with scl-70 antibody. J Am Acad Dermatol 1990; 22:695–696.
38. Clements PJ, Lachenbruch PA, Sterz M, et al. Cyclosporine in systemic sclerosis. Arthritis Rheum 1993; 36:75–83.
39. Zacchariae H, Hansen HE, Olsen T, Steen VD. Haemolytic uraemic syndrome in a patient with systemic sclerosis treated with cyclosporin-A. Acta Derm Venereol (Stockh) 1992; 72:307–309.
40. Denton CP, Abdullah A, Sweny P, Black CM. Acute Renal Failure occurring in scleroderma treated with cyclosporin A—a report of three cases. Br J Rheumatol. (1994). 33:90–92.
41. Sibley RK, Rynariewicz J, Ferguson RM, et al. Morphology of cyclosporine nephrotoxicity and rejection in patients immunosuppressed with cyclosporine and prednisolone. Surgery 1983; 94:225.
42. Bunchmann TE, Brookshire CA. Cyclosporine-induced synthesis of endothelin by cultured endothelial cells. J Clin Invest 1991; 88:310–314.
43. Bode BY, Yocum DE, Gail EP, et al. Methotrexate in scleroderma: experience in ten pateints (abstr). Arthritis Rheum 1990; 33(Suppl):S66.
44. Van den Hoogen FHJ, Boerbooms AMT, van de Putte LBA, et al. Low dose methotrexate in systemic sclerosis. J Rheumatol 1991; 18:1763–1764.
45. Seibold JR, McCloskey DA, Furst DE. Pilot trial of methotrexate in the treatment of early diffuse scleroderma (abstr). Arthritis Rheum 1994; 37(Suppl):R35.

46. Rook AH, Freundlich B, Jegasothy BV, et al. Treatment of systemic sclerosis with exytracorporeal chemotherapy: results of a multicentre trial. Arch Dermatol 1992; 128:337-346.
47. Zacheriae H, Bjerring P, Heickendorff L, et al. Photopheresis in systemic sclerosis: clinical and serological studies using markers of collagen metabolism. Acta Derm Venereol (Stockh): 1993; 73:356-361.
48. Di Spalto FX, Cottrill C, Cahill C, et al. Extrascorporeal photochemotherapy in progressive systemic sclerosis. Int J Dermatol 1993, 32:417-421.
49. Goronzy JJ, Weyand CM. Long term immunomodulatory effects of T-lymphocyte depletion in patients with systemic sclerosis. Arthritis Rheum 1990; 33:511-519.
50. Balabam EP, Zashin SJ, Geppert TD, Lipsky PE. Treatment of systemic sclerosis with antithymocyte globulin. Arthritis Rheum 1991; 34:244-245.
51. Tarkowski A. Andersson-Gare B. Aurell M. Use of anti-thymocyte globulin in the management of refractory systemic autoimmune diseases. Scand J Rheum 1993; 22:261-266.
52. Sinclair HD, Williams JD, Rahman MA, et al. Clinical efficacy of anti-thymocyte globulin in systemic sclerosis: results of a placebo controlled trial (abstr). Arthritis Rheum 1993; 36(Suppl):C175.
53. Nimni M. A defect in the intramolecular and intermolecular cross-linking of collagen caused by penicillamine. I. Metabolic and functional abnormalities in soft tissues. J Biol Chem 1968; 243:1457-1466.
54. Jayson MIV, Lovell C, Black CM. Penicillamine therapy in systemic sclerosis. Proc R Soc Med 1977; 70:80-82.
55. Asboe-Hansen G. Treatment of progressive systemic sclerosis with inhibitors of collagen synthesis. In: Black CM, Myers AR, eds. Current Topics in Rheumatology, Systemic Sclerosis (Scleroderma). New York: Gower, 1985:405-410.
56. Ivanova MM, et al. Treatment of systemic sclerosis with D-penicillamine. Ther Arch 1977; 7:91-99.
57. Steen VD, Medsger TA JR, Rodnan GP. D-penicillamine therapy in progressive systemic sclerosis (scleroderma). Ann Intern Med 1984; 97:652-659.
58. Steen VD. Systemic sclerosis—management. In: Dieppe, Klippel, eds. Textbook of Rheumatology. Vol. 6. 1993:10.1-10.8.
59. Jimenez S, Sigal S. A 15-year prospective study of treatemnt of rapidly progressive systemic sclerosis with D-peicillamine. J Rheumatol 1991:1496-1503.
60. Steen VD, D-penicillamine treatment in systemic sclerosis J Rheumatol 1991:1435-1437.
61. Jimenez SA, Freundlich B, Rosenbloom J. Selective inhibition of human diploid fibroblast collagen synthesis by interferons. J Clin Invest 1984; 74:1112-1116.
62. Czaja MJ, Weiner FR, Eghbali M, et al. Differential effects of gamma interferon on collagen and fibronectin gene expression. J Biol Chem 1987; 262:1348-1351.
63. Varga J, Olsen A, Herhal J, et al. Interferon gamma reverses the stimulation of collagen but not fibronectin gene expression by transforming growth factor-beta in normal human fibroblasts. Eur J Clin Invest 1990; 20:487-493.
64. Gruschwitz M, Muller PU, Sepp N, et al. Transcription and expression of transforming growth factor type beta in the skin of progressive systemic sclerosis: a mediator of fibrosis?. J Invest Dermatol. 1990; 94:197-203.
65. Castilla A, Prieto J, Fausto N. Transforming growth factor beta and alpha in chronic liver disease: Effects of interferon alpha therapy. New Engl J Med 1990; 324:933-940.
66. Duncan MR, Berman B. γ-Interferon is the lymphokine and β-interferon the monokine responsible for inhibition of fibroblast collagen production and late but not early fibroblast proliferation. J Exp Med 1985; 162:516-527.
67. Skurkovich S, Skurkovich B, Eghbali M, et al. A unifying model of the immunoregulatory role of the interferon system: can interferon produce disease in humans? Clin Immunol Immunopathol 1987; 43:362-373.

68. Mahrle G, Schulze HJ. Recombinant interferon-γ in dermatology. J Invest Dermatol 1990; 95(Suppl):132S–137S.
69. Hein R, Behr J, Hundgen M, et al. Urbanski A, Kreig T. Treatment of systemic sclerosis with γ-interferon. Br J Dermatol 1992; 126:496–501.
70. Freundlich B, Jimenez SA, Steen VD, et al. Treatment of systemic sclerosis with recombinant interferon-gamma. Arthritis Rheum 1992; 35:1134–1141.
71. Kahan A, Amor B, Menkes CJ, et al. Recombinant interferon gamma in the treatment of systemic sclerosis. Am J Med 1989; 87:273–277.
72. Stevens W. Vancheeswaran R. Black CM. Alpha interferon-2α (Roferon-A) in the treatment of diffuse cutaneous systemic sclerosis: a pilot study. UK Systemic Sclerosis Study Group. Br J Rheumol (1992); 31:683–689.
73. Guttaduaria M, Diamond H, Kaplan D. Colchicine in the treatment of scleroderma. J Rheumatol 1977; 4:272–275.
74. Gruber BL, Kaufman LD. A double-blind randomised controlled trial of ketotifen versus placebo in early diffuse scleroderma. Arthritis Rheum 1991; 34:362–366.
75. Furst DE, Clements PJ, Harris R, et al. Measurement of clinical change in progressive systemic sclerosis: a one year double blind placebo controlled trial of N-acetylcysteine. Ann Rheum Dis 1979; 38:356–361.
76. Gibson T, Grahame R. Cyclofenil treatment of scleroderma: a controlled study. Br J Rheumatol 1983; 22:218–223.
77. Steen VD, Owens GR, Fino JG, et al. Pulmonary involvement in systemic sclerosis (scleroderma). Arthritis Rheum 1985; 28:759–767.
78. Steen VD, Owens GR, Redmond C, et al. The effect of D-penicillamine on pulmonary findings in systemic sclerosis. Arthritis Rheum 1985; 28:882–888.
79. Broll H, Tausch G, Eberl R, Zur Behandlung der Lungen Fibrose mit D-penicillamine/metalcaptase. Munch Med Wochenschr (1969); 111:1580–1584.
80. Dequeker J, Francx L, Mbuyi JM. Effect of long-term D-penicillamine, corticosteroid and no treatment on lung diffusing capacity in progressive systemic sclerosis. In: Maini R, ed. Modulation of Autoimmunity and Disease. New York: Praeger, 1981:283–290.
81. Edelson JD, Hyland RH, Ramsden M, et al. Lung inflammation in scleroderma: clinical, radiographic, physiologic and cytopathological features. J Rheumatol 1985; 12:957–963.
82. Hughes DTD, Lee FI. Lung function in patients with systemic sclerosis. Thorax 1963; 18:16–20.
83. Rossi GA, Bitterman PB, Rennard SI. Evidence for chronic inflammation as a component of the interstitial lung disease associated with progressive systemic sclerosis. Am Rev Respir Dis 1985; 131:612–617.
84. Sullivan MA, Millar DK. Pulmonary manifestations in collagen disease. Arch Intern Med 1962; 110:769–781.
85. Ashba JK, Ghanem MH. The lungs in systemic sclerosis. Dis Chest 1965; 47:52–64.
86. Dines DE. Pulmonary disease of vascular origin. Dis Chest 1968; 54:3–12.
87. Kallenberg CGM, Janssen HM, Elema JD, The TH. Steroid-responsive interstitial lung disease in systemic sclerosis. Chest 1984; 86:489–492.
88. Nice CM, Menon ANK, Rigler L. Pulmonary manifestations in the collagen diseases. Am J Roentgenol 1959; 81:264–279.
89. Harrison NK, Wells AU, Hansell DM, et al. Treatment of lung disease in systemic sclerosis: a clinical comparison of responders and non-responders (abstr). Am Rev Respir Dis (1992); 14:A755.
90. Silver RM, Warrick JH, Kinsella MB, et al. Cyclophosphamide and low dose pednisolone therapy in patients with systemic sclerosis (scleroderma) with interstitial lung disease. J Rheumatol 1993; 20:838–844.
91. Johnson MA, Kwan S, Snell NJ, et al. Randomised controlled trial comparing prednisolone alone with cyclophosphamide and low dose prednisolone in combination in cryptogenic fibrosing alveolitis. Thorax 1989; 44:280–288.

92. Akesson A, Wollheim FA, Thysell H, et al. Visceral improvement following combined plasmapheresis and immunosuppressive therapy in progressive systemic sclerosis. Scand J Rheumatol 1988; 17:313–323.
93. Ferri C, Bernini L, Gremignai G, et al. Lung involvement in systemic sclerosis sine scleroderma treated by plasma exchange. Int J Artif Organs 1992; 15:426–431.
94. Ohar J, Polatty C, Robichaud A, et al. The role of vasodilators in patients with progressive systemic sclerosis. Interstitial lung disease and pulmonary hypertension. Chest 1985; 88:263S–265S.
95. Fudman EJ, Kelling DG, Jr. Transient effect of nifedipine on pulmonary hypertension of systemic sclerosis. J Rheumatol 1985; 12;1191–1192.
96. Glikson M, Pollack A, Dresner-Feigin R, et al. Nifedipine and prazocin in the management of pulmonary hypertension in CREST syndrome. Chest 1990; 98:759–761.
97. Sfikakis PP, Kyriakidis MK, Vergos CG, et al. Cardiopulmonary haemodynamics in systemic sclerosis and response to nifedipine and captopril. Am J Med 1991; 90:541–546.
98. Seibold JR, Moloney RR, Turkevich D, et al. Acute haemodynamic effects of ketanserin in pulmonary hypertension secondary to systemic sclerosis. J Rheumatol 1987; 14:519–524.
99. Alpert MA, Pressly TA, Mukerji V, et al. Acute and long-term effects of nifedipine on pulmonary and systemic haemodynamics in patients with pulmonary hypertension associated with diffuse systemic sclerosis, the CREST syndrome and mixed connective tissue disease. Am J Cardiol 1991; 68:1687–1691.
100. Alpert MA, Pressly TA, Mukerji V, et al. Short and long term haemodynamic effects of captopril in patients with pulmonary hypertension and selected connective tissue disease. Chest 1992; 102:1407–1412.
101. Baron M, Skrinskas G, Urowitz MB, Madras PN. Prostaglandin E therapy for digital ulcers in scleroderma. Can Med Assoc J 1982; 126:42–45.
102. Baron M, Skrinskas G, Hyland R, Urowitz MB. Effects of prostaglandin E and other vasodilators in pulmonary hypertension of scleroderma. Br Heart J 1982; 48:304–305.
103. Robin ED. Some basic and clinical challenges in the pulmonary circulation. Chest 1982; 81:357–363.
104. Thurm CA, Wigley FM, Dole WP, Wise RA. Failure of vasodilatory infusion to alter pulmonary diffusing capacity in systemic sclerosis. Am J Med 1991; 90:547–552.
105. Badouin SV, Bath P, Martin JF, et al. L-arginine infusion has no effect on systemic haemodynamics in normal volunteers, or systemic and pulmonary haemodynamics in patients with elevated pulmonary vascular resistance. Br J Clin Pharmacol 1993; 36:45–49.
106. Follansbee WP. The cardiovascular manifestations of systemic sclerosis (scleroderma). Curr Prob Cardiol 1986; 11:245–298.
107. Rich S, Brundage BH. High dose calcium channel blocking therapy for primary pulmonary hypertension: evidence for long term reduction in pulmonary arterial pressure and regression of right ventricular hypertrophy. Circulation 1987; 76:135–141.
108. Rubin LJ, Mendoza J, Hood M, et al. Treatment of primary pulmonary hypertension with continuous intravenous prostacyclin (epoprostenol). Results of a randomised trial. Ann Intern Med 112:485–491.
109. Black CM, Stephens CO. Scleroderma - systemic sclerosis. In: PJ Maddison PJ, Isenberg DA, Woo P, Glass DN, eds. Oxford Textbook of Rheumatology. Oxford University Press, 1993:771–789.
110. Helfrich DJ, Banner B, Steen VD, Mesdger TA Jr. Renal failure in normotensive patients with systemic sclerosis. Arthritis Rheum 1989; 32:1128–1134.
111. Black CM. Scleroderma—systemic sclerosis In: Cameron JS, Davidson AM, Grunfeld JP, et al., eds. Oxford Textbook of Clinical Nephrology, Oxford University Press, (Oxford UK.) 1990.
112. Steen VD, Constantino JP, Shapiro AP, Medsger TA Jr. Outcome of renal crisis in systemic sclerosis: relation to the availibility of converting enzyme inhibitors (ACE). Ann Intern Med 1990; 113:352–357.

113. Steen VD, Conte C, Medsger TA Jr. Case-control study of corticosteroid use prior to scleroderma renal crisis (abstr). Arthritis Rheum 194; 37(Suppl):S360.
114. Kahan A, Devaux JY, Amor B, et al. Pharmacodynamic effect of dipyridimole on thallium 201 myocardial perfusion in progressive systemic sclerosis with diffuse scleroderma. Ann Rheum Dis 1986; 45:718–725.
115. Kahan A, Devaux JY, Amor B, et al. Pharmacodynamic effect of nicardipine on left ventricular function in systemic sclerosis. J Cardiovasc Pharmacol 1990; 15:249–253.
116. Kahan A, Devaux JY, Amor B, et al. The effect of captopril on thallium-201 myocardial perfusion in systemic sclerosis. Clin Pharmacol Ther 1990; 47:483–489.
117. Turner R, Lipshutz W, Miller W, et al. Esophageal dysfunction in collagen disease. Am J Med Sci 1973; 265:191–199.
118. Akesson A, Wollheim FA. Organ manifestations in 100 patients with progressive systemic sclerosis: a comparison between the CREST syndrome and diffuse scleroderma. Br J Rheumatol 1989; 28:281–286.
119. Hamel-Roy J, Devroede G, Arham P, et al. Comparative esophageal and anorectal motility in scleroderma. Gastroenterology, 1985; 88:1–7.
120. D'Angelo WA, Fries JF, Masi AT, Shulman LE. Pathologic observations in systemic sclerosis (scleroderma). Am J Med 1969; 46:428–440.
121. Kemp-Harper RA, Jackson DC: Progressive systemic sclerosis. Br J Radiol 1965; 38:825–834.
122. Sjogren RW. Review: Gastrointestinal motility disorders in scleroderma. Arthritis Rheum 1994; 37:1265–1282.
123. Greydanus MP, Camilleri M. Abnormal post-cibal gastric and small bowel motility due to neuropathy or myopathy in systemic sclerosis. Gastroenterology 1989; 96:110–115.
124. Di Trapani G, Pocchiara M, Masullo C, et al. Peripheral neuropathy in the course of progressive systemic sclerosis; a light and ultrastructural study. Ital J Neurol Sci 1982; 3:341–348.
125. Petrokubi RJ, Jeffries GH. Cimetidine versus antacid in scleroderma with reflux esophagitis: a randomised double blind controlled study, Gastroenterology 1979; 77:691–695.
126. Hendel L, Aggestrup S, Sentoft P. Long term ranitidine in progressive systemic sclerosis (scleroderma) with gastroesophageal reflux. Scand J Gastroenterol 1986; 21:799–805.
127. Hendel L. Hydroxyproline in the esophageal mucosa of patients with progressive systemic sclerosis during omeprazole induced healing of reflux eosphagitis. Aliment Pharmacol Ther 1991; 5:471–480.
128. Olive A, Maddison PJ, Davis M. Treatment of oesophagitis in scleroderma with omeprazole (letter). Br J Rheumatol 1989; 28:553.
129. Hendel L, Hage E, Hendel J, Stentoft P. Omeprazole in the long term treatment of severe gastroesophageal reflux disease in patients with systemic sclerosis. Aliment Pharmacol Ther 1992; 6:565–577.
130. Johnson DA, Drane WE, Curran J, et al. Metoclopramide response in patients with progressive systemic sclerosis. Effect on esophageal and gastric motility abnormalities. Arch Intern Med 1987; 147:1597–1601.
131. Ramirez B, Richter JE. Review article: promotility drugs in the treatment of gastroesophageal reflux disease. Aliment Pharmacol Ther 1993; 7:5–20.
132. Orringer MB, Orringer JS, Dabich L, Zarafonetis CJ. Combined Collis gastroplasty fundoplication operations for scleroderma reflux eosophagitis. Surgery 1981; 90:624–630.
133. Orringer MB. Surgical management of scleroderma reflux esophagitis. Surg Clin North Am 1983; 63:859–867.
134. Johnson DA, Drane WE, Curran J, et al. Metoclopramide response in patients with progressive systemic sclerosis. Arch Intern Med 1987; 147:1597–1601.
135. Jian R, Ducrot F, Piedeloup C, et al. Measurement of gastric emptying in dyspeptic patients: effect of a new gastrokinetic agent (cisapride). Gut 1985; 26:352–358.

136. Soudah HC, Hasler WL, Owyang C. Effect of octreoide on intestinal motility and bacterial overgrowth in scleroderma. N Engl J Med 1991; 325:1461–1467.
137. Grabowski G, Grant JP. Nutritional support in patients with systemic scleroerma. J Parenter Enteral Nutr 1989; 13:147–151.
138. Basilisco G, Barbera R, Vanoli M, Bianchi P. delayed colonic transit in constipated patients with progressive systemic sclerosis (PSS) (abstr). Gastroenterology 1992; 102:A421.
139. Berger RG, Featherstone GL, Raasch RH, et al. Treatment of calcinosis universalis with low dose warfarin. Am J Med 1987; 83:72–76.
140. Fuchs D, Fruchter L, Fishel B, et al. Colchicine suppression of local inflammation due to calcinosis in dermatomyositis and progressive systemic sclerosis. Clin Rheumatol 1986; 5:527–530.

27
Eosinophilic Fasciitis and Eosinophilia Myalgia Syndrome

Daniel J. Clauw
Georgetown University Medical Center, Washington, D.C.

I. INTRODUCTION

This chapter will review the treatment of eosinophilic fasciitis (EF) and the eosinophilia myalgia syndrome (EMS). It is likely that these two disorders are within a spectrum of eosinophilic connective tissue diseases, which also includes the toxic oil syndrome (TOS). To better understand concepts regarding the management of these disorders, it is helpful to review first the epidemiology, clinical features, and potential pathogenic mechanisms that may be operative in these conditions.

II. EPIDEMIOLOGY

EF was the first of the diseases in this spectrum to be described; initially by Shulman in 1974 and later by Rodnan and colleagues [1,2]. The early descriptions of EF were of a disorder characterized by peripheral eosinophilia and fasciitis, which could be differentiated from scleroderma by the distinctive pattern of skin involvement (sparing the digits and involving the fasci rather than the derms). In these early reports of EF, this disorder was considered to be clinically and histopathologically localized to the fascia.

However, larger series of cases of EF revealed a widening spectrum of findings [3,4]. Clinical and histopathological evidence of muscle involvement was noted, as evidenced by an increased frequency of myalgias, as well as evidence of myopathy (documented by electromyography [EMG] and of inflammation of the epimysium and perimysium. A number of other symptoms were noted to occur frequently, including arthritis, entrapment neuropathies, and occasional visceral involvement and concurrent lymphoproliferative conditions.

In 1989, an epidemic of an eosinophilic connective tissue disease was recognized in the United States, and it was termed the eosinophilia myalgia syndrome [5–7]. Because of the rapid work of public health officials, it became clear that most of these individuals were consuming L-tryptophan, an amino acid that was available in the United States as an over-the-counter nutritional supplement. Subsequent epidemiological studies suggested that most individuals who developed EMS during the epidemic had consumed L-tryptophan manufactured by a single Japanese company [8,9]. Although only approximately 1700 individuals were reported to the Centers for Disease Control and Prevention (CDC) who met surveillance criteria established for this diagnosis (an absolute eosinophil count >1000 cells/mm^3, severe incapacitating myalgias, and the absence of other conditions to explain these findings), it has been estimated that the true number of cases was severalfold greater. The clinical spectrum of EMS includes fasciitis indistinguishable from that seen in EF, but neuromuscular and visceral involvement is more common, and the rapid response to corticosteroid therapy initially reported in EF is not typically observed in EMS [10,11].

The EMS epidemic led to a reexamination of the toxic oil syndrome (TOS); a similar epidemic of an eosinophilic connective tissue disorder than afflicted approximately 20,000 Spaniards in 1981 [5,12]. TOS was clinically and histopathologically similar to EMS, and, in this case, the inciting agent appeared to be adulterated rapeseed oil [13,14]. Chemically similar trace constituents have been found in the implicated samples of rapeseed oil and tryptophan, raising the possibility that a single toxin, or a group of related substances, may have been responsible for these two epidemics [15].

The recognition that both EMS and TOS were likely induced by toxins also led to a reexamination of earlier cases of EF. Several studies retrospectively examined EF cases that occurred prior to the EMS epidemic, and they found that a significant percentage of these individuals had been consuming L-tryptophan [16,17]. These early cases of EMS associated with L-tryptophan ingestion, which were characterized as EF until 1989, likely contributed to the widening of the spectrum of EF in the late 1980s. Further reports have demonstrated that EMS or clinically indistinguishable conditions can occur in association with exposure to several substances other than L-tryptophan or rapeseed oil, including other nutritional supplements or chemicals (Table 1) [18–20]. Although only the associations with rapeseed oil and L-tryptophan have been confirmed by epidemiological studies, the distinct clinical features of EF as well as the rarity of this condition strengthen the weight of case reports as proof of the potential causation.

Epidemiological studies into EMS have given some insight into potential mechanisms by which toxin exposure may lead to the development of a connective tissue disease [21]. Most such studies in EMS suggested that only a small percentage of those who ingested implicated L-tryptophan became ill; thus suggesting that host factors may

Table 1 Environmental Agents Associated with Development of EF- or EMS-like Disorders

Rapeseed oil
5-Hydroxytryptophan
L-tryptophan
Lysine
Niacin
Trichloroethylene

be important in the development of disease [6,7,22]. Although several studies suggest that the likelihood of developing EMS was related to the quantity of L-tryptophan ingested (and perhaps increased age), it is clear than many afflicted individuals took a very small quantity, and that many individuals who consumed large quantities of implicated L-tryptophan did not become ill [23,24]. Similarly, low attack rates are seen in most other types of environmentally induced connective tissue diseases. There are data to suggest that individuals with abnormal xenobiotic (P450) metabolism may have been predisposed to develop of EMS, either because these individuals could not properly eliminate a toxin, or perhaps because they converted a "protoxin" to a toxin [25]. This is analogous to that seen with other drug- or toxin-induced connective tissue diseases, such as drug -induced systemic lupus erythematosus (SLE) and idiopathic scleroderma [26,27].

To summarize, the accumulated evidence suggests that there is a continuum between EF, which is a *localized* inflammation of the fascia, and EMS and TOS, where the inflammation (and perhaps other pathogenic features) extend into other organs and tissues. It is likely that most of the diseases within this spectrum may be associated with the ingestion or exposure to environmental agents. Because the discrete toxin(s) which may have triggered these outbreaks has not yet been identified, it is likely that similar epidemics will occur in the future. Therefore, when confronted with a patient with EF or EMS, a careful history of potential environmental exposure(s) is critical.

III. CLINICAL FEATURES AND POTENTIAL PATHOGENIC MECHANISMS

In this section, the clinical features of EF and EMS are discussed concurrently with potential pathogenic mechanisms. This approach allows for a better understanding of the therapy of these disorders, which is symptom directed and is discussed in the final section.

Table 2 lists the clinical features that are typically associated with EF, as well as the additional features that may occur in association with EMS. For simplicity, in this chapter, EF will be considered to be a disorder localized to the fascia, whereas individuals with systemic features will be considered to have EMS. In reality, this semantic distinction between EF and EMS may be relatively unimportant, since the treatment of these entities is symptom directed, and no global treatments can be recommended for all patients with either entity.

A. Skin and Fascia Involvement

Skin and fascial involvement can be a significant cause of morbidity in these conditions EF and EMS [28,29]. Although peau d'orange ("orange peel") skin, along with venous furrowing of the uplifted arm ("groove sign"), are the classically described manifestations of the fasciitis seen in EF or EMS, most individuals with these entities have slightly less impressive findings. In many cases, individuals with fasciitis may present with either induration or nonpitting edema of the affected area. This involvement is typically most prominent in the distal leg and forearm, but it can occur anywhere in the body, with prominent truncal involvement being seen relatively frequently. Pigmentation changes and joint contractures are late consequences of fasciitis. Other

Table 2 Clinical Features of EF and Features Associated with EMS

Clinical features of EF	Other features seen in EMS
Cutaneous	Cutaneous
fasciitis / induration	urtcaria
edema	maculopapular rash
pigmentation changes	mucinosis
Rheumatic	dermatographism
joint contractures	alopecia
Neurologic	Rheumatic
carpal tunnel syndrome	myalgias / myopathy
Other	Neurologic
fevers	distal sensorimotor neuropathy
lymphoproliferative disorders	mononeuritis multiplex
Laboratory	cognitive symptoms
eosinophilia	Cardiopulmonary
hypergammaglobulinemia	pneumonitis
	respiratory muscle dysfunction
	pulmonary hypertension
	Other
	severe fatigue
	sicca symptoms
	gastrointestinal
	Laboratory
	elevated serum aidolase
	antinuclear antibodies

cutaneous findings, seen more frequently in EMS than EF, include early maculopapular pruritic eruptions, morphea, urticaria, alopecia, mucinous papules, dermatographism, and subcutaneous nodules [30,31]. It is important to note that neither Raynaud's phenomenon nor digital skin involvement (e.g., sclerodactyly) occur in EMS or EF, and these clinical features remain the best manner to distinguish these conditions from scleroderma.

Common histopathological features seen within the skin of both EF and EMS patients are inflammatory infiltrates involving the dermis (especially prominent in the perivascular regions), dermal fibrosis, and increased deposition of mucin/glycosaminoglycans [29,30,32–34]. The inflammatory infiltrates in these regions contain primarily mononuclear cells and eosinophils, and mast cells may also be increased in number. Qualitatively similar inflammatory infiltrates extend into the fascia, and in EMS the inflammation may also involve the connective tissue surrounding muscle fibers (epimysium, perimysium, and perivascular regions) and nerves. It is important to note that the primary location of the inflammatory infiltrates in these entities differs from those seen in inflammatory muscle disease, where more prominent endomysial inflammation is seen.

Considerable effort has been expended in further delineating the nature of the inflammatory response in EF and EMS. There is good evidence for a central role for T cells in these disorders, as this is the predominant cell type in the affected tissues, and a significant percentage of the T cells are activated [35,36]. There are also data suggesting that fibroblasts play a prominent role in the pathogenesis of these conditions, as one would expect in a fibrosing illness. Varga and colleagues have extensively studied the fibroblast in EMS, and they have established that these cells exhibit increased collagen synthesis, as well as increased expression of both $\alpha 1(1)$ procollagen and transforming growth factor-β_1 genes [31,37]. Although both peripheral and tissue eosinophilia are frequently seen in these disorders, the role of these cells in the pathogenesis of these entities is less certain. It is clear that even when eosinophils are not detected in tissues, there is frequently evidence of eosinophil degradation, as measured by elevations in concentrations of major basic protein and/or eosinophil-derived neurotoxin in serum and tissues [28].

B. Neuromuscular Symptoms

Neuromuscular symptoms arguably lead to the greatest morbidity in EF and EMS, and the pathogenesis of these symptoms is poorly understood. Neurological and muscular symptoms are discussed concurrently, because it is likely that there are overlapping mechanisms responsible for these symptoms.

Muscle pain is common, and likely has several different causes. Constant diffuse myalgias that are present at rest and worsen with exertion may be indicative of concurrent fibromyalgia. Many individuals who developed EMS were consuming L-tryptophan as self-medication for insomnia, premenstrual syndrome, or depression. It should not be surprising, then, that many of these individuals had fibromyalgia prior to developing EMS, and they continue to experience fibromyalgia symptoms after the inflammatory phase of EMS has resolved [38]. It is important to emphasize that the symptom of muscle pain should not be interpreted as evidence for active fascial or muscle inflammation, since myalgias are not prominent in either "pure" EF or inflammatory muscle disease [1,2,9].

Diffuse muscle pain and weakness in EMS may also be due to the development of a metabolic myopathy. EMS patients display evidence of a unique and selective lowering of intramuscular adenosine triphosphate (ATP) levels, as determined ^{31}P magnetic resonance spectroscopy [39]. There are additional data that suggest that the administration of parenteral magnesium can lead to both improvement in symptoms and ATP levels [40].

There are other potential causes of neuromuscular symptoms in both EF and EMS. Entrapment neuropathies, particularly carpal tunnel syndrome, occur commonly in both EF and EMS; presumably because of fibrosis or inflammation causing compression of the median nerve. A distal sensorimotor neuropathy also can occur in EMS, and this may be partly responsible for the symptomatology, especially that involving the distal extremities [41–43]. Other potential causes for chronic muscle pain and weakness have been postulated but are less well established. Some investigators have suggested the term *downslope claudication* to describe a type of compartment syndrome which may result from fascial fibrosis and the resultant restricted blood flow to the extremities in these conditions [44]. In addition to the potential restriction of blood flow that might occur at the level of the large vessels from fascial inflammation and/or fibrosis, ischemia may also result from impeded microvascular flow from the occlusive microangiopathy seen pathologically in EMS. Although rare cases of a Guillian-Barre–like illness have been reported in EMS, it is also possible that a more proximal motor neuropathy, perhaps at the spinal cord level (as is seen in anterior horn cell disorders; e.g., amyotrophic lateral sclerosis), may occur in EMS and contribute to neuromuscular dysfunction [41,42,45].

C. Hematological Symptoms

In nearly all cases of EF and EMS, peripheral eosinophilia resolves with time, and it is typically quite corticosteroid responsive [46]. When eosinophilia persists or is unresponsive to steroid therapy, then it is more likely that the underlying disorder falls within the spectrum of the hypereosinophilic syndrome (HES).

D. Cardiopulmonary Symptoms

There are a variety of cardiopulmonary symptoms that occur in EF and EMS. Early pulmonary involvement, which was most commonly characterized by a transient pneumonitis that resolves spontaneously or with corticosteroid therapy, was commonly seen in EMS [47]. The early pulmonary involvement seen in TOS was more fulminant, and this is one of the principal clinical differences between these two entities [5,12]. Chronic pulmonary symptoms are common in EMS. The most common cause of these chronic symptoms appears to be respiratory muscle dysfunction [48]. Pulmonary function testing, including maximal static inspiratory and expiratory pressures, should be performed, with the latter determinations frequently being the sole abnormality when the dyspnea is due to pain or dysfunction of the chest wall musculature. In more severe cases of neuromuscular chest wall disease (due to neuropathy, weakness, or fasciitis of the chest wall region), a restrictive pattern may be seen on pulmonary function testing. A low diffusing capacity that does not correct for decreased alveolar ventilation or infiltrates or fibrosis on imaging studies (chest radiograph or high-resolution chest computed tomography), may suggest pulmonary hypertension or interstitial lung disease, both of which may occur in EMS [47,49,50].

Direct cardiac inflammation as well as coronary artery spasm have been noted as rare complications of EMS [51,52]. A much more frequent symptom in EMS is noncardiac chest pain. This may be due to muscular chest wall involvement or esophageal dysmotility. Another frequent symptom in EMS is resting tachycardia and postural hypotension; this is likely due to unrecognized autonomic neuropathy (unpublished observation).

E. Other Symptoms

Severe debilitating fatigue, cognitive dysfunction, recurrent fevers, and xerostomia are among the other symptoms that have been reported frequently in EMS [53]. The pathogenic mechanisms remain unclear. There are several potentially identifiable causes, all of which may occur in a higher than expected frequency in patients with EF and EMS. By far the most common is concurrent fibromyalgia, which may not only contribute to fatigue and cognitive dysfunction, but it may also be accompanied by headaches, irritable bowel and sicca symptoms, and esophageal dysmotility [45]. Other potential concurrent conditions which may contribute to these symptoms include depression, hypothyroidism, and sleep apnea.

IV. TREATMENT

In approaching the management of EF and EMS, there are two principles which should be observed. The first is that these conditions are typically characterized by an early inflammatory phase, which commonly lasts approximately 6–12 months, followed by a protracted noninflammatory phase. The second important concept is that therapy must be symptom directed, as with most rheumatological disorders. Unlike other rheumatic diseases, however, there are no controlled studies to guide therapy. Therefore, a general approach to this group of diseases is presented followed by specific examples of therapeutic options.

A. General Considerations

1. Remove the Inciting Agent

Because many of the eosinophilic connective tissue diseases are likely to be associated with exposure to environmental agents, this is particularly important. Patients should be thoroughly questioned regarding *all* substances they are ingesting. The EMS epidemic illustrated that individuals rarely report ingestion of over-the-counter or nutritional supplements to physicians unless specifically queried. A careful history of potential occupational exposures is also essential. Other potential considerations include analysis of drinking water in individuals without a municipal supply and contacting the local or state health department to determine if there are other reports of similar diseases in a given region.

2. Determine What Organs or Tissues Are Clinically Involved and Whether There Is Active Inflammation Present

The first step is easily accomplished with a thorough review of systems and initial screening laboratory tests, whereas the second is frequently difficult with EF and EMS. As noted previously, the natural history of these disorders is for active inflammation to be present early followed by a chronic, noninflammatory phase. This is a quite analogous to the situation that occurs in diffuse scleroderma. Just as with scleroderma, anti-inflammatory or immunosuppressive medications should only be considered during the active inflammatory phase and when the potential consequences of untreated inflammation in a given tissue exceed the toxicity of the drug.

3. Consider Noninflammatory Mechanisms of Symptoms and Address These Concurrently

Once again, these are concepts are similar to the treatment of other rheumatic diseases, but noninflammatory symptoms may be more common in EMS and related disorders than in other connective tissue diseases. The potential noninflammatory mechanisms of symptomatology have been discussed and management suggestions are noted below.

B. Specific Recommendations

1. Skin and Fascia Involvement

Skin and fascial involvement can be a significant cause of morbidity in EF and EMS, with severe joint contractures being the most debilitating resultant feature. Thus, regardless of the pharmacological treatment chosen, an aggressive program of stretching and strengthening is a vital adjunct to the care of affected individuals [54].

Although the physical examination can typically determine whether fasciitis is present, palpation is not generally helpful in differentiating active inflammation from residual fibrosis. This determination is essential when one is contemplating therapy except perhaps in the early phase of the disease when active inflammation is almost invariably present if there is fascial involvement. Although in research settings there may be noninvasive modalities such as magnetic resonance imaging (MRI) which may aid in assessing whether fascia is actively inflamed, a full-thickness (skin/fascia/muscle) biopsy is typically necessary to make this determination [55]. Before performing a biopsy, however, the practitioner should contemplate whether the finding of active inflammation will affect therapy. Although the reflexive response is aggressively to treat inflammation in the fascia, as noted above, fasciitis per se is probably responsible for only skin tightening and joint contractures (not the other neuromuscular symptoms sometimes seen). Also, the natural history of fasciitis in most cases is for spontaneous regression with or without therapy. Thus, a conservative approach to inflammatory disease only involving the skin and fascia may be reasonable in many instances.

If a biopsy is performed and active inflammation is documented, there are a variety of regimens which may be employed. Low-dose or alternate-day corticosteroids or hydroxychloroquine are the least toxic alternatives. Weekly oral methotrexate (in dosages similar to used for rheumatoid arthritis) and cyclosporin are probably likewise effective, but they may be best reserved for patients with recalcitrant fasciitis or inflammation of other tissues [56,57].

2. *Neuromuscular Symptoms*

As previously discussed, neuromuscular symptoms are among the most problematic in EMS and related disorders both because there may be multiple pathogenic mechanisms and also because these symptoms are frequently difficult to ameliorate.

Muscle pain is common in affected patients, and it may have several different causes, some of which can be elucidated with the history and physical examination. *Constant diffuse* myalgias, especially when migratory, are most suggestive of concurrent fibromyalgia or perhaps an acquired metabolic myopathy. When concurrent fibromyalgia is suspected, treatment with low nighttime doses of amitriptyline or cyclobenzaprine can be quite effective, as can a graded low-impact aerobic exercise program. The recognition and treatment of an acquired metabolic myopathy is more complex. As noted, there are preliminary data suggesting that EMS patients may develop a tissue magnesium deficiency despite normal serum levels, and they may benefit from parenteral magnesium repletion. *Muscle spasms and cramping*, which are sometimes severe and debilitating in this condition, seem to be particularly responsive to this treatment modality, when they were studied on an open basis. A multicenter trial is presently underway to determine the efficacy of this treatment regimen in a large cohort of EMS patients. Until these data are available for patients with unremitting neuromuscular symptoms, especially if cramping is prominent, an empiric trial of 1 g of magnesium sulfate administered intramuscularly twice weekly for 12 weeks may be worthwhile. There have been anecdotal reports of success with numerous therapeutic modalities for these symptoms, including anticonvulsants (e.g., phenytoin, valproic acid), sodium dantrolene, and quinine sulfate.

Other neuromuscular symptoms may suggest a different or concurrent problem, and they may respond to appropriate therapy. *Distal pain* is most suggestive of a peripheral sensory neuropathy, and it may respond to treatment with low doses of tricyclic compounds. Ongoing trials using nerve growth factors or other biological compounds in similar types of neuropathy may suggest a role for these agents in the spectrum of eosinophilic connective tissue diseases in the future.

The role of conservative corticosteroid regimens (e.g., <10 mg per day, or alternate-day prednisone) or "pulse" monthly regimens for neuromuscular symptoms remains controversial. The mechanism for symptomatic improvement from corticosteroids in some individuals with corticosteroids is unclear, especially given the paucity of tissue inflammation seen histologically in the chronic phase of this disease. Since it is frequently difficult to discontinue corticosteroids in this setting once they are started, and because of the associated morbidity (albeit low with the above regimens), a prudent approach would be to reserve this form of therapy for patients unresponsive to the potentially less toxic modalities outlined.

3. *Hematological Symptoms*

In most eosinophilic connective tissue diseases, peripheral eosinophilia typically resolves with time. It does not appear as though the degree eosinophilia in EF or EMS relates to the severity of the underlying disease, so it should be emphasized that *treatment of the eosinophilia per se is not necessary* in either of these conditions. When significant eosinophilia persists for more than 6–12 months, however, then it is more likely that the individual falls within the spectrum of HES. In this setting, aggressive therapy directed toward reducing the peripheral eosinophilia is warranted, since prolonged eosinophilia of any cause may lead to severe and irreversible organ damage, especially of the endomyocardial surface, vasculature, and peripheral nerves [58]. Corticosteroids may be of benefit in this setting, but there is some concern that the thrombogenic effects of these drugs may be more prominent in blood vessels that have already been damaged by inflammation, as has also been suggested in the vasculitides.

There are several other regimens that have also been employed in the treatment of EF and EMS. Cyclosporin may be effective in this setting, since it is likely that T lymphocytes play a significant role in maintaining eosinophilia via the release of cytokines (e.g., interleukins IL-3 and IL-5). Alkalating agents such as hydroxyurea may also be useful in this setting. The regimen most recently employed for the treatment of prolonged eosinophilia in HES is interferon-α (IFN-α). IN this study, six patients with HES refractory to other forms of therapy all responded well to daily subcutaneous recombinant IFN-α, with minimal toxicity [59].

Other rare associated hematological findings, such as autoimmune thrombocytopenia or lymphoproliferative disorders, should be treated using standard approaches.

4. *Cardiopulmonary Symptoms*

As noted, the most common cause of pulmonary symptoms appears to be respiratory muscle dysfunction. This symptom may improve with a graded aerobic exercise program or with effective treatment of myalgias using any of the modalities noted above. Pulmonary hypertension and interstitial lung disease may occur rarely in EMS. Perhaps the best guide of appropriate therapy for these findings may come from the scleroderma experience, since the underlying pathological processes may be similar. Vasodilators may be of some benefit in the treatment of the pulmonary hypertension, and aggressive treatment of interstitial lung disease may be warranted if an active alveolitis is identified by bronchoalveolar lavage [60].

5. Other Symptoms

It is difficult to make specific recommendations for the management of the variety of other symptoms seen in EMS such as fatigue or cognitive complaints. A therapeutic trial of low-dose antidepressants and aerobic exercise should be considered even if the patient does not exhibit cardinal manifestations of fibromyalgia. It is most important to stress that there are no data to suggest that these symptoms result from chronic inflammation, so aggressive immunosuppressive regimens should not be utilized to treat these symptoms unless active inflammation is identified. Obviously, if other concurrent problems such as depression, hypothyroidism, or sleep apnea are identified, then appropriate therapy should be initiated.

V. SUMMARY

EF and EMS are both relatively rare disorders. There are considerable data to suggest that most (if not all) of these cases may be due to toxin exposure, although the precise etiological agent(s) has yet to be identified. The approach to the management of these individuals most closely resembles that for diffuse scleroderma in that anti-inflammatory or immunosuppressive regimens are most likely to be effective during the early inflammatory phase of the disease and not in the chronic stage. There are a variety of pharmacological and nonpharmacological treatment regimens that can be effective during the chronic noninflammatory phase of these disorders; these are symptom based and need to be tailored to the clinical features in individual patients.

REFERENCES

1. Shulman LE. Diffuse fasciitis with hypergammaglobulinemia and eosinophilia: A new syndrome? J Rheumatol 1974; 1(Suppl):46.
2. Rodnan GP, DiBartolomeo A, Medsger TA, Barnes EL. Eosinophilic fasciitis: report of six cases of a newly recognized scleroderma-like syndrome. Arthritis Rheum 1975; 18:525.
3. Lakhanpal S, Ginsburg WW, Michet CJ, et al. Eosinophilic fasciitis: clinical spectrum and therapeutic response in 52 cases. Semin Arthritis Rheum 1988; 17:221–231.
4. Michet CJ, Doyle JA, Ginsburg WW. Eosinophilic fasciitis: report of 15 cases. Mayo Clin Proc 1981; 56:27–34.
5. Philen RM, Posada M. Toxic oil syndrome and eosinophilia-myalgia syndrome: May 8–10, 1991, World Health Organization meeting report. Sem Arthritis Rheum 1993; 23:104–124.
6. Belongia EA, Hedberg CW, Gleich GJ, et al. An investigation of the cause of the eosinophilia-myalgia syndrome associated with tryptophan use. N Engl J Med 1990; 323:357–365.
7. Hertzman PA, Falk H, Kilbourne EM, et al. The eosinophilia-myalgia syndrome: the Los Alamos Conference. J Rheumatol 1991; 18:867–873.
8. Belongia EA, Mayeno AN, Osterholm MT. The eosinophilia-myalgia syndrome and tryptophan. Ann Rev Nutr 1992; 12:235–256.
9. Slutsker L, Hoesley FC, Miller L, et al. Eosinophilia-myalgia syndrome associated with exposure to tryptophan from a single manufacturer. JAMA 1990; 264:213–217.

10. Culpepper RC, Williams RG, Mease PJ, et al. Natural history of the eosinophilia-myalgia syndrome. Ann Intern Med 1991; 115:437–442.
11. Silver RM. Eosinophilia-myalgia syndrome, toxic-oil syndrome, and diffuse fasciitis with eosinophilia. Curr Opin Rheumatol 1992; 4:851–856.
12. Kilbourne EM, Posada de la Paz M, Abaitua Borda I, et al. Toxic oil syndrome: a current clinical and epidemiologic summary, including comparisons with the eosinophilia-myalgia syndrome. J Am Coll Cardiol 1991; 18:711–717.
13. Alonso-Ruiz A, Calabozo M, Perez-Ruiz F, Mancebo L. Toxic oil syndrome. A long-term follow-up of a cohort of 332 patients. Medicine (Baltimore) 1993; 72:285–295.
14. Aldridge WN. The toxic oil syndrome (TOS, 1981): from the disease towards a toxicological understanding of its chemical aetiology and mechanism. Toxicol Lett 1992; 59–70.
15. Hill RH Jr, Caudill SP, Philen RM, et al. Contaminants in L-tryptophan associated with eosinophilia myalgia syndrome. Arch Environ Contam Toxicol 1993; 25:134–142.
16. Hibbs JR, Mittleman B, Hill P, Medsger TA Jr. L-tryptophan-associated eosinophilic fasciitis prior to the 1989 eosinophilia-myalgia syndrome outbreak. Arthritis Rheum 1992; 35:299–303.
17. Blauvelt A, Falanga V. Idiopathic and L-tryptophan-associated eosinophilic fasciitis before and after L-tryptophan contamination. Arch Dermatol 1991; 127:1159–1166.
18. Patmas MA. Eosinophilia-myalgia syndrome not associated with L-tryptophan. N Engl J Med J 1992; 89:285–286.
19. Farinelli S, Mariani A, Grimaldi A, et al. Eosinophilia-myalgia syndrome associated with 5-OH-tryptophan. Description of a case. Recenti Prog Med 1991; 82:381–384.
20. Waller PA, Clauw DJ, Cupps T, et al. Fasciitis (not scleroderma) following prolonged exposure to an organic solvent (trichloroethylene). J Rheumatol 1994; 21:1567–1570.
21. Kilbourne EM. Eosinophilia-myalgia syndrome: coming to grips with a new illness. Epidemiol Rev 1992; 14:16–36.
22. Clauw DJ, Nashel DJ, Umhau A, Katz P. Tryptophan-associated eosinophilia connective tissue disease. A new clinical entity? JAMA 1990; 263:1502–1507.
23. Back EE, Henning KJ, Kallenbach LR, et al. Risk factors for developing eosinophilia myalgia syndrome among L-tryptophan users in New York. J Rheumatol 1993; 20:666–672.
24. Kamb ML, Murphy JJ, Jones JL, et al. Eosinophilia-myalgia syndrome in L-tryptophan-exposed patients. JAMA 1992; 267:77–82.
25. Flockhart DA, Clauw DJ, Buchert E, et l. Pharmacogenetic characteristics of the eosinophilia myalgia. Clin Pharm Ther 1994; 56:398–405.
26. Hess EV. Drug-related lupus. Curr Opin Rheumatol 1991; 3:809–814.
27. May DG, Black CM, Olsen NJ, et al. Scleroderma is associated with differences in individual routes of drug metabolism: a study with dapsone, debrisoquin, and mephenytoin. Clin Phamacol Ther 1990; 48:286–295.
28. Martin RW, Duffy J, Engel AG, et al. The clinical spectrum of the eosinophilia-myalgia syndrome associated with L-tryptophan ingestion. Ann Intern Med 1990; 113:124–134.
29. Oursler JR, Farmer ER, Roubenoff R, et al. Cutaneous manifestations of the eosinophilia-myalgia syndrome. Br J Dermatol 1992; 127:138–146.
30. Kaufman LD, Seidman RJ, Phillips ME, Gruber BL. Cutaneous manifestations of the L-tryptophan-associated eosinophilia-myalgia syndrome: a spectrum of sclerodermatous skin disease. J Am Acad Dermatol 1990; 23:1063–1069.
31. Varga J, Jimenez SA, Uitto J. L-tryptophan and the eosinophilia-myalgia syndrome: current understanding of the etiology and pathogenesis. J Invest Dermatol 1993; 100:97S–105S.
32. Valicenti JM, Fleming MG, Pearson RW, et al. Papular mucinosis in L-tryptophan–induced eosinophilia-myalgia syndrome. J Am Acad Dermatol 1991; 25:54–58.
33. Rongioletti F, Rebora A. Cutaneous toxic mucinoses. J Am Acad Dermatol 1992; 26:789–790.

34. Feldman SR, Silver RM, Maize JC. A histopathologic comparison of Shulman's syndrome (diffuse fasciitis with eosinophilia) and the fasciitis associated with the eosinophilia-myalgia syndrome. J Am Acad Dermatol 1992; 26:95–100.
35. Emslie-Smith AM, Engel AG, Duffy J, Bowles CA. Eosinophilia myalgia syndrome: I. Immunocytochemical evidence for a T-cell-mediated immune effector response. Ann Neurol 1991; 29:524–528.
36. McKinley KL, Harati Y, Schneider LW. Chronic immune activation in the eosinophilia-myalgia syndrome. Muscle Nerve 1993; 16:947–951.
37. Peltonen J, Varga J, Sollberg S, et al. Elevated expression of the genes for transforming growth factor-beta 1 and type VI collagen in diffuse fasciitis associated with the eosinophilia-myalgia syndrome. J Invest Dermatol 1991; 96:20–25.
38. Hudson JI, Pope HG Jr, Daniels SR, Horwitz RI. Eosinophilia-myalgia syndrome or fibromyalgia with eosinophilia? JAMA 1993; 269:3108–3109.
39. Clauw DJ, Hewes B, Nelson M, et al. 31-P magnetic resonance spectroscopy of skeletal muscle in the Eosinophilia Myalgia Syndrome. J Rheumatol 1994; 21:654–657.
40. Clauw DJ, Ward K, Wilson B, et al. Magnesium deficiency in the eosinophilia myalgia syndrome: report of clinical and biochemical improvement with repletion. Arthritis Rheum 1994; 37:1331.
41. Donofrio PD, Stanton C, Miller VS, et al. Demyelinating polyneuropathy in eosinophilia-myalgia syndrome. Muscle Nerve 1992; 15:796–805.
42. Satsangi J, Donaghy M. Multifocal peripheral neuropathy in eosinophilic fasciitis. J Neurol 1992; 239:91–92.
43. Freimer ML, Glass JD, Chaundhry V, et al. Chronic demylelinating polyneuropathy associated with eosinophilia-myalgia syndrome. J Neurol Neurosurg Psychiatry 1992; 55:352–358.
44. Naschitz JE, Yeshurun D, Misselevitch I, Boss JH. Downslope claudication in eosinophilic fasciitis: a fourth type of claudication-case presentations. Angiology 1991; 167–171.
45. Slotkoff A, Woodward M, Manz H, et al. Eosinophilia myalgia syndrome: case report of possible spinal cord involvement. Arthritis Rheum 1994; 37(Suppl 6):25.
46. Wallace DJ. Persistent eosinophilia in 2 patients with eosinophilia-myalgia syndrome. Arthritis Rheum 1993; 36:1488.
47. Tazelaar HD, Myers JL, Strickler JG, et al. Tryptophan-induced lung disease: an immunophenotypic, immunofluorescent, and electron microscopic study. Mod Pathol 1993; 6:56–60.
48. Read CA, Clauw D, Weir C, et al. Dyspnea and pulmonary function in the L-tryptophan-associated eosinophilia-myalgia syndrome. Chest 1992; 101:1282–1286.
49. Chauhan D, Mengel CE. Eosinophilia-myalgia syndrome and fasciitis with an active alveolitis. Kans Med 1993; 94:175–177.
50. Cheng TO. Pulmonary hypertension in patients with eosinophilia-myalgia syndrome or toxic oil syndrome. Mayo Clinic Proc 1993; 68:823–824.
51. Hertzman PA, Maddoux GL, Sternbert EM, et al. Repeated coronary artery spasm in a young woman with the eosinophilia-myalgia syndrome. JAMA 1992; 267:2932–2934.
52. James T, Kamb M, Sandberg GA, et al. Postmortem studies of the heart in three fatal cases of the eosinophilia-myalgia syndrome. Ann Intern Med 1991; 115:102–106.
53. Krupp LB, Masur DM, Kaufman LD. Neurocognitive dysfunction in the eosinophilia-myalgia syndrome. Neurology 1993; 43:931–936.
54. Marchman HB, Gleason CB, Shaw JC. Upper extremity contractures in a patient with eosinophilia-myalgia syndrome. Arch Phys Med Rehabil 1991; 72:1029–1030.
55. Marcus RW. Magnetic resonance imaging in eosinophilic fasciitis. J Rheumatol 1991; 18:636–637.
56. Martinez-Osuna P, Wallach PM, Seleznich MJ, et al. Treatment of the eosinophilia-myalgia syndrome. Semin Arthritis Rheum 1991; 21:110–121.

57. Clauw DJ, Alloway JA, Katz P. Use of cyclosporin A in the eosinophilia myalgia syndrome. Ann Rheum Dis 1993; 52:81–82.
58. Fauci AS, Harley JB, Roberts WC, et al. The idiopathic hypereosinophilia syndrome. Ann Intern Med 1982; 97:78–92.
59. Butterfield JH, Gleich GJ. Interferon-alpha treatment of six patients with the idiopathic hypereosinophilic syndrome. Ann Intern Med 1994; 121:638–653.
60. Silver RM, Miller KS, Kinsella MB, et al. Evaluation and management of scleroderma lung disease using bronchalveolar lavage. Am J Med 1990; 88:470–476.

28

Collagen Vascular Diseases: Polymyositis, Dermatomyositis, and Inclusion Body Myositis

Robert F. Spiera and Lawrence Kagen
The Hospital for Special Surgery–Cornell University Medical College, New York, New York

I. INTRODUCTION

The inflammatory myopathies include a group of disorders characterized by chronic inflammation primarily of skeletal muscle. Specific diagnoses generally accepted as constituting distinct disease entities within this group include idiopathic polymyositis (PM), dermatomyositis (DM), and inclusion body myositis (IBM). DM, and on occasion PM and IBM, may occur in association with an underlying malignancy. Myositis can also occur in the setting of an established connective tissue disease, most commonly systemic lupus erythematosus (SLE) or scleroderma.

The clinical features of PM, DM, and myositis of malignancy or connective tissue disease share certain similarities. There is symmetrical proximal muscle weakness of the limb girdles and trunk, pharyngeal muscular weakness with resultant dysphagia, pulmonary disease (related to restriction of ventilation secondary to respiratory muscle weakness or to interstitial alveolitis), and rarely myocardial involvement. Myalgia may be manifest early in the disease course. DM is diagnosed when there is the presence of a characteristic skin rash, and in its childhood form, it may be accompanied by calcinosis as a prominent clinical feature. IBM constitutes a distinct clinical syndrome, generally of an older population, with an insidious onset, distal weakness, and at times an asymmetrical distribution of muscles affected [1–3].

II. DIAGNOSIS

The treatment of inflammatory myopathy utilizes potentially toxic pharmacological agents which may require prolonged administration. It is therefore essential to establish the diagnosis with the greatest degree of certainly possible. The diagnosis is based on a compatible history, physical examination, and laboratory, electromyographic, and histological evidence of muscle inflammation. Other potential etiologies of myopathy, including endocrine disorders, neurological disease, metabolic abnormalities, toxins, and infections, should be excluded.

The hallmark of inflammatory myopathy is proximal muscle weakness, manifested as difficulty with activities of daily living such as combing of the hair or arising from a seated position. Weakness can be quantified by manual muscle strength testing, functional assessment scores, or more precisely by biomechanical testing of individual muscle groups. Constitutional features, fatigue in particular, are common. Muscle soreness may be seen early in the disease course. Laboratory test abnormalities include increased serum concentrations of muscle-derived enzymes, the most sensitive and specific being creatine kinase (CK), but including aldolase, transaminases, lactate dehydrogenase, and myoglobin [4,5]. Electromyography demonstrates findings of muscle irritability on needle insertion at rest and short-duration, low-amplitude, complex potentials on contraction. Biopsy of affected muscles demonstrating chronic inflammation, myonecronosis, and myofibril regeneration is the most specific diagnostic indicator but this may be limited in sensitivity owing to the spotty nature of muscle involvement and consequent potential for sampling error. The development of percutaneous needle biopsy and appreciation of its acceptable sensitivity (approaching that of the open surgical procedure) allows for histological support of the diagnosis to be obtained in a minimally invasive and inexpensive manner [6]. The biopsy can further help in subclassification of the inflammatory myopathies. Perifascicular atrophy is suggestive of DM; IBM has characteristic histopathological features appreciable even on light microscopy. Recently, the role of magnetic resonance imaging and ultrasonography in the diagnosis and localization of myositis has been explored, and the utility of these modalities in diagnosis and assessment is under current development.

A. Classification

The importance of diagnostic accuracy further extends to the appropriate classification of the inflammatory myopathies (Table 1). There is, however, at present, considerable debate as to which classification scheme best distinguishes disease entities with unique clinical, prognostic, and therapeutic implications. At a minimum, DM, PM, and IBM are appreciated as distinct syndromes. The course of IBM is often indolent and pro-

Table 1 Classification of Inflammatory Myopathies

Polymyositis
Dermatomyositis
Inclusion body myositis
Myositis associated with connective tissue disease
Myositis associated with malignancy
Myositis in relation to infection
viral agents (e.g., influenza, Coxsackie, HIV)
bacterial (e.g., pyomyositis, leprous myositis)
parastic (e.g., toxoplasma, trichinellosis)
spirochetal (Lyme disease)
Drug-related myositis (e.g., penicillamine, eosinophilia myalgia syndrome)

gressive, and the response to treatment poor. Correct diagnosis at the outset allows for more accurate prognosis and may help to establish better goals and expectations of planned interventions. Although myositis overlapping other connective tissue disorders or myositis with malignancy is usually separately classified, it is not clear whether these associations always predict a favorable or unfavorable response to therapy. It is nevertheless important to consider these possibilities in a patient with newly diagnosed inflammatory muscle disease.

Recently, antibodies directed against a variety of protein components involved in protein synthesis termed *myositis-specific antibodies* (MSAs) have been detected in a portion of patients with idiopathic inflammatory myopathy. The presence of MSAs seems to be associated with specific clinical features, including an increased prevalence of interstitial lung disease, Raynaud's phenomenon, fever, arthritis, and "mechanic's hands" [7,8]. It has been suggested that antibody status may have implications for prognosis and response to therapy [9]. This further subclassification of idiopathic DM and PM may prove to be useful in prognostication and selection of therapy in the future.

B. Activity of Disease

Treatment of inflammatory muscle disease is guided by the patient's clinical status and response to therapy. Effective management, therefore, requires precision in the assessment of disease activity (Table 2). A number of parameters must be considered in formulating an impression of disease activity. Perhaps foremost is the patient's level of function in activities of daily living. This information can be elicited by history, and it can further be quantified at the time of examination. The patient's overall subjective impression is of importance but may be confounded by a number of emotional factors. Muscle strength can be assessed either manually or, more precisely, but biomechanical testing of individual muscle groups. Other techniques such as the "timed-stands" test have been used to follow progression of disease [2,10]. As in diagnosis, laboratory evidence of muscle inflammation is useful in assessing disease activity. All of these parameters are taken into consideration in formulating a global impression of disease activity. This, in turn, will determine the clinician's assessment of therapeutic efficacy and guide decisions for further therapy. Manifestations other than weakness, such as rash in DM, interstitial lung disease, or arthralgia, must be evaluated independently, and they may or may not correlate with disease activity in skeletal muscle.

III. THERAPY

Treating patients with inflammatory myopathy is a challenge (Table 3). In part due to its rarity and difficulties with diagnosis, there is a paucity of data on the natural his-

Table 2 Successful Therapy

1.	Accuracy of diagnosis rule out metabolic, toxic- or drug-associated, infectious, endocrine, traumatic, ischemic, genetic, or other causes of myopathy
2.	Accuracy of assessment of activity of disease evaluation of changes in function, physiological findings, laboratory tests

Table 3 Goals of Therapy

1.	Halt inflammation
2.	Preserve muscle function
3.	Prevent complications

tory of disease and few controlled trials of specific therapies. As in the other rheumatic diseases, it is important to define the goals of therapy in specific relation to the individual patient. The general therapeutic aim is to halt the inflammatory process, preserve muscle function and strength, and prevent complications. To do so effectively requires a broad approach, of which pharmacotherapy is just one arm (Table 4).

Physical measures play an important role in the management of patients with myositis. During periods of active inflammation, a program of passive range of motion exercises may be employed to prevent contractures. Active range of motion and strengthening exercises are generally instituted once the inflammatory process comes under control as reflected by stabilization or an increase in muscle strength and a decrease in serum concentrations of muscle enzymes [11]. Assistive devices maximize patient independence in activities of daily living and are often quite helpful. In patients with dysphagia, precautions should be taken to prevent aspiration, including instruction in swallowing and selection of appropriate foods. When severe, temporary nasogastric feeding tube placement to assure adequate enteral nutrition may be required. Surgical myotomy has been used with success in patients with myositis with cricopharyngeal spasm.

Attention to psychosocial issues is a vital part of caring for the patient with myositis. The disease can be debilitating, limiting the ability to function adequately at work or at home. Clinicians must be particularly sensitive to elderly patient ability to care for themselves, and try to provide an adequate support system to help with hygiene, nutrition, and administration of medicines if necessary. The lifestyle limitations and occasional loss of independence experienced by patients with myositis can be devastating to their sense of self-esteem. The impact of corticosteroid therapy on emotions, sleep, and mood can further affect psychological well-being. Patient education also plays a critical role. These disorders are rare and unfamiliar to most patients. Moreover, they are chronic and unpredictable with flares being common, particularly during the early course of the disease. All of this may heighten frustration and anxiety. Communication, reassurance, and a sense of mutual trust and regard are therefore crucial, so that patients can overcome exacerbations of disease and understand that these are usually surmountable.

A. Pharmacotherapy

The etiology and pathogenesis of the inflammatory myopathies are not fully understood. As in other autoimmune disorders, it is suspected that an environmental trigger, possi-

Table 4 Approach to Therapy

1.	Pharmacological agents
2.	Physical therapy
3.	Psychosocial assistance

bly infectious or toxic, creates a sustained immune response in a genetically susceptible host leading to the disease manifestations. Although there is overlap, different mechanisms seem important in effecting muscle damage among the categories of myositis. In PM and IBM, cellular immunity seems prominent, as evidenced by the preponderance of $CD8^+$ cytotoxic T cells in the inflammatory infiltrate in muscle, increased major histocompatibility complex (MHC) class I expression on myocytes in close relation to inflammatory cells, and evidence of activated T cells in muscle and peripheral blood [3,12–14]. In DM, there is evidence of complement component (C5b-9 or membrane attack complex)-mediated microangiopathy, leading to capillary loss, fiber ischemia and necrosis, and perifascicular atrophy [15,16]. The inclusions of IBM contain amyloid protein and other components reminiscent of what is seen in the neurofibrillary tangles in the brains of patients with Alzheimer's disease [17]. Humoral immunity is hypothesized as being possibly pathogenic in patients with MSAs [18]. These variations in mechanisms of disease notwithstanding, the general pharmacotherapeutic approach at present is to control and suppress inflammation and hence preserve myofiber number and function (Table 5).

There is uncertainty concerning what constitutes optimal pharmacotherapy in these disorders. More data from adequate controlled blinded trials are needed. There is nonuniformity in diagnostic criteria and classification schemes, as well as debate over what are the most appropriate outcomes to measure, leading to difficulty in comparing and interpreting published clinical trials and patient series. Our knowledge of the natural history of these diseases is limited, although certain characteristics are generally predictive of a poor prognosis, including disease severity [19,20], cardiopulmonary involvement [19,21,22,23], presence of dysphagia and aspiration [19,20,24], the presence of a skin rash on the torso in DM, and a delay in the diagnosis and institution of therapy [21,25,26,27]. Nevertheless, these disorders are treatable, and many patients respond to therapy.

1. Glucocorticoids

Corticosteroids presently constitute the first-line of therapy. Our use of these agents is not based on scientific data derived from controlled clinical trials but rather on the empiric observation of their efficacy. The vast and successful experience with glucocorticoids would make a placebo-controlled trial unacceptable for most investigators at this point. Scant data on the mortality of the myositis disorders in the presteroid era suggest a much higher death rate than what is seen now; however, this is difficult to interpret given concurrent advances in other areas of medical therapeutics and in the sensitivity of diagnosis [28]. It is known, however, that the response rate to corticosteroids is high, with as many as 90% of treated patients responding and perhaps as many

Table 5 Commonly Used Pharmacological Agents

1. Corticosteroids
    - oral (daily or alternate-day dose schedules)
    - parenteral (bolus therapy)
2. Immunomodulating or cytosuppressive agents
    - methotrexate
    - azathioprine
    - others (cyclosporin, chlorambucil, cyclophosphamide)
3. Immune globulin-intravenous IgG

as 50–70% achieving complete remissions as manifested by stabilization of strength and normalization of serum muscle enzyme levels [2].

The general therapeutic approach is to institute high-dose daily glucocorticoids initially and then to taper dosage gradually guided by clinical and laboratory evidence of improvement. Different recommendations have been made on the specifics of administration. Oddis et al. have advocated initial treatment with oral prednisone 1 mg/kg/day in divided doses until normalization of serum CK is achieved. The dose is then consolidated to a single morning dose and then tapered by 25% each month to a 5-10-mg daily maintenance dose, which is then continued for 1 year [29]. We among others, have advocated a less focused emphasis on normalization of serum CK, treating initially with 40–60 mg/day of prednisone for 4–6 weeks or until maximum benefit or remission is achieved. The dose is then gradually tapered with careful monitoring of symptoms, physical findings, and laboratory tests. The employment of alternate-day glucocorticoid therapy either initially [30], or more usually during the period of taper [31], has been advocated in these disorders and may decrease the incidence of steroid side effects. The successful use of high-dose intravenous methylprednisone pulse therapy has been reported in adults with DM refractory to conventional therapy [32], as well as a first-line therapy in juvenile DM [33]. There are no prospective trials comparing the various steroid regimens.

Side effects of glucocorticoids are of major concern in patients with inflammatory muscle disease. The course of therapy is relatively prolonged even in patients with excellent responses, making the potential of steroid complications loom large in the management of these diseases. The large number of potential adverse effects of steroids, including cushingoid appearance, hirsuitism, weight gain, emotional lability, insomnia, hypertension, diabetes, susceptibility to infection, skin fragility, cataract formation, osteoporosis, and avascular necrosis are all relevant and are discussed in detail elsewhere in this text. Corticosteroid-induced myopathy is a particularly vexing problem in patients with myositis. This entity causes predominantly symmetrical proximal musculature weakness and can therefore be mistaken for increase of activity of the underlying disease [34,35]. Distinction between these two entities is difficult. Electromyography is nonspecific, and even muscle biopsy cannot reliably demonstrate steroid myopathy to be the cause of the current episode of weakness. Serum levels of muscle-derived enzymes are generally not elevated in steroid myopathy, but these may also be normal in some patients with active inflammatory myopathy. If the suspicion of steroid myopathy is great, it may be necessary to withdraw steroids and observe the clinical course. Steroid myopathy should improve, whereas inflammatory myopathy should worsen during cessation of therapy. In the unusual patient in whom myositis flare is not accompanied by an increase in muscle enzymes, it has been suggested that the measurement of urinary creatine can be helpful in distinguishing disease activity from steroid myopathy. In the latter, although serum muscle-derived enzymes are normal, urinary creatine excretion is increased, and creatinuria should decrease and strength increase with steroid reduction [35]. In general practice, however, steroid myopathy is infrequently encountered, and increased weakness is more commonly indicative of increased disease activity.

2. *Immunosuppressives*

Although the inflammatory myopathies re generally steroid responsive, at times it is necessary to employ additional agents to treat patients with these disorders. The indications for adding immunosuppressives include a lack of efficacy of steroid therapy despite an adequate trial (several weeks of therapy) or a need for a "steroid-sparing" effect in patients with intolerable side effects at doses of corticosteroids needed to control disease. It has also been suggested that severe progressive disease and organ involvement warrant earlier institution of immunosuppressive therapy. A variety of agents have been used successfully, but they have not been compared with each other in clinical trials. The specific selection of a particular immunosuppressive depends largely on the disease features and comorbid conditions in the individual patient and the clinician's experience and familiarity with these medications.

Methotrexate is perhaps the most frequently used drug in this category at present. There now has been over two decades of experience with this agent in myositis, and numerous uncontrolled trials demonstrating its efficacy and steroid-sparing properties [36,37]. With the expanded use of methotrexate in other areas of rheumatological practice, rheumatoid arthritis in particular, clinicians have become familiar with it and may be using it earlier in inflammatory myopathies. Generally, it is given concomitantly with steroids, reducing the steroid dose as the methotrexate dose is increased and disease control is achieved. It can be administered intravenously, subcutaneously, orally, or intramuscularly, although the latter route is frequently avoided in myositis, as it may cause elevation of muscle enzymes and hamper the already difficult task of assessing disease activity. Response rates of 75% [37] have been reported with intravenous use, which is generally given weekly at doses of 0.5–0.8 mg/kg/day. Oral administration is more commonly used because of its greater convenience. The starting dose is 7.5 mg/week, and this can be increased by 2.5-mg weekly increments up to 30–50 mg/week as needed to control disease. A response is usually seen only after several weeks on therapy, so care should be taken not to escalate the dose too hastily.

Hepatotoxicity has been the greatest concern in patients treated with methotrexate. Preexisting liver disease or alcoholism represent situations mitigating its use. No guidelines have been established for monitoring liver function specifically in myositis patients on methotrexate, but clinicians have generally followed those used for rheumatoid arthritis. Routine pretreatment liver biopsy is probably not necessary, and there is debate over whether biopsy needs to be done after a 1.5-g cumulative dose. Assessing complete blood counts for signs of bone marrow toxicity (leukopenia, anemia, macrocytosis) is routine. Gastrointestinal toxicity in the form of stomatitis, diarrhea, or colitis can be seen as well. As with other immunosuppressives, there is concern regarding increased susceptibility to infection. The pulmonary toxicity of methotrexate, albeit rare, can be problematic in DM and PM patients, since it can be difficult to distinguish from the interstitial lung disease of myositis. We nevertheless do not feel that methotrexate is contraindicated in myositis with lung involvement, but its use requires clinical skill in this setting. Reports of non–Hodgkin's lymphoma in rheumatoid arthritis patients treated with methotrexate [38,39], as well as reversible Epstein-Barr virus–associated Hodgkin's lymphoma in a patient with DM [40], raise concerns regarding immunosuppression-related neoplasms with even low-dose methotrexate therapy.

Azathioprine, in conjunction with corticosteroids, has also ben successfully used in treating inflammatory myopathy, and it is the only such drug that has been tested in a controlled trial. Patients were treated with prednisone 60 mg daily and either azathioprine 2 mg/kg/day or placebo. Results reported at 3-month follow-up failed to show benefit in the treatment group in terms of strength or improvement in the histopathological features on muscle biopsy [41]. Assessment at 1-year and 3-year follow-up, however, showed that the azathioprine-treated patients had better function and required less prednisone than the control group [42]. The dosage used in myositis is 2–3 mg/kg/day. When remission is achieved and patients are on relatively lower doses of corticosteroids, the dose of azathioprine can be tapered by 25 mg/month to a 50- 75-mg daily maintenance dose. Major toxicities include gastrointestinal intolerance, bone marrow suppression, increased susceptibility to infection, rare hepatotoxicity, and the possible increased likelihood of developing malignancies, usually lymphoproliferative. The strength of this possibility remains uncertain. One study of its use in patients with rheumatoid arthritis found a modestly increased frequency of lymphatic malignancies compared with untreated patients [43], although both of these groups had greater frequencies than did a normal comparison group. Reversible lymphoma in a patient with inflammatory bowel disease receiving azathioprine has been reported [44].

Although there are no prospective trials directly comparing methotrexate and azathioprine in inflammatory muscle disease, it is the impression of many clinicians that methotrexate may be the more effective agent. A retrospective analysis of 113 consecutive patients seen at the U.S. National Institutes of Health (NIH) with inflammatory muscle disease suggested that methotrexate may be more effective than azathioprine in patients refractory to corticosteroid therapy. In this study, methotrexate was particularly effective in male patients and patients with antisynthetase antibodies [9].

Therapy with alkylating agents has not been widely used in inflammatory myopathy. A small open-label trial of intravenous monthly cyclophosphamide in patients with severe disease showed a lack of efficacy and significant toxicity [45]. However, cases of improvement in progressive interstitial lung disease with intravenous or oral cyclophosphamide treatment in patients with myositis have been reported [46]. More recently, chlorambucil has been reported as being beneficial in relatively low doses (4 mg/day) in five patients with recalcitrant DM [47]. All patients improved and four of the five achieved sustained remission and were able to discontinue the drug after 13–30 months of treatment. Combination therapy with cytotoxic agents has also been reported as being beneficial in some corticosteroid-resistant patients [48,49]. The potential oncogenicity of these agents and questions of efficacy to date has tempered enthusiasm for their routine use.

Cyclosporin, an immunosuppressive commonly used in renal allograft recipients, has received attention as being potentially useful in myositis. A mechanism of its action is through inhibition of T-cell activation and proliferation [50], and hence it is a reasonable therapeutic candidate in disorders such as myositis where cytotoxic and helper T lymphocytes are felt to play important roles. Numerous descriptions of clinical responses in juvenile [51] and adult [52,53] myositis have been reported. A recently published open-label trial demonstrated its efficacy at low doses (5 mg/kg/day) as a first-line agent in patients with DM [54]. Comparison with historical controls suggested a more rapid clinical response with cyclosporin than with conventional therapy. It has been proposed that a controlled trial comparing cyclosporine with corticosteroids as first-line therapy in myositis may be warranted. The side effects of cyclosporin are significant, including dose-dependent nephrotoxicity, hypertension, hypertrichosis, gingival hypertrophy, and anemia. Furthermore, there is concern regarding the development of lymphoid malignancies [55,56]. The ability to monitor serum levels combined with its reported efficacy at low doses may mitigate these concerns about cyclosporin, and it is likely that this drug and others (e.g., tacrolimus) will be further explored in the treatment of inflammatory myopathies in the future.

3. Intravenous Immune Globulin

A relatively recent and exciting development in the treatment of inflammatory muscle disease is the use of intravenous immune globulin (IVIg). IVIg had previously been recognized as effective in a number of immune-mediated diseases, including immune thrombocytopenic purpura [57], Kawasaki's disease [58], and Guillan-Barré syndrome [59]. The mechanism of action of this therapy is unclear, but a number of hypotheses have been suggested, including blockade of Fc receptors on vascular endothelium and/or on phagocytic cells, interference with complement-mediated damage to endothelium or myocytes, and inhibition of T-cell effector function and cytokine production [60]. In an open-label study of 20 adults with refractory DM or PM treated with monthly IVIg (either 1 g/kg/day for 2 days or 0.4 g/kg/day for 5 days) for a mean of 4 months, clinical improvement was seen in 75% of patients as manifested by increased muscle strength, decreased CK, and a reduction in steroid dose [61]. Side effects were infrequent, mild, and transient. The success of therapy was particularly encouraging, given the refractory nature of disease in these patients. Most had failed at least one immunosuppressive agent and had a long duration of active disease prior to therapy (>3 years); a factor known to predict a poor response to therapy. More recently, a double-blind placebo-controlled trial of IVIg in DM was reported by Dalakis et al. from the NIH [62]. Using a crossover design, a total of 12 patients with previously documented therapy-resistant, biopsy-proven DM were treated with monthly IVIg (2 mg/kg as a single infusion) for 3 months, with continuation of daily prednisone. The response to therapy was impressive; 9 of the 12 patients with severe disability had dramatic clinical responses with near normalization of function and symptomatic relief. Two of the remaining three patients had mild improvement. Of the 11 placebo-treated patients, only 3 had mild improvement, with the others showing a deterioration or no change. The investigators were further able to correlate clinical remission with histological improvement in all five of the responders who underwent pre- and posttreatment muscle biopsies. In general, the response to therapy was rapid, with a noticeable improvement within 2 weeks of the first infusion and a maximal response between the second and third infusions. Although the study conclusively demonstrated the clinical efficacy of this therapy, it also suggested likely limitations of IVIg in clinical practice. The beneficial effects of therapy were short-lived; even patients who had major improvement with therapy regressed to baseline within 3 months of cessation of infusions. There are no good data at present about long-term follow-up of patients on "maintenance" monthly IVIg, although it is the impression of some that its efficacy seems to wane with time. The high cost of infusional IVIg may also be prohibitive. Nevertheless, the impressive clinical response even in refractory patients and benign side effect profile make this a promising therapy in inflammatory muscle disease. Results of ongoing trials of IVIg in patients with PM and IBM are eagerly awaited. It may be reasonable to consider IVIg earlier in the disease course, perhaps prior to the use of the more toxic immunosuppressive and cytotoxic agents, or even as first-line therapy in conjunction with corticosteroids to reduce the total steroid dose necessary to control the disease. However, one recent open-label study of IVIg as initial sole therapy in 11 adult patients with DM or PM was disappointing in terms of efficacy [63]. Further studies will better define the role of IVIg in these diseases. In the meantime, high costs coupled with the present status of myositis as non-FDA (Food and Drug Administration) approved indication for the use of IVIg make access difficult for many patients.

IVIg has been generally safe and well tolerated. Serious side effects are rare, but they have included acute renal failure [64], thromboembolic events [65], and anaphylactic reactions [66]. Quantitation of serum immunoglobulins to rule out individuals with congenital IgA deficiency (which can be present in approximately 1/300 of the general population) prior to initiating this therapy may avoid allergic reactions to the small amounts of IgA present in some preparations. Aseptic meningitis has generally been considered a rare complication of IVIg, although one recent study reported a high frequency (11%) of this adverse effect in a group of patients with neuromuscular disease [67]. However, this side effect has usually been transient. It should also be noted that IVIg consists of pooled human immunoglobulins, making transmission of infectious agents a concern. In fact, recent cases of hepatitis C virus transmission by preparations from one manufacturer of IVIg were recently reported [68]. The more common side effects, however, including headache, backache, nausea, and fever are generally mild, transient, and possibly related to rapidity of infusion. They do not necessarily recur with subsequent infusions; however, prophylaxis against recurrences with nonsteroidal anti-inflammatory drugs (NSAIDs) or even corticosteroids has been used by some clinicians.

4. *Other Modalities*

A number of other modalities have been explored in the treatment of inflammatory muscle disease. Several uncontrolled trials of plasmapheresis suggested a possible role for this treatment in myositis. However, a double-blinded trial of 39 patients with PM or DM failed to support its use [69]. Patients underwent plasma exchange, leukapheresis, or sham apheresis 12 times over a 1-month period. The corticosteroid dose was held constant (approximately 30 mg/day on average) and no concomitant immunosuppressive therapy was administered. Although the plasma exchange–treated patients showed a decrease in CK, no beneficial effect on strength or function could be demonstrated. The question of whether concurrent immunosuppressive therapy would have been essential or whether patients selection was optimal still remains open.

Total body irradiation (TBI) has similarly been reported as being beneficial in some patients with refractory myositis in small case series [70]. Failures of this potentially toxic and expensive therapy have also been reported [71]. No clinical trials have systemically evaluated the efficacy of TBI, and with the attendant concerns of bone marrow suppression and induction of later malignancy, this modality is not indicated in the routine management of DM or PM.

Antimalarial agents may have a role in the treatment of DM. In an open-label prospective study of patients with DM, the addition of hydroxychloroquine to ongoing corticosteroid therapy resulted in improvement in cutaneous disease, with complete resolution of rash in some patients [72]. No benefit on muscle strength was found. A retrospective evaluation of nine children with DM treated with hydroxychloroquine (at 2.5 mg/kg/day) in conjunction with steroids did suggest a beneficial effect on muscle disease and a possible steroid-sparing effect [73]. The treatment was well tolerated and safe. Retinal toxicity, the major feared complication, is extremely rare and probably avoidable through frequent ophthalmological examinations. More common adverse effects include skin rash and occasional abdominal pain and diarrhea. Regular monitoring of hepatic and renal function tests is advised.

IV. SPECIAL CONSIDERATIONS

A. Cutaneous Complications of DM

The response of skin disease in DM can be discordant from the response of skeletal muscle inflammation to systemic therapy. The typical rash of DM involves areas of the hands and face and is therefore visible and an important cosmetic concern. Topical steroids have afforded minimal benefits. Antimalarials are useful in treating the rash of DM.

Calcinosis can be distressing in patients with juvenile DM. This complication can range in severity from an asymptomatic radiographic finding to being diffuse and disabling [74]. Calcific deposits can break through overlying skin causing draining sinuses which may then become secondarily infected. There are at present no predictably effective specific therapeutic strategies for calcinosis in DM. Corticosteroids, ethylenediaminetetra-acetic acid (EDTA), and bisphosphonates seem to be ineffective [75]. One report suggested a very modest efficacy of low-dose oral warfarin in reducing the extent of calcinosis [76]. Colchicine has also been used successfully in suppressing cutaneous inflammation at sites of calcific deposits [77,78]. Aggressive management of infection, local hygenic measures, and even surgical debulking of painful calcific deposits can be helpful. It should be noted that even extensive calcinosis can regress spontaneously with remission of inflammatory disease in DM [74,79].

B. Treatment of Inclusion Body Myositis

The therapeutic approach to patients with IBM is sufficiently distinct to warrant a separate discussion. This disease typically occurs in an older population and often in males. Muscle atrophy may be prominent, CK elevations more modest, and the pattern of muscle involvement more asymmetrical and distal than what is commonly found in the other inflammatory myopathies. Extraskeletal musculature manifestations are rare, although a mild peripheral neuropathy with diminished deep tendon reflexes can be present. The disease course is generally indolent and slowly progressive. IBM is widely appreciated as being resistant to therapy [80,81], so much so that, in the past, some had advocated not subjecting patients with this form of disease to the risk of therapy. It should be noted, however, that this consideration may have been confounded by a number of factors. In many patients in case series reported, the diagnosis of IBM was made only after resistance to therapy was observed, prompting a stronger consideration of IBM and closer examination of muscle specifically searching for evidence of that disorder. This may have led to a selection bias, so that responsive patients were less likely to have the diagnosis of IBM made. Furthermore, as previously mentioned, a delay between the onset of weakness and the institution of therapy is a predictor of poor response to therapy in inflammatory muscle disease. With the insidious nature of IBM and long duration of disease prior to diagnosis, it is possible that the poor responses to therapy may be in part attributable to this factor rather than being inherent to the underlying pathophysiology of IBM per se.

Specific trials of therapy in IBM are few. Most of our information regarding treatment is derived from retrospective studies. The general approach is the same as that for other inflammatory myopathies, with the same agents being used in similar doses. The earlier pessimism regarding the treatment of IBM has been tempered by observations that although therapy may not result in improvement in muscle function, treated patients may have a slower rate of strength decline compared with untreated patients. One retrospective analysis [82] of 32 patients with IBM compared outcomes of patients who received no therapy ($n = 4$) with those who received either prednisone alone ($n = 13$) or prednisone plus another immunosuppressive drug ($n = 15$). All untreated patients deteriorated, whereas in the prednisone group, four patients stabilized and two transiently improved. In the immunosuppressive-treated group, one patient stabilized, five transiently improved, and three patients had long-term remissions (all of whom received oral methotrexate). In a prospective trial comparing azathioprine plus oral methotrexate to high-dose intravenous methotrexate with leucovorin rescue [14], both regimens similarly showed therapeutic benefit in terms of stabilization or improvement of strength in a majority of patients. Although weakened by a lack of placebo controls, this study suggested a benefit to therapy. An open-label trial of IVIg in four patients with IBM showed improvement in 3 [83].

Overall, it seems that therapy should be considered in patients with IBM. What constitutes optimal therapy for this disorder remains to be defined, but immunosuppressive therapy with methotrexate in particular may be beneficial. IVIg also remains a promising possible therapy for this disorder. The treating clinician and patient must recognize that expectations of therapy may need to be somewhat limited and that perhaps stabilization of the course or halting of disease progression may constitute acceptable goals of therapy.

REFERENCES

1. Dalakas MC. Polymyositis, dermatomyositis, and inclusion body myositis. N Engl J Med 1991; 325:1487–1498.
2. Wortman RL. Inflammatory disease of the muscle. In: Kelley, Harris, Ruddy, Sledge, eds. Textbook of Rheumatology. Philadelphia: Saunders, 1993:
3. Plotz PH, Dalakas M, Leff RL, et al. Current concepts in the idiopathic inflammatory myopathies: polymyositis, dermatomyositis, and related disorders, Ann Intern Med 1989; 111:143–157.
4. Vignos PJ, Goldwin J. Evaluation of laboratory tests in diagnosis and management of polymyositis. Am J Med 1972; 263:291–308.
5. Kroll M, Otis J, Kagen L. Serum enzyme, myoglobin, and muscle strength relationships in PM and DM. J Rheum 1986; 13:349–355.
6. O'Rourke KS, Blaivis M, Ike R.Utility of needle muscle biopsy in a university rheumatology practice. J Rheum 1994; 21:413–424.
7. Love LA, Leff RL, Fraser DD, et al. A new approach to the classification of idiopathic inflammatory myopathy: Myositis-specific autoantibodies define useful homogeneous patient groups. Medicine (Baltimore) 1991; 70:360–374.
8. Oddis CV. Therapy for myositis. Curr Opin in Rheumatol 1993; 5:742–748.
9. Joffe MM, Love LA, Leff RL, et al. Drug therapy of the idiopathic inflammatory myopathies: predictors of response to prednisone, azathioprine, and methotrexate and a comparison of their efficacy. Am J Med 1994; 94:379–387.
10. Csuka M, McCarty DJ. Simple method for measurement of lower extremity muscle strength. Am J Med 1985; 78:77–81.
11. Hicks JE. Rehabilitation of patients with myositis. In: Rheumatology, Klippel, Dieppe, eds. St. Louis: Mosby-Year Book, 1994:
12. Engel AG, Arahata K. Mononuclear cells in myopathies: quantitation of functionally dis-

tinct subsets, recognition of antigen-specific cell-mediated cytotoxicity in some diseases, and implications for the pathogenesis of the different inflammatory myopathies. Hum Pathol 1986; 17:704-721.

13. Emslie-Smith AM, Arahata K, Engel AG. major histocompatibility complex class I antigen expression, immunolocalization of interferon subtypes, and T cell-mediated cytotoxicity in myopathies. Hum Pathol 1989; 20:224-231.
14. Leff RL, Miller FW, Hicks J, et al. The treatment of inclusion body myositis: a retrospective review and a randomized, prospective trial of immunosuppressive therapy. Medicine (Baltimore) 1993; 72:225-235.
15. Kissel JT, Mendell JR, Rammohan KW. Microvascular deposition of complement membrane attack complex in dermatomyositis. N Engl J Med 1986; 314:329-334.
16. Emslie-Smith AM, Engel AG. Microvascular changes in early and advanced dermatomyositis: a quantitative study. Ann Neurol 1990; 27:343-356.
17. Askanas V, Engel WK. New advances in inclusion body myositis. Curr Opin Rheumatol 1993; 5:732-741.
18. Miller FW, Waite KA, Biswas T, Plotz PH. The role of an autoantigen, histidyl-tRNA synthetase, in the induction and maintenance of autoimmunity. Proc Natl Acad Sci USA 1990; 87:9993-9937.
19. Medsger TA, Robinson H, Masi AT. Factors affecting survivorship in polymyositis, life table study of 124 patients. Arthritis Rheum 1971; 14:249-258.
20. Carpenter JR, Bunch TW, Engel AG, et al. Survival in polymyositis: Corticosteroids and risk factors. J Rheum 1977; 4:207-214.
21. Henriksson KG, Sandstedt P. Polymyositis treatment and prognosis: a study of 107 patients. Acta Neurol Scand 1982; 65:280-300.
22. Hochberg MC, Feldman D, Stevens MB. Adult onset polymyositis/dermatomyositis: an analysis of clinical and laboratory features and survival in 76 patients with a review of the literature. Semin Arthritis Rheum 1986; 15:168-178.
23. Asura EL, Greenberg AS. Adverse impact of interstitial pulmonary fibrosis on prognosis in polymyositis and dermatomyositis. Sem Arthritis Rheum 1988; 18:29-37.
24. Benbassat J, Gefel D, Larholt K, et al. Prognostic factors in PM-DM: A computer-assisted analysis of 92 cases. Arthritis Rheum 1985; 28:249-255.
25. Bohan A, Peter JB, Bowman RI, Pearson CM. A computer-assisted analysis of 153 patients with polymyositis and dermatomyositis. Medicine 1976; 55:89-104.
26. Tymms KE, Webb J. Dermatopolymyositis and other connective tissue disease. A review of 105 cases. J Rheumatol 1986; 12:1140-1148.
27. Fafalak RG, Peterson MGE, Kagen LJ. Strength in polymyositis and dermatomyositis: best outcome in patients treated early. J Rheumatol 1994; 21:643-648.
28. Ehrenstein MR, Snaith ML, Isenberg DA. Idiopathic myositis: a rheumatological view. Ann Rheum Dis 1992; 51:41-44.
29. Oddis CV, Medsger T. Current management of polymyositis and dermatomyositis. Drugs 1989; 37:382-390.
30. Uchino M, Araki S, Yoshida O, et al. High single-dose alternate-day corticosteroid regimens in treatment of polymyositis. J Neurol 1985; 232:175-178.
31. Dalakas MC. Current treatment of the inflammatory myopathies. Curr Opin Rheum 1994; 6:595-601.
32. Yanagisawa T, Sueishi M, Nawata Y, et al. Methyl prednisolone pulse therapy in dermatomyositis. Dermatologica 1983; 167:47-51.
33. Laxer RM, Stein LD, Petty RE. Intravenous pulse methylprednisolone treatment of juvenile dermatomyositis. Arthritis Rheum 1987; 30:328-234.
34. Afifi AK, Bergman RA, Harvey JC. Steroid myopathy. Clinical, histologic, and cytologic observations. J Hopkins Med J 1968; 123:158.

35. Askari A, Vignos PJ, Moskowitz RW. Steroid myopathy in connective tissue disease. Am J Med 1976; 61:485.
36. Malaviya AN, Many A, Schwartz RS. Treatment of DM with methotrexate. Lancet 1968; 2:485–488.
37. Metzger AL, Bohan A, Goldberg LS, et al. Polymyositis and dermatomyositis: Combined methotrexate and corticosteroid therapy. Ann Intern Med 1974; 81:182–189.
38. Ellman MH, Hurwitz H, Thomas C, Kozloff M. Lymphoma developing in a patient with rheumatoid arthritis taking low-dose weekly methotrexate. J Rheumatol 1991; 18:1741–1743.
39. Kingsmore SE, Hall BD, Allen NB, et al. Association of methotrexate, rheumatoid arthritis, and lymphoma: report of 2 cases and literature review. J Rheumatol 1992; 19:1462–1465.
40. Kamel OW, van de Rijn M, Weiss LM, et al. Reversible lymphomas associated with Epstein-Barr virus occurring during methotrexate therapy for rheumatoid arthritis and dermatomyositis. N Engl J Med 1993; 328:1317–1321.
41. Bunch TW, Worthington JW, Combs JJ, et al. Azathioprine and prednisone for polymyositis: a controlled clinical trial. Ann Intern Med 1980; 92:365–369.
42. Bunch TW. Prednisone and azathioprine for polymyositis. Arthritis Rheum 1981; 25:45–48.
43. Silman AJ, Petrie J, Hazleman B, Evans SJW. Lymphoproliferative cancer and other malignancy in patients with rheumatoid arthritis treated with azathioprine: a 20-year follow-up study. Ann Rheum Dis 1988; 47:988–992.
44. Larvol L, Soule J, Tourneau A. Reversible lymphoma in the setting of azathioprine therapy for Crohn's disease. N Engl J Med 1994; 331:883–884.
45. Cronin ME, Miller FE, Hicks JE, et al. The failure of intravenous cyclophosphamide therapy in refractory idiopathic inflammatory myopathy. J Rheumatol 1989; 16:1225-1228.
46. Al-Janadi M, Smith CD, Karsh J. Cyclophosphamide treatment of interstitial pulmonary fibrosis in polymyositis/dermatomyositis. J Rheumatol 1989; 16:1592.
47. Sinoway PA, Callen JP. Chlorambucil: an effective corticosteroid-sparing agent for patients with recalcitrant DM. Arthritis Rheum 1993; 36:319–324.
48. Wallace DJ, Metzger AL, White KK. Combination immunosuppressive treatment of steroid-resistant dermatomyositis/polymyositis. Arthritis Rheum 1985; 28:590–592.
49. Tiliakos NA. Low-dose cytotoxic combination therapy in intractable dermatopolymyositis. Arthritis Rheum 1987; 30:S14.
50. Shevach EM. The effect of cyclosporin on the immune system. Annu Rev Immunol 1985; 3:397.
51. Dantzig P. Juvenile dermatomyositis treated with cyclosporine. J Am Acad Dermatol 1990; 22:310–11.
52. Pugh MT, Collins NA, Rai A, et al. A case of adult DM treated with cyclosporin A. Br J Rheum 1992; 31:855.
53. Lueck CJ, Trend P, Swash M. Cyclosporin in the management of PM and DM. J Neurol Neurosurg Psychiatr 1991; 54:1007–1008.
54. Grau JM, Herrero C, Casademont J, et al. Cyclosporin A as first choice therapy for DM. J Rheumatol 1994; 21:381–382.
55. Starzl TH, Nalesnik MA, Porter KA, et al. Reversibility of lymphomas and lymphoproliferative lesions developing under cyclosporine-steroid therapy. Lancet 1984; 1:583–587.
56. Masouye I, Salomon D, Saurat JH. B cell lymphoma after cyclosporin for keratosis lichenoides chronica. Arch Dermatol 1993; 129:914–915.
57. Imbach P, Barundun S, d'Apuzzo V, et al. High-dose intravenous gammaglobulin for idiopathic thrombocytopenic purpura in childhood. Lancet 1981; 1:228–231.
58. Newburger JW, Takahashi M, Burns JC, et al. The treatment of Kawasaki syndrome with intravenous gammaglobulin. N Engl J Med 1986; 315:341–347.

59. van der Meche FG, Schmitz PI. A randomized trial comparing intravenous immune globulin and plasma exchange in Guillain-Barre syndrome: Dutch Guillain-Barre Study Group. N Engl J Med 1992; 326:1123–1129.
60. Dwyer JM. Manipulating the immune system with immune globulin. N Engl J Med 1992; 326:107–116.
61. Cherin P, Herson S, Wechsler B, et al. Efficacy of intravenous gammaglobulin therapy in chronic refractory polymyositis and dermatomyositis: an open study with 20 adult patients. Am J Med 1991; 91:162–168.
62. Dalakas MC, Illa I, Dambrosia JM, et al. A controlled trial of high-dose intravenous immune globulin infusions as treatment for dermatomyositis. N Engl J Med 1993; 329:1993–2000.
63. Cherin P, Piette JC, Wechsler B, et al. Intravenous gammaglobulin as first line therapy in polymyositis and dermatomyositis: an open study in 11 adult patients. J Rheumatol 1994; 21:1092–1097.
64. Tan E, Hajinazarian M, Bay W, et al. Acute renal failure resulting form intravenous immunoglobulin therapy. Arch Neurol 1993; 50:136–139.
65. Dalakas MC. High-dose intravenous immunoglobulin and serum viscosity: Risk of precipitating thromboembolic events. Neurology 1994; 44:223–226.
66. Buckley RH, Schiff RI. The use of intravenous immune globulin in immunodeficiency diseases. N Engl J Med 1991; 325:110–117.
67. Sekul EA, Cupler EJ, Dalakas MC. Aseptic meningitis associated with high-dose intravenous immunoglobulin therapy: Frequency and risk factors. Ann Intern Med 1994; 121:259–262.
68. Outbreak of hepatitis C associated with intravenous immunoglobulin administration - United States, October 1993-June 1994. MMWR 1994; 43:505–509.
69. Miller FW, Leitman SF, Cronin ME, et al. Controlled trial of plasma exchange and leukapheresis in polymyositis and dermatomyositis. N Engl J Med 1992; 326:1380.
70. Kelly JJ, Madoc-Jones H, Adelman LS, et al. Response to total body irradiation in dermatomyositis. Muscle Nerve 1988; 11:120–123.
71. Cherin P, Heson S, Coutellier A, et al. Failure of total body irradiation in polymyositis: report of three cases (letter). Br J Rheumatol 1992; 31:282–283.
72. Woo TY, Callen JP, Voorhees JJ, et al. Cutaneous lesions of dermatomyositis are improved by hydroxychloroquine. J Am Acad Dermatol 1984; 10:592–600.
73. Olson NY, Llindsley CB. Adjunctive use of hydroxychloroquine in childhood dermatomyositis. J Rheumatol 1989; 16:1545–1547.
74. Bowyer SL, Blane C, Sullivan DB, Cassidy JT. Childhood dermatomyositis: Factors predicting functional outcome and development of dystrophic calcification. J Pediatr 1983; 103:882–888.
75. Metzger A, Singer F, Bluestone R, Pearson C. Failure of disodium etidronate in calcinosis due to dermatomyositis and scleroderma. N Engl J Med 1974; 291:1294–1296.
76. Berger RG, Featherstone GL, Raasch RH, et al. Treatment of calcinosis universalis with low-dose warfarin. Ann J Med 1987; 83:72–76.
77. Taborn J, Bole GG, Thompson GR. Colchicine suppression of local and systemic inflammation due to calcinosis universalis in chronic dermatomyositis. Ann Intern Med 1978; 89:648–649.
78. Fuchs D, Fruchter L, Fishel B, et al. Colchicine suppression of local inflammation due to calcinosis in dermatomyositis and progressive systemic sclerosis. Clin Rheum 1986; 5:527–530.
79. Ostrov BE, Goldsmith DP, Eichenfield AH, Arthreya BH. Hypercalcemia during the resolution of calcinosis universalis in juvenile dermatomyositis. J Rheumatol 1991; 18:1730–1734.
80. Calabrese LH, Misumoto H, Chou S. Inclusion body myositis presenting as treatment-resistant polymyositis. Arthritis Rheum 1987; 30:397–403.

81. Cohen MR, Sulaiman AR, Garancis JC, Wortmann RL. Clinical heterogeneity and treatment response in inclusion body myositis. Arthritis Rheum 1989; 32:734–740.
82. Sayers ME, Chou SM, Calabrese LH. Inclusion body myositis: Analysis of 32 cases. J Rheumatol 1992; 19:1385–1389.
83. Soueidan SA, Dalakas MC. Treatment of inclusion body myositis with high-dose intravenous immunoglobulin. Neurology 1993; 43:876–879.

29

Taxonomy of the Vasculitis Syndromes

C. G. M. Kallenberg
University Hospital Groningen, Groningen, The Netherlands

I. INTRODUCTION

Vasculitis can be defined as an inflammatory process affecting blood vessels. As such the keystone for a diagnosis of vasculitis is the histopathology of the affected tissue. However, the demonstration of vasculitis in a particular patient is, in itself, insufficient for diagnosis, treatment, and prognosis. The vasculitic process may be localized or widespread, may be secondary to other conditions or constitute a primary idiopathic process, and may constitute a transient self-limiting phenomenon or a progressive life-threatening condition. In order to assess the prognosis and treatment of vasculitis, the classification of vasculitis is mandatory in every patient in whom this diagnosis is made or supposed. The classification of vasculitis is based, on the one hand, on the presence or absence of an underlying condition (i.e., secondary or primary vasculitis) and, on the other, on the histopathology of the inflammatory process, the site of the vessels involved, and the clinical symptomatology. Although many proposals for the classification of vasculitis have been formulated [1–4], a uniform consensus has not been reached until now. In this chapter, I will distinguish the secondary vasculitides from the primary ones. This distinction is of utmost importance, as the recognition of the underlying condition in the secondary vasculitides in many cases gives the clue to a causal way of treatment. In clinical practice, secondary vasculitides frequently present as palpable purpura histopathologically manifest as leukocytoclastic vasculitis. This category will be dealt with in detail. Next, I will discuss the classification of the primary vasculitides. Definitions for those disorders have recently been proposed by the Chapel Hill Consensus Conference [5], whereas criteria for the classification based on clinical and histopathological findings have been formulated by the American College of Rheumatologists (ACR) [6]. Finally, one should realize that a number of conditions mimick vasculitis but do not show inflammatory processes of the vessel wall. These pseudovasculitic syndromes, or vasculitis look-alike disorders, will be discussed separately.

II. SECONDARY VASCULITIDES

The designation *secondary vasculitis* implies that the vasculitic process is secondary to another condition. A classification of the secondary vasculitides is given in Table 1. The secondary vasculitides are, in many cases, characterized by the presence of immune deposits within the vessel wall suggesting that immune complexes are involved in their pathophysiology. Indeed, the nature of the antigen(s) participating in the formation of immune complexes is frequently suggested by the underlying disease. Exogenous antigens, either microbial constituents or heterologous proteins as in serum sickness, as well as endogenous/autologous antigens such as DNA or nucleosomes in systemic lupus erythematosus, are associated with the secondary vasculitides (Table 2). Searching for the antigens involved not only gives insight into the pathophysiology of the disorder but may also provide tools for its treatment. The secondary vasculitides affect small-sized vessels in most of the cases, in particular venules as in leukocytoclastic vasculitis. Clinically, this is frequently apparent as palpable purpura. Thus, a search for an underlying disorder should be done in every patient presenting with purpura. One should, however, realize that palpable purpura and leukocytoclastic vasculitis may also be a manifestation of a primary form of vasculitis. A differential diagnostic approach to leukocytoclastic vasculitis is given in Table 3.

III. VASCULITIS LOOK-ALIKE SYNDROMES

Disseminated processes that result in vascular obstruction can simulate vasculitis. This is particular true for embolic phenomena that may also develop palpable purpura. Emboli may arise from cholesterol-containing atheromatous plaques, left atrial myxoma, or valvular vegetations in bacterial endocarditis. Septic infarction is another condition that may mimic vasculitis. Besides, hyperviscosity syndromes sometimes may simulate vasculitis. Proteinaceous material may be deposited in the vessel lumina in conditions such as paraproteinemia. Also, an excessive increase of blood cell elements may result in symptoms or signs that suggest vasculitis, particularly in the extremities. Systemic microangiopathy, as in diffuse intravascular coagulation and thrombotic thrombocytopenic purpura, is a condition that should be distinguished from vasculitis and requires prompt diagnosis and specific treatment. A particular category is the antiphospholipid antibody syndrome (APS). Although a discussion on this syndrome

Table 1 Secondary Vasculitis

Infection-related vasculitis (see also Tables 2 and 3)
Vasculitis secondary to connective tissue disease
Drug hypersensitivity-related vasculitis
Vasculitis secondary to mixed essential cryoglobulinemia (hepatitis C virus?)
Malignancy-related vasculitis
Hypocomplementemic urticarial vasculitis
Post-organ transplant vasculitis

Source: From ref. 8.

Table 2 Antigens that Might Be Involved in Secondary Forms of Vasculitis

- Exogenous antigens
  - microbial antigens
    - bacterial
      - streptococci
      - staphylococci
      - *mycobacterium leprae*
      - *treponema pallidum*
      - others
    - viral
      - hepatitis B/C virus
      - human immunodeficiency virus
      - cytomegalovirus
      - Epstein-Barr virus
      - others
    - protozoal
      - plasmodia
      - nonmicrobial antigens
      - heterologous proteins, e.g. heterologous sera
      - allergens
      - drugs
      - tumor antigens (?)
- Autologous antigens
  - nuclear antigens (antinuclear antibodies)
  - immunoglobulin G (rheumatoid factor, cryoglobulins)
  - others

is beyond the scope of this chapter, it should be remembered that thrombotic conditions and livedo reticularis may occur as part of the APS. Finally, necrosis of the fingertips or toes can occur in severe cases of vasculitis, but it can also occur in the aforementioned disorders and in vasospastic conditions such as (primary) Raynaud's phenomenon and as a result of the use of ergotamines or other drugs. The occurrence of all those vasculitis look-alike syndromes underscores the importance of obtaining a histopathological diagnosis in all cases where vasculitis is suspected.

IV. PRIMARY OR IDIOPATHIC VASCULITIDES

The primary vasculitides constitute a heterogeneous group of disorders, especially with respect to their clinical presentation and symptomatology. As a consequence, the diagnosis of a specific type of vasculitis is not always easy. In many cases, there is a considerable time interval between the initial symptoms and the moment of diagnosis. A diagnosis of vasculitis should be considered in the presence of visible lesions suggestive of vasculitis such as palpable purpura; when characteristic clinical symptoms are present, such as hypereosinophilia and polyneuropathy in the context of a history of asthma as in Churg-Strauss syndrome; in any case of glomerulonephritis; and in the conditions of fever, myalgia, malaise, and raised erythrocyte sedimentation rate (ESR)

Table 3 Leukocytoclastic Vasculitis (LCV): Differential Diagnosis and Associated Conditions

Entities which are manifest by palpable purpura and LCV histopathologically:
idiopathic
Henoch-Schönlein purpura (IgA-related LCV)
non-IgA vasculitis
acute haemorrhagic oedema of infancy
infectious: any infection can be associated, the following are perhaps more common:
streptococcus
hepatitis B/C
influenza
mononucleosis
otitis media
meningococcaemia
gonococcaemia
human immunodeficiency virus
systemic disease:
lupus erythematosus
rheumatoid arthritis
dermatomyositis
chronic active hepatitis
paraproteinaemia
Sjögren's syndrome
scleroderma
inflammatory bowel disease
Wegener's granulomatosis
cystic fibrosis
malignancy ("paraneoplastic vasculitis")
leukemia and lymphoma
multiple myeloma
Hodgkin's disease
solid tumours
drugs and chemicals: any drug can be associated, the following are perhaps more common:
penicillin
quinidine
propylthiouracil
sulfonamides
allopurinol
food additives
Entities which demonstrate LCV histopathologically but may not exhibit palpable purpura:
hypocomplementemic (urticarial) vasculitis
Degos' disease
Erythema elevatum diutinum
Entities which may demonstrate palpable purpura but are not LCV histopathologically:
antiphospholipid syndrome
purpura fulminans
coumarin necrosis
cryofibrinogenemia
atrophie blanche (livedoid vasculitis)
disseminated intravascular coagulopathy
embolic phenomenon:
bacterial endocarditis
atheroemboli
cholesterol emboli
left atrial myxoma

Table 4 Names and Definitions of Vasculitis Adopted by the Chapel Hill Conference on the Nomenclature of Systemic Vasculitis

Large vessel vasculitis[a]	
Giant cell (temporal) arteritis	Granulomatous arteritis of the aorta and its major branches, with a predilection for the extracranial branches of the carotid artery. *Often involves the temporal artery. Usually occurs in patients older than age 50 and often is associated with polymyalgia rheumatica.*
Takayasu's arteritis	Granulomatous inflammation of the aorta and its major branches. *Usually occurs in patients younger than age 50.*
Medium-sized vessel vasculitis[a]	
Polyarteritis nodosa[b] (classic polyarteritis nodosa)	Necrotizing inflammation of medium-sized or small arteries without glomerulonephritis or vasculitis in arterioles, capillaries, or venules
Kawasaki disease	Arteritis involving large, medium-sized, and small arteries, and associated with mucocutaneous lymph node syndrome. *Coronary arteries are often involved. Aorta and veins may be involved. Usually occurs in children.*
Small vessel vasculitis[a]	
Wegener's granulomatosis[c]	Granulomatous inflammation involving the respiratory tract, and necrotizing vasculitis affecting small to medium-sized vessels (e.g., capillaries, venules, arterioles, and arteries). *Necrotizing glomerulonephritis is common.*
Churg-Strauss syndrome[c]	Eosinophil-rich and granulomatous inflammation involving the respiratory tract, and necrotizing vasculitis affecting small to medium-sized vessels, and associated with asthma and eosinophilia.
Microscopic polyangiitis[b] (microscopic polyarteritis)	Necrotizing vasculitis, with few or no immune deposits, affecting small vessels (i.e., capillaries, venules, or arterioles). *Necrotizing arteritis involving small and medium-sized arteritis may be present. Necrotizing glomerulonephritis is very common. Pulmonary capillaritis often occurs.*
Henoch-Schönlein purpura	Vasculitis, with IgA-dominant immune deposits, affecting small vessels (i.e., capillaries, venules, or arterioles). *Typically involves skin, gut, and glomeruli, and is associated with arthralgias or arthritis.*

(*continued*)

Table 4 Continued

Essential cryoglobulinemic vasculitis	Vasculitis, with cryoglobulin immune deposits, affecting small vessels (i.e., capillaries, venules, or arterioles), and associated with cryoglobulins in serum. *Skin and glomeruli are often involved.*
Cutaneous leukocytoclastic angiitis	Isolated cutaneous leukocytoclastic angiitis without systemic vasculitis or glomerulonephritis.

[a]Large vessel refers to the aorta and the largest branches directed toward major body regions (e.g., to the extremities and the head and neck); medium-sized vessel refers to the main visceral arteries (e.g., renal, hepatic, coronary, and mesenteric arteries); small vessel refers to venules, capillaries, arterioles, and the intraparenchymal distal arterial radicals that connect with arterioles. Some small and large vessel vasculitides may involve medium-sized arteries, but large and medium-sized vessel vasculitides do not involve vessels smaller than arteries. Essential components are represented by normal type; italicized type represents usual, but not essential components.
[b]Preferred term.
[c]Strongly associated with antineutrophil cytoplasmic autoantibodies.
Source: From ref. 5.

Table 5 Classification Criteria for Polyarteritis Nodosa

Criterion	Definition
1. Weight loss ≥4 kg	Loss of 4 kg or more of body weight since illness began not due to dieting or other factors.
2. Livedo reticularis	Mottled reticular pattern over the skin of portions of the extremities or torso
3. Testicular pain or tenderness	Pain or tenderness of the testicles not due to infection, trauma, or other causes.
4. Myalgias, weakness, or leg tenderness	Diffuse myalgias (excluding shoulder and hip girdle) or weakness of muscles or tenderness of leg muscles.
5. Mononeuropathy or polyneuropathy	Development of mononeuropathy, multiple mononeuropathies, or polyneuropathy.
6. Diastolic BP >90 mmHg	Development of hypertension with the diastolic BP higher than 90 mmHg.
7. Elevated BUN or creatinine	Elevation of BUN >40 mg/dL or creatinine >1.5 mg/dL not due to dehydration or obstruction.
8. Hepatitis B virus	Presence of hepatitis B surface antigen or antibody in serum.
9. Arteriographic abnormality	Arteriogram showing aneurysms or occlusions of the visceral arteries, not due to arteriosclerosis, fibromuscular dysplasia, or other noninflammatory causes
10. Biopsy of small or medium-sized artery containing PMN	Histological changes showing the presence of granulocytes and/or mononuclear leukocytes in the artery wall

BP, blood pressure; BUN, blood urea nitrogen; PMN, polymorphonuclear neutrophils.
For classification purposes, a patient shall be said to have polyarteritis nodosa if at least 3 of these 10 criteria are present. The presence of any 3 or more criteria yields a sensitivity of 82.2% and a specificity of 86.6%.
Source: From ref. 9.

Table 6 Classification Criteria for Churg-Strauss Syndrome

Criterion	Definition
1. Asthma	History of wheezing or diffuse high-pitched rales on expiration.
2. Eosinophilia	Eosinophilia >10% on white blood cell differential count.
3. Mononeuropathy or polyneuropathy	Development of mononeuropathy, multiple mononeuropathies, or polyneuropathy (i.e., glove/ stocking distribution) attributable to a systemic vasculitis.
4. Pulmonary infiltrates, nonfixed	Migratory or transitory pulmonary infiltrates on radiographs (not including fixed infiltrates), attributable to a systemic vasculitis
5. Paranasal sinus abnormality	History of acute or chronic paranasal sinus pain or tenderness or radiographic opacification of the paranasal sinuses.
6. Extravascular eosinophils	Biopsy including artery, arteriole, or venule showing accumulations of eosinophils in extravascular areas.

For classification purposes, a patient shall be said to have Churg-Strauss syndrome if at least four of these criteria are positive. The presence of any four or more of the six criteria yields a sensitivity of 85% and a specificity of 99.7%.
Source: From ref. 11.

of unknown origin. As discussed before, histopathological proof of vasculitis should be obtained in order to make a diagnosis. Once vasculitis has been demonstrated histopathologically or, in a few cases, by angiography, the vasculitic process should be classified into one or another category.

Recently, an international consensus group [5] has defined the various vasculitides based, in general, on the more or less specific histopathological findings (Table 4). In particular, the size of the vessels involved as well as the character of the inflammatory process underly those definitions. For example, classic polyarteritis nodosa is defined as necrotizing inflammation of medium-sized or small arteries without glomerulonephritis or vasculitis in arterioles, capillaries, or venules. However, in clinical practice, it is almost impossible to rule out the presence of vasculitis in arterioles in a patient suspected of polyarteritis nodosa in whom, for example, biopsy-proven arteritis is found in a muscle biopsy. Thus, although strict definitions for the various vasculitides seem attractive for classification, they are not always applicable in clinical practice. The ACR criteria for the classification of the primary vasculitides are based both on clinical symptoms and histopathology [6,9–15]. Diverse degrees of sensitivity and specificity are reached when those criteria are used to classify patients with vasculitis who were classified in a certain category by expert opinion. Examples of ACR criteria for polyarteritis nodosa and Churg-Strauss syndrome are given in Tables 5 and 6, respectively. It should be realized that many patients with vasculitis present with a few or overlapping symptoms of the various vasculitides and cannot be accurately classified in one of those categories. This underscores the limitations of classification.

V. CONCLUSION

In every patient suspected of vasculitis, histopathological proof of vasculitis should be obtained. Vasculitis look-alike syndromes should be distinguished from real vasculitis. Next, one should approach the question as to whether the vasculitic process is secondary to another condition or a primary idiopathic condition. In the secondary vasculitides, which frequently are immune complex diseases, a search for the antigen(s) involved is of crucial importance for the diagnosis and treatment. When the vasculitic process is considered to be primary, it should be classified in one or another category based on histopathological data and clinical symptoms. Finally, the extension of the process and its activity should be assessed as has been discussed in Chapter 30 on Wegener's granulomatosis. This enables a rational approach to treatment.

REFERENCES

1. Fauci AS, Haynes BF, Katz P. The spectrum of vasculitis: clinical, pathologic, immunologic, and therapeutic considerations. Ann Intern Med 1978; 89:660–676.
2. Alarcón-Segovia D. Classification of the necrotizing vasculitides in man. Clin Rheum Dis 1980; 6:223–231.
3. McCluskey RT, Fienberg R. Vasculitis in primary vasculitides, granulomatoses, and connective tissue diseases. Hum Pathol 1983; 14:305–315.
4. Lie JT. Vasculitis, 1815 to 1991: classification and diagnostic specificity. J Rheumatol 1991; 19:83–89.
5. Jennette JC, Falk RJ, Andrassy K, et al. Nomenclature of systemic vasculitides: the proposal of an international consensus conference. Arthritis Rheum 1994; 37:187–192.
6. Hunder GG, Arend WP, Bloch DA, et al. The American College of Rheumatology 1990 criteria for the classification of vasculitis. Arthritis Rheum 1990; 33:1065–1067.
7. Callen JP, Kallenberg CGM. The vasculitides: relationship of cutaneous vasculitis to systemic disease. In: Kater L, Baart de la Faille H, eds.; Multi-systemic auto-immune diseases: an integrated approach. Amsterdam: Elsevier, 1995:267–297.
8. Lie JT. Nomenclature and classification of vasculitis: plus ça change, plus c'est la même chose. Arthritis Rheum 1994; 37:181–186.
9. Lightfoot Jr RW, Michel BA, Bloch DA, et al. The American College of Rheumatology 1990 criteria for the classification of polyarteritis nodosa. Arthritis Rheum 1990; 33:1088–1093.
10. Leavitt RY, Fauci AS, Bloch DA, et al. The American College of Rheumatology 1990 criteria for the classification of Wegener's granulomatosis. Arthritis Rheum 1990; 33:1101–1107.
11. Masi T, Hunder GG, Lie JT et al: The American College of Rheumatology 1990 criteria for the classification of Churg-Strauss syndrome (allergic granulomatosis and angiitis). Arthritis Rheum 1990; 33:1094–1100.
12. Calabrese LH, Michel BA, Bloch DA, et al: The American College of Rheumatology 1990 criteria for the classification of hypersensitivity vasculitis. Arthritis Rheum 1990; 33:1108–1113.
13. Mills JA, Michel BA, Bloch DA, et al: The American College of Rheumatology 1990 criteria for the classification of Henoch-Schönlein purpura. Arthritis Rheum 1990; 33:1114–1121.
14. Hunder GG, Bloch DA, Michel BA, et al: The American College of Rheumatology 1990 criteria for the classification of giant cell arteritis. Arthritis Rheum 1990; 33:1122–1128.
15. Arend WP, Michel BA, Bloch DA, et al: The American College of Rheumatology 1990 criteria for the classification of Takayasu arteritis. Arthritis Rheum 1990; 33:1129–1135.

30

Therapy of Wegener's Granulomatosis

C. G. M. Kallenberg
University Hospital Groningen, Groningen, The Netherlands

I. INTRODUCTION

Wegener's granulomatosis (WG) belongs to the group of idiopathic systemic vasculitides (see Chapter 29). Its incidence has been estimated as 10 per million per year. The disease owes its name to Friedrich Wegener, a German pathologist, who described the histopathology in 1937 [1]. In its classic, extended form,WG is characterized by necrotizing granulomatous inflammation of the upper and lower airways, systemic vasculitis, and necrotizing crescentic glomerulonephritis without immune deposits. Limited forms of the disease do, however, also occur. In limited WG, renal lesions are not apparent and the disease may manifest with (upper) airway symptoms only. Although the symptomatology of the full-blown disease is highly characteristic and enables it diagnosis in many cases, the diagnosis frequently is not apparent in its initial phase, during which the disease generally follows an indolent course [2]. Recurrent or persistent sinusitis or otitis, arthralgia, and mononeuritis, frequently accompanied by general malaise, may be presenting symptoms not recognized as being manifestations of WG in evolution.

The diagnosis of WG is based on characteristic histopathological findings in combination with clinical symptoms. As part of an attempt to define the idiopathic systemic vasculitides, an international consensus conference recently has described WG as a condition with granulomatous inflammation involving the respiratory tract in combination with necrotizing vasculitis affecting small to medium-sized vessels; necrotizing glomerulonephritis, to be considered as small vessel vasculitis of the kidney, frequently occurs [3]. In order to establish a diagnosis that strictly fullfils this definition, biopsy specimens displaying pathognomonic findings should be obtained both from the respiratory tract (showing granulomatous inflammation) and from other sites (showing necrotizing vasculitis or glomerulonephritis). In clinical practice, this goal cannot be accomplished in many of the patients. For this reason, the American College of

Rheumatologists (ACR) has proposed a set of classification criteria for WG which are based on clinical symptoms as well as on histopathological findings compatible with WG [4] (Table 1). One should, however, realize that the ACR classification criteria are based on the assumption that vasculitis has already been demonstrated in the patient either by histopathology or by angiography. Thus, the ACR criteria should not be used as diagnostic criteria but only for the purpose of classifying a patient with proven vasculitis.

The diagnosis of WG has been facilitated by the discovery of autoantibodies that occur in the sera of most of the patients with active disease. The antibodies are directed to cytoplasmic constituents of myeloid cells and are designated as antineutrophil cytoplasmic antibodies (ANCAs) [5]. By indirect immunofluorescence on ethanol-fixed neutrophils, most WG sera (85%) show a characteristic cytoplasmic fluorescence pattern (c-ANCA) which is produced by antibodies to proteinase 3, a serine protease from the azurophilic granule (Fig. 1). A minority (15%) of WG sera produce a perinuclear fluorescence pattern on the aforementioned substrate (p-ANCA) which, in almost all of the cases, is produced by antibodies to myeloperoxidase and, incidentally, to elastase or bactericidal permeability increasing protein [5–7] (Fig 1; Table 2). The specificity of antibodies to proteinase 3 has been found as high as 98% for WG when sera were studied from patients with a wide variety of renal, autoimmune, vasculitic, infectious, or lymphoproliferative disorders. It should, however, be realized that anti–proteinase 3 antibodies are also detected in patients with overlapping symptoms of WG and other forms of vasculitis and in some patients with idiopathic necrotizing glomerulonephritis without systemic involvement [5]. Some of these patients will evolve into definite, extended WG suggesting that the autoantibodies are already present in an early phase of the disease. In addition, levels of anti–proteinase 3 antibodies in many cases rise preceding a relapse of WG [8], and changes in levels of those antibodies may be a guideline for treatment [9]. These and other in vitro and in vivo experimental data suggest that the antibodies are directly involved in the pathophysiology of WG [5,10]. This fact will be dealt with in more detail later on in this chapter when experimental ways of treatment are discussed.

Table 1 1990 ACR Criteria for the Classification of Wegener's Granulomatosis[a]

Criteria	Definition
1. Nasal or oral inflammation	Development of painful or painless oral ulcers or purulent or bloody nasal discharge.
2. Abnormal chest radiograph	Chest radiograph showing the presence of nodules, fixed infiltrates, or cavities.
3. Urinary sediment	Microhematuria (>5 red blood cells per high power field) or red cells casts in urine sediment
4. Granulomatous inflammation on biopsy	Histological changes showing granulomatous inflammation within the wall of an artery or in the perivascular or extravascular area (artery or arteriole)

[a]For purposes of classification, a patient shall be said to have Wegener's granulomatosis if at least two of the four criteria are present. The presence of any two or more criteria yields a sensitivity of 88.2% and a specificity of 92.0%.

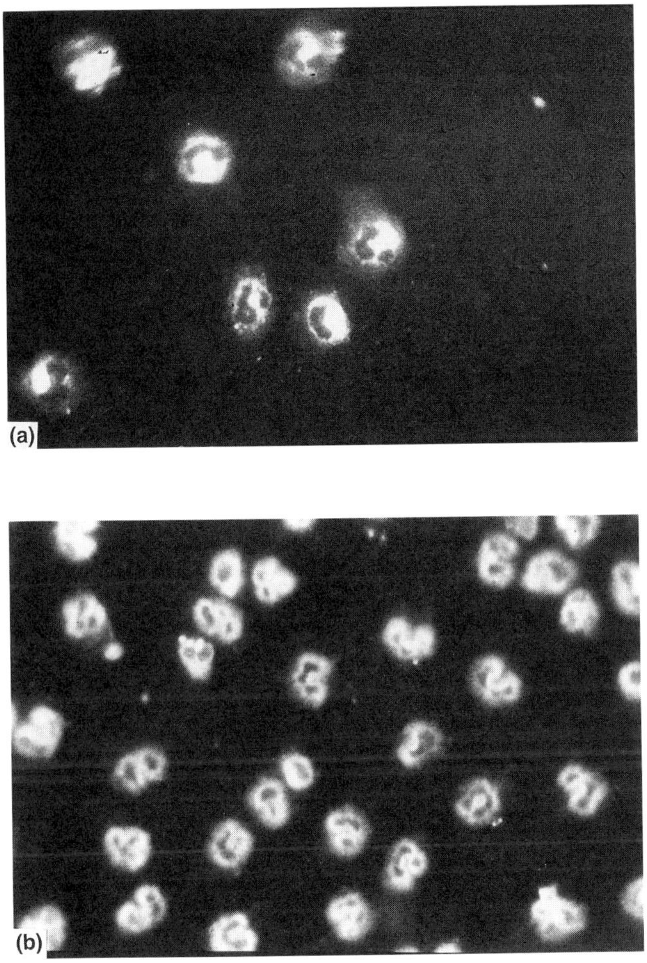

Figure 1 Staining of ethanol-fixed neutrophils by indirect immunofluorescence by sera producing (a) a characteristic cytoplasmic staining pattern with accentuation of the fluorescence intensity in the area within the nuclear lobes (c-ANCA) and (b) a perinuclear staining pattern (p-ANCA).

Table 2 Disease Associations of Antiproteinase 3 Antibodies and Antimyeloperoxidase Antibodies

	Sensitivity of	
Disease entity	Antiproteinase 3 (%)	Antimyeloperoxidase (%)
Wegener's granulomatosis	85	10
Microscopic polyangiitis	45	45
Idiopathic crescentic glomerulonephritis	25	65
Churg-Strauss syndrome	10	60
Polyarteritis nodosa	5	15

Taken together, WG can, at present, be considered to be an idiopathic systemic inflammatory disease with a probably autoimmune background characterized by granulomatous and necrotizing inflammation and widespread vasculitis frequently involving the kidneys as well. Untreated, the disease follows a rapid down-hill course with an average survival of only 5 months after diagnosis [11]. This forms the rationale for current treatment modalities which aim not only at the induction of remission but also at maintenance of remission once induction has been successful. In this chapter I will focus on established treatment modalities for the induction and maintenance of remission, the treatment of refractory cases as well as on experimental ways of treatment based on new insights into the pathophysiology of the disease. Before doing so, I will discuss the assessment of disease activity, which is important for the evaluation of the effects of treatment.

II. ASSESSING DISEASE ACTIVITY IN WG

When evaluating treatment in idiopathic systemic diseases like WG, it is not only important to use strict criteria for diagnosis but also to define the extent and activity of the disease in a standardized way. In a number of previous studies relating serological data to clinical disease activity, we have used definitions for relapses of the disease, in fact, based on the intention to treat (Table 3) [8,9,12-15]. The manifestations in question had to be new or recurrent findings not related to infection, side effects of drugs, or other identifiable causes. However, in clinical practice, it is not always easy to distinguish between disease activity of WG and infection; in particular when the manifestations are localized in the (upper) airways. Specialized ear, nose, and throat (ENT) examinations, including biopsies and cultures, may be necessary in order to establish or exclude the disease activity of WG. Besides disease activity, remission has to be defined. In the aforementioned studies [8,9,12–15], it was described as the absence of

Table 3 Definitions for Major and Minor Relapses of Wegener's Granulomatosis

Major relapses[a]: The patient should fulfill one or more of the following factors
- decrease of creatinine clearance of more than 30% within a period of 3 months or less in combination with erythrocyturia
- pulmonary infiltrates on chest radiograph in combination with dyspnea and rising CRP
- cerebral vasculitis
- motor and sensory nerve disturbances with rising CRP
- cranial nerve palsy with rising CRP
- orbital pseudotumor
- necrotizing scleritis
- tracheal stenosis with severe dyspnea
- myocardial infarction due to vasculitis
- acute abdomen or massive gastrointestinal hemorrhage due to vasculitis
- progressive disease despite treatment of minor relapses with prednisolone 30 mg and cyclophosphamide 75 mg for at least 2 weeks

Minor relapses[a]: Increase of the disease activity index [12] score of five points or more within a period of 3 months and without fulfilling the criteria for a major exacerbation

[a]Any manifestation is considered only in the absence of other concomitant conditions that may be related to that manifestation and should occur as a new or recurrent finding.

signs or symptoms attributable to active vasculitic disease in combination with a normal C-reactive protein (CRP) level.

In order to evaluate the effects of treatment, disease activity criteria have been defined in which scores are given to individual symptoms and signs. The sum of those scores is considered as the disease activity score. Those scoring systems should be validated by comparing their results with the global assessment of a number of physicians highly experienced in the treatment of patients with the given disorder. As for WG, we have proposed a disease activity score that is based both on the extent of the disease and the severity of the individual manifestations [12]. This scoring system, which was particularly developed for WG, is based on objective findings only and tries to distinguish between infection and disease activity by requiring histological proof of disease activity in certain organs. It proved to be useful in assessing disease activity in a number of studies [13,16]. Other groups have used different activity scores. The ELK-classification (ENT-lung-kidney) proposed by De Remee et al. [17] particularly focuses on the localization of the disease symptoms. As for systemic vasculitis in general, Luqmani et al. [18] have developed the Birmingham Vasculitis Activity System (BVAS), which now has been validated by different centers. This scoring system has now been applied to multicenter therapeutic studies in systemic vasculitis that have been started within a European network sponsored by the European community [19]. The value in clinical practice of the various disease activity indices should be proven in further studies. In order to assess damage resulting from previous episodes of disease activity, side effects of drugs, and from other conditions, the Birmingham group also has proposed a chronicity index.

Also, laboratory tests may prove to be useful as parameters of disease activity during long-term follow-up of patients with WG. Levels of acute phase proteins such as CRP reflect the systemic inflammatory process of WG but are not specific for the disease (Fig. 2). They also rise in response to infection. Many other laboratory tests, such as soluble interleukine-2 receptor levels [14] and levels of soluble adhesion molecules [13], have been shown to reflect changing patterns in disease activity. In general, they are neither sensitive nor specific. A number of studies have shown that levels of c-ANCA parallel or even precede disease activity of WG [8,9,20,21] (see Fig. 2), although this association has not been confirmed by others [22]. Taken together, the disease activity of WG should be assessed clinically, the distinction between infection and disease activity needs careful consideration, and rising titers of c-ANCA or proteinase 3 antibodies should alert the clinician to a possibly ensuing relapse.

III. INDUCTION OF REMISSION

Once active WG, either in its initial presentation or in relapse, has been diagnosed, treatment should be instituted immediately, as the disease frequently runs a rapid downhill course. Indeed, before corticosteroids and immunosuppressives were available, the average survival time of patients with WG amounted no more than 5 months [11]. Although giving subjective improvement and definite amelioration of extrarenal symptoms, corticosteroids alone have improved the average survival time only from 5.0 to 12.5 months [11], as many cases progress to end-stage renal failure or show a fatal outcome due to extrarenal, particularly pulmonary, involvement. The introduction of cyclophosphamide has been a major advance in the treatment of the systemic necrotiz-

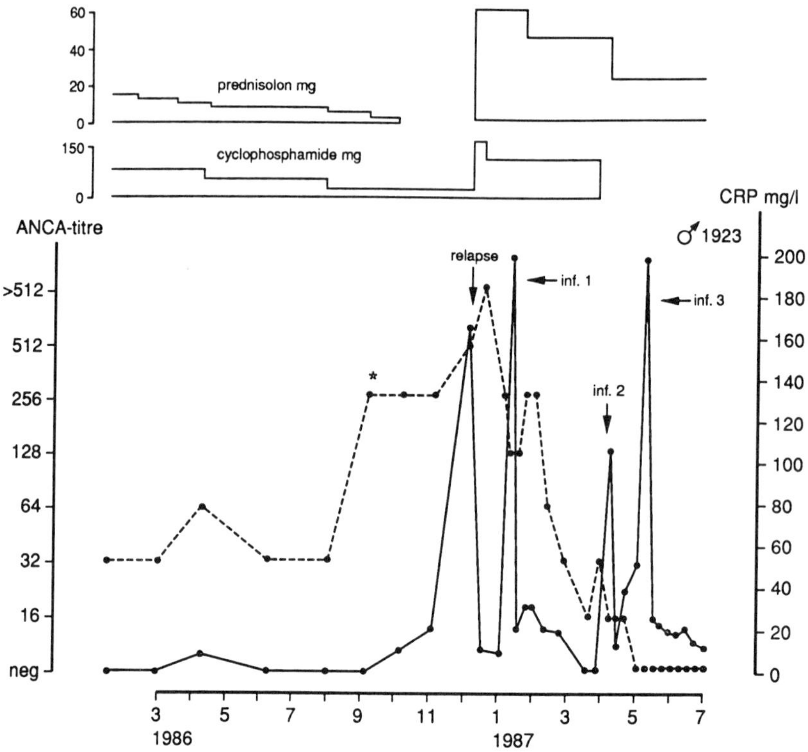

Figure 2 Antineutrophil cytoplasmic antibody (ANCA) titers (dotted line), levels of C-reactive protein (CRP; solid line), and relapsing disease activity in a patient with Wegener's granulomatosis. After a significant rise in the ANCA titer occurred in September 1986, a clinical relapse was diagnosed in December 1986, coinciding with a rise in level of C-reactive protein. During immunosuppressive treatment, ANCA titers decreased, whereas levels of C-reactive protein increased another three times concomitantly with three episodes of infection. In March 1987, cyclophosphamide treatment was discontinued because of *Pneumocystis carinii* pneumonia and cytomegalovirus infection. Asterisk indicates significant rise of ANCA titer.

ing vasculitides as shown by the studies of the US National Institutes of Health (NIH) [23,24]. In its first report NIH mentioned complete remission in 14 of 17 patients with severe vasculitis [23]. With respect to WG, the NIH regimen, consisting of oral cyclophosphamide in combination with prednisone, resulted in complete remission in 79 of 85 patients [24]. Based on these studies, the standard regimen for induction of remission in WG now consists of cyclophosphamide 2–3 mg/kg/day orally in combination with prednisone 1 mg/kg/day orally. Besides the well-known side effects of high-dose corticosteroids (which necessitates careful observation and the prophylactic use of H_2-receptor antagonists such as ranitidine as well as calcium suppletion), special attention should be given to the development of cytopenias, in particular leukopenia, as a result of cyclophosphamide treatment. As the median age of presentation of WG is rather high (around 55 years of age), leukopenia may develop in many patients and constitutes, together with high-dose corticosteroids, a major risk factor for the occurrence of opportunistic infections. Indeed, a recent study from France [25] showed serious infections with *Pneumocystis carinii* or, to a lesser extent, cytomegalovirus infection, in 9 of 16 patients with WG during induction treatment. Based on these findings, the investigators advocated the prophylactic use of trimethoprim-sulfamethoxazole 960 mg twice daily during treatment with cyclophosphamide in patients with WG. Although this high rate of opportunistic infections has not been mentioned by the NIH group [11] and others [26], careful monitoring of the peripheral blood leukocyte count is of utmost importance. Dose adjustments for cyclophosphamide have to be made to maintain the white blood cell count above 4×10^9/L.

The occurrence of life-threatening opportunistic infections during oral cyclophosphamide treatment [25,26], as well as the other side effects such as hemorrhagic cystitis, occurring in 15% of patients [27], the late development of bladder carcinoma (in 3% of patients [27]) and other malignancies, and the induction of infertility, have caused physicians to use intermittent intravenous pulse cyclophosphamide instead of oral cyclophosphamide. In proliferative lupus nephritis, intravenous pulse cyclophosphamide has been proven to be as effective as its oral administration, whereas the frequency of adverse effects appeared to be reduced considerably [28]. In WG, however, the NIH group described a less favorable therapeutic effect of intravenous versus oral cyclophosphamide [29]. In ANCA-positive glomerulonephritis and systemic vasculitis, including WG, Falk et al. [30] found no differences in renal or patient survival between both regimens. A controlled study from the United Kingdom also showed that pulse and oral cyclophosphamide are equally effective in inducing remission in patients with systemic vasculitis [31]. It is, nevertheless, our impression that oral cyclophosphamide is superior to intravenous pulse cyclophosphamide when the NIH lupus nephritis protocol (i.e., 0.5–1.0 g/m^2 every 4 weeks) is used. Future studies should prove whether a more intense schedule with intravenous pulses every 2 weeks is equally effective as the oral administration and still has the advantage of fewer side effects.

Both the NIH group [11] and most European groups reach remission with the oral cyclophosphamide/corticosteroid regimen in some 75% of the patients with (generalized) WG (European Community Concerted Action Group for the Study of Therapeutic Trials in Systemic Vasculitis [19], personal communication). Thus, 25% of the patients require additional treatment in order to induce remission. Whereas the treatment of refractory cases will be discussed later on in this chapter, two additional treatment modalities will be discussed here. The first relates to the use of high-dose intravenous corticosteroids (1 g of methylprednisolone on 3 consecutive days). Although controlled studies are lacking, many clinicians consider pulse steroids to be useful in severe cases of WG. The second modality concerns plasmapheresis. A controlled study on the additional role of plasma exchange in the initial treatment of patients with necrotizing glomerulonephritis without anti-GBM antibodies (many of whom had generalized WG) was published in 1991 [32]. Included were patients with impaired renal function, crescentic necrotizing glomerulonephritis in the biopsy, and a clinical diagnosis of either WG, microscopic polyangiitis, or idiopathic rapidly progressive glomerulonephritis. Forty-eight cases could be analyzed, of whom 23 were treated with immunosuppressives only and 25 with additional plasma exchange. Only in patients who were dialysis dependent at presentation ($n = 19$) was an additional benefit of plasma exchange observed: 10 of 11 patients treated with additional plasma exchange recovered from renal failure, whereas only 3 patients recovered of 8 patients treated with immunosuppressives alone. A comparable beneficial effect has been found for the additional use of methylprednisolone in patients with rapidly progressive glomerulonephritis, either idiopathic or WG associated, who were dialysis dependent at presentation [33]. Thus, either plasma exchange or pulse methylprednisolone can be added to the oral regimen described before in patients with WG who present with acute renal failure.

A number of other, less toxic treatment modalities have been proposed for WG. None, however, is based on prospective controlled studies. Two regimens will be discussed briefly, as they may prove important in the future. Trimethoprim-sulfamethoxazole has been mentioned as being an effective agent in the treatment of WG, particularly in those with airway involvement as the main finding [34]. A prospective study in 17 patients with limited WG recently showed a response rate of 65% [35]. This means of treatment is not advocated in generalized WG. The use of trimethoprim-sulfamethoxazole in the prevention of relapses of WG will be discussed later on. The NIH recently reported on the results of prednisone combined with methotrexate for the treatment of patients with WG without life-threatening disease [36]. Weekly administration of methotrexate in a dosage up to 20–25 mg in combination with prednisone 1 mg/kg daily resulted in remission in 30 of the 42 patients. The median time to remission was 4.2 months. Further studies should demonstrate whether methotrexate is a good alternative for cyclophosphamide in a selected group of WG patients.

IV. MAINTENANCE TREATMENT

In the original reports from the NIH, prolonged courses of cyclophosphamide for up to 2 years were advocated in order to prevent the occurrence of relapses. Corticosteroids are tapered by most clinicians once a remission is induced. Our own approach [9] consists of tapering cyclophosphamide by 25-mg decrements every 3 months. The dosage of prednisolone is tapered by 5-mg decrements every 2 weeks. In some cases, a low dose of prednisolone (5–10 mg/day) is continued; in particular when constitutional symptoms and other minor signs of disease activity persist. It has already been mentioned that long-term cyclophosphamide treatment is associated with serious toxicities. For this reason, conversion from cyclophosphamide to azathioprine 2 months after induction of remission has been proposed by clinicians in the United Kingdom. In their experience, relapse rates are not higher with azathioprine compared with cyclophosphamide. Recently, the European Community Concerted Action Group for the Study of Therapeutic Trials in Systemic Vasculitis (ECSYSVASTRIAL) has started a randomized trial of cyclophosphamide versus azathioprine for the maintenance of remission in systemic vasculitis. Besides immunosuppressives, trimethoprim-sulfamethoxazole (TS) has been used in WG to prevent the occurrence of relapses. The use of this antibiotic drug is first based on its therapeutic effect in a number of cases of WG [34], especially when symptoms are restricted to the extrarenal regions [35]. Second, it is based on the observation that relapses of WG occur more frequently in patients who are chronic nasal carriers of *Staphylococcus aureus* [15]. In a prospective randomized placebo-controlled study with TS, 800/160 mg bid, during 24 months in 81 patients with WG, it proved that 7 of 41 patients assigned to TS relapsed compared with 16 of 40 patients assigned to placebo (relative risk 0.40) [37]. In addition, a reduction in the number of respiratory and nonrespiratory infections was found with TS as compared with placebo [37]. Thus, prolonged treatment with TS is effective in reducing the incidence of relapses in

WG. Whether treatment should only be directed at the elimination of *Staphylococcus aureus* carriage is still under investigation.

Another way to prevent relapses has been suggested by Cohen Tervaert et al. [9]. As discussed before, the majority of patients with WG have autoantibodies directed against proteinase 3 which produce a cytoplasmic fluorescence pattern on ethanol-fixed neutrophils (c-ANCA). Rises of c-ANCA titers precede the development of clinical relapses of WG in many cases. Based on these findings, a controlled prospective study was performed in which patients were assigned to treatment or no treatment once a significant rise of ANCA had occurred [9]. Treatment based on rises of ANCA titer appeared to prevent relapses of WG in this study on a small number of patients. These data have to be confirmed by studies on a larger group of patients.

V. TREATMENT OF REFRACTORY CASES

As stated before, conventional treatment of active WG with cyclophosphamide and corticosteroids may not be sufficient in fulminant cases. In those conditions, particularly when acute renal failure develops, either intravenous methylprednisolone pulses or plasma exchange can be added to the aforementioned regimen [32,33]. In some 10–20% of cases, however, this combined treatment also fails to induce remission either because the complete regimen is not effective or because the patient does not tolerate this regimen owing to leukopenia or other causes. Several new approaches have recently been proposed for those refractory cases. Two of them will be described here; namely, the use of high-dose intravenous immunoglobulin and the administration of monoclonal antibodies to lymphocytes.

A. Intravenous Gamma Globulin

Intravenous gamma globulin (IVIg) therapy has been tried in an increasing number of autoimmune diseases. Originally used in autoimmune thrombocytopenia in order to block or saturate Fc receptor–mediated clearance of antibody-coated platelets, IVIg might also exert its effect by the presence in the preparation of anti-idiotypic antibodies which interact with the idiotypic network. Anti-idiotypic antibodies reactive to ANCA have indeed been detected in pooled human immunoglobulin and in the sera from patients with ANCA-positive vasculitis drawn during remission [38]. Preliminary data on seven patients suggest that IVIg infused at 0.4 g/kg/day on five consecutive days may have a beneficial effect in patients with ANCA-positive vasculitis resulting not only in clinical improvement but also in some 50% reduction in levels of ANCAs [39]. It should be mentioned that none of the seven patients had rapidly progressive glomerulonephritis. Very recently, Jayne and Lockwood (personal communication) have treated 26 patients with systemic vasculitis refractory to conventional treatment with IVIg [40]. By 2 months, 50% of the patients had full remission and the remainder had partial remission. After 1 year of follow-up, 19 of 26 patients were in remission, 6 were in partial remission, and 1 had died as a result of sepsis. Thus, at present, IVIg may be used as compassionate treatment in selected cases of WG, but its clinical usefulness should be demonstrated by future controlled prospective studies.

B. Monoclonal Antibodies

Inflammatory lesions of the lung and kidney in WG are characterized by large mononuclear infiltrates containing monocytes and T lymphocytes, with a majority of CD4-positive cells [41,42]. The antigenic specificities of those T cells are not known, but peripheral blood lymphocytes reactive to ANCA antigens such as proteinase 3 and myeloperoxidase (MPO) have been described [43,44]. In a patient with long-standing unclassified vasculitis, treatment with the combination of two monoclonal antibodies, one directed against an antigen present on all mononuclear cells (CDw52) and the other against the CD4 molecule, resulted in long-lasting clinical remission, whereas injection of the first antibody alone induced a short-lived remission only [45]. Two additional patients with microscopic polyangiitis unresponsive to conventional treatment were treated with a comparable regimen; long-lasting remission was reached in one patient and the other developed antibodies to the humanized anti-CDw52 monoclonal antibody [46]. At present, 11 patients with either T-cell–associated vasculitis or ANCA-associated vasculitis have been treated. Improvement of vasculitic lesions without serious side effects was reported. Prospective, controlled studies are awaited. Besides this regimen, antithymocyte globulin has been used in refractory cases of WG [47]. Improvement of granulomatous lesions was observed, but again the value of this treatment should be demonstrated by further studies.

VI. CONCLUSIONS

Standard induction treatment of WG still consists of cyclophosphamide (2 mg/kg/day orally) in combination with prednisone (1 mg/kg/day orally). When the patient presents with acute renal failure, either intravenous pulses of methylprednisolone (1 g on 3 consecutive days) or plasma exchange should be added to this regimen. Maintenance treatment consists of cyclophosphamide, but conversion to azathioprine might prove to be effective and less toxic. For limited WG localized to the (upper) airways, only either methotrexate in combination with prednisone or, possibly, trimethoprim-sulfamethoxazole may be an alternative. The latter drug also is effective in reducing the number of relapses. Otherwise, relapses may be prevented by instituting (low-dose) immunosuppressive drugs once a rise in levels of ANCA has occurred. For cases of WG refractory to the aforementioned treatment, several regimens are now available, which, however, should prove their value in prospective controlled studies. These as well as other therapeutic studies are presently performed within the European network for the study of vasculitis.

REFERENCES

1. Wegener F. Über eine eigenartige rhinogene Granulomatose mit besonderen Beteiligung des Arteriensystems und der Nieren. Beitr Path Anat 1939; 102:36–68.
2. Cohen Tervaert JW, van der Woude FJ, Kallenberg CGM. De ziekte van Wegener: een ernstige aandoening met een sluipend begin. Ned Tijdschr Geneesk 1987; 131:1391–1394.
3. Jennette JC, Falk RJ, Andrassy K, et al. Nomenclature of systemic vasculitides: the proposal of an international consensus conference. Arthritis Rheum 1994; 37:187–192.
4. Leavitt RY, Fauci AS, Bloch DA, et al. The American College of Rheumatology 1990 cri-

teria for the classification of Wegener's granulomatosis. Arthritis Rheum 1990; 33:1101–1107.
5. Kallenberg CGM, Brouwer E, Weening JJ, Cohen Tervaert JW. Anti-neutrophil cytoplasmic antibodies: current diagnostic and pathophysiological potential. Kidney Int 1994; 46:1–15.
6. Cohen Tervaert JW, Mulder AHL, Stegeman CA, et al. The occurrence of autoantibodies to human leukocyte elastase in Wegener's granulomatosis and other inflammatory disorders. Ann Rheum Dis 1993; 52:115–120.
7. Zhao MH, Jones SJ, Lockwood CM. Bactericidal/permeability-increasing protein (BPI) is an important antigen for anti-neutrophil cytoplasmic autoantibodies (ANCA) in vasculitis. Clin Exp Immunol 1995; 99:49–56.
8. Cohen Tervaert JW, van der Woude FJ, Fauci AS, et al. Association between active Wegener's granulomatosis and anticytoplasmic antibodies. Arch Intern Med 1989; 149:2461–2465.
9. Cohen Tervaert JW, Huitema MG, Hené RJ, et al. Prevention of relapses in Wegener's granulomatosis by treatment based on antineutrophil cytoplasmic antibody titre. Lancet 1990; 336:709–711.
10. Kallenberg CGM, Brouwer E, Mulder AHL, et al. ANCA—pathophysiology revisited (review). Clin Exp Immunol 1995; 100:1–3.
11. Hoffman GS, Kerr GS, Leavitt KY, et al. Wegener granulomatosis: an analysis of 158 patients. Ann Intern Med 1992; 116:488–498.
12. Kallenberg CGM, Cohen Tervaert JW, Stegeman CA. Criteria for disease activity in Wegener's granulomatosis: a requirement for longitudinal clinical studies. APMIS 1990; 98 (Suppl 19):37–39.
13. Stegeman CA, Cohen Tervaert JW, Huitema MG, et al. Serum levels of soluble adhesion molecules intercellular adhesion molecule 1, vascular cell adhesion molecule 1, and E-selectin in patients with Wegener's granulomatosis. Relationship to disease activity and relevance during follow-up. Arthritis Rheum 1994; 37:1228–1235.
14. Stegeman CA, Cohen Tervaert JW, Huitema MG, Kallenberg CGM. Serum markers of T-cell activation in relapses of Wegener's granulomatosis. Clin Exp Immunol 1993; 91:415–420.
15. Stegeman CA, Cohen Tervaert JW, Manson WL, Kallenberg CGM. Chronic nasal carriage of Staphylococcus aureus in Wegener's granulomatosis: identification of a subgroup more prone to relapses. Ann Intern Med 1994; 120:12–17.
16. Dolman KM, Stegeman CA, Wiel BA van de, et al. Relevance of classic anti-neutrophil cytoplasmic autoantibody (c-ANCA)-mediated inhibition of proteinase 3-α_1-antitrypsin complexation to disease activity in Wegener's granulomatosis. Clin Exp Immunol 1993; 93:405–410.
17. DeRemee RA, McDonald TJ, Harrison EG Jr, Coles DT. Wegener's granulomatosis: anatomic correlates, a proposed classification. Mayo Clin Proc 1976; 51:777–781.
18. Luqmani RA, Bacon PA, Moots RJ, et al. Birmingham Vasculitis Activity Score (BVAS) in systemic necrotizing vasculitis. Q J Med 1994; 87:671–678.
19. Rasmussen N on behalf of the European Community Study Group on Clinical Trials in Systemic Vasculitis. Consensus therapeutic regimens for ANCA-associated systemic vasculitis. Lancet 1997; 349:1029–1030.
20. Egner W, Chapel HM. Titration of antibodies against neutrophil cytoplasmic antigens is useful in monitoring disease activity in systemic vasculitides. Clin Exp Immunol 1990; 82:244–249.
21. Jayne DRW, Gaskin G, Pusey CD, Lockwood CM. ANCA and predicting relapse in systemic vasculitis. Q J Med 1995; 88:127–133.
22. Kerr GR, Fleischer THA, Hallahan CW, et al. Limited prognostic value of changes in

antineutrophil cytoplasmic antibody titer in patients with Wegener's granulomatosis. Arthritis Rheum 1993; 36:365–371.
23. Fauci AS, Katz P, Haynes BF, Wolff SM. Cyclophosphamide therapy of severe systemic necrotizing vasculitis. N Engl J Med 1979; 301:235–238.
24. Fauci AS, Haynes BF, Katz P, Wolff SM: Wegener's granulomatosis: prospective clinical and therapeutic experience with 85 patients for 21 years. Ann Intern Med 1983; 98:76–85.
25. Quillevin L, Lhote F, Jarrousse B, et al. Treatment of severe Wegener's granulomatosis: a prospective trial in 50 patients comparing prednisone (CS), pulse cyclophosphamide (CY) versus CS and oral CY. Clin Exp Immunol 1995; 101 (Suppl 1):43.
26. Bradley JD, Brandt KD, Katz BP. Infectious complications of cyclophosphamide treatment for vasculitis. Arthritis Rheum 1989; 32:45–53.
27. Stillwell ThJ, Benson RC, DeRemee RA, et al. Cyclophosphamide-induced bladder toxicity in Wegener's granulomatosis. Arthritis Rheum 1988; 31:465–470.
28. Balow JE, Austin HA, Tsokos CG, et al. Lupus nephritis. Ann Intern Med 1987; 106:79–94.
29. Hoffman GS, Leavitt RY, Fleisher THA, et al. Treatment of Wegener's granulomatosis with intermittent high-dose intravenous cyclophosphamide. Am J Med 1990; 89:403–410.
30. Falk RJ, Hogan S, Carey TS, Jennette JC. Clinical course of anti-neutrophil cytoplasmic autoantibody-associated glomerulonephritis and systemic vasculitis. Ann Intern Med 1990; 113:656–663.
31. Adu D, Pall A, Luqmani RA, et al. Controlled trial of treatment of vasculitis. Q J Med 1995;
32. Pusey CD, Rees AJ, Evans DJ, et al. Plasma exchange in focal necrotizing glomerulonephritis without anti-GBM antibodies. Kidney Int 1991; 40:757–763.
33. Bolton WK, Sturgill BC. Methylprednisolone therapy for acute crescentic rapidly progressive nephritis. Am J Nephrol 1989; 9:368–375.
34. DeRemee RA. The treatment of Wegener's Granulomatosis with trimethoprim/sulfamethoxazole: illusion or vision? Arthritis Rheum 1988; 31:1068–1072.
35. Reinhold-Keller E, De Groot K, Rudert H, et al. Response to trimethoprim/sulfamethoxazole in Wegener's granulomatosis depends on the phase of disease Q J Med 1996; 89:15–23.
36. Hoffman GS, Leavitt RY, Kerr GS, Fauci AS. The treatment of Wegener's granulomatosis with glucocorticoids and methotrexate. Arthritis Rheum 1992; 35:1322–1329.
37. Stegeman CA, Cohen Tervaert JW, de Jong PE, Kallenberg CGM. Trimethoprim/sulfamethoxazole (cotrimoxazole) for the prevention of relapses of Wegener's granulomatosis. New Eng J Med 1996; 335:16–20.
38. Rossi F, Jayne DRW, Lockwood CM, Kazatchkine MD. Anti-idiotypes against antineutrophil cytoplasmic antigen autoantibodies in normal human polyspecific IgG for therapeutic use and in the remission sera of patients with systemic vasculitis. Clin Exp Immunol 1991; 83:298–303.
39. Jayne DRW, Davies MJ, Fox CJV, et al. Treatment of systemic vasculitis with pooled intravenous immunoglobulin. Lancet 1991; 337:1137–1139.
40. Lockwood CM. New treatment strategies for systemic vasculitis: the role of intravenous immune globulin therapy. Clin Exp Immunol 1996; 104(Suppl 1): 77–82.
41. Gephardt GN, Ahmed M, Tubbs RR. Pulmonary vasculitis (Wegener's granulomatosis). Immunohistochemical study of T and B cell markers. Am J Med 1983; 74:700–704.
42. ten Berge RJM, Wilmink JM, Meyer CJLM, et al. Clinical and immunological follow-up in patients with severe renal disease in Wegener's granulomatosis. Am J Nephrol 1985; 5:21–29.
43. Brouwer E, Stegeman CA, Huitema MG, et al. T-cell reactivity to proteinase 3 and myeloperoxidase in patients with Wegener's granulomatosis. Clin Exp Immunol 1994; 98:448-453.
44. Mathieson PW, Oliveira DBG. The role of cellular immunity in systemic vasculitis. Clin Exp Immunol 1995; 100:183–185.

45. Mathieson PW, Cobbold SP, Hale G, et al. Monoclonal-antibody therapy in systemic vasculitis. N Engl J Med 1990; 323:250–254.
46. Lockwood CM, Thiru S, Isaacs JD, et al. Long-term remission of intractable systemic vasculitis with monoclonal antibody therapy. Lancet 1993; 341:1620–1622.
47. Hagen EC, de Keizer RJW, Andrassy K, et al. Compassionate treatment of Wegener's granulomatosis with rabbit anti-thymocyte globulin. Clin Nephrol 1995; 43:351–359.

31

Therapy of Other Vasculitis Syndromes

George D. Kitas
Dudley NHS Trust, and the University of Birmingham, Birmingham, United Kingdom

Paul A. Bacon and Raashid Luqmani*
The University of Birmingham, Birmingham, United Kingdom

I. INTRODUCTION

Interest—and advances—in the therapy of vasculitis has followed behind the increased clinical recognition of these syndromes and ideas about their pathogenesis. Once it was easy to dismiss vasculitis as "so rare it is not worth bothering about." Over the past 100 years, the accelerating frequency of diagnosis has been accompanied by improved recognition of different syndromes split off from the bulk label of "polyarteritis." The concept of vasculitis as an autoimmune disease has led to more successful attempts to control its high mortality, and induction of remission is now the norm. This encourages study of the differences in treatment response between the various conditions and allows time to devise rational long-term therapies. In time, this should lead to specific treatment based on the activity and range of organ involvement in a particular syndrome; that is, tailored to the individual patient. To achieve this, we require detailed assessment of disease status and better understanding of disease mechanisms.

II. HISTORICAL PERSPECTIVE

Vasculitis in the 19th century was regarded as a rare disease with high mortality. It is not a coincidence that the first descriptions of both polyarteritis nodosa (PAN) and Wegener's granulomatosis (WG) were from postmortem studies. In the early 20th century, the increasing use of routine pathology and the recognition of small vessel involvement led to descriptions of far more cases, often of diverse presentation. This led to the initial attempts of classification, with some separation of milder cases such as cu-

**Current affiliation*: Western General Hospital, South Edinburgh, United Kingdom

taneous vasculitis. However, the therapeutic approach to the different syndromes was similar, and mortality remained high. For example, Walton documented only a 20% survival in 1 year and 7% in 2 years [1]. Treatment remained symptomatic and was in effect, as in Kussmaul and Maier's original case [2], terminal care. The introduction of steroids [3] represented the first serious advance in the treatment of vasculitis. Short-term survival improved but long-term outcome remained unaffected. However, the improvement in immediate prognosis emphasized the importance of attention to such factors as hypertension and renal function, which remains a major aspect of therapy. In the second half of the 20th century, the outlook has brightened considerably. Major advances occurred in four main areas: disease classification, control of acute mortality, understanding of etiopathogenesis, and accurate disease assessment.

A. Classification

The increased recognition of vasculitis has led to separating many conditions from the once all-encompassing label of polyarteritis. Indeed, classic PAN is now extremely rare. More detailed classification has been associated with recognition of minor, but important, differences in treatment responses between the various syndromes. This is slowly evolving into regimens tailored for each syndrome and should eventually lead to disease-specific therapy.

Unfortunately, classification is not easy, particularly in the early stages of the disease, since it is not based on the full knowledge of the pathogenesis. In the absence of rational classification systems, a consensus may be the best approach. That achieved at the Chapel Hill Meeting [4] provides a simple, usable, and widely accepted approach. This chapter concentrates on primary systemic necrotizing vasculitis (1°SNV) requiring aggressive therapy, excluding WG, which is dealt with elsewhere. The important subgroups are those that involve large and/or medium-sized arteries, including giant cell arteritis (GCA) and Takayasu's arteritis, classic PAN, Churg-Strauss syndrome, and microscopic polyangiitis (MPA). Juvenile polyarteritis is treated as the adult disease, apart from Kawasaki's syndrome, which is clinically different and treated in a different way. In contrast, diseases confined to small vessels—such as Henoch-Schönlein purpura (HSP), essential cryoglobulinemia, and cutaneous vasculitis—rarely require aggressive therapy unless there is severe renal disease. However, some of the alternative therapy used in the latter conditions may provide important lessons for maintenance therapy in 1°SNV.

The secondary necrotizing vasculitis complicating connective tissue diseases (CTDs) is rare but serious and may also require aggressive therapy, particularly in rheumatoid arthritis (RA), Systemic lupus erythematosus (SLE), and Behçet's disease. However, this should probably be of limited duration and followed by milder maintenance therapy appropriate to the underlying disease. It is interesting that in CTDs, therapy may alter the balance between local and systemic features. In RA, for example, steroids, gold, or methotrexate used to control synovitis may induce vasculitis [5–9], whereas pulse cyclophosphamide used to treat systemic rheumatoid vasculitis (SRV) may lead to a recurrence of synovitis [7,10]. These phenomena are reminiscent of those seen during the treatment of leprosy, and they may be due to a shift from TH1 to TH2 type of T-cell responses, providing interesting insights into the pathogenesis of rheumatoid disease.

B. Control of Acute Mortality

The most important overall achievement in the treatment of systemic vasculitis in recent years has been the control of acute mortality. Aggressive therapy has converted 1°SNV from acute life-threatening conditions to chronic relapsing diseases. Cyclophosphamide was the first significant therapeutic intervention in 1°SNV [11,12]. Longer term experience from the US National Institutes of Health (NIH) suggested that continuous cyclophosphamide could achieve an 80% 5-year survival in WG, with cures in some cases [13]. Unfortunately, not all syndromes do so well. For example, the therapeutic response in MPA is significantly lower than in WG [14,15], which is mainly due to renal involvement, and this has a significant impact on mortality. Thus the specific disease label, and the type and pattern of major organ involvement are important considerations in deciding the nature and intensity of treatment.

Despite these differences, cyclophosphamide has represented a great advance across the entire field of systemic vasculitis. Our own interest was directed not at whether, but at how, it should be used, and we started experimenting with various regimens [16]. Intermittent intravenous (IV) pulses were initially introduced in SRV [17] but were subsequently applied successfully in 1°SNV [18]. Three years ago, we set up a formal study of pulse versus continuous cyclophosphamide in our unit. Analysis of the first 50 patients showed more than 85% survival at 1 year in both patient groups despite a significant proportion of patients with MPA. There was no major difference in terms of treatment response between the two regimens [19]. We conclude that cyclophosphamide in an adequate dose, whatever regimen is used, produces significant improvement in survival. It is important to emphasize that the pulse regimens we have used differ from the monthly pulse favored in SLE and sometimes applied to vasculitis. Our most recent regimen is outlined in Table 1.

Unfortunately, longer term follow-up has revealed major problems of relapse and toxicity. The first controlled trial of cyclophosphamide [20] showed a definite short-

Table 1 Dose Schedule for High-dose Intermittent Cyclophosphamide and Prednisolone with Alterations for Age, Renal Function, and Marrow Toxicity

	Cyclophosphamide 15 mg/kg (up to 1000 mg/bolus)	Prednisolone 10 mg/kg (up to 1000 mg/bolus)
Renal impairement		
Serium creatinine		
<150 μmol/L	15	10
151–250 μmol/L	10	10
251–500 μmol/L	7.5	10
>501 μmol/L	5.0	7
Marrow toxicity	Stop until blood count returns to within normal; reduce dose by 25%	10
Previous cytotoxics	Stop; commence bolus after 2 weeks	10
Age >70 years	10	10

Each bolus is given either as an intravenous infusion in 1 day (prednisolone followed by cyclophosphamide) or orally (same total dose divided over 3 days). Bolus doses are given at increasing intervals according to clinical response.

term improvement and diminished early relapse when this drug was added to high-dose prednisolone plus plasma exchange. However, the 10-year survival showed no significant differences between the groups; probably due to the high relapse rate. A longitudinal study of 150 patients presenting over a 10-year period to the Queen Elizabeth Hospital, Birmingham with vasculitis, including classic PAN, MPA, and WG, documented an up to 40% incidence of relapse [21]. This was not limited to the early years, so that unlike survival, the Kaplan-Maier curve for the probability of *disease-free survival* does not flatten out. This analysis would predict that as many as three quarters of the patients will relapse if followed over a 10-year period and emphasizes the need for long-term follow-up. Relapse is not necessarily as severe as the initial disease episode, and it is usually controlled early, since the patients are already under observation. Mortality is lower in relapse, but significant disease-induced damage can still occur. It is interesting that classic PAN and WG were once regarded as "one-shot" diseases, but they are now seen to have a high relapse rate. In contrast, SRV, classically regarded as a relapsing-remitting condition, has a significantly lower relapse rate with aggressive cytotoxic therapy [22].

At first glance, this high relapse rate suggests a requirement for prolonged cyclophosphamide therapy, but this has considerable disadvantages. In continuous oral cyclophosphamide regimens, the dose is limited by toxicity according to a recent review of the NIH series [23]. Relapses also occurred in half of these patients, so that less than half of the total patient years of follow-up were spent in remission. The investigators concluded that "survival in vasculitis comes at great cost." Therefore, maintenance of remission with low toxicity should be our next important goal.

C. Etiopathogenesis

It is not the purpose of this chapter to elaborate on the etiopathogenesis of vasculitis. Better understanding of the factors involved in the initiation and perpetuation of vasculitis will allow the development of more rational therapy and even cure of these conditions. We believe that treatment of systemic vasculitis should have two major aims: (a) control of the acute inflammatory phase, which is currently achieved by the use of steroids and cytotoxics, but alternative drugs and immunotherapy may be useful and should be explored further; and (b) prevention and treatment of alterations in blood vessel physiology and the development of occlusive vasculopathy which may follow the acute inflammatory phase. This may be of greater importance to the long-term morbidity and mortality; more so now that survival has improved.

D. Assessment of Disease Status

The need for assessment of disease status has come to the fore with the shift in systemic vasculitis from acute, fatal conditions to chronic disorders. Mortality is no longer an acceptable endpoint for assessing treatment efficacy. Proper studies require detailed assessment of disease status in order to estimate the degree of improvement together with the effect of any damage accumulated either due to the disease itself or its treatment. Both contribute to the functional ability and long-term outcome of patients. Assessment of disease activity is necessary for monitoring the response to treatment and identifying relapses. Assessment of damage (long-term scarring) is also important, as this will not be amenable to aggressive immunosuppression. Treatment to prevent or retard end-organ damage may have to be instituted instead, and measures toward appropriate rehabilitation may have to be taken. Finally, an overall assessment of the patient's physical, psychological, and social function will help in the provision of supportive care. These issues have been approached recently in several centers, but the field is still in its infancy. A complete assessment package (VITAL, Vasculitis Integrated Assessment Log) was initially devised by the Birmingham Vasculitis Group and further developed by the disease assessment subcommittee of the ECSYSVAS Trial. This has now been accepted for general use in multicenter trials of therapy for vasculitis.

III. FUTURE DIRECTIONS OF THERAPY

There is a need to refine therapy for vasculitis to produce a maximum effect over a short time and to minimize long-term drug toxicity. There may be many strategies to this end, but we have used two with some success. The first is to use pulse regimens, which have the advantage of delivering a high individual dose with an interval for recovery. With cyclophosphamide, this appears to be important for bladder toxicity. It is also associated with a lower long-term infection rate, which may reflect the far lower total dose given with pulses compared with continuous oral therapy. The second approach is to use relatively short regimens of aggressive therapy. Our current randomized controlled trial comparing pulse and continuous cytotoxic regimens suggests that with either of them, the maximum benefit is seen in the first 3 months, with only a slow consolidation of improvement thereafter. It is not clear whether the latter phase requires aggressive immunosuppression. We have been experimenting with 6-month or even 3-month cyclophosphamide regimens with some success, but this has to be confirmed in large series.

The underlying principle is to divide therapy of the inflammatory component of vasculitis into three phases based on the need for both high-dose immunosuppression at presentation and long-term therapy to avoid relapse. *The first phase is a remission-induction regimen*, which should be aggressive but could be brief. Cyclophosphamide is the best individual drug at present, usually combined with steroids, although other potent cytotoxics such as chlorambucil could serve a similar purpose. Less potent and possibly safer drugs such as methotrexate could be used in not immediately life-threatening disease. In contrast, additional adjuvant therapy may be required in particularly severe cases, especially those with advanced renal involvement at presentation. Regimens incorporating plasma exchange or intravenous immunoglobulin or new experimental therapies such as monoclonal antibodies or cytokine inhibitors may have a role here. *The second phase should be maintenance of remission*, which may require a prolonged but milder regimen. Indeed, indefinite therapy may be necessary, certainly indefinite follow-up, given the problems with relapse. For this phase, there is currently no single drug which can be confidently recommended for all cases; possible candidates are discussed later on. *The third phase is the management of relapse*. The options here are to use a short induction regimen again or use newer experimental therapies. Meticulous attention to blood pressure and renal function is critically important throughout, whereas attempts to retard occlusive vasculopathy are also necessary.

As our knowledge of the etiopathogenesis of vasculitis increases, disease-specific regimens should become increasingly possible. However, even in the absence of full understanding of disease processes, specific therapies can be developed. For example, in Kawasaki's disease, the adverse influence of steroids on the development of coronary aneurysms, the reluctance of pediatricians to give cyclophosphamide to young children, and the suspicion (but no definite evidence) that this is an infection-triggered condition led to the trials of intravenous immunoglobulin which proved a great success. Currently, the only truly disease-specific regimen appears to be the antiviral treatment of hepatitis B-associated PAN. In this case, combination of nonspecific treatment of the disease (inflammatory vasculitis) with specific treatment of the underlying causative factor (hepatitis B virus) seems to lead to cure in many cases—that is, prolonged drug-free remission [24]. This is an important stimulus for future research.

IV. CURRENT THERAPY

A. Management of Inflammation

The management of inflammation in vasculitis involves mainly the use of glucocorticoids and cytotoxic—immunosuppressive drugs. Many other drugs have been used on an empirical basis, and they may have a place particularly as maintenance therapy. Recent advances in immunotherapy are continuously being explored.

1. *Glucocorticoids and Immunosuppressives*

Glucocorticoids. The glucocorticoids have universal effects on nucleated cells by forming complexes with specific cytoplasmic receptors, which bind to specific sites on the chromatin and regulate transcription of various genes [25]. They exert their anti-inflammatory effects by decreasing the chemotaxis of polymorphonuclear cells (PMNs), monocytes and macrophages, suppressing monocyte bactericidal activity and lymphocyte cytokine production or immunoglobulin synthesis, and causing at least transient lymphopenia, monocytopaenia, and eosinopenia—they also reduce the inflammatory dilatation and increased permeability of the microcirculation [26–30]. Unfortunately, vasoconstriction, mediated probably by their effects on arachidonic acid metabolism, may activate a cascade of thrombotic events leading to vascular occlusion and ischemic organ damage.

Side effects of steroids are well known, and they represent a significant problem in patients with vasculitis. They include suppression of the hypothalamic-pituitary-adrenal axis, osteopenia, avascular necrosis, susceptibility to infections, cataracts, proximal muscle weakness, and thinning of the skin. Steroids may aggravate hypertension and diabetes mellitus, and long-term use may induce accelerated artherosclerosis. Side effects appear to be related to initial and total cumulative dose [31], so unless the disease is well controlled with moderate doses, most clinicians will use concurrent cytotoxic treatment in order to minimize steroid requirement and improve efficacy.

Glucocorticoids alone are still the mainstay of treatment in GCA, polymyalgia rheumatica (PMR), and Takayasu's arteritis [31–34]. Their place in the initial management of GCA is universally accepted, and their use results in most cases in rapid resolution of symptoms. However, the optimal dose, exact regimen, and duration of treatment are highly controversial. Common practice is to treat minor symptoms with lower doses (10–20 mg/day of prednisolone) and use higher doses (40–60 mg/day) for major threatening complications such as blindness [35]. A retrospective study from a French hospital suggests, however, that patients with GCA who were started on low-dose prednisolone (10–20 mg/day) developed fewer side effects and had no more visual or neurological complications than those who were started on higher doses (20–60 mg/day) [36]. As to the duration of treatment, at least 2 years are usually considered necessary, following which treatment can be cautiously withdrawn. Yet, two studies from Sweden [37,38], also retrospective, appear to suggest that any attempt to withdraw treatment, regardless of the time since diagnosis, resulted in relapse in almost half the cases—the conclusion was that it was often necessary to continue with a modest dose of corticosteroids for many years. Retrospective studies have built-in flaws, and any conclusions drawn from them cannot be definite. Prospective studies are therefore necessary, and the effects of concomitant treatment with cytotoxic drugs should also be assessed. Such studies are now underway.

Steroids are often the primary treatment in the Churg-Strauss syndrome, although in cases with extensive systemic involvement, such as renal, neurological, or cardiac disease, additional treatment with cyclophosphamide or azathioprine may be required [39–41]. Glucocorticoids are an integral part of the initial management of all systemic vasculitic syndromes but are inadequate alone in the management of WG [13,23], PAN, or MPA. If used orally, initial doses of 40–60 mg of prednisone per day may be required if there is extensive disease. As the clinical syndrome and inflammatory markers improve, tapering of the dose should be started—initially by decrements of 5–10 mg every 1–2 weeks but more progressively as the dose decreases. When this is down to 10 mg/day, decrements should not exceed 1.0–2.5 mg every few weeks. The rationale for using megadoses of glucocorticoids is a matter of debate. This is probably not more immunosuppressive than 80 mg of oral prednisone in terms of their effects on lymphocyte number and function [42], although large doses may last longer.

Cyclophosphamide. This is an alkylating agent derived from nitrogen mustard. It is not bound to plasma protein, but many of its metabolites are. It is soluble in both aqueous and lipid compartments and its plasma half-life varies from 2 to 10 h. Cyclophosphamide is metabolized mainly in the liver, and because it is a potent stimulator of hepatic microsomal enzymes, its half-life is shortened after chronic use. This may not be of biological importance in view of the increased production of active metabolites such as phosphoramide mustard. The main renal metabolite of cyclophosphamide is acrolein, which is not therapeutically useful but may be responsible for bladder toxicity [43–45]. Renal failure may impair drug excretion [42], in which case high-dose IV cyclophosphamide can be dangerous [47].

Cyclophsphamide is beneficial, if not the mainstay of treatment, in many types of systemic vasculitis, but its mechanism of action remains unclear. It is unlikely that cyclophosphamide affects the underlying trigger factors, but it may interfere with many of the pathogenetic mechanisms involved in vascular inflammation. It appears to act predominantly on the premitotic phase (G_2) of the cell cycle, but it also interferes with several metabolic pathways [48,49]. Cyclophosphamide may have both immunosuppressive and immunostimulatory effects [50]—the latter may be due to differential effects on T-cell subsets, which on occasions may help eradicate bacterial infections [51]. The mode of administration and dose of the drug may also have a bearing on its mechanism of action. Low-dose intravenous cyclophosphamide appears to be more toxic to B cells, whereas higher doses may affect cytotoxic T cells, occasionally causing a paradoxical increase of their function; $CD4^+$ T cells appear to be quite resistant to the effects of the drug [52], but a permanent decrease of T-cell numbers may occur at very high doses [53]. Some studies suggest that pulse therapy may have more of an effect on humoral immunity, whereas continuous low-dose oral cyclophosphamide may affect predominantly cell-mediated immunity [54]. Potential targets of cyclophosphamide therapy may also include natural killer (NK) cells, neutrophils, and endothelial cells, but convincing evidence for this is currently lacking.

Short- and long-term cyclophosphamide toxicity represents a serious problem. Nausea and vomiting are common, particularly during pulse therapy, but this is usually well controlled with adequate antiemetic therapy. Gastric perforation has occurred with pulse cyclophosphamide and prednisolone; thus we favor the use of prophylactic H_2 antagonists or proton pump inhibitors. Alopecia and myelodysplasia have been reported in 17 and 2% of patients, respectively [23], whereas sterility probably occurs in all patients treated with long-term cyclophosphamide. Acrolein, its main urinary metabolite, can cause hemorrhagic cystitis in up to 45% of patients, and it is associated with the development of bladder carcinoma in 2.8%—this represents a 33-fold increased risk of developing bladder tumors [55]. Bladder toxicity however appears to be far higher in patients treated with continuous oral cyclophosphamide regimens than in those receiving pulse treatment [23,55,56]; indeed we have never seen it with pulse therapy. We recommend a high fluid intake on days of pulse therapy, and methylcysteine may also be used as a bladder protectant. Immunosuppression may increase the risk of serious infections. In a recent series of 15 patients treated with daily oral cyclophosphamide, 10 developed significant infections, 2 of whom died [57]. This was not associated with the dose or the degree of leukopenia induced. Although this is a cause for concern, the proportion of patients with severe infections was considerably higher than our own experience and that of others [58]. The oncogenic potential of long-term cyclophosphamide therapy is well known. In vitro studies have shown a variety of mutations in T cells [59,60], the clinical consequences of which are not clearly established, but there are many case reports of leukemia and lymphoma occurring with cyclophosphamide treatment for rheumatic diseases [61]. The incidence of late-onset malignancy in such patients appears to be associated with the total dose and duration of therapy [62]. Although only time will tell, it is probable that intermittent instead of continuous administration of cyclophosphamide will reduce both short- and long-term toxicity. This is one of the main reasons that we favor high-dose intermittent regimens whether intravenous or oral.

Cyclophosphamide has been used extensively for the treatment of many vasculitic syndromes, and several relevant issues have already been discussed in the introduction to this chapter. Its use in WG is described elsewhere in this book (Chapter 30), and its impact on the improvement of prognosis in PAN has been reviewed recently [7]. A group of patients that appears to have a less favorable response to cyclophosphamide is that of MPA. In our patients with MPA and significant renal impairment, the mortality was previously 38% despite aggressive therapy [15]; this is not a unique experience, since the mortality in this group of patients ranges between 20 and 50% [14,63,64]. Risk factors for poor outcome include age, serum creatinine of more than 500 μmol/L at presentation, oliguria, and the presence of crescents on renal histology. The current early mortality in our patients is definitely lower.

Cyclophosphamide has been used in cases of Behçet's disease with central nervous system involvement [65] and in primary angiitis of the nervous system with promising results [66,67], but the numbers are too low to draw definite conclusions. Its use in the Churg-Strauss syndrome also requires further investigation. In a recent large study combining data on PAN and the Churg-Strauss syndrome—which the investigators considered to be inseparable—there was no significant improvement in terms of long-term (10-year) outcome from cyclophosphamide therapy [68]. In the early stages, however, mortality was high in the steroid-only group, and cyclophosphamide was probably not used at sufficient doses. In our limited experience of four cases with a poor response to steroids alone, all four did well on intermittent high-dose cyclophosphamide and prednisolone. The use of cyclophosphamide in lupus nephritis, neuropsychiatric lupus, and rheumatoid vasculitis has been reviewed comprehensively [69,70].

Chlorambucil. Like cyclophosphamide, chlorambucil is an alkylating agent possessing two chloroethyl radicals with a high affinity for DNA, resulting in cross linking of DNA strands, and thus cell death during division. Unlike cyclophosphamide, chlorambucil is active in an unchanged state; intravenous administration results in rapid hydrolysis, so the drug is given orally, being absorbed rapidly (within 15 min) and reaching peak plasma levels within 1 h. It has a short half-life of approximately 90 min and little is still detectable after 6 h. Phenylacetic mustard, its main metabolite, is also an alkylating agent, and it is excreted via the kidney together with the parent drug [71–74).

Chlorambucil can cause nausea and vomiting, but it is generally better tolerated than cyclophosphamide. Hypersensitivity reactions are uncommon [75] and cross reactivity to cyclophosphamide has been reported [76]. Marrow suppression is well described, but at low(er) doses, chlorambucil appears to exert a more selective effect on lymphopoiesis rather than granulopoiesis [77]; thus it may be safer than cyclophosphamide from the aspect of infection. Children with nephrotic syndrome may develop oligospermia or azoospermia with abnormal sex hormone levels [78,79], and testicular damage may be seen on biopsy [80]. There are theoretical reasons for which chlorambucil may have a lesser oncogenic potential than cyclophosphamide [59], and the expected incidence of myelodysplastic leukemia is estimated at approximately 1% [81]. There are however several case reports of malignancies, particularly acute leukemia, in adults or children with CTD treated with chlorambucil [82,83]. In a retrospective survey of 39 patients with RA receiving chlorambucil for a mean of 2 years, approximately 20% developed cutaneous malignancies and 7.5% hematological malignancies. In the control group of 30 cases treated with azathioprine or 6-mercaptopurine, only 1 (0.3%) developed skin cancer [84]. These figures are obviously a cause for concern, but as with cyclophosphamide, toxicity may relate to the length of administration and cumulative dose of the drug.

Most of the experience with chlorambucil in vasculitis is from the treatment of patients with Behçet's disease, particularly when severe eye or central nervous system involvement has occurred [65]. The drug is considered superior to azathioprine in such cases [85,86], although no direct comparisons have been performed. Good results have been achieved when treating Behçet's disease with posterior uveitis or meningoencephalitis using chlorambucil at a dose of 0.1 mg/kg/day and reducing the dose after uveitis has been controlled or neurological events have subsided [87,88]. Similar responses have been seen by starting chlorambucil at a total dose of 2 mg/day and increasing weekly by 2 mg to the maximum tolerable dosage; remission of severe uveitis was achieved in less than 9 months [89]. There are reports of the use of chlorambucil in patients with SRV [90] and other vasculitic syndromes with generally promising results. Chlorambucil is also the only drug which has consistently been reported to prolong long-term survival in amyloidosis secondary to connective tissue disease [81,91,92]. Chlorambucil might be an equally effective but less toxic drug to use than cyclophosphamide for the induction of remission in systemic vasculitis. Concerns over its oncogenic potential may be overcome by using the drug only for short periods (e.g. 3–6 months) until remission has been achieved and then changing to alternative medication for maintenance.

These issues should be addressed in prospective comparative studies with cyclophosphamide.

Azathioprine. This is an oral purine analogue that interferes with the biosynthesis of adenine and guanine and inhibits DNA synthesis. It is biologically active only after metabolism in the liver to 6-thioinosinic acid and 6-thioguanyllic acid, and it is excreted in the kidney [93]. Azathioprine is used widely in transplant recipients and also in the treatment of many autoimmune conditions; mainly when corticosteroid therapy alone has not provided adequate control. There is less evidence for its effectiveness in vasculitis, and its mechanism of action remains unknown. Azathioprine appears to reduce the rate of cell division, acting predominantly on cells in the S phase of the mitotic cycle [93]. Some reports suggest that it inhibits T-cell function [94], B-cell proliferation, and effector functions [95], including antibody production [96] and the number and function of natural killer (NK) cells [93].

The usual dose of azathioprine in vasculitis is 2.0–2.5 mg/kg per day, often combined with prednisolone. The commonest side effects are gastrointestinal and bone marrow suppression. The latter tends to be dose related and may warrant dose adjustment with or without a short period of discontinuation of treatment. Hepatotoxicity occurs rarely [97], and since the drug is metabolized to mercaptopurine, the dose should be reduced when concurrent therapy with allopurinol is given. The risk of azathioprine-induced lymphoproliferative disorders in connective tissue diseases is not well defined; probably there is no significant increase over that expected by the disease itself [71,98,99]. The drug has been used safely in pregnancy [100] despite the fact that it crosses the placental barrier [101]; it also appears in breast milk [102].

Azathioprine may be useful, and is often used empirically, as a steroid-sparing agent in the treatment of refractory PMR/GCA [103] and in the elderly with polymyalgic onset of RA [104], but its effects have not been studied in a systematic fashion in these conditions. It has been used in a study setting in small vessel vasculitis complicating RA [105,106] and recalcitrant cutaneous lupus erythematosus or cutaneous leukocytoclastic vasculitis [107], but it did not provide any particular benefit; it does not appear to be beneficial in urticarial vasculitis occurring with a variety of CTDs [108]. There have been isolated reports of treatment of Behçet's disease with azathioprine, and there has been a single controlled study which suggests that the drug is effective at preventing new ocular disease and maintaining visual acuity but not at improving it [109]. Although used successfully in the induction of remission of PAN in early studies [110], azathioprine has been superseded by cyclophosphamide in the treatment of necrotizing vasculitis. In these cases, it is still being used as maintenance therapy following cyclophosphamide, but its real value remains to be established [7].

Methotrexate. This is a structural analogue of folic acid and aminopterin which binds to the enzyme dihydrofolate reductase and prevents the reduction of folic acid to the metabolically active folates dihydrofolate and tetrahydrofolate. This results in inhibition of thymidylate biosynthesis, protein biosynthesis, and both DNA and RNA production [111]. Its mechanism of action in autoimmune diseases is not known, but again it is likely to reflect diminished cellular activation and proliferation. Methotrexate has been reported to suppress antibody production [112], suppress primary and secondary immune responses [113,114], alter circulating lymphocyte phenotype and function [115–117], and inhibit neutrophil chemotaxis and the release of inflammatory mediators such as leukotriene B_4 [118–121]; all of these may reduce the inflammatory component of vasculitis. Methotrexate however may also inhibit vascular proliferation induced by factors arising from macrophages, platelets, and endothelial cells in a manner analogous to that described in atherosclerosis. Indeed, it has been shown to inhibit proliferation of human umbilical cord endothelial cells in vitro and rabbit corneal neovascularization in vivo [122]. This effect may be more important in terms of long-term outcome in systemic vasculitis.

Methotrexate is used at a starting dose of 7.5 mg weekly and, increasing up to 15 or 20 mg if necessary. Absorption of the oral compound is incomplete, but it is usually high enough to induce efficacy; intramuscular administration ensures better bioavailability. The drug and its metabolites are primarily excreted by the kidney, thus it is not recommended in renal failure, and care should be taken if compounds affecting renal function are administered concurrently. Data on the toxicity of methotrexate in rheumatic diseases is mainly available from studies in RA. Toxicity occurs frequently but is generally mild; the commonest side effects are gastrointestinal [123]. Cutaneous reactions include thinning of the hair and urticaria. Bone marrow toxicity is rare, but the risk increases in renal failure, folate deficiency, acute infections (including viral), and the concomitant use of co-trimoxazole (septrin) [124]. Pulmonary toxicity includes acute pneumonitis [125,126] and an increased incidence of chest infections. Concerns over the development of hepatic fibrosis may have been overstated, and currently most physicians do not find liver biopsies to be justified as routine follow-up; high-risk patients include those with alcohol abuse, obesity, and preexisting liver disease [99]. Methotrexate is teratogenic, and therefore contraception is mandatory in women of child-bearing age [127]. Its use in men is also of concern because of the prolonged maturation of sperm.

Studies in small numbers of patients suggest that methotrexate may be useful in polymyositis, SLE, and vasculitis [128]. It has been used for the treatment of Behçet's disease, particularly in cases with severe oral ulcerations, skin disease, or arthritis [65]. In two patients with Behçet's disease and cutaneous neutrophilic vascular reactions which had not responded to other treatment (including steroids, dapsone, colchicine, azathioprine, and chlorambucil), the skin lesions cleared completely with 15–20 mg of methotrexate weekly [129]. A case of urticarial vasculitis unresponsive to any other treatment apart from systemic corticosteroids also responded completely to low-dose weekly methotrexate, allowing withdrawal of steroids [130]. An interesting situation occurs in RA, where although methotrexate may be useful in the treatment of cutaneous ulceration [131], it may also induce vasculitis [8,9]. It may be useful in the treatment of GCA, but proper studies have not yet been performed; an international study comparing steroids alone versus steroids and methotrexate in biopsy-proven GCA is currently underway. The use of methotrexate in WG is discussed in detail elsewhere in this book (Chapter 30); it is however important to mention here that low-dose methotrexate with glucocorticoids has shown promising results in WG [132] and may be a valuable, less toxic alternative to treatment with cyclophosphamide in patients with not immediately life-threatening disease (e.g., without severe renal involvement). Thus, methotrexate may be of value in the initial treatment of mild or moderately severe vasculitis and for maintenance therapy in severe disease.

Cyclosporin A. This is a cyclic polypeptide composed of 11 amino acids. It was originally isolated from the arctic fungus Tolypocladium inflatum gams and was found to have major immunomodulating properties. It is used for the treatment of various immunologically mediated diseases, including RA, psoriasis, Behçet's disease, ocular inflammation, SLE, inflammatory bowel disease, and insulin-dependent diabetes mellitus. The mechanism of action of cyclosporin A (and another immunosuppressive agent, FK506, with similar properties) has been the subject of intensive research over the last few years. This work and the clinical applications of cyclosporin have been comprehensively reviewed recently [69,133–135). Cyclosporin A mainly suppresses T-cell activation, maintaining T cells in the G_0 or early G_1 phase of the cell cycle. Both cyclosporin and FK506 bind to intracellular enzymes (immunophilins: cyclophilin A and FKBP, respectively) forming complexes that selectively bind the calcium- and calmodulin-dependent protein phosphatase calcineurin, reducing its phosphorylase activity. This inhbiits translocation of specific nuclear binding proteins (such as NF-ATc) from the cytoplasm to the nucleus, thus inhibiting interleukin-2 (IL-2) gene transcription. In addition to IL-2, cyclosporin also inhibits indirectly other cytokines, such as IL-3, IL-4, IL-5, tumor necrosis factor-α (TNF-α) and interferon-γ (IFN-γ), and interferes to a lesser extent with the function of other cell types, such as mast cells, B cells and PMNs. Thus it has the theoretical potential to interfere with many of the processes thought to be involved in the pathogenesis of vasculitis, but the general impression is that it is less useful than cyclophosphamide in 1°SNV.

Cyclosporin is metabolized in the liver by the cytochrome P450-dependent mixed-function oxidase CYP3A3/Y and eliminated via bile. Enzyme inhibitors, including many calcium antagonists (but not nifedipine or isradipine), will increase cyclosporin levels, whereas enzyme inducers will decrease them. Clearance of prednisolone may be inhibited by cyclosporin, whereas cyclosporin levels may increase when used in conjunction with high-dose methylprednisolone. Serum levels of nonsteroidal anti-inflammatory drugs may increase as a result of the use of cyclosporin, and the reduced renal blood flow due to cyclooxygenase inhibition by these drugs may increase the potential of cyclosporin nephrotoxicity. Cyclosporin may decrease the efficacy of live attenuated vaccines, and it enters breast milk.

The side effects of cyclosporin are usually dose dependent. Nephrotoxicity and hypertension are the most important and quite common. Nephrotoxicity occurs both on the account of tubulopathy and vasculopathy. The mechanisms resulting in hypertension are obscure; changes in renal blood flow are important but other factors may also contribute. Other side effects (tremor, hypertrichosis, fatigue, gingival hypertrophy, gastrointestinal disturbance, skin rashes, weight gain, neuromyopathy, confusion, menstrual irregularities) appear to be transient and idiosyncratic and reverse on stopping treatment.

Many vasculitic conditions have been treated with cyclosporin A; mostly in an open setting. Patients with autoimmune inflammatory disorders of the eye in isolation or as part of Behçet's disease or other systemic vasculitides probably represent the largest group. Early open studies and preliminary controlled studies showed promising results [136,137], which appear to have been confirmed later [138,139]. In general, the use of cyclosporin in Behçet's disease has been reserved for severe or refractory cases, particularly with ocular involvement [140], but a recent case report described good results in a patient with Behçet's disease and generalized myositis only [141]. Cyclosporin does not appear to be useful in the treatment of central nervous system abnormalities and intestinal involvement in Behçet's disease [142], but a single report suggests that it may be effective in combination with coumarin in rapidly progressing pulmonary thromboembolism [143]. Cyclosporin is now established in the treatment of RA. Two recent reports suggest that it may be useful in the treatment of rheumatoid vasculitis with predominant eye disease [144,145], but we have not been impressed by its effectiveness in SRV. The use of cyclosporin in WG has been summarized by Schollmeyer and Gross [146]. It may be appropriate in combination with cyclophosphamide for patients who do not respond to standard regimens, instead of cyclophosphamide for patients with leukopenia or thrombocytopaenia and for maintenance treatment instead of azathioprine.

2. Miscellaneous Drugs

Hydroxychloroquine. This agent has been used for a long time in SLE with skin and joint involvement with generally good results and little toxicity; it may be helpful in cutaneous vasculitis complicating systemic rheumatic disorders. Indeed it has been reported to be beneficial in a case of hypocomplemententemic urticarial vasculitis [147]. Although hydroxychloroquine has anti-inflammatory effects and reduces platelet aggregation [148], its exact mechanism of action is unknown.

Colchicine. This is an anti-inflammatory antimitotic drug derived from the roots of the autumn crocus (Colchicum autumnale) and is used for the treatment of gout. It interferes with PMN chemotaxis and phagocytic activity [148,150]. These effects were thought to be useful in the treatment of vasculitic conditions, particularly Behçet's disease, which is characterized by neutrophil hyperfunction. Colchicine has been used successfully in Behçet's disease, particularly in cases with orogenital ulcerations, skin disease, and arthritis, but also in severe uveitis [65,151]. Indeed it has been shown that in Behçet's disease colchicine reduces inflammation by inhibiting both the cyclooxygenase and lipoxygenase pathways [152]. The drug has been used empirically in HSP, and it may be useful in cutaneous leukocytoclasic vasculitis [153,154] and urticarial vasculitis [155,156], although a small study in 13 patients with chronic recurrent small vessel vasculitis did not demonstrate any efficacy [157].

Dapsone. This antileprotic drug has also been used for the treatment of dermatitis herpetiformis. It has been reported to be of help alone or with steroids in cases with leukocytoclastic or PAN-type vasculitis, subacute cutaneous lupus erythematosus, and urticarial vasculitis [158–160]. Side effects, including nausea and vomiting, neuropathy, allergic dermatitis, hepatitis, anemia and agranulocytosis, are rare and dose related. Agranulocytosis has been reported in a case with leukocytoclastic vasculitis treated with dapsone [161], and may respond to treatment with recombinant granulocyte colony-stimulating factor (G-CSF) [162].

Pentoxifylline. This is a peripheral vasodilator which has been shown to inhibit various cytokines that may be involved in vasculitis [163]. In particular, the administration of pentoxifylline in HIV-infected patients [164,165] or bone marrow recipients [166] has been shown to inhibit production of TNF-α in vivo and reduce TNF-associated morbidity and mortality. Inhibition of TNF-α may be of importance in most inflammatory processes, since this may subsequently inhibit the production of IL-1, granulocyte-macrophage CSF (GM-CSF), and G-CSF, IL-6, and IL-8 and the expression of adhesion molecules. Evidence from in vivo studies in transgenic mice overexpressing the TNF-α gene [167] and in RA [168] suggests that TNF inhibition using anti-TNF monoclonal antibodies (mAbs) leads to suppression of inflammatory responses in the joint, and pentoxifylline is currently being evaluated as an alternative to mAbs in RA. Similar cytokine networks may be involved in the pathogenesis of vasculitis. In this context, two recent case reports showing effective control of leukocytoclastic vasculitis with this drug alone [169] or in combination with dapsone [170] may be of significance. An alternative to pentoxifylline may be *thalidomide*, which modulates degradation of TNF-α mRNA [171,172]. Thalidomide is currently used for the treatment of erythema nodosum leprosum with good results. It has been used successfully in a patient with vasculitis resistant to prednisone/azathioprine. Both pentoxifylline and thalidomide appear to have some promise, and we are currently evaluating them alone or in combination as maintenance therapy in several vasculitic syndromes.

Dialyzable Leukocyte Extract and 5-Fluouracil. Subconjunctivally injected dialyzable leukocyte extract and the antimetabolite 5-fluouracil have been used as alternatives to steroid therapy in chronic uveitis with good results, but these need to be confirmed [173].

Nafamostat Mesilate and Camostat Mesilate. Nafamostat [174] and camostat mesilate [175] are inhibitors of complement serine proteases. They have been used in patients with heavy proteinuria due to various conditions, including vasculitis, resulting in prompt, significant decreases of urinary protein excretion and an increase in serum C_3 but no significant change in serum creatinine. The investigators suggest that these agents cause a beneficial change in glomerular capillary permeability for macromolecules through their inhibitory effects on the kallikrein-kinin system, complement system, coagulation system, and platelet function and can contribute to the treatment of immune-mediated nephropathies.

3. Immunotherapy

The major problem of cytotoxic treatment is that it has wide ranging, and probably uncontrolled, effects on many arms of the immune system. More selective therapeutic approaches may be more specific, thus diminishing side effects and also providing important information about the pathogenetic mechanisms involved.

Plasmapheresis. This is currently the best studied apheretic treatment. It is considered to have almost immediate beneficial effects by removing from the circulation agents involved in the inflammatory process, but its effects may last even longer by improving reticuloendothelial function and thus immune complex clearance [176]. It can be lifesaving in urgent situations of immune complex disease such as mixed cryoglobulinemia not controlled with steroids and/or cytotoxics by reducing high titers of cryoglobulin [177]. However, there are no large, controlled studies to prove its efficacy in other systemic vasculitides. Although plasmapheresis is generally well tolerated, with hypotension being the commonest side effect, its use in combination with cytotoxic therapy should be carefully balanced against the risk of lethal sepsis, which is reported to occur in 5% or more of patients [178,179]. Hind et al., in 1983 [180], showed that dialysis-dependent patients with rapidly progressive glomerulonephritis (without anti-GBM antibodies) recovered renal function better if steroids and immunosuppressives were combined with plasma exchange, but there was considerable mortality that was often due to sepsis. Similar results were seen in a study of 20 such patients by other investigators [181]. The first group confirmed these findings more recently in a randomized controlled trial with stratification for renal function on entry in 48 patients [182]. Patients who were initially dialysis dependent were more likely to recover renal function if treated with plasma exchange and drugs than with drugs alone. This improvement was generally maintained on long-term follow-up. Thus plasmapheresis appears to have a place at least as adjuvant therapy in the induction of a remission regimen of primary systemic vasculitis with severe renal impairment at presentation. Its use in other vasculitic syndromes is less well defined. Isolated case reports suggest improvement with plasmapheresis in aseptic meningoencephalitis in primary Sjögren's syndrome [183] or SRV [184]. Larger, although still uncontrolled, studies in SRV from our group indicate only a transient response to plasmapheresis, with some halting of the development of new lesions, but no healing of old lesions, and a high relapse rate unless cyclophosphamide is added to the treatment regimen. This occurs despite a prompt fall of complement-fixing immune complexes and IgG (but not IgM) rheumatoid factors [185]. It appears, however, that although addition of cytotoxic drugs to the regimen delays relapse, the combination predisposes to a very high risk of serious sepsis.

Alternative apheresis methods are currently being evaluated for the treatment of systemic vasculitis. These include synchronization of plasma exchange with pulse cyclophosphamide [186], combination with steroid and antiviral therapy (discussed in detail below), heparin cryoprecipitation of plasma proteins [187], and specific immunoadsorption of relevant autoantibodies [188–190]. The results are in general very preliminary and need confirmation before more widespread use.

Intravenous Immunoglobulin (IVIg). As replacement therapy, IVIg is well established in the treatment of immunodeficiency disorders and infectious diseases. It has been used prophylactically in potentially life-threatening CMV infections in transplanted patients. Since its efficacy was shown in immune thrombocytopenic purpura (ITP) [191], IVIg has been used at high doses as an immunomodulator in many conditions known or suspected to have an autoimmune pathogenesis. These include severe asthma, juvenile chronic arthritis and dermatomyositis, demyelinating polyneuropathies, and the vasculitides, most notably Kawasaki's disease [192]. Studies in ITP and Kawasaki's disease, suggest that it may increase T cells with suppressor function and decrease helper cells, inhibit B-cell antibody and autoantibody synthesis, neutralize autoantibodies by anti-idiotypic antibodies, block Fc (IgG) receptors on macrophages, particularly in the spleen and liver, and decrease cytokine production [191,193].

Kawasaki's disease is the only vasculitic condition where IVIg therapy has been assessed in a controlled setting [194] with impressive results. The use of IVIg in other systemic vasculitides looks promising but as yet is entirely based on case reports [195–198] and small, uncontrolled studies [199,200]. Jayne and Lockwood have recently reviewed their results of an open study of 26 patients with active systemic vasculitis treated with Sandoglubolin: Two months after IVIg,half of the patients were in complete and the other half in partial remission. The clinical benefit was reflected by a fall of C-reactive protein (CRP) and antineutrophil cytoplasm antibody (ANCA), and was maintained for up to a year in 70% of patients [201]. A controlled trial is now in progress.

Adverse reactions to IVIg are well described; mainly from its used as replacement therapy. They include immediate hypersensitivity reactions related to the dose and frequency of previous infusions; the risk of viral contamination with older generation products [202,203] (recent, fourth-generation products may be safer, since a specific viral inactivation step is included in the manufacture); transient, short-lived increases of serum creatinine in patients with nephrotic syndrome [204], and acute renal failure in a patient with mixed essential cryoglobulinaemia [205]. Small changes in plasma viscosity also occur which may be clinically insignificant but suggest cautious use in elderly individuals with preexisting ischemic disease [206]. High-dose IVIg has also been associated with intravascular hemolysis and aseptic meningism [207].

In view of its relative safety but considerable cost, IVIg may be appropriate to use as adjuvant therapy for the induction of remission in patients with systemic vasculitis who are intolerant or unresponsive to other treatment or have a coexisting infection, or it may be appropriate as adjuvant treatment for maintenance in patients with frequent relapses despite standard therapy.

Monoclonal Antibodies (mAbs). These promise a more specific manipulation of the immune response than that achieved by immunosuppressive therapy. The therapeutic value of various mAbs has already been studied in autoimmune states in animal models and humans, with most data on human rheumatological conditions arising from work in RA. In general, the use of murine or rat mAbs is limited by cross-species sensitization resulting in a high incidence of anaphylaxis and diminished efficacy on repeat treatment. Several chimeric and humanized mAbs have been developed, and although less antigenic, they may still cause significant systemic side effects (high fever, hypotension) and an antihuman antibody response. More recently, mAb conjugates have been developed in order to deliver drugs or toxins to specific targets; aiming to reduce systemic side effects. However, nondepleting anti–T-cell antibodies appear to be more effective than cytotoxic ones.

The first case of vasculitis treated with mAbs was reported in 1990 by Mathieson et al. [208]. A humanized anti-CDw52 antibody (Campath 1H), which recognizes most T cells and macrophages, was administered several times with considerable but transient improvement. Further use of an anti-CD4 mAbs resulted in remission lasting for more than a year. The same group has now reported a further four cases (MPA, Behçet's disease, Sjögren's syndrome) unresponsive to immunosuppressive therapy who benefited from treatment with Campath 1H and anti-CD4 [209]. There have been two more reports from other groups of the successful use of mouse [210] and chimeric [211] anti-CD4 mAbs in the treatment of relapsing polychondritis with vasculitis. Another murine mAb (CD5 Plus) recognizing most T cells and a particular subset of B cells thought to be involved in autoantibody production has been used in four patients with refractory lupus nephritis [212]. This mAb was amplified by conjugation to ricin A, an inhibitor of protein synthesis, the role of which is not clear. Three of the four patients showed a partial response, particularly if prolonged T-cell suppression was induced, but cross sensitization occurred which could preclude further treatment.

In the future, more mAbs will no doubt be evaluated in the treatment of systemic vasculitis. Relevant targets would be adhesion molecules and cytokines and their receptors, such as IL-1β, IL-2 and TNF-α. Naturally occurring cytokine inhibitors, such as IL-1 receptor antagonist and soluble IL-1 receptor, have also been described. These have been or are currently being characterized [213], and they could also be evaluated in the treatment of systemic vasculitis.

Antiviral Therapy. This represents one of the most exciting developments in the investigation of the etiopathogenesis and treatment of vasculitis. Evidence is accumulating that viral infections are not only associated with classic PAN but also with mixed cryoglobulinemia, hypersensitivity vasculitis, angiitis of the central nervous system, and even PMR [214]. Two recent studies from a French group pursued the principle of attacking both the probable trigger and the resulting immunological response in PAN associated with hepatitis B virus. In the first prospective nonblinded study, 33 patients were treated with short-term steroids, the antiviral agent vidarabine and plasma exchange, with complete recovery and no clinical or laboratory evidence of vasculitis in the long term in approximately 75% of the patients [24]. In the second smaller study of six patients, plasma exchange was combined with IFN-α2b with effective cure of systemic vasculitis in all of them, although two still required IFN owing to chronic active hepatitis [215]. Several groups have suggested at least some benefit from treatment with IFN-α in mixed cryoglobulinemia associated with hepatitis C infection [216–220]. In the largest open study of 21 patients with severe mixed cryoglobulinaemia, approximately 75% achieved complete or partial response to recombinant IFN-α2a or natural IFN-b, with a significant drop in cryocrit levels. The only major side effect was severe neutropenia, which occurred in two patients [221]. In a more recent prospective randomized controlled trial of IFN-α2a, 53 patients with hepatitis C virus–associated mixed cryoglobulinemia were investigated [222]. Treatment was generally well tolerated and discontinued only in two patients owing to atrial fibrillation and depression. IFN-treated patients had significantly superior clinical, virological and biochemical responses compared with controls. This was closely related to the antiviral activity of the drug; supporting the conjecture of an infectious aetiology of the disease. Isolated reports also suggest benefit from IFN treatment in vasculitis associated with hairy cell leukemia [223] and human T lymphotropic virus type I myelopathy [224]. Clearly, this form of therapy merits further evaluation in relevant vasculitic syndromes both in terms of uncovering important etiopathogenic mechanisms and of designing more effective and even curative treatment regimes.

B. Management of Chronic Vasculopathy

Several lines of evidence suggest that the acute inflammatory stage of vasculitis and consequent endothelial cell damage may have long-term sequelae with the development of an occlusive vasculopathy. This may be of great significance in the long-term morbidity and mortality of patients with systemic vasculitis, and therapeutic intervention to control this stage of the disease should become a major area of interest.

Studies in RA suggest a two- to five-fold higher risk of cardiovascular death compared with the general population. It appears that subclinical vasculitis in RA may be much commoner than previously thought, and necropsy studies suggest an even higher rate of cardiovascular death in patients with RA known or found to have vasculitis [225]. Indeed chronic occlusive arterial lesions associated with fibrin deposition are seen in involved nerves in rheumatoid vasculitis [226]. In PAN, blood vessel occlusion due to clots or intimal and smooth muscle proliferation, with little evidence of inflammation, is a common finding; this may be related to steroid treatment [3,227]. Occlusive vasculopathy complicates human allograft transplantation following immunological phenomena involving blood vessels similar to those occurring in vasculitis [228]. Finally, recent studies suggest that the same factors that influence long-term outcome in atherosclerosis may determine outcome in temporal arteritis [229]; suggesting at least some common mechanisms between the two conditions.

The possible pathogenetic mechanisms leading to occlusive vasculopathy have not been studied in systemic vasculitis. Work in animal models and some human diseases suggests a sequence of events that may be applicable to vasculitis. Endothelial cell injury through the inflammatory process may lead to the decreased production of potent vasodilators such as nitric oxide or prostacyclin and the increased production of vasoconstrictors such as the endothelins, thus altering blood vessel wall contractility and allowing platelet aggregation to occur [230]. It is of concern that glucocorticoids can also inhibit endothelial cell–derived prostacyclin [231]; thus although they control vascular inflammation, they may promote vasospasm [3]. Coagulation abnormalities may follow resulting in arterial occlusion. Indeed, such abnormalities, including elevated fibrinogen and thromboglobulin levels, the defective release of tissue plasminogen activator, and decreased fibrinolytic activity have been described in Takayasu's arteritis [232], Kawasaki's disease [233], and some cases of cutaneous or systemic vasculitis [234,235]. Finally, the release of growth factors such as IL-1, IL-6, TNF-α, MCP-1, and PDGF, may result in smooth muscle cell proliferation and luminal occlusion [236].

Management of this component of systemic vasculitis is entirely empirical. *Antiplatelet drugs*, particularly *aspirin*, are commonly used, and in theory may modify the possible vasospastic and cellular proliferative effect of steroids. *Dipyridamole* and *ticlopidine hydrochloride* have also been used on an empirical basis [237], whereas *calcium channel blockers* are commonly prescribed in order to counteract vasospasm.

Iloprost, a prostacyclin (prostaglandin I_2) analogue, may represent the most significant recent advance from this point of view. It is a potent vasodilator, but prolonged clinical responses, extending beyond the 3- to 5-day infusion regimens used, suggest that it may in addition have a nonvasodilatory mechanism of action, presumably by interfering with platelet activation and adherence. Several studies have now established that iloprost may be of real value in refractory Raynaud's phenomenon, Buerger's disease, digital vasculitis associated with CTD, and ulcerating livedo reticularis [238-242]. Intravenous prostaglandin E_1 may be of similar value but requires further evaluation [243].

The possible effects of *pentoxifylline* and *thalidomide* on the cytokine network involved in vasculitis have already been discussed in detail. By inhibiting TNF-α, IL-1, and IL-6, these drugs may also prevent smooth muscle proliferation in addition to their anti-inflammatory effects [163,166,171]. *Methotrexate* may also inhibit smooth muscle proliferation as already mentioned [122], but this needs further assessment.

A very interesting concept is the use of *thrombolytic therapy* in vasculitis complicated by occlusive vasculopathy [244]. Thrombolysis has the potential of dissolving microvascular thrombi, restoring circulation, and promoting wound healing. Experience of its use in myocardial infarction is extensive, and its use in ischemic strokes is expanding. In a study of six patients with livedoid vasculitis who had nonhealing ulcers despite numerous conventional therapies, low-dose tissue plasminogen activator (10 mg) was given intravenously over four h daily for 2 weeks [245]. Five of the six patients showed dramatic improvement with almost complete healing of the ulcers during hospitalization and significant improvement of tissue oxygenation. The only treatment failure was due to microvascular rethrombosis: This patient was subsequently treated with t-PA and concurrent anticoagulation, with full healing of her leg ulcers.

V. SUMMARY

In the last 20 years, considerable advances have occurred in the recognition and management of systemic vasculitis. More rational classification has helped recognize important differences in treatment responses, which will hopefully evolve to disease-specific therapy. Acute mortality has been controlled with aggressive immunosuppressive therapy but relapse continues to be a major problem together with drug toxicity and long-term morbidity and mortality. Treatment regimens in the future should be more rationally devised and be based on our increasing understanding of etiopathogenesis and better assessment of the disease status so as to relate directly to the individual patient.

We suggest that therapy in general should have three main objectives: (a) induction of remission by controlling the acute inflammatory component of the vasculitic process—the intensity and length of this initial treatment should be balanced against the potential of life-threatening side effects, whereas recent advances in immunotherapy and antiviral therapy could be incorporated in the regimes at this stage; (b) maintenance of remission, possibly with less potent but also less toxic immunosuppressive drugs or alternative medication with immunomodulatory properties; and (c) prevention and treatment of long-term occlusive vasculopathy and its complications.

REFERENCES

1. Walton EW. Giant cell granuloma of the respiratory tract (Wegener's granulomatosis). Br Med J 1958; 2:265–270.
2. Kussmaul A, Maier R. Uber eine bisher nicht bescreibene eigenthumliche Arteriener Krankung (periarteritis nodosa), Die mit Morbus Brightii und rapid fortscreitender allgemeiner Muskellahmung einhergeth. Deutsches Arch Klin Med 1866; 1:484–517.
3. Baggenstoss AH, Shick RM, Polley HF. The effect of cortisone on the lesions of periarteritis nodosa. Am J Pathol 1951; 27:537–551.
4. Jennette JC, et al. Nomenclature of systemic vasculitides—proposal of an international consensus conference. Arthritis Rheum 1994; 37:187–192.
5. Kemper JW, Baggenstoss AH, Slocum CH. The relationship of therapy with cortisone to the incidence of vascular lesions in rheumatoid arthritis. Ann Intern Med 1957; 46:831–851.
6. Vollertsen RS, et al. Rheumatoid vasculitis: survival and associated risk factors. Medicine (Baltimore) 1986; 65:365–375.
7. Bacon PA, et al. Immunopharmacology of vasculitic syndromes. In: Rugstad, et al., eds. Immunopharmacology in Autoimmune Diseases and Transplantation. New York: Plenum Press; 1992;273–290.
8. Segal R, et al. Accelerated nodulosis and vasculitis during methotrexate therapy for rheumatoid arthritis. Arthritis Rheum 1987; 21:186–195.
9. Combe B, et al. Accelerated nodulosis and systemic manifestations during methotrexate therapy for rheumatoid arthritis. Eur J Med 1993; 2:153–156.
10. Bacon PA. Extraarticular rheumatoid arthritis. In: Arthritis and Allied Conditions, 12th ed., McCarty, Koopman, eds. Philadelphia: Lea & Febiger, 1993:811–840.
11. Novack SNA, Pearson CM, Cyclophosphamide therapy in Wegener's granulomatosis. N Engl J Med 1971; 284:938–942.
12. Fauci AS, Wolff SM. Wegener's granulomatosis: studies in eighteen patients and review of the literature. Medicine (Baltimore) 1973; 52:535–561.
13. Fauci, AS, et al. Wegener's granulomatosis: prospective clinical and therapeutic experience with 85 patients for 21 years. Ann Intern Med 1983; 98:76–85.
14. Savage CO, et al. Microscopic polyarteritis: presentation, pathology and prognosis. Q J Med 1985; 56:467–483.
15. Adu D, et al. Polyarteritis and the kidney. Q J Med 1987; 62:221–237.
16. Hall ND, et al. A combined clinical and immunological assessment of four cyclophosphamide regimes in rheumatoid arthritis. Agents Actions 1979; 9:97–102.
17. Scott DGI, Bacon PA. Intravenous cyclophosphamide plus methylprednisolone in the treatment of systemic rheumatoid vasculitis. Am J Med 1984; 76:377–384.
18. Bacon PA. Vasculitis: clinical aspects and therapy. Act Med Scand 1987; 715(Suppl.):157–163.

19. Adu D, et al. Controlled trial of treatment of vasculitis. Clin Exp Immunol 1993;(Suppl.1):39.
20. Guillevan L, et al. Long term follow up after treatment of polyarteritis nodosa and Churg-Strauss angiitis with comparison of steroids, plasma exchange and cyclophosphamide to steroids and plasma exchange. A prospective randomised trial of 71 patients. J Rheumatol 1991; 18:567–574.
21. Gordon M, et al. Relapses in patients with systemic vasculitis. Q J Med 1993; 86:779–789.
22. Bacon PA. Vasculitis from the rheumatologist's viewpoint. Adv Exp Med Biol, 1993; 336:185–195.
23. Hoffman GS, et al. Wegener's granulomatosis: an analysis of 158 patients. Ann Intern Med 1992; 116:448–498.
24. Guillevin L, et al. Treatment of polyarteritis nodosa related to hepatitis B virus with short term steroid therapy associated with antiviral agents and plasma exchanges. A prospective trial in 33 patients. J Rheumatol 1993; 20:289–298.
25. Cupps TR, Fauci AS. Corticosteroid-mediated immunoregulation in man. Immunol Rev 1982; 65:133–155.
26. Yu DTY, et al. Human lymphocyte subpopulations: effect of corticosteroids. J Clin Invest 1974; 53:565–571.
27. Haynes BF, Fauci AS. The differential effect of in vivo hydrocortisone on the kinetics of subpopulations of human peripheral blood thymus-derived lymphocytes. J Clin Invest 1978; 61:703–707.
28. Ebert RH, Barclay WR. Changes in connective tissue reaction induced by cortizone. Ann Intern Med 1952; 37:506–518.
29. Rinehart JJ, et al. Effects of corticosteroids on human monocyte function. J Clin Invest 1974; 54:1337–1343.
30. Butler WT, Rossen RD. Effects of corticosteroids in immunity in man. I. Decreased serum IgG concentration caused by 3 or 5 days of high doses of methylprednisolone. J Clin Invest 1973; 52:2629–2640.
31. Kyle V, Hazleman B. Treatment of polymyalgia rheumatica and giant cell arteritis: I. Steroid regimens in first two months. Ann Rheum Dis 1989; 48:658–661.
32. Huston KA, et al. Temporal arteritis: a 25-year epidemiologic, clinical and pathologic study. Ann Intern Med 1978; 88:162–169.
33. Hall S, et al. Takayasu arteritis. A study of 32 North American patients. Medicine (Baltimore) 1985; 64:89–94.
34. Shelhamer JH, et al. Takayasu's arteritis and its therapy. Ann Intern Med 1985; 103:121–128.
35. Huston KA, Hunder GG. Giant cell (cranial) arteritis: a clinical review. Am Heart J 1980; 100:99–107.
36. Delecoeullerie G, et al. Polymyalgia rheumatica and temporal arteritis: a retrospective analysis of prognostic features and different corticosteroid regimes. Ann Rheum Dis 1988; 47:733–739.
37. Anderson R, et al. Long term survival in giant cell arteritis, including temporal arteritis and polymyalgia rheumatica. Acta Med Scand 1986; 220:361–364.
38. Anderson R, Malmvall BE, Bengtsson BA. Long term corticosteroid treatment in giant cell arteritis. Act Med Scand 1986; 220:465–469.
39. Clutterback EJ, Evans DJ, Pusey CD. Renal involvement in Churt-Strauss syndrome. Nephrol Dial Transplant 1990; 5:161–167.
40. Haas C, et al. L'Angeite allergicue avec granulomatose: Syndrome de Churg et Strauss. Ann Med Interne (Paris) 1991; 142:335–342.
41. Scully R, et al. Case records of the Massachusetts General Hospital: weekly clinicopathological exercises, Case 188, 1992. N Engl J Med 1992; 326:1204–1212.

42. Webel ML, et al. Cellular immunity after intravenous administration of methylprednisolone. J Lab Clin Med 1974; 83:383–392.
43. Arnold H, Bourseaux F. Synthese und Abbau cytostatisch wirksamer cyclischer N-Phosphamidester des Bis-(B-chlorathyl)-amins. Angew Chem 1958; 70:530–544.
44. Bagley CM Jr, Bostick FW, De Vita VT. Clinical pharmacology of cyclophosphamide. Cancer Res 1973; 33:226–233.
45. Friedman OM, Myles A, Colvin M. Cyclophosphamide and related phosphoramide mustards: current status and future prospects. Adv Cancer Chemother 1979; 1:143–204.
46. Mouridsen HT, Jacobsen E. Pharmacokinetics of cyclophosphamide in renal failure. Acta Pharmacol Toxicol 1975; 36:409–414.
47. Cheigh JS, Reidenberg MM. Cyclophosphamide dose in renal failure. Am J Med 1978; 64:726.
48. Wheeler G, Alexander JA. Effects of nitrogen mustard and cyclophosphamide upon the synthesis of DNA in vivo and in cell-free preparations. Cancer Res 1969; 29:98–109.
49. Hengst JCD, Kempf RA. Immunomodulation by cyclophosphamide. Clin Immunol Allergy 1984; 4:199–216.
50. Turk JL, Parker A. The effect of cyclophosphamide on the immune response. J Immunopharmacol 1979; 1:127–137.
51. Miller TE, North DK. Clinical infections, antibiotics and immunosuppression. A puzzling relationship. Am J Med 1981; 71:334–336.
52. Bast RC Jr, et al. Contrasting effects of cyclophosphamide and prednisolone on the phenotype of human peripheral blood lymphocytes. Clin Immunol Immunopathol 1983; 28:101–114.
53. Uitdehaag BM, Nielsen UM, Hommes OR. Long lasting effects of cyclophosphamide on lymphocytes in peripheral blood and spinal fluid. Acta Neurol Scand 1989; 79:12-17.
54. Hersh EM, Wong VG, Friedrich EJ. Inhibition of the local inflammatory response in man by antimetabolites . Blood 1966; 27:38–48.
55. Stillwell TJ, et al. Cyclophosphamide-induced bladder toxicity in Wegener's granulomatosis. Arthritis Rheum 1988; 31:465–470.
56. Austin HA, et al. Therapy of lupus nephritis: controlled trial of prednisolone and cytotoxic drugs. N Engl J Med 1986; 314:614–19.
57. Bradley JD, Brandt KD, Katz BP. Infectious complications of cyclophosphamide treatment for vasculitis. Arthritis Rheum 1989; 32:45–53.
58. Fauci AS, et al. Cyclophosphamide therapy of severe systemic necrotising vasculitis. N Engl J Med 1979; 301:235–238.
59. Palmer RG, Dore S, Denman AM. Cyclophosphamide induces more chromosome damage than chlorambucil in patients with connective tissue diseases. Q J Med 1986; 59:395–400.
60. Palmer RG, et al. Use of T cell cloning to detect in vivo mutations induced by cyclophosphamide. Arthritis Rheum 1988; 31:757–761.
61. Nashel DJ. Mechanisms of action and clinical applications of cytotoxic drugs in rheumatic disorders. Med Clin North Am 1985; 69:817–840.
62. Baker GL, et al. Malignancy following the treatment of rheumatoid arthritis with cyclophosphamide. Long term case control follow up study. Am J Med 1987; 83:1–9.
63. Droz D, et al. Glomerulonephritis and necrotising angiitis. In: Advanced Nephrology. Vol. 8. Chicago: Year Book, 1979:343–363.
64. Serra A, et al. Vacsulitis affecting the kidney: presentation, histopathology and long term outcome. Q J Med 1984; 53:181–207.
65. Allen NB. Miscellaneous vasculitic syndromes including Behçet's disease and central nervous system vasculitis. Curr Opin Rheumatol 1993; 5:51–56.
66. Sigal L. The neurologic presentation of vasculitic and rheumatological syndromes: A review. Medicine (Baltimore) 1987; 66:157–179.

67. Calabrese LH, Mallek JA. Primary angiitis of the central nervous system. Medicine (Baltimore) 1987; 67:20–39.
68. Guillevin L, et al. Clinical findings and prognosis of polyarteritis nodosa and Churg-Strauss angiitis: a study of 165 patients. BR J Rheumatol 1988; 27:258–264.
69. McCune WJ, Friedman AW. Immunosuppressive drug therapy for rheumatic diseases. Curr Opin Rheumatol 1993; 5:282–292.
70. Luqmani RA, et al. Treatment of vasculitis in rheumatoid arthritis. Ann Int Med (Paris) 1995;
71. Clements PJ, Davis J. Cytotoxic drugs: their clinical application to the rheumatic diseases. Semin Arthritis Rheum 1986; 15:231–254.
72. McLean A, et al. Pharmacokinetics and metabolism of chlorambucil in patients with malignant disease. Cancer Treat Rev 1979; 6(Suppl.):33–42.
73. McLean A, Newell D, Baker G, Connors T. The metabolism of chlorambucil. Biochem Pharmacol 1980; 29:2039–2047.
74. Luqmani RA, Palmer RG, Bacon PA. Azathioprine, cyclophosphamide and chlorambucil. Baillieres Clin Rheumatol 1990; 4:595–619.
75. Hitchins RN, Hockger S, Thomson DB. Chlorambucil allergy—a series of 3 cases. Aust NZ J Med 1987; 17:600–602.
76. Kritharides L, Lawrie K, Varigos GA. Cyclophosphamide hypersensitivity and cross-reactivity with chlorambucil. Cancer Treat Rep 1987; 71:1323-1324.
77. Brooks PM, Buchanan WW, Grove M, Downie WW. Effects of enzyme induction on metabolism of prednisolone. Clinical and laboratory study. Ann Rheum Dis 1976; 35:339–343.
78. Guesry P, Lenoir G, Broyer M. Gonadal effects of chlorambucil given to prepubertal boys for nephrotic syndrome. J Paediatr 1978; 92:299–303.
79. Callis L, Nieto J, Vila A, Rende J. Chlorambucil treatment in minimal lesion nephrotic syndrome. A reappraisal of its gonadal toxicity. J Paediatr 1980; 97:653–656.
80. Reichter P, Calamera JC, Morgenfeld MC, et al. Effect of chlorambucil on spermatogensis in a human with malignant melanoma. Cancer 1970; 25:1026–1030.
81. Berglund K, Hultquist R. The treatment of renal AA amyloidosis secondary to rheumatic diseases. Rheumatol Eur 1994; 23:148–150.
82. Kakn MF, Arlet J, Bloch-Michel J, et al. Acute leukaemia after treatment with cytotoxic drugs in rheumatology. Nouv Presse Med 1979; 8:1393–1397.
83. Buriot D, Prieur A, Lebranchu Y, et al. Acute leukaemia in 3 children after treatment of juvenile chronic arthritis with chlorambucil. Arch Franc Pediatr 1979; 36:92–98.
84. Patapanian H, Graham S, Sambrook PN, et al. The oncogenicity of chlorambucil in rheumatoid arthritis. Br J Rheumatol. 1988; 27:44–47.
85. O'Duffy JD. Vacsulitis in Behçet's disease. Rheum Dis Clin North Am 1990; 16:423–431.
86. McCalmont TH, Jorizzo JL. Behçet's disease. In: Systemic Vasculitides. Churg A, Churh J, eds. New York: Igaku-Shoin; 1992;212–228.
87. O'Duffy JD, Bowles CA, O'Fallon WM. The immunosuppressive treatment of Behçet's disease with emphasis on chlorambucil. In: Recent Advances in Behçet's Disease. Congress and Symposium Series No. 103, London: Royal Society of Medicine Service, 1986:301-306.
88. O'Duffy JD, Robertson DM, Goldstein NP. Chlorambucil in the treatment of uveitis and meningoencephalitis of Behçet's disease. Am J Med 1984; 77:75–84.
89. Tessler H2, Jennings T. High dose, short term chlorambucil for intractable sympathetic ophthalmia and Behçet's disease. Br J Ophthalmol 1990; 74:353–357.
90. Kahn MF, Bedoiseau M, deSeze S. Immunosuppressive drugs in the management of malignant and severe rheumatoid arthritis. Proc R Soc Med 1967; 60:130–133.
91. Schnitzer TJ, Ansell BM. Amyloidosis in juvenile chronic polyarteritis. Arthritis Rheum 1977; 20:242–252.

92. Berglund K, Keller C, Thysell H. Alkylating cytostatic treatment in renal amyloidosis secondary to rheumatic disease. Ann Rheum Dis 1987; 46:757–762.
93. Spina CA. Azathioprine as an immune modulating drug: clinical applications. Clin Immunol Allergy 1984; 4:415–446.
94. Yu DT, et al. Lymphocyte characteristics in rheumatic patients and response to therapy. Arthritis Rheum. 1974; 17:37–45.
95. Levy J, et al. The effect of azathioprine on gammaglobulin synthesis in man. J Clin Invest 1972; 51:2233–2238.
96. Abdou NI, Zweimann B, Casella R. The effects of azathioprine on bone marrow dependent and thymus dependent cells in man. Clin Exp Immunol 1973; 13:55–64.
97. Zarday Z, et al. Irreversible liver damage after azathioprine. JAMA 1972; 222:690–691.
98. Silman AJ, et al. Lymphoproliferative cancer and other malignancy in patients with rheumatoid arthritis treated with azathioprine: a 20 year follow up study. Ann Rheum Dis 1988; 47:988–992.
99. Urowitz MB, Lee P. The risks of antimalarial retinopathy, azathioprine lymphoma and methotrexate hepatotoxicity during the treatment of rheumatoid arthritis. Baillieres Clin Rheumatol 1990; 4:193–206.
100. Schein PS, Winocur ST. Immunosuppressive and cytotoxic chemotherapy: Long term complications. Ann Intern Med 1975; 82:84–95.
101. Saarikoski S, Seppala M. Immunosuppression during pregnancy: transmission of azathioprine and its metabolites from the mother to the fetus. Am J Obstet Gynaecol 1973; 115:1100–1106.
102. Platzker ACD, Lew CD, Stewart D. Drug "administration" via breast milk. Hospital Pract 1980; 15:111–122.
103. DeSilva M, Hazleman BL. Azathioprine in giant cell arteritis/polymyalgia rheumatica in a double blind study. Ann Rheum Dis 1986; 45:136–138.
104. Mason M, et al. Azathioprine in rheumatoid arthritis. Br Med J 1969; 1:420-422.
105. Heurkens AH, Westedt ML, Breedveld FC. Prednisolone plus azathioprine treatment in patients with rheumatoid arthritis complicated by vasculitis. Arch Intern Med 1991; 151:2249–2254.
106. Nicholls A, et al. Controlled trial of azathioprine in rheumatoid vasculitis. Ann Rheum Dis 1973; 32:589–591.
107. Callen JP, et al. Azathioprine. An effective corticosteroid sparing therapy for patients with recalcitrant cutaneous lupus erythematosus or with recalcitrant cutaneous leukocytoclastic vasculitis. Arch Dermatol 1991; 127:515–522.
108. Asherson RA, et al. Urticarial vasculitis in a connective tissue disease clinic: patterns, presentations and treatment. Semin Arthritis Rheum 1991; 20:285–296.
109. Yaziki H, et al. A controlled trial of azathioprine in Behçet's disease. N Engl J Med 1990; 322:281–285.
110. Leib ES, Restivo C, Paulus HE. Immunosuppressive and corticosteroid therapy of polyarteritis nodosa. Am J Med 1979; 67:941–947.
111. Weinblatt ME, Maier AL. Methotrexate in rheumatoid arthritis. Eur J Rheumatol Inflamm 1991; 11:148–161.
112. Sterzl J. Effect of some metabolic inhibitors in antibody formation. Nature 1961; 189:1022–1023.
113. Mitchell MS, et al. Immunosuppressive effects of cytosine arabinoside and methotrexate in man. Ann Intern Med 1969; 70:535–546.
114. Olsen NJ, Callahan LF, Pincus T. Immunologic studies of rheumatoid arthritis patients treated with methotrexate. Arthritis Rheum 1987; 30:481–488.
115. Weinblatt ME, et al. Efficacy of low dose methotrexate in rheumatoid arthritis. N Engl J Med 1985; 312:818-822.
116. Andersen PA, et al. Weekly pulse methotrexate in rheumatoid arthritis. Clinical and im-

munologic effects in a randomised double blind study. Ann Intern Med 1985; 103:489–496.

117. Weinblatt ME, et al. Long term prospective trial of low dose methotrexate in rheumatoid arthritis. Arthritis Rheum 1988; 31:167–175.
118. Suarez CR, et al. Effect of low dose methotrexate on neutrophil chemotaxis induced by leukotriene B4 and complement C5a. J Rheumatol 1987; 14:9–11.
119. Ternowitz T, et al. Methotrexate inhibits the human C5a induced skin response in patients with psoriasis. J Invest Dermatol 1987; 89:192–196.
120. van DeKerkhof CM, et al. Methotrexate inhibits the leukotriene B4 induced intraepidermal accumulation of polymorphonuclear leucocytes. Br J Dermatol 1985; 113:251a-255a.
121. Sperling R, Benincaso AI, Anderson RJ, et al. Acute and chronic supression of leukotriene B4 synthesis ex vivo in neutrophils from patients with rheumatoid arthritis beginning treatment with methotrexate. Arthritis Rheum 1992; 35:376–384.
122. Hirata S, et al. Inhibition of in vitro vascular endothelial cell proliferation and in vivo neovascularisation by low dose methotrexate. Arthritis Rheum 1989; 32:1065–1073.
123. Weinblatt ME. Toxicity of low dose methotrexate in rheumatoid arthritis. J Rheumatol 1985; 12 (Suppl):35–39.
124. Mackinnon SK, Starkebaum G, Wilkens RF. Pancytopaenia associated with low dose pulse methotrexate in the treatment of rheumatoid arthritis. Sem Arthritis Rheum 1985; 15:119–126.
125. Carson CW, et al. Pulmonary disease during the treatment of rheumatoid arthritis with low dose pulse methotrexate. Sem Arthritis Rheum 1987; 16:186-195.
126. St Clair EW, Rice JR, Synderman P. Pneumonitis complicating low dose methotrexate therapy in rheumatoid arthritis. Arch Intern Med 1985; 145:2035–2038.
127. Milunski A, Graef JW, Gaynor MF. Methotrexate-induced congenital malformations. J Paediatr 1968; 72:790–795.
128. Jeurissen ME, Boerbooms AM, van de Putte LB. Methotrexate therapy in connective tissue diseases: a review of the literature. Neth J Med 1989; 35:44–58.
129. Jorizzo JL, et al. Low-dose weekly methotrexate for unusual neutrophilic vascular reactions: cutaneous polyarteritis nodosa and Behçet's disease. J Am Acad Dermatol 1991; 24:973–978.
130. Stacks PS. Methotrexate for urticarial vasculitis. Ann Allergy 1994; 72:36–38.
131. Williams HC, Pembroke AC. Methotrexate in the treatment of vasculitic cutaneous ulceration in rheumatoid arthritis. J R Soc Med 1989; 82:763.
132. Hoffman GS, Leavitt RY, Kerr GS, Fauci AS. The treatment of Wegener's granulomatosis with glucocorticoids and methotrexate. Arthritis Rheum 1992; 35:1322–1329.
133. McKeon F. When worlds collide: immunosuppressants meet protein phosphatases. Cell 1991; 66:823–826.
134. Schreiber SL, Crabtree GR. The mechanism of action of cyclosporin A and FK506. Immunol Today 1992; 13:136–142.
135. Shreiber SL. Immunophilin-sensitive protein phosphatase action in cell signalling pathways. Cell 1992; 70:365–368.
136. Klein S, et al. Cyclosporin A therapy in chronic uveitis. Ophthalmologe 1992; 89:411–415.
137. Nussenblatt RB. The expanding use of immunosuppression in the treatment of non-infectious eye disease. J Autoimmun 1992; 5(Suppl. A):247–257.
138. Nussenblatt RB, et al. Effectiveness of cyclosporin therapy for Behcet's disease. Arthritis Rheum 1985; 28:671–679.
139. Masuda K, et al. Double masked trial of cyclosporin versus colchicine and long term open study of cyclosporin for Behcet's disease. Lancet 1989; 1:1093–1096.
140. Yaziki H, Barnes CG. Practical treatment recommendations for pharmacotherapy of Behçet's syndrome. Drugs 1991; 42:796–804.

141. Lingenfelser T, et al. Generalised myositis in Behçet's disease: treatment with cyclosporin. Ann Intern Med 1992; 116:651–653.
142. Hashimoto T, Takeuchi A. Treatment of Behçet's disease. Curr Opin Rheumatol 1992; 4:31–34.
143. Vansteenkiste JF, et al. Cyclosporin treatment in rapidly progressive pulmonary thromboembolic Behcet's disease. Thorax 1990; 45:295–296.
144. McCarthy JM, et al. Cyclosporin A for the treatment of necrotising scleritis and corneal melting in patients with rheumatoid arthritis. J Rheumatol 1992; 19:1358–1361.
145. Kervick GN, et al. Paracentral rheumatoid corneal ulceration. Clinical features and cyclosporin therapy. Ophthalmology 1992; 99:80–88.
146. Schollmeyer P, Gross W. Cyclosporin in the treatment of Wegener's granulomatosis and APMIS (Copenhagen) related diseases. 1990; 19(Suppl):54–55.
147. Lopez LR, et al. The hypocomplementemic urticarial vasculitis syndrome; therapeutic response to hydroxychloroquine. J Allergy Clin Immunol 1984; 73:600–603.
148. Loudon JR. Hydroxychloroquine and postoperative thromboembolism after total hip replacement. Am J Med 1988; 85:57–61.
149. Ahern MJ, et al. Does colchicine work? The results of the first controlled study in acute gout. Aust NZ J Med 1987; 17:301–304.
150. Wallace SL, Singer JZ. Therapy in gout. Rheum Dis Clin North Am 1988; 14:441–457.
151. Hashimoto T, Takeuchi A. Treatment of Behçet's disease. Curr Opin Rheumatol 1992; 4:31–34.
152. Gurer MA, et al. Arachidonic acid metabolites and colchicine in Behçet's disease. Prostaglandins Leukot Essent Fatty Acids 1991; 43:257–259.
153. Plotnick S, Huppert AS, Kantor G. Colchicine and leucocytoclastic vasculitis. Arthritis Rheum 1989; 32:1489–1490.
154. Callen JP. Colchicine is effective in controlling chronic cutaneous leucocytoclastic vasculitis. J Am Acad Dermatol 1985; 13:193–200.
155. Gimenez-Garcia R, Gimenez-Garcia MC, Llorente-de-la-Fuente A. Urticarial vasculitis. Response to treatment with colchicine. Rev Clin Esp 1990; 187:96.
156. Asherson RA, et al. The normocomplementemic urticarial vasculitis syndrome. Report of a case and response to colchicine. Clin Exp Dermatol 1991; 16:424–427.
157. Cupps TR, Springer RM, Fauci AS. Chronic recurrent small vessel cutaneous vasculitis: clinical experience in 13 patients. JAMA 1982; 247:1994–1998.
158. Uetrecht J. Dapsone and sulphapyridine. Clin Dermatol 1989; 7:11–120.
159. Holtman JH, et al. Dapsone is an effective therapy for the skin lesions of subacute cutaneous lupus erythematosus and urticarial vasculitis in a patient with C2 deficiency. J Rheumatol 1990; 1222–1225.
160. Gonzalez-Quijada S, et al. Gastrointestinal involvement and the response to dapsone in a case of the urticarial vasculitis syndrome. Med Clin Barc 1991; 97:706–708.
161. Woodbury GR Jr, et al. Dapsone-associated agranulocytosis and severe anaemia and in a patient with leucocytoclastic vasculitis. J Am Acad Dermatol 1993; 28:781–783.
162. Miyagawa S, et al. Recombinant granulocyte colony-stimulating factor for dapsone-induced agranulocytosis in leucocytoclastic vasculitis. J Am Acad Dermatol 1993; 28:659–661.
163. Zabel P, Schlaak M, Schade FU. Inhibition of cytokines by pentoxifylline.Immunobiology 1993; 187:447–463.
164. Dezube BJ. Pentoxifylline for the treatment of infection with human immunodeficiency virus. Clin Infect Dis 1994; 18:285–287.
165. Landman D, Sarai A, Sathe SS. Use of pentoxifylline therapy for patients with AIDS-related wasting. Pilot study. Clin Infect Dis 1994; 18:97–99.
166. Bianco JA, et al. Phase I–II trial of pentoxiphylline for the prevention of transplant-related toxicities following bone-marrow transplantation. Blood 1991; 78:1205–1211.

167. Keffer J, et al. Transgenic mice expressing human tumour necrosis factor: a predictive model of arthritis. EMBO J 1991; 10:4025–4031.
168. Elliott MJ, et al. Treatment of rheumatoid arthritis with chimaeric monoclonal antibodies to tumour necrosis factor alpha. Arthritis Rheum 1993; 36:1681–1690.
169. Wahba-Yahav AV. Chronic leucocytoclastic vasculitis associated with polycythaemia vera: effective control with pentoxifylline. J Am Acad Dermatol 1992; 26:1006–1007.
170. Nurnberg W, Grabbe J, Czarnetzki BM. Synergistic effects of pentoxifylline and dapsone in leucocytoclastic vasculitis. Lancet 1994; 343:491.
171. Sampaio EP, et al. Thalidomide selectively inhibits tumour necrosis factor alpha production by stimulated human monocytes. J Exp Med 1991; 173:699–703.
172. Moreira AL, et al. Thalidomide exerts its inhibitory action on tumour necrosis factor alpha by enhancing mRNA degradation. J Exp Med 1993; 177:1675–1680.
173. Klein S, et al. Alternatives to steroid therapy in chronic uveitis. Fortschr Ophthalmol 1990; 87:355–358.
174. Miyata T, et al. Effectiveness of nafamostat mesilate on glomerulonephritis in immune complex disease. Lancet 1993; 341:1353.
175. Matsubara M, et al. Effect of camostat mesilate on heavy proteinuria in various nephropathies. Clin Nephrol 1989; 32:119–123.
176. Lockwood CM, et al. Reversal of impaired splenic function of patients with nephritis or vasculitis (or both). N Engl J Med 1979; 300:524–530.
177. Campion EW. Desperate diseases and plasmapheresis. N Engl J Med 1992; 326:1425–1427.
178. Wing EJ, et al. Infectious complications with plasmapheresis in rapidly progressive glomerulonephritis. JAMA 1980; 244:2423–2426.
179. Lhote F, et al. Combination of plasma exchange in the treatment of polyarteritis nodosa and Churg-Strauss angiitis and the contribution of adjuvant immunosuppressive therapy: A randomised trial in 72 patients. Artif Organs 1988; 12:27–32.
180. Hind CRK, et al. Prognosis after immunosuppression of patients with crescentic nephritis requiring dialysis. Lancet 1983; 1:263–265.
181. Milovanov IuS, Komiagin IuV, Nikolaev AIu. Plasmapheresis in the treatment of rapidly progressive glomerulonephritis. Ter Arkh 1993; 65:27–30.
182. Pusey CD, et al. Plasma exchange in focal necrotising glomerulonephritis without anti-GBM antibodies. Kidney Int. 1991; 40:757–763.
183. Gerraty RP, McKelvie PA, Byrne E. Aseptic meningoencephalitis in primary Sjogren's syndrome. Response to plasmapheresis and absence of CNS vasculitis at autopsy. Acta Neurol Scand 1993; 88:309–311.
184. Ushiyama O, et al. A case of malignant rheumatoid arthritis with long-term improvement by regular use of cryofiltration plasmapheresis. Ryumachi 1993; 33:149–155.
185. Scott DGI, et al. Plasma exchange in rheumatoid vasulitis. J Rheumatol 1981; 8:433–439.
186. Jarrousse B, et al. Synchronisation of plasma exchange and cyclophosphamide in severe systemic diseases. A consecutive study of 10 patients. Presse Med 1993; 22:293–298.
187. Margulis EIa, Savchenco VG. The results of 5 years use of a method for heparin cryoprecipitation of plasma proteins (selective plasmapheresis) in patients with an immune complex pathology. Ter Arkh 1989; 61:65–69.
188. Esnault VL, et al. Influence of immunoadsorption on the removal of immunoglobulin G autoantibodies in crescentic glomerulonephritis. Nephron 1993; 65:180–184.
189. Suzuki K, et al. Continuous removal of anti-DNA antibody using a new extracorporeal immunoadsorption system in patients with systemic lupus erythematosus. Arthritis Rheum 1991; 34:1546–1552.
190. Kobayashi S, et al. Immunoadsorbent plasmapheresis for a patient with antiphospholipid syndrome during pregnancy. Ann Rheum Dis 1992; 51:399–401.
191. Newland AC, Macey MG, Keys PA. IVIG: mechanisms of action and their clinical application. In: Imbach P, ed. Immunotherapy with Intravenous Immunoglobulins. London: Academic Press, 1991:15–26.

192. Permin H, et al. Clinical use of intravenous immunoglobulin IgG. Ugeskr-Laeger 1992; 154:3411–3416.
193. Leung DYM. Immunomodulation by intravenous immune globulin in Kawasaki's disease. J Allergy Clin Immunol 1989; 84:588–594.
194. Newburger JW, et al. The treatment of Kawasaki syndrome with intravenous gamma globulin. N Engl J Med 1986; 315:341–347.
195. Tuso P, et al. Treatment of antineutrophil cytoplasmic antibody-positive systemic vasculitis and glomerulonephritis with pooled intravenous gammaglobulin. Am J Kidney Dis 1992; 20:504–508.
196. Antonelli A, Agostini G, Agostini S. Preliminary results of intravenous immunoglobulins in treating patients with vasculitis. Clin Ter 1992; 141:33–36.
197. Armentia A, et al. Asthma and vasculitis. Response to intravenous immunoglobulins. Allergol Immunopathol Mad 1993; 21:47–52.
198. Pirner K, et al. Intravenous administration of immunoglobulins in systemic lupus erythematosus: review of the literature and initial clinical experiences. Infusionther Transfusionmed 1993; 20:(Suppl. 1):131–135.
199. Jayne DR, et al. Treatment of systemic vasculitis with pooled intravenous immunoglobulin. Lancet 1991; 337:1137–1139.
200. Richter C, et al. Treatment of Wegener's granulomatosis with intravenous immunoglobulin. Adv Exp Med Biol 1993; 336:487–489.
201. Jayne DR, Lockwood CM. Pooled intravenous immunoglobulin in the management of systemic vasculitis. Adv Exp Med Biol 1993; 336:469–472.
202. Bjorkander J, et al. Intravenous immunoglobulin prophylaxis causing liver damage in 16 of 77 patients with hypogammaglobulinaemia or IgG subclass deficiency. Am J Med 1988; 84:107–111.
203. Williams PE, et al. Transmission of non-A and non-B hepatitis by pH4 treated intravenous immunoglobulin. Vox Sang 1989; 57:15–18.
204. Schifferli J, et al. High dose IVIg treatment and renal function. Lancet 1991; 337:457–458.
205. Barton J, et al. Acute cryoglobulinaemic renal failure after intravenous infusion of gammaglobulin. Am J Med 1987; 82:624–629.
206. Reihart WH, Berchtold PE. Effect of high dose intravenous immunoglobulin therapy on blood rheology. Lancet 1992; 339:662–664.
207. Chapel H. Intravenous immunoglobulin as a therapeutic tool. Hosp Update Plus 1993; 19:46–54.
208. Mathieson PW, et al. Monoclonal antibody therapy in systemic vasculitis. N Engl J Med 1990; 323:250–254.
209. Lockwood CM, et al. Long-term remission of intractable systemic vasculitis with monoclonal antibody therapy. Lancet 1993; 341:1620–1622.
210. Van Der Lubbe PA, Miltenburg AM, Breedveld FC. Anti-CD4 monoclonal antibody for relapsing polychondritis. Lancet 1991; 337:1349.
211. Choy EHS, et al. Chimaeric anti-CD4 monoclonal antibody for relapsing polychondritis. Lancet 1991; 338:450.
212. Wacholtz MC, Lipsky PE. Treatment of lupus nephritis with CD5 Plus, an immunoconjugate of an anti-CD5 monoclonal antibody and ricin A chain. Arthritis Rheum 1992; 35:837–838.
213. Arend WP, Dayer JM. Cytokines and cytokine inhibitors or antagonists in rheumatoid arthritis. Arthritis Rheum 1990; 33:305–315.
214. Mader R, Keystone EC. Infections that cause vasculitis. Curr Opin Rheumatol 1992; 4:35–38.
215. Guillevin L, et al. Treatment of polyarteritis nodosa related to hepatitis B virus with interferon alpha and plasma exchanges. Ann Rheum Dis 1994; 53:334–337.

216. Bonomo L, et al. Treatment of idiopathic mixed cyroglobulinaemia with alpha interferon. Am J Med 1987; 83:726–730.
217. Taillan B, et al. Is interferon alpha 2b effective in cryoglobulinaemia related to hepatitis C virus. Clin Rheumatol 1992; 11:579.
218. Durand JM, et al. Effect of interferon alpha 2b on cryoglobulinaemia associated with hepatitis C infection. J. Infect Dis 1992; 165:778–779.
219. Boyer N, et al. Recombinant interferon alpha for chronic hepatitis C in patients positive for antibody to human immunodeficiency virus. J Infect Dis 1992; 165:723–726.
220. Ferri C, et al. Antibodies to hepatitis C virus in patient with mixed cryoglobulinaemia. Arthritis Rheum 1991; 34:1606–1610.
221. Bonomo L, Casato M. Clinical use of interferons in rare haematological diseases: Type II cryoglobulinaemia and essential thrombocythemia. In: Baron S, Coppenhaver DH, Dianzani F, et al., eds. Interferon: Principles and Medical Applications. Galveston, TX: University of Texas 1992:575–580.
222. Misiani R, et al. Interferon alpha 2a therapy in cryoglobulinaemia associated with hepatitis C virus. N Engl J Med 1994; 330:751–756.
223. Gomez-Almaguer D, et al. Vacsulitis in hairy cell leukaemia: rapid response to interferon alpha. Am J Haematol 1989; 30:216–222.
224. Ishimoto S, et al. Interferon alpha for the treatment of retinal vasculitis associated with human T lymphotropic virus type I myelopathy (HAM). Nippon Ganka Gakkai Zasshi 1990; 94:769–773.
225. Bacon PA, Kitas GD. The significance of vascular inflammation in rheumatoid arthritis. Ann Rheum Dis 1994; 53:621–623.
226. Conn DL, McDuffie FC, Dyck PJ. Immunopathologic study of sural nerves in rheumatoid arthritis. Arthritis Rheum 1972; 15:135–143.
227. Conn DL, Tompkins RB, Nichols WL. Glucocorticoids in the management of vasculitis—a double-edged sword? J Rheumatol 1988; 15:1181–1183.
228. Muller-Hermelink HK, Dammrich JR. Die obliterative transplantvasculopathie: pathogenese und pathomechanismen. Verh Dtsch Ges Pathol 1989; 73:193–206.
229. Machado EBV, et al. A population based case controlled study of temporal arteritis: evidence for an association between temporal arteritis and degenerative vascular disease? Int J Epidimiol 1989; 18:836–841.
230. Vane JR, Anggard EE, Botting RM. Regulatory functions of the vascular endothelium. N Engl J Med 1990; 323:27–36.
231. Lewis GD, Campbell WB, Johnson AR. Inhibition of prostaglandin synthesis by glucocorticoids in human endothelial cells. Endocrinology 1986; 119:62–69.
232. Kanaide H, Takeshita A, Nakamura M. Etiologic aspects of coagulopathy in Takayasu's aortitis. Am Heart J 1982; 104:1039–1045.
233. Burns JC, et al. Coagulopathy and platelet activation in Kawasaki syndrome: identification of patients at high risk of development of coronary artery aneurysms. J Pediatr 1984; 105:206–211.
234. Jordan JM, Allen NB, Pizzo SV. Defective release of tissue plasminogen activator in systemic and cutaneous vasculitis. Am J Med 1987; 82:397–400.
235. Sun NCJ, et al. Skin fibrinolytic complement deposition in skin of rheumatoid arthritis and systemic lupus erythematosus. Ann Rheum Dis 1976; 35:321–326.
236. Wick G, et al. Is atherosclerosis an immunologically mediated disease? Immunol Today 1995; 16:27–33.
237. Yamamoto M, et al. Antithrombotic treatment of livedo vasculitis. J Am Acad Dermatol 1988; 18:57–62.
238. Wigley FM, et al. Intravenous iloprost treatment of Raynaud's phenomenon and ischaemic ulcers secondary to systemic sclerosis. J Rheumatol 1992; 19:1407–1414.
239. Torley HI, et al. A double blind randomised multicentre comparison of two doses of intra-

venous iloprost in the treatment of Raynaud's phenomenon secondary to connective tissue diseases. Ann Rheum Dis 1991; 50:800–804.
240. De Stefano R, et al. Efficacy and tolerability of iloprost in the treatment of digital vasculitis secondary to connective tissue diseases. Rec Prog Med 1992; 83:510–514.
241. Hoogenberg K, et al. Successful treatment of ulcerating livedo reticularis with infusions of prostacyclin. Br J Dermatol 1992; 127:64–66.
242. Fiessinger JN, Schafer M. Trial of iloprost versus aspirin treatment for critical limb ischaemia of thromboangiitis obliterans. Lancet 1990; 335:555–557.
243. Hauptman HW, Ruddy S, Roberts WN. Reversal of the vasospastic component of lupus vasculopathy by infusion of prostaglandin E1. J Rheumatol 1991; 18:1747–1752.
244. Curwin J, Jang IK, Fuster V. Expanded use of thrombolytic therapy. Mayo Clin Proc 1992; 67:1004–1005.
245. Klein KL, Pittelkow MR. Tissue Plasminogen activator for treatment of livedoidvasculitis. Mayo Clin Proc 1992; 67:923–933.

32
Therapy of Sjögren's Syndrome

Panayiotis G. Vlachoyiannopoulos and Haralampos M. Moutsopoulos
National University of Athens, Athens, Greece

I. INTRODUCTION

Sjögren's syndrome (SS) is a chronic autoimmune disorder primarily affecting females. SS can occur alone (primary SS, pSS) or in association with almost all of the autoimmune diseases (secondary SS, sSS). It usually appears in the fourth or fifth decade of life, and it is the second most common autoimmune rheumatic disorder after rheumatoid arthritis (RA). The autoimmune hallmarks of SS are lymphoid cell infiltration of the exocrine glands and overproduction of various autoantibodies [1]. The manifestations of the disease can be divided in glandular and extraglandular. Glandular manifestations include keratoconjunctivitis sicca (KCS) (leading to erosion of the corneal epithelium, filamentary keratitis, and cornea ulcers); xerostomia (leading to severe periodontal disease, dental caries, oral candidiasis, and loss of teeth); parotid gland enlargement, which is usually a self-limited condition; and dryness of upper airways mucosa and skin. The extraglandular manifestations comprise a wide variety of features, such as arthralgias, myalgias, low-grade fever, fatigue, Raynaud's phenomenon, pulmonary and kidney involvement, vasculitis, and B-cell lymphomas [1,2].

Despite the efforts to understanding the pathogenesis of SS the etiology of the disease still remains unknown. Therefore, the therapy remains empirical and symptomatic. Several therapeutic modalities however have been tested in recent years in placebo-controlled trials.

II. GENERAL CONSIDERATIONS

Regular outpatients visits; close collaboration with the outpatient clinics of rheumatology, ophthalmology, and oral medicine; and concentration on simple measures to relieve desiccation give the most satisfactory results in the therapy of SS [1,2].

Follow-up of disease laboratory parameters such as serum creatinine, C-reactive protein, rheumatoid factor, antinuclear antibodies, cryoglobulins, C3 and C4 levels, complete blood count, and urinalysis may allow early diagnosis of the extraglandular complications, side effects of the drugs, or malignancy [1–3].

Treatment of the patients with SS is divided into two parts: treatment of glandular manifestations and their consequences and treatment of the extraglandular manifestations. Treatment of the associated rheumatic disorders such as rheumatoid arthritis or systemic lupus erythematosus remains the same as it would if SS was not present [1–3].

III. GLANDULAR MANIFESTATIONS

Glandular manifestations of SS are due to decreased glandular secretions. The principal goal in treating the impaired lacrimal and salivary production associated with SS is the successful replacement of the glandular secretions. Immunotherapy does not relieve desiccation.

A. Opthalmological Manifestations—Keratoconjunctivitis Sicca

Patients with keratoconjunctivitis sicca (KCS) may complain of a "foreign body sensation" in the eye, accumulation of thick ropy secretions along the inner canthi, photosensitivity, or blurred vision [1].

Three tests are helpful to assess KCS: Shirmers I test, which measures tear production; the brake-up time, which measures tear quality; and rose bengal staining of the cornea (Figure 1), which may reveal superficial erosions of the corneal epithelium, filamentary keratitis, or ulcers of the cornea (Tables 1 and 2) [4,5].

1. Treatment of Dry Eyes

Therapeutic measures for dry eyes are [3,6,7,8]:

1. Local stimulators of tear secretion
2. Protective bicarbonate-buffered solutions
3. Replacement therapy
4. Supportive operative procedures

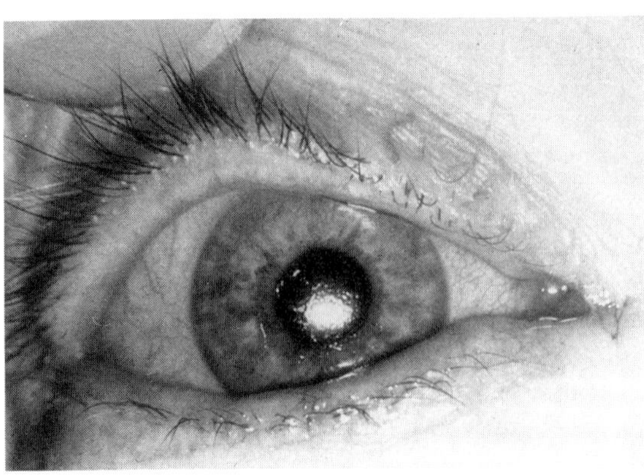

Figure 1 Injected conjunctiva, keratitis sicca, and crusted, dry eyelashes of a patient with Sjögren's syndrome.

Table 1 Tests to Assess Keratoconjunctivitis Sicca and Xerostomia

Test	Description	Positive if	Examines
Schirmer's I	Strips of filter paper 30 mm in length. One end of the paper is bent and the paper is slipped beneath the interior lid with the remainder of paper hanging out. Measure the length of paper wet by the tears.	≤5 mm in 5 min	Tear production
Break-up time	A drop of fluorescein is instilled in the eye. Measure the time between the last blink and the appearance of nonfluorescent areas in the tear film.	≤10 s	Tear quality
Rose bengal score	Rose bengal is an aniline dye which can stain only damaged epithelium of the cornea or conjunctiva. The pattern of staining is examined and scored according to Bijsterveld's scoring system [4].	≥4	Ocular surface condition
Stimulated parotid flow rate	Flow rate of the saliva after stimulation using citric acid.	≤7 mL/10 min	Amount of saliva as a reflection of the fucntional integrity of the parotid glands.
Unstimulated parotid flow rate	Measurement of the spontaneous saliva secretion.	≤1.5 mL/15 min	

Table 2 Imaging Techniques to Assess Functional and Anatomical Integrity of the Parotid Glands

Test	Description	Examines
Parotid gland scintigraphy	99^{m} Tc sodium pertechnate is injected intravenously. Observe the rate and density of label uptake and time of appearance of label in the mouth.	Functional integrity of the major salivary glands
Parotid sialography	Water-based contrast media are injected in the salivary gland duct system.	Anatomical integrity of the salivary gland duct system

A rapid worsening of complaints or excessive mucous production may denote infection and require treatment with proper antibiotics. The use of corticosteroids locally or systemically is not recommended, because corneal and conjunctival lesions may worsen, immune resistance is impaired, and the risk of infection increases [1–3].

Topical Stimulators. These include the following preparations, although none is commercially available [6,7]:

1. A cyclic, adenosine monophosphate (AMP) stimulator, 3-isobutyl-1-methylxanthine, administered as eye drops, has been found to decrease tear film osmolality and rose bengal staining [9].
2. A bromhexine derivative such as N-cyclohexyl-N-methyl-2-phenylethylamine HCI increases tear and protein secretion in rabbit eyes [6,7].
3. Cyclosporin A 2% in olive solution, in the form of eye drops, has been shown to be relatively effective in treating KCS in a recent placebo-controlled trial [10]. Cyclosporin A is a hydrophobic peptide, and it penetrates very easily the intact hydrophobic corneal epithelium to accumulate on the stroma. It has been shown that the topical cyclosporin eye solution increases significantly the break-up time and decreases the rose bengal score, but it does not affect Shrimer's I test [10]. The above results indicate that cyclosporin A is effective on the ocular surface where the goblet cells are abundant, but its effect on the lacrimal secretory/drainage system is rather remote. Major side effects of cyclosporin A eye solution are a mild discomfort due to local irritation, which can be decreased by concomitant use of artificial tears [10]. Scanning electron microscopic studies of rabbit corneas treated with topical cyclosporin revealed local areas of epithelial cell loss; probably due to the oil used as a vehicle and not to the cyclosporin A [11].

Bicarbonate-Buffered Electrolyte Solutions. These contain electrolytes which mimic the electrolyte composition of human lacrimal gland fluids enriched in a bicarbonate buffer. The preparation of such solutions was based on the hypothesis that bicarbonate interacts with mucin secreted by the conjunctival goblet cells to form a mucin-bicarbonate gel which protects the ocular surface in a mode of action well known in the physiology of gastric mucosa [7]. Such products are under evaluation at present, but an open pilot study has shown encouraging results. A nonpreserved bicarbonate-bufferred solution containing NaCl, KCl, CaCl2, MgCl2, NaCO3, and ZnCl2 is commercially available (BION Tears, Alcon Laboratories, Forth Worth, TX).

Artificial Lubricants. A number of artificial lubricants are available for the treatment of dry eyes (Table 3). These products only mimic the physical properties (pH, osmolarity) and not the chemical or the biological properties of the tears. They consist of a polymer, electrolytes, buffers, and EDTA, and some contain preservatives [6,7]. As a rule, the lubricating agents which contain preservatives are rather toxic to the ocular surface and cause local burning. If this is the case, they should be replaced by another preparation without preservatives [1–3,6–8]. A reasonable strategy for the alleviation of dry eye symptoms is as follows: If the patient has tears, she or he may use sustained-release carboxymethylpropylcellulose capsules placed in each eye twice daily. If the patient does not have tears, the capsules act as irritants and the use of lubricants in the

Table 3 Artificial Tear Preparations

Commercial name	Major component	Manufacturer
Preservative free		
Lacrisert	Hydroxypropylcellulose	Merck Sharp & Dohme
Cellufresh (0.5%)	Carboxymethylcellulose	Allergan (Irvine, CA)
Celluvisc (1%)	Carboxymethylcellulose	Allergan
Gum cellulose (0.3,0.625,0.9%)	Carboxymethylcellulose	Dessel's Pharmacy (San Francisco, CA)
Refresh	Polyvinyl alcohol and providone	Allergan
Hypotears PF	Other polymeric systems	IOLAB
Tears Naturale free	Other polymeric systems	Alcon
Unisol	Steril saline	Cooper Vision
With preservatives		
Tear Guard [a]	Hydroxymethylcellulose	Bio-Products (Westport, CT)
Lacril [b]	Hydroxypropylmethylcellulose	Allergan (Irvine, CA)
Moisture drops (0.5%)[c]	Hydroxypropylmethylcellulose	Bausch & Lomb
Tears Renewed [d]	Hydroxypropylmethylcellulose	Akon (Abita Springs, LA)
Liquifilm Tears [b]	Polyvinyl alcohol	Allergan (Irvine, CA)
Liquifilm Forte [e]	Polyvinyl alcohol	Allergan
Dwelle [f]	Polyvinyl alcohol	Dakryon (Lubbock, TX)
Dakrina [f]	Polyvinyl alcohol	Dakryon (Lubbock, TX)
Nutratear [g]	Polyvinyl alcohol	Dakryon (Lubbock, TX)
Tears plus [b]	Polyvinyl alcohol	Allergan
Hypotears [d]	Other polymeric systems	IOLAB
Tears Naturale [d]	Other polymeric systems	Alcon
Tears Naturalle II [h]	Other polymeric systems	Alcon

The products included here reflect merely the experience of the authors. Many other products may be of help to SS patients. No mention of a product in this table in no way reflects on its efficacy.
[a]Sorbic acid and edatade disodium.
[b]Chlorobutanol.
[c]Benzalkonium chloride.
[d]Benzalkonium chloride and edetate disodium.
[e]Thimerosal and edetate disodium.
[f]Potassium sorbate and EDTA.
[g]Benzalkonium 0.04% + 0.8% EDTA.
[h]Polyquard.

form of eye drops is to be preferred. If vision is blurred, a preparation with lower viscosity should be used [2,3,6,8].

The majority of the preparations used to treat KCS have been chosen on an empirical basis. Three preparations of eye lubricants meet the standards used in randomized, controlled clinical trials [6,7]:

1. A solution of 1% carboxymethylcellulose containing CaCl2, KCl, NaCl, and sodium lactate (Celluvisc, Allergan Pharmaceuticals, Irvine, CA) [7,12]
2. A preparation containing propyethyleneglycol 400 (PEG 400), dextran, and polycorbophil in an NaCl solution containing EDTA (Aquasite, Civa Vision, Duluth, GA) [7,13].
3. Topical sodium hyaluronate and topical fibronectin preparations, which at least are as good as other commercially available lubricants [14,15]

If the patient has found an appropriate eye lubricant and applies it more frequently than once an hour, a combination of a lubricating ointment (Table 4) during the night with eye drops during the day should be tried (2,6,8).

Supportive Operative Procedures. These may have to be done if the patient has to apply a lubricating agent more frequently than once an hour. If this is the case, the patient has severe dry eyes, and punctual cauterization is the procedure of choice. In case the patient has a mild dry eyes, cauterization may result in tearing, which would require reopening of the canaliculus puncta. Thus it is important to use the above procedure first on a temporary basis in order to determine whether the patient receives some symptomatic relief. Finally, in a case of severe dryness, lateral tarsorrhaphy is indicated in order to decrease the ocular surface. In cases of corneal perforation, a corneal transplant is necessary [2,6,8].

B. Oral Manifestations

Oral symptoms of SS are due to decreased saliva and vary widely from patient to patient. Patients may experience difficulties in eating dry foods without sufficient moisture, frequent ingestion of liquids, carrying water bottles in the pocket, oral soreness, adherence of food to buccal surfaces, dysphagia, and loss of taste and smell. The clinical examination may reveal fissuring of the tongue, angular cheilitis (Figure 2), dental caries, or painful white patchy lesions on the tongue or oral mucosa, which usually rep-

Table 4 Ocular Ointments

Commercial name	Preservative	Manufacturer
Duratears	Methylparaben/polyparaben	Alcon
Acrilube S.O.P.	Chlorobutanol	Allergan
Thilogel	Thiomersal	THILO & Co. GmbH
Refresh P.M.	Free	Allergan
Duolube	Free	Bausch & Lomb
Hypotears	Free	IOLAB
Akwa-Tears ointment	Free	Akorn (Abita Springs, LA)

The products included here reflect merely the experience of the authors. Many other products may be of help to SS patients. No mention of a product in this table in no way reflects on its efficacy.

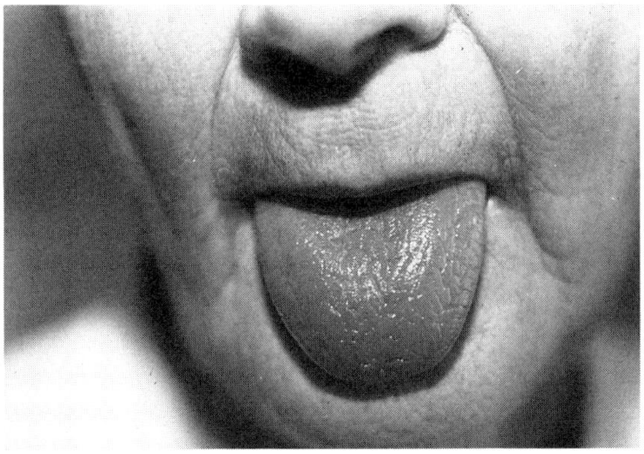

Figure 2 Atrophic, dry, deeply fissured tongue of a patient with Sjögren's syndrome.

resent oral candidiasis [1,2]. Tests to assess xerostomia on an objective basis are stimulated and unstimulated parotid flow rate, which measure the production of the saliva; and parotid gland scintigraphy and parotid gland sialography, which assess the functional and anatomical integrity of the salivary ducts of the parotid glands.

1. Treatment of Xerostomia and Prevention of Related Problems

The treatment xerostomia should meet the following aims [3,6,8,16]:

1. Oral hygiene to prevent dental caries
2. Careful examination to diagnose and treat oral candidiasis
3. Systemic therapy to stimulate glandular secretions
4. Use of saliva substitutes

Prevention of Dental Caries. To prevent or significantly reduce dental caries, the patients should avoid dietary sugar and use topical fluorides both as a fluoride-containing toothpaste or as a mouth rinse (e.g., 0.05% sodium fluoride for 2 min at bedtime). Chlorhexidine mouth rinse or gel may reduce cariogenic microorganisms, but it can cause taste disturbances and dental staining and is not well tolerated by patients with severe dryness, since it contains alcohol [16–18].

Therapy of Candidiasis. Candidiasis, seen as erythematous plaques on the tongue or gums, occurs in 30% of SS patients and causes mucosal burning and intolerance to acidic foods. Eradication is often difficult. The therapy of choice is application of topical nystatin 200,000-unit pastilles four to five times daily or 10 mg clotrimazole oral lozenges five times daily. Since the above preparations contain sugar, they are not indicated for maintenance therapy in cases of recurrent candidiasis. In such cases, 100,000-unit nystatin vaginal tablets, which can be slowly dissolved over 20 min two to three times daily for weeks or even months, are recommended [16].

Stimulation of Salivary Secretion. Local methods to stimulate secretion from residual salivary tissue include chewing sugarless gum or electrical stimulation with a Salitron R for 3 min, three times a day. If the salivary hypofunction is severe, the above measures are ineffective. Pilocarpine used systemically 5 mg three times daily increases salivary secretion with mild side effects, such as flushing and sweating. Pilocarpine for oral use is not commercially available at present, but it can be prescribed as pilocarpine hydrochloride aqueous solution 1 mg/mL [21]. Contraindications of pilocarpine include pregnancy, history of gastrointestinal ulcer, arrhythmias, severe, nonwell controlled hypertention [16]. Bromhexine orally at a high dose 48 mg/day (divided into three doses) may change the consistency of secreted saliva and decrease the feeling of dryness, but it has no effect on increasing the salivary secretion [16].

Saliva Substitutes. The best saliva substitute is water; therefore the best preventive measure against dryness is sipping fluids throughout the day. Saliva substitutes (Table 5) contain sorbitol as lubricant, electrolytes, calcium, phosphorus, and a preservative [16]. They should be prescribed in cases of severe dryness without any residual salivary gland function. However, the available products are effective only for a short duration. Drugs with antidepressant, anticholinergic, antihistaminic, and antidiuretic properties should be eliminated if possible [1–3,6,8].

C. Parotid Gland Enlargement

Parotid or other major salivary gland enlargement occurs very frequently in patients with primary SS (Figure 3), whereas lacrimal gland enlargement is very uncommon [1,2]. The volume of the parotid gland increases because of cellular infiltration and/or ductal obstruction. Therefore, the enlargement can be asymptomatic and self-limited. However, sometimes it can be more permanent and is associated with pain and erythema. In that case, a superinfection of the gland or the development of lymphoma should be suspected [1,2]. If the gland remains tender or enlarged, rule out lymphoma by biopsy. Recent studies have shown that the biopsy of the superficial lobe of the parotid gland has no side effects [3].

1. Treatment

There is no effective treatment for parotid gland swelling, which is a mild, self-limited condition. If the gland becomes tender with persistent enlargement, tetracycline orally (500 mg four times daily) should be tried. Local moist heat and nonsteroidal anti-inflammatory drugs may be helpful. Corticosteroids, although helpful, are not recom-

Table 5 Saliva Substitutes

Commercial name	Manufacturer
Mouthkote	Parnell Pharmaceuticals Inc. (Foster city, CA)
Oral Balance	Laclede (Cardena, CA) Heather Dental Supplies (Vancouver, BC, Canada)
Salivart	Cebauer Co. (Cleveland, OH)
Xero-Lube	Colgate Hoyt/Gel-Kam (Dallas, TX)

The products included here reflect merely the experience of the authors. Many other products may be of help to SS patients. No mention of a product in this table in no way reflects on its efficacy.

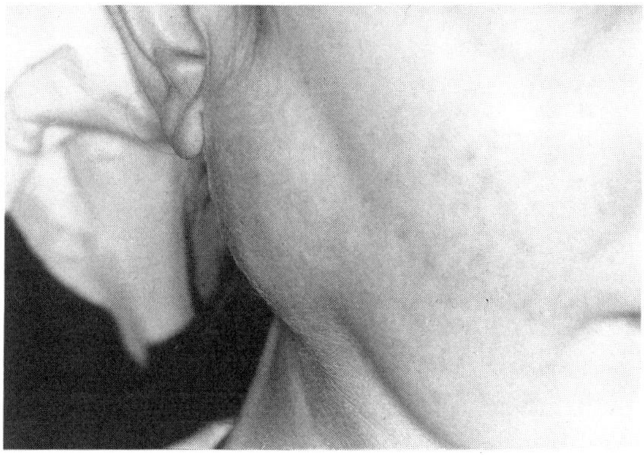

Figure 3 Patient with primary Sjögren's syndrome and persisting, firm enlargement of the parotid gland.

mended, because they may exacerbate an infection. Local radiation treatment and/or cytotoxic drugs are not recommended, because the risk for developing lymphoma increases from 40- to 100-fold [1–3].

D. Other Glandular Manifestations

Involvement of other exocrine glands, such as those of the upper airways, gastrointestinal tract, and skin occurs less frequently in SS. Dryness of the upper respiratory tract mucosa attributed to lymphocytic inflammation and an alteration in secretion as a result of gland damage can cause dry, crusted secretions in the nose, epistaxis, hoarseness, and, as described previously, bronchial hyperresponsiveness [23].

Among gastrointestinal manifestations of SS, chronic atrophic gastritis is the most common finding. Gastric discomfort and anemia due to loss of gastric mucosal function associated with the loss of intrinsic factor may be the most common complications [1,2,24].

When pancreatic function testing was carried out in primary or secondary SS patients, exocrine pancreatic impairment was found to be present in 63% of them [24]. This abnormality tended to be more severe in patients with longer disease duration and to be related to the degree of salivary flow reduction.

1. Treatment of the Dryness of the Airways

If there is nasal dryness or severe xerotrachea, a home humidifier to moisten the air and/or bromhexine at a dose of 48 mg/day may be effective measures. The following supportive measures are also of importance: immunization with pneumococcal polysaccharide vaccine to prevent pneumococcal pneumonia, antibiotic treatment of sinusitis, and removal of dry, crusted secretions to leave the sinuses clear [3,8].

2. Treatment of Atrophic Gastritis

Atrophic gastritis and esophagitis are usually mild and require no therapy. Anemia in primary SS should be evaluated with serum vitamin B_{12} levels and treated properly. In severe cases of epigastric discomfort and/or pain, antacids are of some value [3,8].

IV. EXTRAGLANDULAR MANIFESTATIONS

A. Musculoskeletal Manifestations

Extraglandular manifestations (systemic) are seen in one third of primary SS patients. The most common are easy fatigue, low-grade fever, myalgias, arthralgias, Raynaud's phenomenon, and nonerosive arthritis.

1. Raynaud's Phenomenon

Raynaud's phenomenon occurs in one third of SS patients. Primary SS patients with Raynaud's phenomenon had a greater tendency to develop extraglandular manifestations despite similar autoantibody profiles to that of patients without Raynaud's phenomenon and usually precedes sicca manifestations by many years [25].

Treatment of Musculoskeletal Manifestations and Raynaud's Phenomenon. Nonsteroidal anti-inflammatory drugs are helpful in the treatment of arthralgias/myalgias associated with SS. Hydroxychloroquine 200 mg per day can be effective in a subgroup of patients with arthalgias, anemia, and thrombocytopenia [8]. Avoidance of physical (cold exposure) or emotional stress together with nifedipine 5–10 mg three times daily are indicated to decrease the severity and frequency of Raynaud's phenomenon [2,3,6].

B. Pulmonary Manifestations

Pulmonary symptoms of SS are due to lymphocytic infiltration of the lung parenchyma and manifest radiologically as interstitial lung disease; pulmonary infiltrates, especially in perialveolar areas [22]; and rarely as nodular or cavitary lesions, which may represent lymphoma. It has been shown by a controlled study that over 30% of unselected primary SS patients have interstitial lung disease, which in the majority of cases was subclinical. When pulmonary involvement is symptomatic, it manifests as exertional dyspnea, recently developed cough, and bibasilar crackles on auscultation [26].

1. Treatment

If solid or cavitary lung nodules or hilar adenopathy are present, open biopsy is necessary to establish the diagnosis. Diffuse interstitial lung disease is usually mild and requires no therapy. However, follow-up of the patient with pulmonary function tests every year is recommended. In case the interstitial lesion is progressive, it must be treated with prednisone in: an initial dose of 1 mg/kg/day for 1 month following by progressive tapering of dosage according to the improvement in the pulmonary function and diffusion capacity parameters. [1–2,3,6].

C. Hepatic Manifestations and Their Treatment

Liver involvement in SS is rather rare, affecting 7% of patients. It has two forms: (a) primary biliary cirrhosis (PBC, usually stage I, in patients with antimitochondrial antibodies (AMAs) [27]; and (b) autoimmune chronic hepatitis. In addition, hepatitis related to the hepatitis C virus has been described in a limited number of patients [28]. Patients with SS and PBC can be treated with ursodeoxycholic acid, whereas SS patients with hepatitis C can be treated with interferon-α.

D. Renal Involvement

Two types of renal involvement are seen in primary SS patients [3]: (a) Glomerulonephritis, which is considered a consequence of systemic vasculitis, is manifested as proteinuria and raised creatinine levels [29], (b) interstitial nephritis, which is considered to be a consequence of lymphocytic infiltration of the renal interstitial space, is manifested as oliguria and renal tubular dysfunction with or without acidosis and Fanconi's syndrome. It occurs in 30% of primary SS patients. Untreated renal tubular acidosis usually leads to renal calculi and nephrocalcinosis [30].

1. Treatment

Glomerulonephritis is treated with prednisone at a dose of 0.5–1.0 mg/kg/day, with the dose being reduced according to the clinical situation. If the disease is refractory to prednisone, pulse intravenous cyclophosphamide (0.5–0.75 g/m^2) should be given at intervals of 1–2 months. In case of interstitial nephritis, the major problem is acidosis, which may be corrected with oral potassium and sodium bicarbonate. The administration of $NaHCO_3$ should begin with 1 g three times daily, but up to 12 g daily may be required. If the patient has gastrointestinal discomfort, a 10% sodium citrate solution may be given instead of $NaHCO_3$ [1–3,6,8].

E. Vasculitis and Its Treatment

Vasculitis in pSS can occur in two forms [1–3]: (a) Vasculitis limited to the skin (20% of pSS patients), which manifests as palpable purpura (leukoclastic vasculitis). (b) Systemic necrotizing vasculitis and endarteritis obliterans involving small and medium-sized arteries. It occurs in a minority of pSS patients, and usually involves the skin, peripheral nerves, and gastrointestinal tract, as well as the kidney, and is often associated with fever, cryoglobulinemia, and high titers of rheumatoid factor. It manifests as ulcerative skin lesions, digital gangrene, mononeuritis multiplex, mesenteric arteritis, myositis, and glomerulonephritis [1,3,6]. Leukoclastic vasculitis requires no specific therapy. Systemic necrotizing vasculitis can be treated with steroids, pulses of cyclophosphamide, as mentioned previously, and plasmapheresis [2].

F. Obstetrical and Gynecological Problems and Their Treatment

The fertility, parity, and sexual activity of women with pSS does not differ from that of the healthy women. In a recent report, dyspareunia was observed in 40% of premenopausal women with pSS compared with 3% observed in premenopausal controls. The histological picture of the patients' vaginal tissues revealed perivascular infiltration. It is well known that vaginal lubrication is not related to the production of fluids from the local glands, but it is mainly a transudate from the vaginal walls. Therefore, the small vessel vasculitis of the pelvis may be the explanation for the vaginal dryness [31].

1. Treatment of Vaginal Dryness

Vaginal dryness is a cause of painful intercourse. Vaginal lubricants such as K-Y jelly or recently available vaginal inserts are helpful. The patients should avoid cortisone creams. In postmenopausal women, estrogen preparations are recommended. It is important to explain that dyspareunia does not mean an "organic" failure of sexual activity [1–3,6]. In fact, the intercourse frequency did not diminish with age nor with the presence of dyspareunia in pSS patients unlike what has been observed in a control population [31].

G. Clinical Manifestations of Lymphoma in SS

Lymphomas in SS develop 43 times more commonly than in the general population and are of B-cell origin [1,2,32–34]. Further enlargement of the parotid glands, with the glandular tissue becoming firmer and tender, the recent development of lymph nodes or hepatosplenomegaly, cough, dyspnea on exertion, mediastinal or hilar lymph nodes, and nodular lung lesions may herald lymphoma development. There is some agreement that bilateral small reticulondular opacities are more compatible with lymphocytic pneumonitis, whereas larger, unilaterally localized nodules are more compatible with lymphoma [1–3,6,26].

1. Treatment

The treatment of lymphoma is based on the histological grading. Patients with low-grade lymphomas affecting exocrine glands should be completely evaluated for the extent of the disease, and if the disease is localized, a wait and watch policy should be undertaken [3,6,35]. In the case of advanced low-grade lymphomas with no symptoms, a conservative policy is also recommended. If the lymphomas are histologically high grade and clinically aggressive, combination chemotherapy is advised in close collaboration with the oncology department [36].

REFERENCES

1. Talal N, Moutsopoulos HM, Kassan SS. Sjogren's Syndrome. Clinical and Immunological aspects. Berlin: Springer 1987.
2. Moutsopoulos HM, Tzioufas AG. Sjögren's syndrome. In: Klippel JH, Dieppe PA, eds. Rheumatology. Mosby-Year Book, 1994:6.27.1–6.27.2.
3. Moutsopoulos HM, Vlachoyiannopoulos PG. What would I do if I had Sjogren's syndrome? Rheumatol Rev 1993; 2:17–23.
4. Workshop on Diagnostic Criteria for Sjögren's syndrome. I. Questionnaires for dry eye and dry mouth. II. Manual of Methods and procedures. Clin Exp Rheumatol 1989; 7:212–219.
5. Vitali C, Bombardieri S, Moutsopoulos HM, et al. Diagnostic criteria for Sjögren's syndrome. Results of a European prospective multicentre study. Arthritis Rheum 1993; 36:340–347.
6. Vlachoyiannopoulos PG, Moutsopoulos HM. Therapy of Sjögren's syndrome. Rheumatol Eur 1995; 24:63–64.
7. Nelson DJ. What's new in the treatment of dry eye? In: Homma M, Sugai S, Toyo T, et al., eds. Sjogren's Syndrome—State of the Art. Tokyo: Kugler, 1994:33–36.
8. Fox RI Treatment of the patient with Sjogren's syndrome. Rheum Dis Clin North Am 1992; 18:699–709.
9. Gilbard JP, Rossi SR, Heyda KG, Dartt DA. Stimulation of tear secretion and treatment of dry-eye disease with 3-isobutyl-1-methylxanthine. Arch Ophthalmol 1991; 109:672–676.
10. Gündüz K, Ozdemir O. Topical cyclosporin treatment of keratoconjunctivitis sicca in secondary Sjogren's syndrome. Acta Ophthalmo 1994; 72:438–442.

11. Yersuza P, Cellini M, Zucchini PG, et al. Ultrastructural and immunohistochemical study on the effect of topical cyclosporin A in the rabbit eye. Cornea 1989; 8:81–89.
12. Adams J, Wilcox MJ, Mordaunt J, et al. Unpreserved corboxymethylcellulose artificial tears evaluated in patient with keratoconjunctivitis sicca. Cornea 1992; 11:294–301.
13. Tauber J, Crosser VA, Mardelli PG. Improvement of squamous metaplasia following Aquasite TM treatment in patients with dry eye syndrome and in normal volunteers. Invest Ophthalmol Vis Sci 1993; 34:(Suppl.):1742.
14. Nelson JD, Farris RL. Sodium hyaluronate and polyvinyl alcohol artificial tear preparations: a comparison in patients with keratoconjunctivitis sicca. Arch Ophthalmol 1988; 106:484–487.
15. Nelson JD, Gordon JF. Topical fibronectin in the treatment of keratoconjunctivitis sicca. Am J Ophthalmol 1992; 114:441–447.
16. Daniels TE. New approaches to treating dry mouth. In: Homma M, Sugai S, Toyo T, et al., eds. Sjogren's Syndrome—State of the Art. Tokyo: Kugler, 1994:61–65.
17. Newbrun E, Preventing dental caries: current and prospective strategies. J Am Dent Assoc 1992; 123:68–73.
18. Newbrun E. Preventing dental caries: breaking the chain of transmission. J Am Dent Assoc 1992; 123:55–59.
19. Stellez M, Chou L, Daniels TE. Electrical stimulation of salivary flow in patients with Sjögren's syndrome. J Dent Res 1988; 657:1334–1337.
20. Talal N, Quin JH, Daniels TE. The clinical effects of electrostimulation on salivary function of Sjögren's syndrome patients. Rheumatol Int 1992; 12:43–45.
21. Fox PC, Atkinson JC, Macynski AA, et al. Pilocarpine treatment of salivary gland hypofunction and dry mouth (xerostomia). Arch Intern Med 1991; 151:1149–1152.
22. Papiris SA, Skopouli FN, Maniati MA, et al. Bronchiolitis in primary Sjögren's syndrome. In: Homma, M, Sugai, S, Tojo, T, et al., eds. Sjögren's syndrome—State of the Art. Amsterdam: Kugler, 1994:431.
23. La Corte R, Potena A, Bajocchi G, et al. Increased bronchial responsiveness in primary Sjögren's syndrome: a sign of tracheo-bronchial involvement. Clin Exp Rheumatol 1991; 9:125–130.
24. Tsianos EB, Moutsopoulos HM: Sjogren's syndrome and the gut. Baillieres Clin Rheumatol 1989; 3:357–370.
25. Skopouli FN, Talal A, Galanopoulou V, et al. Raynaud's phenomenon in primary Sjogren's syndrome. J Rheumatol 1990; 17:618–620.
26. Constantopoulos SH, Tsianos EV, Moutsopoulos HM. Pulmonary and gastrointestinal manifestations of Sjogren's syndrome. Rheum Dis Clin North Am 1992 18:617–635.
27. Skopouli FN, Barbatis C, Moutsopoulos HM. Liver Involvement in primary Sjogren's syndrome. Br J Rheum 1994; 33:745–748.
28. Haddad J, Deny P, Munz-Gotheil C, et al. Lymphocytic sialoadenitis of Sjögren's syndrome associated with chronic hepatitis C virus liver disease. Lancet 1992; 321–323.
29. Moutsopoulos HM, Balow JE, Lawley TJ, et al. Immune complex glomerulonephritis in sicca syndrome. Am J Med 1978; 64:955–960.
30. Siamopoulos KC, Elisaf M, Drosos AA, et al. Renal tubular acidosis in primary Sjogren's syndrome. Clin Rheumatol 1992; 11:1–5.
31. Skopouli FN, Papanikolaou S, Malamou-Mitsi V, et al. Obstetric and gynecologic profile in primary Sjogren's syndrome patients. Ann Rheum Dis 1994; 53:569–573.
32. Talal N, Sokoloff L, Barth WF. Extrasalivary lymphoid abnormalities in Sjögren's syndrome (reticulum cell sarcoma, "pseudrolymphoma, macroglobulinemia) Am J Med 1967; 43:50–65.
33. Zulman J, Jaffe R, Talal N. Evidence that the malignant lymphoma of Sjögren's syndrome is a monoclonal B-cell neoplasm. N Engl J Med 1978; 299:1215–1220.

34. Kassan SS, Thomas TL, Moutsopoulos HM, et al. Increased risk of lymphoma in sicca syndrome. Ann Intern Med 1978; 89:888-892.
35. Pavlidis NA, Drosos AA, Papadimitriou C, et al. Lymphoma in Sjogren's syndrome can regress spontaneously. Med Paediatr Oncol 1992; 20:279–283.

33
Management of the Antiphospholipid Syndrome

E. Nigel Harris*
University of Louisville, Louisville, Kentucky

I. ANTIPHOSPHOLIPID SYNDROME

A. Case Report and Discussion

A 38-year-old woman was admitted to the hospital because of sudden confusion. On the day of admission, she was performing her usual job as an assembly worker when she slumped forward, started mumbling incoherently, and appeared confused. She was rushed to the emergency room of this hospital, but by the time of arrival, she was talking normally and was fully oriented with respect to time, person, and place. She had no memory of the event at work. Three similar events had occurred during the last 6 months, but these lasted only a few seconds and were noticed only by her spouse. The patient had been otherwise well and was taking no medications. She had two children, ages 15 and 10 years of age, both of whom were well. Her third child (age 4 years) was delivered at 30 weeks because of intrauterine growth retardation. She developed deep vein thrombosis 2 weeks after delivery of her second child and was treated with heparin and then Warfarin for 3 months. Subsequently, there were no other problems. The patient has had no family history of unexplained thrombosis, stroke, or myocardial infarction. Review of systems and past medical history revealed no symptoms of systemic lupus erythematosus (SLE).

Physical examination, including a thorough neurological evaluation, was normal. Laboratory tests were significant for low platelet count (65,000/mm^3), and a prolonged partial thromboplastin time (38 s; control 27 s). Master chemistry, urinalysis, and electrocardiogram (EKG) were normal. Antinuclear antibody (ANA) was positive at 1:40. ECHO cardiogram showed slightly thickened mitral valves with trivial mitral insufficiency. Electroencephalogram (EEG) was normal. A magnetic resonance imaging (MRI) showed three discrete areas of infarction, one in the cerebellum, another in the right parietal lobe, and a third in the left temporal lobe.

Additional laboratory studies were ordered. Plasma levels of protein C, S, antithrombin III, and homocysteine were normal. IgG anticardiolipin was high positive (250

**Current affiliation*: Morehouse School of Medicine, Atlanta, George

GPL units), and IgM anticardiolipin moderate positive (50 MPL units). A lupus anticoagulant test was also positive. A diagnosis of the antiphospholipid syndrome (APS) was made.

The patient was started on Coumadin at a dose adjusted to achieve an INR (International Normalized Ratio) of 3.0. Half an aspirin daily was also begun. Issues of contraception, management of any future pregnancies, and any future surgical procedures were discussed. Six months after discharge from the hospital, the patient remains asymptomatic. The IgG and IgM anticardiolipin tests remain high positive.

1. Case Discussion

The above history is fairly typical of the APS. Few other disorders would explain postpartum venous thrombosis, multiple cerebral infarcts, and intrauterine growth retardation in this woman's last pregnancy. However, APS is not the only diagnosis that should be considered. Venous thrombosis is not infrequent in the postpartum period, and intrauterine growth retardation in her third pregnancy may have had an explanation other than APS, given that her first two pregnancies were normal. All these events could have occurred too in the context of SLE without the patient having APS. Cerebral vasculitis as a complication of SLE could have accounted for multiple cerebral lesions, and venous thrombosis might have been a complication of the nephrotic syndrome. This patient did not have sufficient clinical and laboratory features for a diagnosis of SLE. A high positive IgG anticardiolipin antibody and positive lupus anticoagulant test clinched the diagnosis of APS. Prophylactic treatment was started with Coumadin and aspirin to prevent recurrences of venous and arterial thrombosis. As is typical in these patients, anticardiolipin tests remained high positive several months after treatment was initiated. Features of APS as well as its laboratory diagnosis and medical management are the subjects discussed in this chapter.

II. ANTIPHOSPHOLIPID SYNDROME: DEFINITION AND CLINICAL PRESENTATIONS

The antiphospholipid syndrome may be defined as a disorder of recurrent venous and/or arterial thromboses, pregnancy losses, and thrombocytopenia associated with positive anticardiolipin and lupus anticoagulants tests (Table 1) [1]. A number of other ("minor") clinical features have been recognized in these patients [2–6], but none is frequent or specific enough to enable diagnosis, nor is it known the extent to which they are predictive for recurrent thrombosis or pregnancy losses. However, the presence of "minor" features such as livedo reticularis, cardiac valvular vegetations, chronic leg ulcers, and transverse myelitis (Table 1) in patients with unexplained thrombosis or pregnancy loss help strengthen a diagnosis of APS. A significant percentage of APS patients seen by rheumatologists also have SLE or, less frequently, other connective tissue diseases. Some authorities have subcategorized APS into a "secondary" antiphospholipid syndrome (SAPS) when the patient also has SLE or other connective tissue disease, and "primary" antiphospholipid syndrome (PAPS) if this is the only disorder present [7–10]. Thus far, characteristic features of APS appear to be essentially the same in both PAPS and SAPS [11], and a recent retrospective collaborative study [166] suggests that the risks of recurrent thrombosis and pregnancy loss are also the same. Hence, although distinctions between PAPS and SAPS may be important for

Table 1 Features of APS[a]

Clinical	
major features	
venous thrombosis	
arterial thrombosis	
recurrent loss of pregnancy	
thrombocytopenia	
minor features	
livedo reticularis	
Libman-Sacks endocarditis and cardiac valve dysfunction	
chronic leg ulcers	
transverse myelopathy	
avascular necrosis	
Laboratory	
IgG anticardiolipin (>20 GPL units)	
IgM anticardiolipin (>40 MPL units)	
IgA anticardiolipin (?)	
lupus anticoagulant	

[a]A diagnosis of APS is based on the presence of one major clinical and one laboratory feature. The laboratory test should be positive on more than one occasion more than 8 weeks apart. The more clinical and laboratory features present, the more likely the diagnosis.

clinical and laboratory investigators interested in studying this disorder, the management of features characteristic of the syndrome is the same.

A. Thrombosis

Veins and arteries of all sizes are subject to thrombosis in patients with APS. These events usually occur intermittently and at single sites. Since thrombotic events are intermittent, but antiphospholipid antibodies persist at high levels for prolonged periods of time, it seems likely that some triggering event must also occur in the vasculature to induce thrombosis. Antiphospholipid antibodies probably induce only a hypercoaguable state. It should be noted that like APS, patients with other hypercoaguable states such as hereditary protein C, protein S, or antithrombin III deficiency are also subject to discrete thrombotic events that are often triggered by factors such as surgery or pregnancy [12]. There have been reports of thrombosis related to APS occurring in children [13–20].

Patients with thrombosis are subject to recurrent events. Two retrospective series have suggested that patients have thrombotic events only in the venous circulation or only in the arterial circulation [21,22]. However, another recent retrospective series (Krnic et al., submitted) found that about half of the patients studied had histories of both arterial and venous thromboses. Since Coumadin currently appears to be the treatment of choice to prevent either recurrent venous or arterial thrombosis, management to prevent future events is essentially the same regardless of the site of the original thrombus.

Since thrombosis may occur at any venous or arterial site, patients may present in diverse ways. Involvement of the arterial circulation presents most frequently as

Table 2 Causes of Recurrent Arterial Thrombosis Other than APS

Atherosclerosis
Systemic vasculitis
Emboli from cardiac valve vegetations
Protein C deficiency
Protein S deficiency
Antithrombin III deficiency
Buerger's disease
Homocystinuria

cerebral infarction [23–25]. In addition to usual presentations of stroke, patients may come to medical attention because of intellectual deterioration, frank dementia [26,27], or episodic confusion, as exemplified in the case history presented in the introduction of this chapter. About one third of affected patients presenting with features of stroke have normal computerized tomography (CT) and magentic resonance imaging scans and cerebral angiogram may be normal as well [25].

Other presentations secondary to thrombosis of the arterial circulation include myocardial infarction [28,29], peripheral gangrene [30], bowel infarction [31], ophthalmic artery occlusion [32], dermal infarction [33] or Addison's disease [34,35]. Renal abnormalities may be secondary to occlusion of large, medium, or small renal arteries [36–39]. In patients presenting with unexplained arterial thrombotic events, other causes besides APS should be considered (Table 2) [40].

Presentations of venous thrombosis are also diverse. Deep vein thrombosis of the lower extremities with or without pulmonary embolism are described most frequently [41–45]. In a few instances, patients may present with pulmonary hypertension which may be secondary to recurrent pulmonary emboli but might occur because of in situ thrombosis [46,47]. Other presentations include thrombosis of the inferior vena cava [44,48] or thrombosis of the renal [38,49], hepatic (Budd-Chiari syndrome) [50–52], ophthalmic, or saggital veins [53]. Venous thrombosis at the latter sites should prompt consideration of a hypercoaguable state (Table 3) [12].

Table 3 Causes of Recurrent Venous Thrombosis Other than APS

Resistance to activated protein C
Protein C deficiency
Protein S deficiency
Antithrombin III deficiency
Nephrotic syndrome
Malignancy

Source: From Svensson PJ, Dahlback B. Resistance to activated protein C as a basis for venous thrombosis. N Engl J Med 1994; 330:517–522.

B. Pregnancy Loss

Recurrent pregnancy loss is a frequent presenting feature of APS [54–57]. Most reviews emphasize pregnancy loss in the second or third trimester, but recurrent first-trimester recurrences are also common. A thorough obstetrical history is necessary, since patients may have given birth to live babies, but their pregnancies might have been complicated by intrauterine growth retardation, preeclampsia, or prematurity, as exemplified in the case history at the start of this chapter. When fetuses aborted by women with APS are examined, they are usually normal except that they may be small for gestational dates. Placental infarction associated with placental vessel thrombosis is a characteristic finding [58,59]. In evaluating women for recurrent pregnancy losses, physicians should recognize that there are several other causes of recurrent abortion and fetal loss, and APS accounts for only a small minority of these events [60]. A history of venous or arterial thrombosis, false-positive test for syphilis, or the presence of features of SLE should prompt anticardiolipin and lupus anticoagulant tests to be ordered in women who have one or two miscarriages. Otherwise, these tests are appropriate only in women with three or more first-trimester miscarriages, or with one or more second- or third-trimester pregnancy losses. Healthy pregnant women should not be tested [3,61], and the value of the test in women with one or two first-trimester miscarriages is uncertain.

Although there are case reports of thrombosis occurring in neonates born to mothers with APS [12–15], it is clear that the overwhelming majority of these children are normal at birth and can expect an uneventful childhood. Based on limited family studies, mothers can be reassured that the chance of their children developing APS as an adult is probably small.

C. Thrombocytopenia

The third major complication of APS is a low platelet count [8,61,62]. A few patients present only with features of idiopathic thrombocytopenic purpura [63]. However, most patients with thrombocytopenia have only mildly depressed platelet counts (100,000–150,000 mm^3). Thrombocytopenia is often intermittent and does not appear to be related to changes in anticardiolipin antibody levels. Some patients have positive Coombs' tests [62,64], and a small percentage of these suffer hemolytic anemia [64].

Thrombocytopenia may not protect patients against thrombosis. A recent retrospective series of our own [166] found cases of thrombosis occurring in patients with platelet counts of even less than 50,000/mm^3. Prescribing prophylactic anticoagulant treatment in patients who are thrombocytopenic poses a problem, which will be addressed later in this chapter.

III. DIAGNOSTIC TESTS

Diagnosis of APS is based on a characteristic history as well as a positive anticardiolipin or lupus anticoagulant test [1]. Some patients have false-positive tests for syphilis, but standard tests for syphilis are neither sensitive nor specific enough to be useful in the diagnosis of APS. Although both the anticardiolipin and lupus anticoagulant tests are positive in about 60–70% of patients, only one of the two tests is positive in the remainder. Hence, physicians should order *both* tests in patients suspected of APS. However, the lupus anticoagulant test is unreliable in patients on heparin or taking oral anticoagulants; hence, in those instances, reliance has to be placed solely on the anticardiolipin test for diagnosis.

A. Anticardiolipin Test

The anticardiolipin test is a serological test, so the laboratory should be instructed to collect blood in a (red) top tube. Calibrators enabling uniformity in reporting antibody levels have been accepted by many laboratories, and test performance follows standard procedures [65–70].

Briefly, the assay involves coating polystyrene ELISA plates with cardiolipin and then blocking overnight with a 10% adult bovine serum (ABS)/phosphate-buffered saline (PBS) buffer (Fig. 1). Patient samples and calibrators diluted 1/50 in 10% ABS/PBS are then added in duplicate to the ELISA plate wells. After an incubation period of 0.5 to 1.0 h, the plates are emptied and washed with PBS. Then alkaline phosphatase or horseradish peroxidase–labeled antihuman IgG (for IgG anticardiolipin detection), antihuman IgM (for IgM anticardiolipin detection), or antihuman IgA (for IgA anti-

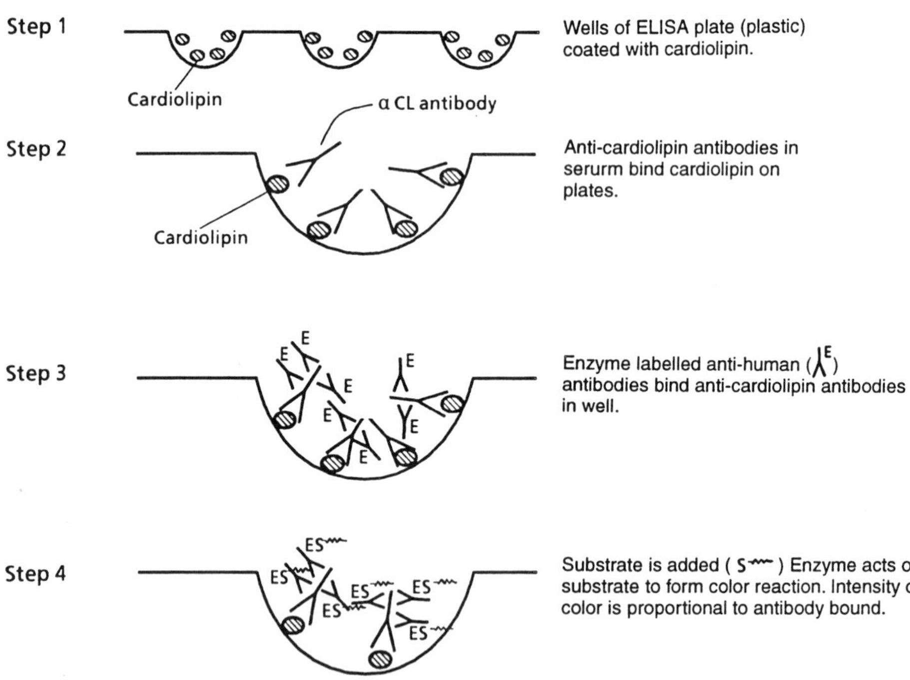

Figure 1 Diagrammatic depiction of the anticardiolipin test. Wells of ELISA plates are first coated with cardiolipin and then the plates are blocked with 10% adult bovine serum (ABS)/PBS. Patient samples diluted in 10% ABS/PBS are added to wells, and after incubation, the wells are washed and enzyme-labeled antihuman antibodies are added. After incubation, plates are washed and enzyme substrate is added. Breakdown of the substrate by enzyme-labeled antibodies in the wells causes a color reaction that is proportional to the amount of anticardiolipin antibodies present.

cardiolipin detection) are added to the wells. After another incubation period, the plates are again emptied and washed with PBS. The final step of the assay involves the addition of appropriate substrates for alkaline phosphatase or horseradish perioxidase depending on the type of conjugate that was used. A color reaction develops, the intensity of which can be measured as an optical density reading by an ELISA reader. By plotting optical density readings of the calibrators against their known anticardiolipin levels (using a log-logit or log-log plot), a calibration curve can be established. Anticardiolipin levels for patient samples can be derived from the calibration curve. Some well-validated anticardiolipin kits are currently being marketed, and these have made performance of the test easier for laboratory technicians.

IgG anticardiolipin results are reported in GPL units, IgM anticardiolipin in MPL units, and IgA anticardiolipin in APL units. Because the error range of test results can be relatively large, we recommend reporting results both quantitatively and semiquantitatively. Thus, values are regarded as "negative" if they fall below 10 GPL units (for IgG), below 10 MPL units (for IgM), or below 15 APL units (for IgA). Low, medium, and high positive results are defined as between 10 and 20, 20 and 80, and above 80 GPL, MPL, or APL units, respectively [68].

A positive anticardiolipin test result requires careful interpretation. These antibodies are induced by a variety of infectious, inflammatory and connective tissue disorders, as well as in normal individuals. In general, medium to high positive IgG anticardiolipin test results are most specific for the diagnosis of APS. Occasionally, patients have been recognized with thrombosis who have only elevated IgM anticardiolipin levels, but the significance of this isotype in predicting pregnancy loss remains in doubt. Rarely, we have seen patients only with high positive IgA anticardiolipin test results who have had thrombosis. Our practice is to run the IgG and IgM anticardiolipin tests routinely. The IgA anticardiolipin test is performed only when the diagnosis of APS is strongly suspected but IgG and IgM anticardiolipin tests are negative.

Anticardiolipin antibodies cross react with negatively charged phospholipids (70,71); hence, some laboratories have introduced ELISA assays with other phospholipids as antigens. Thus, in addition to anticardiolipin test results, these laboratories report antiphosphatidylserine, antiphosphatidylglycerol, and so forth results. Unpublished studies of our own have found few instances of APS sera being high positive for one antigen but not for another. Discrepancies do exist at low levels, but the clinical significance of such results is uncertain. Some laboratories have found that use of an alternative phospholipid such as phosphatidylserine instead of cardiolipin has enabled more specific results [72], and there are functional data to support such a claim [73,74]. A recently introduced diagnostic kit, the APhL ELISA (Louisville APL Diagnostics, Louisville, KY) utilizes a mixture of negatively charged phospholipids as antigen, which reportedly enable more specific detection of APS sera—syphilis and other infectious disease sera do not bind other phospholipid antigens as well as APS; hence, the use of alternative phospholipids as antigens may reduce false-positive results due to infectious disease and other sera.

There is currently much interest in the antigen bound by anticardiolipin antibodies. Although it was originally believed that these antibodies bound negatively charged phospholipids [70–74], many groups now suggest that they bind instead a plasma protein called β_2-glycoprotein 1 (β_2GP1) [75–79]. The basis of the latter hypothesis is the observation that binding by anticardiolipin antibodies from patients with APS is increased when a diluting buffer containing bovine serum (or serum from other animals) is used [80,81]. The serum protein responsible for enhanced binding is β_2GP1. β_2GP1 binds negatively charged molecules avidly (82), and since this protein has been demonstrated to inhibit phospholipid-dependent coagulation reactions [83,84], it has been suggested that it serves as a natural anticoagulant in plasma [83,84]. Interruption of its activity by anticardiolipin antibodies would favor thrombosis. The debate about how β_2GP1 enhances anticardiolipin binding is complex. Some investigators find these antibodies bind β_2GP1 alone, although they disagree about the ELISA plates [78,79] and assay conditions required to demonstrate such binding. Other investigators have not found anticardiolipin binding to β_2GP1 alone [85–89], although all agree that the protein does enhance binding activity. The issue of what anticardiolipin antibodies bind in the ELISA test should not detract from its clinical usefulness in identifying patients with APS. Standard assay procedures contain sufficient β_2GP1 to enable maximal anticardiolipin binding activity [69].

B. Lupus Anticoagulant Test

The lupus anticoagulant test measures a functional characteristic of antiphospholipid antibodies; that is, their ability to inhibit clot formation in a test tube by inhibiting the conversion of prothrombin to thrombin or the activation of factor X (Fig. 2). The latter reactions are both catalyzed by negatively charged phospholipids, and antibodies with lupus anticoagulant activity can inhibit formation of the "prothrombinase" and "tenase" complexes (Fig. 2).

The lupus anticoagulant test is a clotting assay and is performed using patient plasma. Hence, blood should be collected in a citrated (blue-top) tube for testing. Physicians should request a lupus anticoagulant test rather than a specific assay, such as a partial thromboplastin time (PTT) or Russell viper venom time (RVVT). Laboratories performing the lupus anticoagulant test usually do two or three assays to first establish whether the plasma clotting time is prolonged. The most frequently used assays are the PTT, RVVT, or kaolin clotting time (KCT) [89]. One or more of these tests will be prolonged if a lupus anticoagulant is present. However, a clotting factor deficiency can also cause prolonged clotting times. The latter possibility is excluded by mixing equal volumes of patient and normal plasma. If the prolonged clotting time is due to a factor deficiency, the test will correct with mixing, but if the prolonged clotting time is due to a clotting factor inhibitor, such as the lupus anticoagulant, the mixing test will remain abnormal or correct only partially. Finally, to distinguish the lupus anticoagulant from other clotting factor inhibitors, a phospholipid mixture or freeze-dried platelets (a source of membrane phospholipids) is added to the plasma [89]. Normalization of the clotting time by addition of excess phospholipids confirms the presence of the lupus anticoagulant.

Variations in reagents used to perform these clotting assays as well as differences in collection, preparation, and storage of plasma may all account for significant interlaboratory differences in lupus anticoagulant results. In the United States, the College of American Physicians has established a monitoring program for lupus anticoagulant testing, and this may eventually enable greater uniformity in results in the future.

There has been considerable interest in the relationship of antibodies detected in the anticardiolipin test to antibodies detected in the lupus anticoagulant assay. The

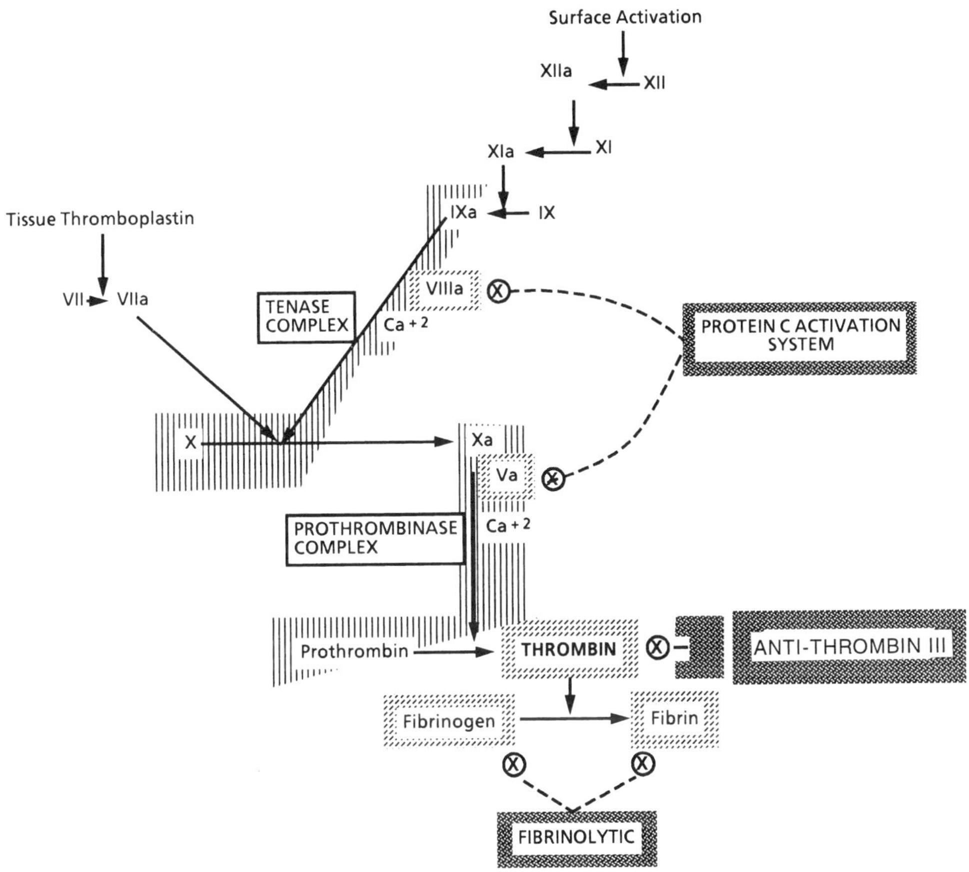

Figure 2 The clotting cascade. There are several steps in the clotting cascade that are catalyzed by phospholipids. These include activation of factor X by the "tenase complex," the prothrombin-thrombin conversion reaction by the "prothrombinase complex," or protein C activation. Any of the phospholipid-dependent coagulation reactions can be inhibited by antiphospholipid antibodies. In the test tube, the main effect of these antibodies is to inhibit either the "prothrombinase" or "tenase" reactions so delaying clot formation—hence, the lupus anticoagulant test is characterized by a prolonged clotting time. In vivo, protein C activation may be inhibited, which may lead to thrombosis, since activation of protein C normally inhibits clotting—neutralization of this effect by antiphospholipid antibodies might cause thrombosis.

anticardiolipin test quantifies antibody bound to cardiolipin in an ELISA plate, whereas the lupus anticoagulant test measures the functional ability of antiphospholipid antibodies to inhibit clotting. Hence, these two tests measure different attributes of antiphospholipid antibodies. It is therefore not surprising that 20–30% of patients with APS will have one test positive and the other negative. Two studies have reported physical separation of antibodies with cardiolipin binding and lupus anticoagulant activities [90,91], but two subsequent groups of investigators could not separate these activities [92–94]. It is currently believed by some investigators that antibodies with lupus anticoagulant activity are specific for prothrombin [95] or a complex of prothrombin and phospholipid

[96], whereas anticardiolipin antibodies bind β_2GP1 with or without cardiolipin. In contrast, other investigators believe both groups of antibodies to be specific for phospholipids; differences between anticardiolipin and lupus anticoagulant being more likely attributable to differences in assays used for their detection [73,92].

IV. MANAGEMENT

In a patient diagnosed as having APS, certain important questions must be addressed. The first involves the risk of thrombosis and management to prevent such events. The second involves the risk of pregnancy loss and management to prevent such losses. Thrombocytopenia, the third frequent complication of APS, is rarely severe enough to cause hemorrhage, but treatment of severe thrombocytopenia and thrombosis prophylaxis in affected patients with platelet counts less than 50,000/mm^3 must also be considered.

A. Thrombosis

Patients with APS who have had one thrombotic event are at risk for recurrent events. This was first documented by Glueck and colleagues, who reported that 13.7% of their patients with venous thrombosis and 6.7% of those with arterial thrombosis were at risk of recurrent events per year [47]. Subsequently, a number of retrospective series reported by neurologists [25,97,98], rheumatologists [99–101,166], hematologists [21], and obstetricians [22] have recognized this high risk of recurrence. Recently, some investigators have addressed treatment to prevent such recurrences [21,100,101,166]. Other issues such as the management of patients with recurrent thrombosis despite adequate anticoagulation therapy, the management of patients with APS undergoing surgery, and whether to treat patients with APS who have never had thrombosis have all become important. These subjects will be addressed below.

1. Prevention of Recurrent Venous Thrombosis

The initial management of venous thrombosis in patients with APS follows standard guidelines. Patients are initially heparinized to achieve a PTT of 1.5–2.5 times normal, and then warfarin can be initiated within a day or two of starting heparin [102]. Some patients with lupus anticoagulant activity already have a prolonged PTT, and there is often uncertainty as to what PTT is appropriate for full anticoagulation. In the latter circumstance, some physicians estimate the patient's need for heparin and administer that dose—for example, an IV bolus of 5000 units followed by 1000–1250 units/h. However, the dose of heparin to achieve full anticoagulation varies between patients, and a better approach might be to measure plasma heparin levels and aiming for 0.2–0.4 units/μL.

Hemorrhage is the most frequent complication of heparin therapy, but the half-life of this agent is short, and PTT returns to normal rapidly once administration of the drug ceases [102]. Heparin may cause thrombocytopenia in 6–15% of treated patients—an idiosyncratic effect [103]. This complication usually occurs within 3 to 5 days of initiation of therapy and resolves with discontinuation of the drug. About 0.5% of patients with heparin-induced thrombocytopenia may develop venous or arterial thrombosis [104]. Distinguishing heparin-induced and APS-induced thrombocytopenia and thrombosis may be difficult. However, if these events occur within 1 week of initiation of heparin, it would be safe to assume that they are drug related; in addition, resolution with discontinuation of the drug will confirm that heparin was the cause.

Once the acute management of venous thrombosis has been accomplished with heparin, the next issue is prophylactic therapy. This is achieved with warfarin. In patients with APS, additional questions that must be asked are what level of anticoagulation is required and for how long must this drug be given?

Three retrospective series [21,100,101] and an unpublished one of our own [166] found that recurrences of venous thrombosis were frequent when warfarin was stopped. In a study of 19 patients with antiphospholipid antibodies and histories of venous thrombosis, Derksen and colleagues [100], reported a 50% probability of recurrence at 2 years and 78% probability of recurrence at 8 years without anticoagulation. Patients receiving warfarin had a 100% probability of no thrombotic recurrences at 8 years. Rosove [21], Khamashta [101], and their respective colleagues as well as our own series [166] also found that use of warfarin significantly reduced the frequency of recurrent venous and arterial thrombotic events.

Two studies have addressed the issue of intensity of warfarin therapy. Rosove and colleagues reported that recurrent thrombotic events were uncommon in patients with INRs above 2.6, and on the basis of their results, suggested aiming for an INR of 3.0 [21]. Khamashta and colleagues reported that thrombotic recurrences were significantly reduced in patients on warfarin therapy whose INRs exceeded 3.0 compared with those with INR values less than 3.0 [101]. Both studies were retrospective and patient data were often collected before the International Normalized Ratio (INR)* was widely used for measuring the intensity of anticoagulation. Our own retrospective series relied on the prothrombin ratio and found that patients with prothrombin ratios of 1.5–2.0 (approximating an INR of 2.5–3.0) seldom had thrombotic recurrences. Given the risk of hemorrhage at INR values above 3.0 [21,101], our present recommendation is to aim for an INR of 2.6–3.0.

Hemorrhage is the major side effect of warfarin. When hemorrhage occurs, or anticoagulation has to be reversed for surgery, the administration of fresh frozen plasma is effective rapidly, and 1–2 mg vitamin K intravenously is effective within 24 h. Skin necrosis is a rare complication of Coumadin therapy and is often associated with protein C deficiency** [105,106].

Women of reproductive age taking warfarin should be warned of the teratogenic effects of this drug [107,108]. Unfortunately, estrogen-containing oral contraceptives

---

*Adoption of the International Normalized Ratio (INR) as a measure of intensity of anticoagulant therapy was required because of variations in thromboplastin reagents used to determine prothrombin time (PT). Traditionally, a prothrombin ratio (PT [patient]/PT [control]) has been used to monitor intensity of anticoagulation. However, variation in thromboplastin reagents resulted in variations of prothrombin ratios between laboratories. To correct for these differences, each reagent is now assigned an International Sensitivity Index (ISI) value and the INR is calculated as $([\text{PT patient}]/\text{mean normal PT})^{\text{ISI}}$.

**Coumadin causes deficiencies of protein C and protein S in addition to factors II, VII, IX, and X. In patients who have partial protein C deficiency, Coumadin therapy can cause further decrease in protein C levels before other factors are lowered, and the patient paradoxically becomes prone to thrombosis—skin infarction may result secondary to thrombosis of dermal arteries.

cannot be recommended to prevent pregnancy, since these drugs may increase the risk of thrombosis [22,100,109]. Hence some other means of contraception must be recommended. For affected women who are taking warfarin and wish to become pregnant, we recommend stopping warfarin about 2 months prior to cessation of contraception and then starting subcutaneous heparin. Subcutaneous heparin can be initiated at 15,000 units sc every 12 h and increased as needed to achieve a PTT of 1.5–2.0 times normal at 6 h after the last heparin dose. These patients will need to maintain heparin therapy at this dosage throughout pregnancy and for a few days postpartum before reinstituting warfarin [108].

2. *Arterial Thrombosis*

Like venous thrombosis, patients with APS who get arterial thrombosis, in particular strokes, appear to be subject to recurrent events [21,42,100,101,110–112]. Options to prevent stroke recurrence include aspirin alone, warfarin alone, warfarin and aspirin, steroids, and immunosuppressive agents. Retrospective series have usually compared aspirin alone, warfarin alone or with aspirin, or none of those agents (regarded as "no treatment") [21,100,101]. Two series have reported that warfarin alone [21,101] or with aspirin [101] was more effective than aspirin alone or no treatment in the prevention of recurrences of arterial thrombosis. Our own series found the same result [166]. The discussion regarding intensity of warfarin therapy in the venous thrombosis section of this chapter is also applicable to that of arterial thrombosis. Aiming for an INR of 3.0 seems to be appropriate, although some authorities suggest that it may be better to aim for INRs above 3.0 [101]. We have made it a practice to add half to one adult aspirin per day to warfarin in patients with arterial thrombosis and, based on small patient numbers, this combination may have been slightly more effective than warfarin alone [166]. However, the addition of aspirin to warfarin does increase the risk of hemorrhage.

There is no basis for the use of prednisone to prevent recurrent arterial thrombosis. There are many reports of patients with APS who have had recurrent thrombosis while on prednisone [110,112]. Our retrospective series found that the use of prednisone alone or prednisone and warfarin were actually associated with an increased risk of venous and arterial thrombosis compared to warfarin alone [166]. Another argument against the use of prednisone is that it would have to be used at high doses for prolonged periods of time to suppress antiphospholipid antibody levels, since these antibodies are present for many years. Complications with the long-term use of steroids are usually substantial.

Immunosuppressive agents such as Imuran (azathioprine) and cydophosphamide are unproven as thrombosis prophylaxis in APS [110]. However, in patients with "catastrophic" antiphospholipid syndrome [113–120] or with recurrent thrombosis despite adequate anticoagulation therapy, the use of these agents may be considered. Long-term use of immunosuppressive agents are associated with severe side effects and should not be considered as first-line thrombosis prophylaxis in APS.

There have been isolated reports suggesting that patients with APS who were taking Plaquenil (hydroxychloroquine) had fewer thrombotic recurrences [121]. High doses of Plaquenil (800–1200 mg) have been reported to be effective in preventing venous thrombosis in patients undergoing hip surgery [122]. However, the latter effect has never been demonstrated in a double-blind, prospective study, and the mode of action of Plaquenil as an anticoagulant is unclear [122]. Further, the doses of

Plaquenil taken by patients with SLE and related disorders are much lower than were used for thrombosis prophylaxis in hip surgery patients, and the use of Plaquenil for prolonged periods of time at high doses may substantially increase the risk of retinal toxicity.

3. *Additional Measures to Prevent Thrombosis*

Although there is no definite evidence to suggest that risk factors for myocardial infarction and stroke will also increase the risk of recurrent arterial thrombosis in patients with APS, prudence suggests that if those factors are present, they should be reduced or eliminated. Patients should be advised to stop smoking. High cholesterol levels should be treated by diet and cholesterol-lowering agents. Diabetes should be controlled with appropriate drugs. Estrogen-containing oral contraceptive agents should not be taken [22,100] and alternative methods of contraception should be advised. Contraceptive agents containing progesterone alone (levonorgestrel implants [Norplant], depomedroxyprogesterone acetate) do not appear to be associated with an increased risk of thrombosis in otherwise healthy women.

4. *Surgery*

Patient with APS undergoing surgery are probably at increased risk for thrombosis, although there are no definite data to confirm this. We make it a practice of prescribing prophylactic heparin 5000 units sc just before induction of anesthesia and then 5000 units sc every 12 h for the first 2–3 postoperative days or for as long as the patient is in bed [107].

5. *"Catastrophic" Antiphospholipid Syndrome*

Some patients with APS develop thrombosis at several sites either simultaneously or over a short period of time [113–120]. Asherson reviewed several published case reports of such patients and suggested the term catastrophic antiphospholipid syndrome [113]. Whether this is a separate disease category or an extreme form of APS is debatable. However, when such patients present, they are often extremely ill, with multiorgan failure sometimes including gangrene and dermal infarction [116]. Thrombotic thrombocytopenia purpura (TTP) and diffuse intravascular coagulation (DIC) should be excluded prior to labeling such patients as APS [115,116]. In cases with which we are acquainted, thrombosis progresses despite full anticoagulation therapy. In these circumstances, the use of high doses of steroids intravenously (Solumedrol), intravenous cyclophosphamide, and plasmapheresis have been instituted with varying success [113,115,116,120–122]. High doses of intravenous gamma globulin, which are useful in the treatment of pregnant women with APS [123], may also be considered in these patients [124]. A fibrinolytic agent (Ancrod) proved to be beneficial in one report [125].

B. Pregnancy Loss

The availability of therapy to prevent pregnancy loss in APS is one of the more rewarding and important achievements in the management of this disorder. Various centers have reported success with a variety of treatment regimens. Unfortunately, the majority of studies are retrospective and involve relatively small numbers of patients. In addition, there are marked variations in criteria for patient entry, and even when the same treatment regimen has been used, doses of drugs as well as the time when treatment has been started and its duration have varied. Although it is difficult to make definite recommendations about treatment, the following sections will briefly review available data, and then guidelines will be suggested.

1. Prednisone and Low-dose Aspirin

There are several series in which the use of prednisone with low-dose aspirin has resulted in successful pregnancy outcome. Lubbe and colleagues first published their experience with six women who were lupus anticoagulant positive [126,127]. These women had histories of recurrent abortion or fetal losses in 25 of 28 previous pregnancies [126,127]. Prednisone was used at doses sufficient to suppress lupus anticoagulant activity ranging from 40 to 60 mg daily. Treatment resulted in live births in five of the six pregnancies, and the investigators reported few side effects. In contrast, Branch and colleagues reported successful outcomes in five of eight women treated with prednisone 50 mg/day and low-dose aspirin, but complication with prednisone therapy were more frequent, and suppression of the lupus anticoagulant test did not necessarily correlate with successful outcome [128]. Concern about the side effects of prednisone in high doses encouraged other investigators to try reduced doses of this drug.

Carp and colleagues used prednisone 30 mg plus aspirin 225–500 mg plus dipyridamole 75 mg thrice daily to treat 27 pregnancies in 19 women with lupus anticoagulant [129]. All of the women had a history of two or more consecutive pregnancy losses. Prednisone was increased from 30 to 40 mg, if necessary, to suppress lupus anticoagulant activity. Thirteen treated pregnancies resulted in live births, nine in first-trimester abortion, and the remainder in second- or third-trimester fetal deaths. Lupus anticoagulant activity was suppressed in all pregnant women studied, but in all instances when fetal death occurred, the lupus anticoagulant test was also normal—hence, normalization of the lupus anticoagulant test did not assure normal pregnancy outcome. Examination of the placentas in women giving birth to live babies appeared normal, unlike their previous pregnancies associated with fetal loss in which placental infarction was frequent [129].

Ordi and colleagues [130] used prednisone at 20 mg daily and increased this by 10 mg daily, if necessary, to suppress lupus anticoagulant activity. They treated seven women with histories of 7 miscarriages and 10 fetal deaths. Lupus anticoagulant activity normalized in two women after 1 month; in three women after increasing the dose to 30 mg daily, and there was no suppression even at 60 mg daily in one woman. They reported a decrease in anticardiolipin titers in all patients. Seven of the nine treated pregnancies ended in live births at 32–36 weeks' gestation, and the average weight of infants born to these mothers were 2500–3500 g [130]. Side effects included cushingoid facies, acne, mycobacterial infection, and adrenal insufficiency. An alternative regimen was reported by Silviera and colleagues [131]. Prednisone was given in doses of 40 mg daily for 4 weeks and then tapered by 10 mg every 4 weeks to a maintenance dose of 5 mg daily. Low-dose aspirin was given daily with prednisone. They treated 11 women with histories of at least one pregnancy loss. All the patients were anticardiolipin positive, but three patients had low IgG levels and two patients were only IgM positive (low positive IgG and IgM anticardiolipin positivity are less frequently associated with poor pregnancy outcome [132,133]). They reported 100% success with their treatment regimen [131]. Other groups have given prednisone at doses of 20–40 mg daily for 5 days each week (Thursday and Sunday termed "rest" days) plus low-dose aspirin and azathioprine [134,135]. The latter regimen was reportedly successful and associated with few side effects [134,135]. Imuran was given concomitantly with prednisone in another treated pregnancy [136], but the use of this drug has a theoretical risk of teratogenicity, although it has been safely administered during pregnancy to women who have had renal transplantation [137].

Some studies have compared prednisone and aspirin treatment with no treatment, low-dose aspirin alone, or heparin and aspirin. Only two of these were prospective and randomized [138,139] and the remainder were retrospective. In one of the retrospective studies, Lockshin and colleagues treated 25 asymptomatic women with SLE who had medium to high positive IgG anticardiolipin antibody levels and histories of prior fetal losses [133]. They found that pregnancy outcome was actually worse with prednisone and low-dose aspirin compared with low-dose aspirin alone. However, the doses of prednisone in that study varied from 10 to 60 mg, and the time of institution and duration of treatment varied markedly. In the largest retrospective study published to date, Branch and colleagues [140] compared pregnancy outcome in women treated with prednisone and aspirin versus heparin and aspirin. Eighty-two treated pregnancies in 54 women were reviewed. All patients fulfilled criteria for the antiphospholipid syndrome. Of 39 pregnancies (33 women) treated with prednisone and aspirin, there were 21 surviving neonates (54%), 8 (21%) spontaneous abortions, 8 (21%) fetal deaths, and 2 (5%) neonatal deaths. Of the 21 surviving infants, 10 were delivered before 32 weeks. Nineteen pregnancies (17 patients) were managed with subcutaneous heparin (given usually as twice daily subcutaneous doses; mean total dose 15,000 units) and low-dose aspirin. Of the 19 pregnancies, 14 (74%) ended in live born infants and 11 delivered after 32 weeks. One (5%) of the 19 pregnancies ended in spontaneous abortion, 2 (10%) in fetal death, and 2 in neonatal death (11%). Although outcome with heparin and aspirin appeared more favorable than with prednisone and aspirin, the differences were not statistically significant [140]. Preeclampsia was present in comparable percentages in both groups of treated patients [140].

Two prospective, randomized treatment trials of pregnant women with positive anticardiolipin or lupus anticoagulant tests have been published. Cowchock and colleagues compared treatment with prednisone and aspirin versus heparin and aspirin [138]. The number of patients actually randomized to each group was small, 12 treated with heparin and 8 treated with prednisone, although data from another 25 patients who either refused or were ineligible for randomization were included and served to bolster conclusions of the study. Patients were included if anticardiolipin tests were positive at any level, and it is likely that a proportion did not fulfill criteria for APS. Cowchock and colleagues found about 75% successful outcome in both treated groups. However, preterm deliveries (before 37 weeks' gestation), premature rupture of membranes, and preeclampsia were more frequent in the prednisone-treated group [138]. Another randomized, prospective study conducted by Silver and colleagues compared treatment with low-dose aspirin and prednisone 20 mg daily (increased if necessary to suppress anticardiolipin level) versus low-dose aspirin alone. Seventeen women were in the prednisone and aspirin group, and 22 were in the low-dose aspirin group. All 34 pregnancies ended in live births, but preterm delivery, low mean birth weight, and premature rupture of membranes or abruptio placentae were more frequent in the prednisone-treated group. The excellent outcome of treated pregnancies in this study may have occurred because a significant proportion of patients had low anticardiolipin levels. Adverse pregnancy outcome is certainly more frequent in patients with medium to high positive IgG anticardiolipin tests [132,133,141,142] and uncommon in patients with

IgM anticardiolipin tests at any level. Hence, it is important that antibody isotype and level be considered in selecting patients for treatment trials.

Despite the shortcomings in studies of prednisone and low-dose aspirin treatment, there are certain general conclusions that seem to be true. Pregnancy outcome appeared to be improved with prednisone and aspirin in most series. Lower doses of prednisone (20–30 mg) appeared as effective as higher doses (40–60 mg). Both maternal and fetal morbidity appeared to be significant with prednisone; cushingoid facies, acne [126,127], gestational diabetes [139], wound dehiscence [130], avascular necrosis [139], mycobacterial infection [130–143], and one death [143] were all reported. The prevalence of prematurity, preeclampsia, premature rupture of membranes, and abruptio placentae may be increased with prednisone treatment and this contributes to morbidity in infants [138,139]. For these reasons, clinicians have turned to the use of alternative agents for treatment of pregnant women with APS.

2. *Heparin*

The first large series of women with APS treated during pregnancy with heparin and low- dose aspirin was reported by Rosove and colleagues [144]. They treated 14 women who were either anticardiolipin or lupus anticoagulant positive. These women received twice daily subcutaneous heparin; in total doses ranging from 10,000 to 36,000 units daily (mean dose was 24,700 $\pm$ 7400 units). The dose of heparin was designed to prolong plasma PTT to 1.5–2.0 times normal 6 hrs after the last dose. Fourteen of the 15 women had live births at a mean gestational age of 36 weeks (range 33–39 weeks), with mean birth weight percentiles of 57 $\pm$ 21 and Apgar scores that were "good to excellent." Although these results are encouraging, it should be noted that all patients had levels below 40 GPL or MPL units and the majority had low anticardiolipin levels ($<$20 GPL or $<$20 MPL units). Only five were lupus anticoagulant positive. In contrast, the majority of women studied in the Lockshin [133] and Branch [140] series had levels above 40 GPL units, and few were included who were only IgM positive. However, the favorable effects of heparin and low-dose aspirin observed by Rosove and colleagues were borne out in subsequent series reported by Branch [140], Cowchock [138], and their respective colleagues. The latter studies were discussed previously, both showing that pregnancy outcome was improved in about 70–75% of women treated with subcutaneous heparin and low-dose aspirin. In contrast to Rosove and colleagues [144], the latter studies [138,140] used lower total doses of heparin that ranged from 10,000 to 20,000 units daily, and no attempt was made to prolong plasma PTT.

Osteoporosis is a complication of heparin given for prolonged periods of time at high doses [103,145]. Other risks include bleeding at the injection site as well as hemorrhage, which can be reduced with lower doses of heparin. Thrombocytopenia and thrombosis are also rare idiosyncratic complications of heparin therapy discussed previously [103,104].

3. *Immunoglobulin Therapy*

There are a number of case reports [146–151] and one series [152] of pregnant women with APS who were successfully treated with intravenous immunoglobulin infusions. As was the case in other studies discussed previously, the criteria for the diagnosis of APS as well as treatment protocols varied. Scott and colleagues [146] first reported successful pregnancy outcome after treatment of a woman with APS who had a history of one previous live birth and seven fetal/neonatal deaths. She had previously failed treatment with prednisone and aspirin. Utilization of two courses of intravenous immunoglobulin 0.4 g/kg/day for 5 days in the 8th and 14th weeks of gestation resulted in a live birth. Then other case reports followed [148–151] in which this therapy was used successfully, usually in women who had failed previous treatment with prednisone and aspirin or heparin and aspirin. Spinnato and colleagues have treated nine women so far with intravenous immunoglobulin, five of whom have been reported [152]. All nine pregnancies have ended in live births, and in only one case has a birth occurred preterm (<37 weeks)—in that case, the infant was delivered at 32 weeks' gestation with a diagnosis of fetal distress, but the child survived without any long-term problems [152]. Each patient in that series received intravenous immunoglobulin 0.4 g/kg/day for 5 days/month from the time of diagnosis of pregnancy to delivery. Several of the patients were also receiving heparin and aspirin because of previous histories of thrombosis, and in one, prednisone therapy was administered from the 20th week of gestation because of a diagnosis of herpes gestationis. The five surviving infants that were reported, as well as an additional four (Spinnato et al. [152]), all had good to excellent Apgar scores. With the exception of the first case, all neonates had birth weights within the normal range. Placentas were either healthy or showed minimal infarction [152].

The mode of action of immunoglobulins in reducing the risk of pregnancy loss in APS is unknown. In two studies [151,152], patients were found to have reduced anticardiolipin antibody levels soon after infusion, but levels rose quickly to pretreatment values within a few days. However, after several months of treatment, there was an overall decrease in anticardiolipin levels. Such a decrease may be attributable to anti-idiotype antibodies present in the immunoglobulin solution which may bind anticardiolipin antibodies and promote their removal from the circulation [151]. Alternatively, high doses of immunoglobulins may suppress the production of anticardiolipin antibodies by B cells. Whether this reduction in anticardiolipin levels contributes to a favorable pregnancy outcome is unclear.

Side effects observed with intravenous immunoglobulin therapy were few and minimal; they included low-grade fever and headache during infusions, which responded to acetaminophen [152]. There is a small risk of transmission of viral infections [153] with immunoglobulin infusions, but treatment of these preparations prior to use makes this unlikely [154]. In addition, patients with IgA deficiency may be at increased risk theoretically of allergic reactions to proteins in the infusion solution. The main drawback to immunoglobulin treatment is its cost. Each 5-day course costs $4000–$5,000. However, the possible benefits in reduced perinatal morbidity or mortality and consequent reduced nursery costs may offset some of the expenses associated with this treatment.

4. Low-dose Aspirin

In nearly all instances where pregnant women with APS were treated, low-dose aspirin has been included in the treatment regimen. This is based on the observation that pregnancy loss in APS resembles that in preeclampsia [155], with placental infarction being a frequent finding in both conditions [57,58]. This complication is explained by a decrease in placental vessel prostacyclin [156] or a relative increase in platelet thromboxane production [157,158]. Prostacyclin generation by endothelial cells of the placenta is believed to be necessary to maintain an adequate blood supply to the fetus [155]. An excess of thromboxane can cause vasoconstriction and placental infarction. Low doses of aspirin inhibit thromboxane synthesis, and this drug has been shown in more than one study to reduce the frequency of preeclampsia and pregnancy-induced hypertension [159,160]. As discussed previously, Silver and colleagues found that low-dose aspirin alone was equally effective to prednisone and low-dose aspirin in a prospective, randomized treatment trial of pregnant women with APS [139]. Other studies have also suggested that low-dose aspirin alone may be effective in promoting successful pregnancy outcome in some affected women [133,143]. However, our anecdotal experience and that of some other centers have been that this treatment has often not been sufficient to enable successful pregnancy outcome in women with high IgG anticardiolipin antibody levels who have had previous pregnancy losses.

5. No Treatment

One study reported that careful monitoring of women during pregnancy utilizing Doppler velocimetry to measure umbilical artery and ductus arteriosus blood flow enabled better timing of delivery and successful pregnancy outcome in six untreated pregnancies in four women [161]. There are other reports of women with APS who have given birth to live babies without treatment. Lockshin [133], Ramsey-Goldman [162], and their respective colleagues suggest that a history of pregnancy loss is probably as important a predictor of adverse pregnancy outcome as is anticardiolipin positivity. Hence, a good case can be made for no treatment of women with APS who are pregnant for the first time. Such women may have a relatively good chance of successful pregnancy outcome [133].

C. An Approach to the Management of Pregnancy in Women with APS

Based on treatment data outlined above, there are certain guidelines that can be followed when managing pregnancies in women with APS. These are discussed below.

1. General Management

A careful history is essential when evaluating patients with APS who wish to become pregnant. Important issues include the number of previous pregnancies and their outcome; a history of previous venous or arterial thrombosis and whether these occurred during pregnancy or the postpartum period or were associated with oral contraceptive use. The tests on which a diagnosis of APS was made should be reviewed; in particular, the isotype and level of anticardiolipin positivity. We routinely repeat those tests if they were done more than 3 months previously, since they may now be negative—reversion to negative values is uncommon in patients with APS, but it can occur. Finally, physicians should assess the emotional stability of the patient and her family and their ability to withstand a difficult pregnancy which might end in fetal loss.

These women are best managed during pregnancy by a high-risk obstetrician and rheumatologist who are acquainted with the APS. Many series monitor fetal heart rate [163] monthly as well as fetal growth using Doppler ultrasonography. Some groups have found that the measurement of umbilical artery and ductus arteriosus blood flow by Doppler velocimetry, starting at 20 weeks of gestation and continuing at 2- to 3-week intervals until delivery, has been useful in monitoring the course of the fetus and in predicting fetal distress [161,164]. Trudinger and colleagues [161] suggested that the appearance of abnormal Doppler readings indicated increased placental vascular resistance, and this helped in the early prediction of fetal distress.

Affected women who have a history of thrombosis and are on warfarin prophylaxis require discontinuation of warfarin 2–3 months before pregnancy contraception is stopped. Warfarin taken during the first trimester of pregnancy is teratogenic [107]; hence, the need for its discontinuance prior to attempting to become pregnant. Once warfarin is discontinued, these women should start subcutaneous heparin in twice daily doses adjusted to prolong plasma PTT to 1.5–2.0 times normal 6 h after the last dose. Heparin should be continued throughout pregnancy and warfarin restarted within a few days of completion of pregnancy.

In the discussion that follows, guidelines about when not to treat affected women during pregnancy, as well as when and how to use low-dose aspirin alone, heparin and aspirin, immunoglobulin infusion, and prednisone and aspirin are suggested.

2. *No Treatment*

The no treatment option might be considered in women who have positive lupus anticoagulant or anticardiolipin tests at any level but no history of pregnancy losses or thrombosis. A substantial number of women with positive anticardiolipin tests or with the lupus anticoagulant have been reported with normal pregnancy outcomes [133,143,161]. Hence, the use of dangerous or expensive drugs to treat these women is not justified.

3. *Low-dose Aspirin*

The low-dose aspirin option seems logical in women with positive anticardiolipin or lupus anticoagulant tests who has had one miscarriage in the past but no history of thrombosis. Some studies have reported a favorable outcome with low-dose aspirin therapy [133,139,143], and this seems to be a relatively safe, cheap option in a group of patients who may have a good chance of successful pregnancy outcome.

4. *Heparin and Low-dose Aspirin*

There are two groups of women with APS in which the heparin and low-dose aspirin option should be considered. The first is women with histories of at least one second- or third-trimester loss or at least three first-trimester losses and a moderate to high positive anticardiolipin test (preferably IgG isotype) or a positive lupus anticoagulant test. Heparin in doses of 10,000 units sc bid plus low-dose aspirin should be used. If the woman has a history of thrombosis, the second treatment option discussed below should be considered.

Women fulfilling criteria for APS who have had a history of thrombosis should probably be treated with sufficient heparin to prevent thrombosis. This is particularly important if thrombosis occurred during a previous pregnancy, the postpartum period, or while on oral contraceptives. Heparin should be administered at doses of 15,000 units sc bid, and the dose adjusted to achieve a PTT (measured at 6 hs after heparin administration) of 1.5–2.0 times normal [107,108]. In women with a baseline prolonged PTT due to the lupus anticoagulant, plasma heparin levels can be measured and adjusted to achieve a concentration of 0.2–0.4 IU/mL [165]. Patients receiving heparin should receive vitamin D (600–800 units) and calcium carbonate (4 g) supplementation. Physicians should be aware of the small risk of idiosyncratic thrombocytopenia and thrombosis with heparin treatment.

5. *Intravenous Immunoglobulin Therapy*

Intravenous immunoglobulin therapy should be considered in women with a definite diagnosis of APS who have had a pregnancy loss despite treatment with heparin and aspirin. Treatment should be started as soon as pregnancy is diagnosed. The regimen is 0.4 g/kg/day for 4–5 days each month for the duration of the pregnancy [152]. Low-dose aspirin should also be given daily. In women with a history of thrombosis, heparin should also be administered as described previously. Side effects and potential risks of immunoglobulin treatment have been discussed previously but these are uncommon. This treatment is expensive, as discussed previously.

6. *Prednisone and Aspirin*

Prednisone and aspirin therapy should be reserved only for women with definite APS who have had pregnancy losses despite treatment with heparin and aspirin and treatment with intravenous immunoglobulin. Prednisone in doses of 20–30 mg and one low-dose aspirin daily would be appropriate. Tapering doses of prednisone, as outlined in some studies [131,138], might be considered, particularly after the 28th week of gestation, providing the pregnancy is proceeding well. Patients should be warned about the side effects of prednisone, including avascular necrosis.

Prednisone will not protect patients from recurrent thrombosis [110], and if the woman has a history of thrombosis, she should also receive full heparin prophylaxis as described previously. Combined prednisone and heparin will substantially increase the risk of osteoporosis and women should receive vitamin D (600–800 IU) and calcium (4 g) supplementation daily.

V. THROMBOCYTOPENIA

In most cases, patients with APS who have thrombocytopenia require no treatment, since platelet counts usually exceed 50,000/mm^3. However, a few may have episodes of severe thrombocytopenia, and since this appears to be autoimmune mediated in most instances, treatment guidelines are the same as for idiopathic thrombocytopenic purpura. High-dose steroids are given to suppress platelet autoantibody production and to increase platelet counts. If steroids are not effective, or need to be given for prolonged periods of time, other immunosuppressive agents such as azathioprine may be useful. Splenectomy is considered in patients with severe thrombocytopenia unresponsive to immunosuppressive therapy. The use of high-dose immunoglobulin treatment has proved to be useful in the acute management of thrombocytopenic patients, but the effect of this agent is short lived.

Patients who are thrombocytopenic may still be at risk for thrombosis [166]. However, the use of anticoagulants will increase the risk of hemorrhage. One approach might be to use immunosuppressive agents and/or gamma globulin to increase platelet levels above 50,000/mm^3 and then to anticoagulate the patients. That such an approach will work has not been proven.

VI. CONCLUSIONS

The diagnosis and management of APS are challenging. We have outlined clinical features of this disorder, tests used for its diagnosis, and management of major complications. There is considerable interest in the disorder, and, in time, guidelines about patient management will be based on a sounder scientific basis than it is at the present time.

REFERENCES

1. Harris EN, Syndrome of the black swan. Br J Rheumatol 1987; 26:324–326.
2. Harris EN, Gharavi A, Asherson RA, et al. Antiphospholipid antibodies—middle aged but robust. J Rheumatol 1994; 21:978–981.
3. Lockshin MD. Antiphospholipid antibody syndrome. Rheum Dis Clin North Am 1994; 20:45–60.
4. Sammaritano LR, Gharavi AE. Antiphospholipid syndrome. Clin Lab Med 1992; 12:41–59.
5. Petri M. Antiphospholipid antibodies: lupus anticoagulant and anticardiolipin antibody. In: Weston WL, ed., Current Problems in Dermatology. St. Louis: Mosby-Year Book, 1992:171–201.
6. McNeil HP, Chesterman CN, Krilis SA. Immunology and clinical importance of antiphospholipid antibodies. Adv Immunol 1991; 49:193–280.
7. Asherson RA. A "primary" antiphospholipid syndrome? J Rheumatol 1988; 15:1742–1746.
8. Alarcon-Segovia D, Sanchez-Guerrero J. Primary antiphospholipid syndrome. J Rheumatol 1989; 16:482–488.
9. Mackworth-Young CG, Loizou S, Walport MJ. Primary antiphospholipid syndrome: features of patients with raised anticardiolipin antibodies and no other disorders. Ann Rheum Dis 1989;48:362–367.
10. Piette JC, Wechsler B, Frances C, Godeau P. Systemic lupus erythematosus and the antiphospholipid syndrome: reflections about the relevance of ARA criteria. J Rheumatol 1992;19:1835–1837.
11. Vianna JL, Khamashta MA, Ordi-Ros J, et al. Comparison of the primary and secondary antiphospholipid syndrome—a European multicenter study of 114 Patients. Am J Med 1994; 96:3–9.
12. Nachman RL, Silvertstein R. Hypercoaguable states. Ann Intern Med 1993; 119:819–827.
13. Sheridan-Pereira M, Porreco RP, Hays T, Burke MS. Neonatal aortic thrombosis associated with the lupus anticoagulant. Obstet Gynecol 1988; 71:1061–1068.
14. Finazzi G, Correlazzo S, Viero P, et al. Maternal lupus anticoagulant and fetal neonatal thrombosis. Thromb Haemost 1987; 57:238.
15. Tabbutt S, Griswold WR, Ogino MT, et al. Multiple thromboses in a prenatal infant associated with maternal phospholipid antibody syndrome. J Perinatol 1994; 14:66–70.
16. Contractor S, Hiatt M, Kosmin M, Kim HC. Neonatal thrombosis with anticardiolipin antibody in baby and mother. Am J Perinatol 1992; 9:409–410.
17. Manco-Johnson MJ, Nuss R. Lupus anticoagulant in children with thrombosis. Am J Hematol 1995; 48:240–243.
18. Olson JC, Konkol RJ, Gill JC, et al. Childhood stroke and lupus anticoagulant. Pediatr Neurol 1994; 10:54–57.
19. Ravelli A, Martini A, Burgio R. Antiphospholipid antibody syndrome as a cause of venous thrombosis in children. J Pediatr 1994; 124:831–832.
20. Saca LF, Szer IS, Henor E, et al. Budd-Chiari Syndrome associated with antiphospholipid antibodies in a child: report of a case and review of the literature. J Rheumatol 1993; 21:545–548.
21. Rosove MH, Brewer PMC. Antiphospholipid thrombosis: clinical course after the first thrombotic event in 70 patients. Ann Intern Med 1992; 17:303–308.

22. Silver RM, Draper ML, Scott JR, et al. Clinical Consequences of antiphospholipid antibodies—an historic cohort study. Obstet Gynecol 1994; 83:372–377.
23. Levine Sr, Deegan MJ, Futrell N, Welch KM. Cerebrovascular and neurologic disease associated with antiphospholipid antibodies: 48 cases. Neurology 1990; 40:1181–1189.
24. Coull BM, Levine SR, Brey RL. The role of antiphospholipid antibodies in stroke. Neurol Clin 1992; 10:125–142.
25. The Antiphospholipid Antibodies in Stroke Study Group. Clinical and laboratory findings in patients with antiphospholipid antibodies and cerebral ischemia. Stroke 1990; 21:1268–1273.
26. Coull BM, Bourdelte DN, Goodnight SH, et al. Multiple cerebral infarctions and dementia associated with anticardiolipin antibodies. Stroke 1987; 18:1107–1112.
27. Asherson RA, Mercey D, Phillips G, et al. Recurrent stroke and multi-infarct dementia in systemic lupus erythematosus: association with antiphospholipid antibodies. Ann Rheum Dis 1987; 46:605–611.
28. Ahserson RA, Mackay IR, Harris EN. Myocardial infarction in SLE associated with deep vein thrombosis and anti-phospholipid antibodies. Br Heart J 1986; 56:190–193.
29. Asherson RA, Khamashta MA, Baguley E, et al. Myocardial infarction and antiphoapholipid antibodies in SLE and related disorders. Q J Med 1989; 73:1103–1117.
30. Asherson RA, Derksen RHMW, Harris EN, et al. Large vessel occlusion and gangrene in SLE and lupus-like disease—report of 6 cases. J Rheum 1986; 13:740–747.
31. Cappell MS, Mikhail N, Gujral N. Gastrointestinal hemorrhage and intestinal ischemia associated with anticardiolipin antibodies. Dig Dis Sci 1994; 39:1359–1364.
32. Johnson MW, Thomley ML, Huang SS, Gass JDM. Idiopathic recurrent branch retinal arterial occlusion: natural history and laboratory evaluation. Ophthalmology 1994; 101:480–489.
33. Alegre VA, Gastineau DA, Winkelmann RD. Skin lesions associated with circulating lupus anticoagulant. Br J Dermatol 1989; 120:419–429.
34. Asherson RA, Hughest GRV. Hypoadrenalism, Addison's disease and antiphospholipid antibodies. J Rheumatol 1991; 18:1-3.
35. Lenaerts J, Vanneste S, Knockaert D, et al. SLE and acute Addisonian crisis due to bilateral adrenal hemorrhage association with antiphospholipid antibodies. Clin Exp Rheumatol 1991; 9:407–409.
36. Amigo MC, Garcia-Torres R, Robles M, et al. Renal involvement in primary antiphospholipid syndrome. J Rheumatol 1992; 19:1181–1185.
37. Laeker B, McGregor A, Griffiths M, et al. Insiduous loss of renal function in patients with anticardiolipin antibodies and absence of overt nephritis. Br J Rheumatol 1991; 30:422–425.
38. Kincaid-Smith P, Fairley M. Lupus anticoagulant associated with renal thrombotic microangiopathy and pregnancy-related renal failure. Q J Med 1988; 69:795–815.
39. D'Agati V, Kunis C, Williams G, Appel GB. Anti-cardiolipin antibody and renal disease: a report of three cases. J Am Soc Nephrol 1990; 1:777–784.
40. Hart RG, Kanter MC. Hematologic disorders and ischemic stroke: a selective review. Stroke 1990; 21:1111–1121.
41. Elias M, Eldor A. Thromboembolism in patients with the "lupus-like" circulating anticoagulant. Arch Intern Med 1984; 144:510–543.
42. Glueck HI, Kant KS, Weiss MA. Thrombosis in systemic lupus erythematosus: relation to the presence of circulating anticoagulants. Arch Intern Med 1985; 145:1389–1395.
43. Lechner K. A new type of coagulation inhibitor. Thromb Diath Haemorrh 1969; 21:482–499.
44. Asherson RA, Khamashta MA, Ordi-Ros J, et al. The "primary" antiphospholipid syndrome: major clinical and serological features. Med 1989; 68:366–374.

45. Alarcon-Segovia D, Deleze M, Oria CV. Antiphospholipid antibodies and the antiphospholipid syndrome in systemic lupus erythematosus: a prospective analysis of 500 consecutive patients. Medicine 1989; 68:353–365.
46. Asherson RA, Mackworth-Young CG, Boey ML, et al. Pulmonary hypertension in systemic lupus erythematosus. Br Med J 1983; 287:1024–1205.
47. Anderson NE, Ali MR. The lupus anticoagulant, pulmonary thromboembolism, and fatal pulmonary hypertension. Ann Rheum Dis 1984; 43:760–763.
48. Terabayashi H, Okuda K, Nomura F, et al. Transformation of inferior vena cava thrombosis to membranous obstruction in a patient with the lupus anticoagulant.Gastroenterology 1986; 91:219–224.
49. Asherson RA, Lanham JG, Hull RG, et al. Renal vein thrombosis in systemic lupus erythematosus: association with the "lupus anticoagulant." Clin Exp Rheumatol 1984; 2:75–79.
50. Pomeroy C, Knodell RG, Swaim WR, et al. Budd-Chiari syndrome in a patient with the lupus anticoagulant. Gastroenterology 1984; 86:158–161.
51. Mackworth-Young CG, Melia WH, Harris EN, et al. The Budd-Chiari syndrome. Possible pathogenetic role of anti-phospholipid antibodies. J Hepatol 1986; 3:83–86.
52. Ouwendijk RJ, Koster JC, Wilson JHP, et al. Budd-Chiari syndrome in a young patient with anticardiolipin antibodies: need for prolonged anticoagulant treatment. Gut 1994; 35:1004–1006.
53. Levine SR, Deegan MJ, Futrell N, Welch KM. Cerebrovascular and neurologic disease associated with antiphospholipid antibodies: 48 cases. Neurology 1990; 40:1181–1189.
54. Reece EA, Gabrielli S, Cullen MT, et al. Recurrent adverse pregnancy outcome and antiphospholipid antibodies. Am J Obstet Gynecol 1990; 163:162–169.
55. Scott JR, Rote NS, Branch DW. Immunologic aspects of recurrent abortion and fetal death. Obstet Gynecol 1987; 70:645–656.
56. Triplett DA. Antiphospholipid antibodies and recurrent pregnancy loss. Am J Reprod Immunol 1989; 20:52–67.
57. Out HJ, Bruinse HW, Derksen RHWM. Antiphospholipid antibodies and pregnancy loss. Hum Repord 1991; 6:889–897.
58. DeWolf F, Carreras LO, Moerman P. Decidual vasculopathy and extensive placental infarction in a patient with thromboembolic accidents, recurrent fetal loss, and a lupus anticoagulant. Am J Obstet Gynecol 1982; 142:829–834.
59. Out HJ, Kooijman CD, Bruinse HW, Derksen RHWM. Histopathological findings in placental from patients with intra-uterine fetal death and anti-phospholipid antibodies. Eur J Obstet Gynecol Reprod Biol 1991; 41:179–186.
60. Pridham DD, Cook CL. Habitual abortion. In: Harris EN, Exner T, Hughes GRV, Asherson RA, eds. Phospholipid Binding Antibodies. Boca Raton, FL: CRC Press, 1991:271–306.
61. Harris EN, Asherson RA, Gharavi AE, Morgan SH, Derue G, Hughes GRV. Thrombocytopenia in SLE and related autoimmune disorders: association with anticardiolipin antibody. Br J Haematol 1985; 59:227–230.
62. Harris EN, Chan JKH, Asherson RA, et al. Thrombosis, recurrent fetal loss and thrombocytopenia. Predictive value of the anti-cardiolipin antibody test. Arch Intern Med 1986; 146:2153–2156.
63. Harris EN, Gharavi AE, Hedge U, et al. Anti-cardiolipin antibodies in autoimmune thrombocytopenia purpura. Br J Haematol 1985; 59:231–234.
64. Deleze M, Alarcon-Segovia D, Oria CV. Hemocytopenia in systemic lupus erythematosus. Relationship to antiphospholipid antibodies. J Rheumatol 1989; 16:926–930.
65. Harris EN, Gharavi AE, Boey ML, et al. Anti-cardiolipin antibodies: detection by radioimmunoassay and association with thrombosis. Lancet 1983; 2:1211–1214.
66. Harris EN, Gharavi AE, Patel S, Hughes GRV. Evaluation of the anti-cardiolipin antibody test: report of an international workshop held 4 April 1986. Clin Exp Immunol 1987; 68:215–222.

67. Harris EN. The Second International Anti-cardiolipin Standardization Workshop/The Kingston Antiphospholipid Antibody Study (KAPS) Group. Am J Clin Pathol 1990; 94:476–484.
68. Harris EN, Pierangeli SS, Birch D. Anticardiolipin Wet Workshop Report: Vth International Symposium on Antiphospholipid Antibodies. Am J Clin Pathol 1994; 101:616–624.
69. Harris EN, Pierangeli SS. Anticardiolipin and lupus anticoagulant testing and significance. J Clin Immunoassay 1994; 17:1–10.
70. Gharavi AE, Harris EN, Ahserson RA, Hughes GRV. Anticardiolipin antibody isotype distribution and phospholipid specificity. Ann Rheum Dis 1987; 46:1–6.
71. Harris EN, Gharavi AE, Tincani A, et al. Affinity purified anti-cardiolipin and anti-DNA antibodies. J Clin Lab Immunol 1985; 17:155–162.
72. Rote NS, Dostal-Johnson D, Branch WD. Antiphospholipid antibodies and recurrent pregnancy loss: correlation between the activated partial thromboplastin time and antibodies against phosphatidylserine and cardiolipin. Am J Obstet Gynecol 1990; 163:575–584.
73. Pierangeli SS, Goldsmith GH, Krnic S, Harris EN. Differences in functional activity of anticardiolipin antibodies from patients with syphilis and the antiphospholipd syndrome. Infect Immun 1994; 62:4081–4084.
74. Campbell AL, Pierangeli SS, Wellhausen S, Harris EN. Comparison of the effects of anticardiolipin antibodies from patients with the antiphospholipid syndrome and with syphilis on platelet activation and aggregation. Thromb Haemost 1995; 73:529–534.
75. Galli M, Comfurius P, Maasen C, et al. Anticardiolipin antibodies (ACA) directed not to cardiolipin but to a plasma protein cofactor. Lancet 1990; 336:1544–47.
76. Arvieux J, Pouzol P, Roussel B, et al. Measurement of anti-phospholipid antibodies by ELISA using $\beta_2$glycoprotein 1 as an antigen. Br J Haematol 1992; 81:568–573.
77. Viard JP, Amoura Z, Bach JF. Association of anti-β_2 glycoprotein with lupus circulating anticoagulant and thrombosis in SLE. Am J Med 1992; 93:181–186.
78. Matsuura E, Igarashi Y, Yasuda T, et al. Anticardiolipin antibodies recognize beta(2)-glycoprotein 1 structure altered by interacting with an oxygen modified solid phase surface. J Exp Med 1994; 179:457–462.
79. Roubey RAS, Pratt CW, Buyon JP, Winfield JB. Lupus anticoagulant activity of autoimmune antiphospholipid antibodies is dependent on β_2 glycoprotein 1. J Clin Invest 1992; 90:1100–1104.
80. Tincani A, Meroni PL, Brucato A, et al. Anti-phospholipid and anti-mitichondrial type M5 antibodies in systemic lupus erythematosus. Clin Exp Rheumatol 1985; 3:321–326.
81. Loizou S, McCrea JD, Rudge AC, et al. Measurement of anticardiolipin antibodies by an enzyme linked immunosorbent assay (ELISA): standardization and quantitation of results. Clin Exp Immunol 1985; 62:738–745.
82. Schousboe I. Characterization of the interaction between β_2-glycoprotein 1 and mitochondria, platelets, liposomes, adn bile acids. Int J Biochem 1983; 15:1393–1397.
83. Nimpf J, Bevers EM, Bomans PHH, Till U. Prothrombinase activity of human platelets is influenced by β_2 glycoprotein 1. Biochim Biophys Acta 1986; 884:142–144.
84. Schousboe I. β_2-glycoprotein 1: a plasma inhibitor of the contact activation of the intrinsic blood coagulation pathway. Blood 1985; 66:1086–1091.
85. McNeil HP, Simpson RJ, Chesterman CN, Krilis S. Anti-phospholipid antibodies are directed against a complex antigen that includes a lipid-binding inhibitor of coagulation: β_2 glycoprotein 1 (apolipoprotein H). Proc Natl Acad Sci USA 1990; 87:4120–4124.
86. Pierangeli SS, Harris EN, Davis SA, DeLorenzo G. β_2 glycoprotein 1 enhances cardiolipin binding activity but is not the antigen for antiphospholipid antibodies. Br J Haematol 1992; 82:565–570.
87. Gharavi AE, Harris EN, Sammaratano LR, et al. Do patients with antiphospholipid syndrome have antibodies to β_2 glycoprotein 1? J Lab Clin Med 1993; 122:426–431.

88. Sammaritano LR, Lockshin MD, Gharavi AE. Antiphospholipid antibodies differ in aPL cofactor requirement. Lupus 1992; 1:51–56.
89. Triplett DA, Brandt J. Laboratory identification of lupus anticoagulant. Br J Haematol 1989; 73:139–142.
90. Exner T, Shaman N, Trudinger B. Separation of anticardiolipin antibodies from lupus anticoagulant by a phospholipdi coated polystyrene column. Biochem Biophys Res Commun 1988; 155:1001–1007.
91. McNeil HP, Chesterman CN, Krilis SA. Anticardiolipin antibodies and lupus anticoagulants comprise separate antibody subgroups with different phospholipid binding characteristics. Br J Haematol 1989; 73:506–510.
92. Goldsmith GH, Pierangeli SS, Branch DW, et al. Inhibition of prothrombin activation by antiphospholipid antibodies and β_2 glycoprotein 1. Br J Haematol 1994; 87:548–554.
93. Pengo V, Heine MJ, Thiagarajan P, Shapiro SS. Immunological specificity and mechanism of action of IgG lupus anticoagulants. Blood 1987; 70:69–76.
94. Walton SP, Pierangeli SS, Campbell A, et al. Demonstration of antiphospholipid antibodies heterogeneity by phospholipid column chromatography and salt gradient elution. Lupus 1995;
95. Permpikul P, Rao LVM, Rapaport SI. Functional and binding studies of the role of prothrombin and β_2 glycoprotein 1 in the expression of lupus anticoagulant activity. Blood 1994; 83:2878–2892.
96. Bevers EM, Galli M, Barbui T, et al. Lupus anticoagulant (LA) IgG's are not directed to phospholipids only but to a complex lipid-bound human prothrombin. Thromb Haemost 1991; 66:629–632.
97. Brey RL, Hart RG, Sherman DG, Tegeler CH. Antiphospholipid antibodies and cerebral ischemia in young people. Neurology 1990; 40:1190–1196.
98. Levine SR, Brey RL, Joseph ClM, Havstad S. Risk of recurrent thromboembolic events in patients with focal cerebral ischemia and antiphospholipid antibodies. Stroke 1992; 23(Suppl 2):I-29–I-32.
99. Asherson RA, Chan JKH, Harris EN, et al. Anticardiolipin antibody, recurrent thrombosis and warfarin withdrawal. Ann Rheum Dis 1985; 44:823–825.
100. Derksen RHWM, deGroot PG, Kater L, Nieuwenhuis HK. Patients with antiphospholipid antibodies and venous thrombosis should receive long term anticoagulant treatment. Ann Rheum Dis 1993; 52:689–692.
101. Khamashta MA, Cuadrado J, Mujic F, et al. The management of thrombosis in the antiphospholipid-antibody syndrome. N Engl J Med 1995; 332:993–997.
102. Heparin therapy: regimens and treatment considerations. Drugs 1992; 44:738–749.
103. Warkentin TE, Kelton JG. Heparin induced thrombocytopenia. Prog Hemost Thromb 1991; 10:1–34.
104. Cines DB, Tomaski A, Tannenbaum S. Immune endothelial cell injury in heparin-associated thrombocytopenia. N Engl J Med 1987; 316:581–589.
105. Dreyfus M, Magny JF, Bridley F, et al. Treatment of homozygous protein C deficiency and neonatal purpura fulminians with a purified protein C concentrate. N Engl J Med 1991; 325;1565–1570.
106. Zauber NP, Start MW. Successful warfarin anticoagulation despite protein C deficiency and a history of warfarin necrosis. Ann Intern Med 1986; 104:659–662.
107. Hall JG, Pauli RM, Wilson KM. Maternal and fetal sequelae of anticoagulation during pregnancy. Am J Med 1990; 68:122–140.
108. Ginsberg JS, Hirsh J. Use of antithrombotic agents during pregnancy. Chest 1992; 102(Suppl.):385S–390S.
109. Vianna JL, Khamashta MA, Ordi-Ros J, et al. Comparison of the primary and secondary

antiphospholipid syndrome—a European multicenter study of 114 Patients. Am J Med 1994; 96:3–9.
110. Babikian VL, Levine SR. Therapeutic considerations for stroke patients with antiphospholipid antibodies. Stroke 1992; 23:(Suppl.1):1-33–I-37.
111. Triplett DA, Brandt JT. Lupus anticoagulants: Misnomer, paradox, riddle, epiphenomenon. Hematol Pathol 1988; 2:121–143.
112. Hart RG, Miller VT, Coull BM, Bril V. Cerebral infarction association with lupus anticoagulants: Preliminary report. Stroke 1984; 15:114–118.
113. Asherson RA, Bagaley E, Khamashta MA, Hughes GRV. Multiple small-vessel occlusions in systemic lupus erythematosus [letter]. Stroke 1989; 20:127–129.
114. Ingram SB, Goodnight SH, Bennett RM. An unusual syndrome of a devastating noninflammatory vasculopathy associated with anticardiolipin antibodies: report of two cases. Arth Rheum 1987; 30:1167–1171.
115. Harris EN, Bos K. An acute disseminated coagulopathy-vasculopathy associated with the antiphospholipid syndrome. Arch Intern Med 1991; 151:231–233.
116. Asherson RA. The catastrophic antiphospholipid syndrome. J Rheumatol 1992; 19:508–512.
117. Wallace D. Does hydroxychloroquine sulfate prevent clot formation in systemic lupus erythematosus? [letter]. Arthr Rheum 1990; 33:1061–1062.
118. Greisman CG, Thayamparan RS, Goodwin TA, Lockshin MD. Occlusive vasculopathy in systemic lupus erythematosus: association with anticardiolipin antibody. Arch Intern Med 1991; 151:389-392.
119. Perez RE, McClendon JR, Lie JT. Primary antiphospholipid syndrome with multi organ arterial and venous thromboses. J Rheumatol 1992; 19:1289–1292.
120. Egan RM, Munn RK. Catastrophic antiphospholipid antibody syndrome presenting with multiple thromboses and sites of avascular necrosis. J Rheumatol 1994; 21:2376–2379.
121. Wallace DJ, Linker-Israeli M, Metzger AL, Stecher VJ. The relevance of antimalarial therapy with regard to thrombosis, hypercholesterolemia and cytokines in SLE. Lupus 1993; 2(Suppl. 1):S13–S15.
122. Johnson R, Orth MC, Charnley JN. Hydroxychloroquine in prophylaxis of pulmonary embolism following hip arthroplasty. Clin Orthop 1979; 144:714–718.
123. Spinnato JA, Clark AL, Pierangeli SS, Harris EN. Intravenous immunoglobulin therapy for the antiphospholipid syndrome. Am J Obstet Gynecol 1995; 172:690–694.
124. Sturfelt G, Mousa F, Jonsson H, et al. Recurrent cerebral infarction and the antiphospholipid syndrome: effect of intravenous gammaglobulin in a patient with systemic lupus erythematosus. Ann Rheum Dis 1990; 49:939–941.
125. Dosekun AK, Pollak VE, Glas-Greenwalt P, et al. Ancrod in systemic lupus erythematosus with thrombosis. Clinical and fibrinolytic effects. Arch Intern Med 1984; 144:37–42.
126. Lubbe WF, Palmer SJ, Butler WS, Liggins GE. Fetal survivial after prednisone suppression of maternal lupus anticoagulant. Lancet 1983; 1:1361–363.
127. Lubbe WF, Butler WS, Palme SJ, Liggins GC. Lupus anticoagulant in pregnancy. Br J Obstet Gynecol 1984; 91:357–363.
128. Branch DW, Scott Jr, Kochenour NK, Hershgold E. Obstetric complications associated with the lupus anticoagulant. N Engl J Med 1985; 313:1322–1326.
129. Carp HJA, Frenkel Y, Many A, et al. Fetal demise associated with the lupus anticoagulant: clinical features and results of treatment. Gynecol Obstet Invest 1989; 28:178–184.
130. Ordi J, Barquinero J, Vilardell M, et al. Fetal loss treatment in patients with antiphospholipid antibodies. Ann Rheum Dis 1989; 48:798–802.
131. Silviera LH, Hubble CL, Jara LJ, et al. Prevention of anticardiolipin antibody-related pregnancy losses with prednisone and aspirin. Am J Med 1992; 93:403–411.
132. Harris EN, Spinnato J. Should anticardiolipin tests be performed in otherwise healthy pregnant women? Am J Obstet Gynecol 1991; 165:1272–1277.

133. Lockshin MD, Druzin ML, Qamar T. Prednisone does not prevent recurrent fetal death in women with antiphospholipid antibody. Am J Obstet Gynecol 1989; 160:439–443.
134. Passaleva A, Massai G, D'Elios MM, et al. Prevention of miscarriage in antiphospholipid syndrome. Autoimmunity 1992; 14:121–125.
135. Tincani A, Faden D, Tarantini M, et al. Systemic lupus erythematosus and pregnancy: a prospective study. Clin Exp Rheumatol 1992; 10:439–446.
136. Chan JKH, Harris EN, Hughes GRV. Successful pregnancy following suppression of anticardiolipin antibody and lupus anticoagulant with azathioprine in systemic lupus erythematosus. 1986; 7:16–17.
137. Rudolph JE, Schweizer RT, Bartus SA. Pregnancy in renal transplant patients. A reviw. Transplantation 1979; 27:26–29.
138. Cowchock FS, Reece EA, Balaban D, et al. Repeated fetal losses associated with antiphospholipid antibodies: a collaborative randomized trial comparing prednisone with low-dose heparin treatment. Am J Obstet Gynecol 1992; 166:1318–1323.
139. Silver RK, MacGregor SN, Sholl JS, et al. Comparative trial of prednisone plus aspirin versus aspirin alone in the treatment of anticardiolipin antibody-positive obstetric patients. Am J Obstet Gynecol 1993; 169:1411–1417.
140. Branch WD, Silver RM, Blackwell JL, et al. outcome of treated pregnancies in women with antiphospholipid syndrome: an update of the Utah experience. Obstet Gynecol 1992; 80:614–620.
141. Harris EN, Chan JKH, Asherson RA, et al. Thrombosis, recurrent fetal loss and thrombocytopenia. Predictive value of the anti-cardiolipin antibody test. Arch Intern Med 1986; 146:2153–2156.
142. Loizou S, Byron MA, Englert HR, et al. Association of quantitative anti-cardiolipin antibody levels with fetal loss. Q J Med 1988; 68:525-531.
143. Englert JH, Derue GM, Loizou S, et al. Pregnancy and lupus: prognostic indicators and response to treatment. Q J Med 1988; 66:125–136.
144. Rosove MH, Tabsh K, Wasserstrum N, et al. Heparin therapy for pregnant women with lupus anticoagulant and anticardiolipin antibodies. Obstet Gynecol 1990; 75:630–634.
145. Ginsberg JS, Kowalchuk G, Kirsh J, et al. Heparin effect on bone density. Thromb Haemostas 1990; 64:286–289.
146. Scott JR, Branch WD, Kochenour NK, Ward K. Intravenous immunoglobulin treatment of pregnant patients with recurrent pregnancy loss caused by antiphospholipid antibodies and Rh immunization. Am J Obstet Gynecol 1988; 159:1055–1056.
147. Francoise A, Freund M, Daffos F, et al. Repeated fetal losses and the lupus anticoagulant. Ann Intern Med 1988; 109:993–994.
148. Parke A, Maier D, Wilson D, et al. Intravenous gammaglobulin, antiphospholipid antibodies, and pregnancy. Ann Intern Med 1989; 110:495–496.
149. Carreras LO, Perez GN, Vega HR, et al. Lupus anticoagulant and recurrent pregnancy loss: successful treatment with gammaglobulin. Lancet 1988; 2:393–394.
150. Wapner RJ, Cowchock S, Shaprio SS. Successful treatment in two women with antiphospholipid antibodies and refractory pregnancy losses with intravenous immunoglobulin infusions. Am J Obstet Gynecol 1989; 161:1271–1272.
151. Arnout J, Spitz B, Wittevrongel C, et al. High-dose intravenous immunoglobulin treatment of pregnant patient with an antiphospholipid syndrome: immunological changes associated with a successful outcome. Thromb Haemostas 1994; 71:741–747.
152. Spinatto JA, Clark AL, Pierangeli SS, Harris EN. Intravenous immunoglobulin therapy for the antiphospholipid syndrome in pregnancy. Am J Obstet Gynecol 1995; 172:690–694.
153. Schiano TD, Bellary SV, Black M. Possible transmission of hepatitis C virus infection with intravenous immunoglobulin. Ann Intern Med 1995; 122:802.
154. Ochs MD. Intravenous immunoglobulin therapy of patients with primary immunodeficiency syndromes: efficacy and safety of a new modified preparation. In: Alving BM, Finlayson

JS, eds. Characteristics and Uses of Intravenous Preparations. Washington DC: Department of Health and Human Services, 1980; 9–14.
155. Gregorini G, Setti G, Remuzzi G. Recurrent abortion with lupus anticoagulant and pre-eclampsia: a common final pathway for two different diseases? Case report. Br J Obstet Gynecol 1986; 93:194–196.
156. Carreras LO, Machin SJ, Deman R. Arterial thrombosis, intrauterine death, and "lupus anticoagulant": detection of immunoglobulin interfering with prostacyclin formation. Lancet 1981; 1:244–246.
157. Kaaja R, Julkunen H, Viinikka L, Ylikorkala O. Production of prostacyclin and thromboxane in lupus pregnancies: effect of small dose of aspirin. Obstet Gynecol 1993; 81:327–331.
158. Martinuzzo ME, Maclouf J, Carreras LO, Levy-Toledano S. Antiphospholipid antibodies enhance thrombin-induced platelet activation and thromboxane formation. Thromb Haemostas 1993; 70:667–671.
159. Wallenberg HCS, Dekker GA, Makovitz JW, Rotmans P. Low-dose aspirin prevents pregnancy-induced hypertension and pre-eclampsia in angiotensin-sensitive primigravidae. Lancet 1986; 1:1–3.
160. Benignc A, Gregorini G, Frusca T, et al. Effect of flow-dose aspirin on fetal and maternal generation of thromboxane by platelets in women at risk for pregnancy-induced hypertension. N Engl J Med 1989; 321:357–362.
161. Trudinger BJ, Stewart GJ, Cook CM, et al. Monitoring lupus anticoagulant-positive pregancies with umbilical artery flow velocity wave forms. Obstet Gynecol 1990; 75:630–634.
162. Ramsey-Goldman R, Kutzer JE, Kuller LH, et al. Pregnancy outcome and anti-cardiolipin antibody in women with systemic lupus erythematosus. Am J Epidemiol 1993; 138:1057–1069.
163. Lockshin MD, Druzin ML, Goei S, et al. Antibody to cardiolipin as a predictor of fetal distress or death in pregnant patients with systemic lupus erythematosus. N Engl J Med 1985; 313:152–156.
164. Forouzan I, Cohen AW, Lindenbaum C, Samuels P. Umbilical artery and ductal blood flow velocities inpatients treated with aspirin and prednisone for presence of anticardiolipin antibody. J Ultrasound Med 1993; 3:135–138.
165. Hahn CLA. Pulsatile heparin administration in pregnancy: a new approach. Am J Obstet Gynecol 1986; 155:283–287.
166. Krnic-Barrie S, O'Connor CR, Looney SW, et al. Retrospective review of 61 patients with autophospholipid syndrome: analysis of factors influencing recurrent thrombosis. Arch Intern Med. 1997 (in press).

34

Second-line Agents in Rheumatic Diseases During Pregnancy

Dafna D. Gladman
The University of Toronto, and Toronto Hospital, Toronto, Ontario, Canada

Gideon Koren
The University of Toronto, and The Hospital for Sick Children, Toronto, Ontario, Canada

I. INTRODUCTION

The treatment of many of the rheumatological diseases is based on the control of inflammation. In many instances, nonsteroidal anti-inflammatory medications are sufficient. However, in a large number of patients, these medications do not adequately control the disease, and "second-line" drugs are introduced. These include gold, antimalarials, penicillamine, and sulfasalazine, which are anti-inflammatory and may be "disease suppressive" but are not considered "immunosuppressive" or "cytotoxic." When the disease-suppressive medications either are inadequate to control disease activity or cause unacceptable side effects or toxic reactions, one may consider the next step in the therapeutic pyramid. There are several drugs in this group that have been used extensively studied in rheumatoid arthritis, psoriatic arthritis, and systemic lupus erythematosus (SLE), including azathioprine, methotrexate, cyclophosphamide, chlorambucil, and cyclosporin A. In this chapter, the use of these second-line drugs during pregnancy will be discussed with regards to their clinical influence and effect on pregnancy and the fetus. It should be noted that many of the disorders for which these drugs are used improve during pregnancy [1]. A more detailed discussion of these second-line agents is undertaken in other chapters within the book.

II. DISEASE-SUPPRESSIVE MEDICATIONS

A. Gold Salts

Gold salts were first used in the treatment of rheumatoid arthritis by Forrestier in 1929, and reports of the efficacy of gold salts in this condition date back to 1935 [2]. Since then there have been numerous studies documenting the clinical use of gold salts, not only in rheumatoid arthritis [3] but also in psoriatic arthritis [4–6] and even in the arthritis of systemic lupus erythematosus [7].

Studies in rheumatoid arthritis have shown the efficacy of gold salts. Thus, the Empire Rheumatism Council study, which was the first double-blind control trial of the agent, demonstrated that patients who received 1 g of gold over 6 months fared better than controls who received a minute amount over the same period of time [8]. It was further demonstrated that gold actually reduced radiographic progression in rheumatoid arthritis [9]. Its clinical effect in psoriatic arthritis is marginal [4–6,10], and in systemic lupus erythematosus gold is not usually considered because of the concern for renal deposition and the development of immune complex disease [7].

The mechanism of action of gold is unclear, but there is evidence that it causes a reduction in titers of rheumatoid factor and in concentrations of other immunoglobulins. It also inhibits the phagocytic function of polymorphonuclear cells. Gold is given intramuscularly as weekly injections of 50 mg for a minimum of 20 weeks. When an improvement is noted, the frequency of injections may be reduced gradually to a maintenance dose of 50 mg once a month. Improvement is usually delayed until about 700 mg has been administered.

Gold is a potentially toxic drug. Its most common side effect is a skin rash, which is classically pruritic. Although gold has been continued in some patients with skin reactions, it should be discontinued in the face of severe reactions and particularly if the mucous membranes are involved. Bone marrow suppression is an infrequent but worrisome complication usually heralded by a drop in the platelet or hemoglobin level or white cell count. These are, therefore, checked routinely before each injection is administered. Immune complex nephritis is another significant complication. Urinalysis is always reviewed for any evidence of proteinuria. The proteinuria is reversible on discontinuation of the drug. Other rare reactions include colitis, lung toxicity, and hepatotoxicity. It had frequently been noted that patients who develop toxic reactions note a coincident remission of the arthritis.

There have been some reports of the successful treatment of pregnant women with gold without harmful fetal effects [11]. Gold is highly protein bound and presumably crosses the placenta poorly. However, there is one report on the passage of gold through the placenta [12]. There is also one report of the transfer of gold to an infant through breast milk, leading to concentrations greater than in maternal serum [13,14]. The only cohort study available to date is from Japan where only two malformations occurred among 93 infants exposed in utero to gold; a rate which is within the normal range [15]. Despite this apparent safe use and because rheumatoid arthritis frequently remits during pregnancy, it is safer to delay initiating gold therapy until after delivery.

B. Antimalarial Drugs

Antimalarial drugs have also been shown in controlled trials to be effective in rheumatoid arthritis and to compare favorably with gold therapy in early disease [16]. They have an advantage over gold in that they are given by mouth once a day and lack the renal and hematological complications of gold therapy. The antimalarial drugs chloroquine and hydroxychloroquine have been shown to be beneficial in treating some forms of skin rash in SLE as well as systemic symptoms [17]. Antimalarials have also been shown to be effective in the treatment of psoriatic arthritis [18].

The major toxicity of antimalarial drugs is gastrointestinal irritation and the ocular damage that results from their deposition in the retina. This appears to be dose related and is usually reversible, although there have been reports of persistent retinopathy [13]. In virtually all cases there is some chloroquine deposition in the cornea, which is of minor clinical significance and does not correlate with retinal deposits. Corneal deposits are not a contraindication to antimalarial therapy. Regular ophthalmological examinations are recommended to detect early retinal toxicity, and antimalarial therapy should be stopped if any evidence of retinal toxicity is found. It is reported that hydroxychloroquine is associated with less toxicity than chloroquine sulfate.

The main concern for the fetus is the effect of antimalarials on retinal development, the development of thrombocytopenia, and central nervous system abnormalities. Indeed, ototoxicity has been sporadically reported after the use of chloroquine during pregnancy [19]. Most of the literature available on antimalarials during pregnancy relates to prophylaxis for malaria, where much lower doses than those used in rheumatic diseases are used. These drugs have been used inadvertently during the first trimester with no adverse effects in some patients with SLE [20,21]. Although there are reports of uncomplicated pregnancies in patients treated with antimalarials, their use in pregnant patients with rheumatic diseases throughout the pregnancy cannot be recommended, because available safety data of high doses relate only to the first trimester. Hydroxychloroquine is found in human milk, but the infant would be exposed to only 2% of the maternal dose per day and therefore breast feeding is not contraindicated [22].

C. Penicillamine

Penicillamine is a more recent addition to the antirheumatic armamentarium [23]. It has been shown to be as effective as gold in the treatment of rheumatoid arthritis, and penicillamine has a similar mode of action with a delayed onset of response. It is thought to work by cleaving disulfide bridges and inhibiting collagen cross linking. Penicillamine has also been associated with a decrease in titers of rheumatoid factor. It is given orally as a 250-mg capsule. The initial dose os penicillamine is one capsule daily, which is to be increased slowly (at monthly intervals) to a dose of 500–750 mg/day. The side effects of penicillamine are similar to those of gold, and the same precautions apply (i.e. regular blood and urine examinations). It has been shown that penicillamine may be effective in patients who have been gold resistant or who have had reactions to gold. Penicillamine has recently been shown to be effective in the treatment of psoriatic arthritis [24].

Although penicillamine has been used successfully in pregnancy in patients with Wilson's disease [25,26], there have been two reports of connective tissue defects developing in infants born to mothers who took penicillamine during pregnancy [27]. Penicillamine does cross the placenta and theoretically may harm the fetus. Endres [27] suggests that although penicillamine it may be necessary in patients with Wilson's disease, it should not be given to patients with rheumatoid arthritis. Penicillamine has a short elimination half-life and is extensively protein bound, so only small amounts should be present in milk. Because of the natural improvement in rheumatoid arthritis and psoriatic arthritis that often occurs during pregnancy, it is advisable to withhold penicillamine until the end of gestation.

D. Sulfasalazine

Sulfasalazine, or salazopyrin, is the only drug which was originally developed for the treatment of rheumatoid arthritis [28]. Although initial studies were not successful, for the past 20 years it has been used effectively in the treatment of rheumatoid arthritis. More recently, sulfasalazine has been reported to be effective in the treatment of spondyloarthropathies, including ankylosing spondylitis, Reiter's disease, and psoriatic arthritis [29–31]. Its effect is usually noted within 8–12 weeks of onset of therapy. The usual therapeutic dose ranges from 2 to 3g/day. The mechanism of action of sulfasalazine is not known. Its side effects include allergic reactions to the sulfa moiety, bone marrow suppression, and diarrhea.

The use of sulfasalazine in pregnancy is reported exclusively in patients with inflammatory bowel disease, where it appears to be safe [32]. Both the sulfonamide and 5-aminosalicylic acid components of this agent have not been associated with increased teratogenic risks in humans. Sulfasalazine passes only in negligible amounts into milk and thus can be given during nursing [33].

III. IMMUNOSUPPRESSIVE AND CYTOTOXIC MEDICATIONS

Since the mechanism of action of these drugs involves a nonselective inhibition of normal DNA synthesis, it has been suggested that these drugs would be particularly toxic to the developing embryo whose growth entails extreme cell division. Indeed, animal studies have suggested that these medications may be toxic to the developing embryo. An in vitro study which exposed embryonic cells to several immunosuppressive drugs revealed that azathioprine, mercaptopurine (a metabolite of azathioprine), and methotrexate caused significant inhibition of cell growth and differentiation, whereas cyclosporin A did not interfere with embryonic development [34].

A. Azathioprine

Azathioprine has been used successfully in the treatment of rheumatoid arthritis, psoriatic arthritis, other seronegative arthropathies, and systemic lupus erythematosus. It is a long-acting drug, with therapeutic effect noticeable at about 4 months of therapy. Effective dose ranges from 1.5 to 2.5 mg/kg body weight/day. Side effects include bone marrow suppression, gastrointestinal irritation, and rarely a granulomatous reaction in the skin and liver.

Azathioprine has been used successfully in pregnancy in renal transplant patients as well as in patients with Crohn's disease [12,35–37]. No congenital malformations were noted in six patients treated with azathioprine for systemic lupus erythematosus during pregnancy [38]. However, there is a report of chromosomal aberrations in a child of a patient with SLE treated with azathioprine and prednisone before and during pregnancy [39]. There is also a report of prenatal cytomegalovirus infection associated with severe brain damage in an infant whose mother was treated with prednisolone and azathioprine for SLE [40]. Compilation of the world literature failed to show teratogenicity among over 70 collected cases [41]. It is not clear whether azathioprine is secreted in breast milk. It is felt by many today that if a patient with rheumatoid arthritis or

SLE has responded well to azathioprine and there is a fear of exacerbation on discontinuation, the drug may be continued during pregnancy.

B. Methotrexate

Methotrexate has been used successfully to treat patients with psoriatic arthritis [42], rheumatoid arthritis [43], and more recently in SLE [44]. The dose required for therapeutic response has varied from 7.5 to 25 mg/week. Its major side effects include gastrointestinal complaints, bone marrow suppression, and liver toxicity. The use of weekly doses seems to reduce toxicity. Its therapeutic effect is usually noted within 6–8 weeks.

Methotrexate has been used to induce abortions, and indeed may lead to spontaneous abortions when used in early pregnancy [12,34,45]. Although there have been a few live births with the children being normal at follow-up for a mean of 11 years [46], its routine use is not recommended. Feltkamp and Carey recently discussed the difficulty in establishing the risk for fetal malformations with methotrexate [47]. They suggest that there is no significant risk for fetal malformation with exposure to less than 10 mg/week of methotrexate, and that the critical time for developing methotrexate fetal toxicity is between 6 and 8 postconception weeks. A collaborative study published recently has concurred with these recommendations [48]. There is a single report of the secretion of methotrexate in milk during lactation, although the amount detected (0.25 μg/100 mL) was nontoxic despite a high intake of 22.5 mg daily by the mother [49].

C. Cyclosporin A

Cyclosporin is a relatively new immunosuppressive drug used in the treatment of rheumatoid arthritis and other rheumatic diseases [50,51]. It has significant side effects, most notably its nephrotoxicity [52]. Most of the information on its use in pregnancy comes from transplantation patients, where it appears that its use has not been associated with an increased risk of birth defects [53]. There are recent reports of the successful use of cyclosporin A in pregnant nontransplant patients [54,55]. No information is available on the secretion of cyclosporin A in breast milk.

D. Cyclophosphamide

Cyclophosphamide has been used for the treatment of a number of rheumatic diseases, including systemic lupus erythematosus, where it is usually given as a monthly intravenous bolus; vasculitis, where it is given as a daily oral dose; and rheumatoid arthritis, where it has been used orally. Its potential toxicity is considerable [56].

Cyclophosphamide has caused fetal malformations in animals, and in humans, there have been several cases of fetal malformations following first-trimester exposure to the drug [10,11]. A recent case report of twins whose mother was treated with cyclophosphamide throughout the pregnancy highlights the pharmacogenetic nature of fetal sensitivity. One twin (a boy) has had multiple malformations, mental deficiency, and two different types of cancer (neuroblastoma and thyroid carcinoma), whereas his sister is totally healthy at 20 years of follow-up. Different metabolism of the drug into toxic metabolites may explain this variability [57]. There are only very few patients with rheumatic diseases given cyclophosphamide during pregnancy [36]. Its use is clearly not recommended during pregnancy.

E. Chlorambucil

Chlorambucil is an alkylating agent which has been used in the treatment of a number rheumatic diseases [56]. There are reports of at least three instances of fetal malformations resulting in death [12] in cases where chlorambucil was given in early pregnancy. However, it seems that the drug is safer when given in late pregnancy.

As mentioned above, since the majority of patients with rheumatoid arthritis improve during pregnancy, it may not be necessary to consider immunoregulatory therapy before delivery. The difficulty arises when one wishes to begin this type of therapy in a patient who would like to become pregnant. In this situation, it appears that it would be safer to use gold, sulfasalazine, or azathioprine than any of the other immunosuppressive medications. Nevertheless, it is advisable to discontinue their use prior to conception. Should a patient become pregnant and require these medications for control of disease, she would have to be counseled on the safety/risk of the drugs in the context of fetal safety and persistence of active illness.

IV. COUNSELING THE RHEUMATIC PATIENT TAKING SECOND-LINE DRUGS

Counseling should be performed by health professionals familiar with the medical condition(s) of the patient, including the dynamics of the illness, her medication, and her obstetrical background. It is important to ensure that the patient understands the concept of teratogenic risk in terms of percentage and in comparison to baseline population risk. It is easier to decrease or discontinue drug therapy in women experiencing remission during pregnancy. When a drug is needed, the minimum effective dose schedule should be used. It is crucial not to overlook other reproductive risks the woman may have. For example, the teratogenic risks of most second-line drugs are far lower than the risk of Down's syndrome in a 40-year-old patient. The latter can be ruled out by amniocentesis, for example. In different institutions such counseling is offered by clinical teratologists, geneticists, toxicologists, or perinatologists.

REFERENCES

1. Gladman DD, Urowitz MB. Rheumatic disease in pregnancy. In: Burrow JN, Ferris TF, eds. Medical Complications During Pregnancy. 4th ed. Philadelphia: Saunders, 1995:501–529.
2. Forrestier I. Rheumatoid arthritis and its treatment by gold salts. J Lab Clin Med 1935; 20:828.
3. Gordon DA: Gold compounds. In: Kelly WN, Harris ED, Ruddy S, Sledge CB, eds. Textbook of Rheumatology, 4th ed. Philadelphia: B. Saunders, 1993:743–759.
4. Dowart BB, Gall EP, Schumacher HR, Krauser RE. Chrysotherapy in psoriatic arthritis: efficacy and toxicity compared to rheumatoid arthritis. Arthritis Rheum 1978; 21:513–515.
5. Carrett S, Calin A. Evaluation of auranofin in psoriatic arthritis: a double blind placebo controlled trial. Arthritis Rheum 1989; 32:158–165.
6. Palit J, Hill J, Capell HA, et al. A multicentre double-blind comparison of auranofin, intramuscular gold thiomalate and placebo in patients with psoriatic arthritis. Br J Rheumatol 1990; 29:280–283.

7. Weisman MH, Albert D, Mueller MR, et al. Gold therapy in patients with systemic lupus erythematosus. Am J Med 1983; 75:157–164.
8. Empire Rheumatism Council. Gold therapy in rheumatoid arthritis: Final report of a multicentre controlled trial. Ann Rheum Dis 1961; 20:315–
9. Siegler JW, Bluhm GB, Duncan H, et al. Gold salts in the treatment of rheumatoid arthritis. A double-blind study. Ann Intern Med 1974; 80:21–26.
10. Mader R, Gladman DD, Long J, et al. Does injectable gold prevent progression of psoriatic arthritis (PsA)—long-term follow up. Clin Invest Med 1995; 18:139–143.
11. Roubenoff R, Hoyt J, Petri M, et al. Effects of antiinflammatory and immunosuppressive drugs on pregnancy and fertility. Semin Arthrit Rheum 1988; 18:88–110.
12. Ostensen MA. Treatment with immunosuppressive and disease modifying drugs during pregnancy and lactation. Am J Reprod Immunol 1992; 28:148–152.
13. Blau SO. Metabolism of gold during lactation. Arthrit Rheum 1973; 16:777–778.
14. Bennett PN, Humphries SJ, Osborne JP, et al. Use of sodium autothiomalate during lactation. Br J Pharmacal 1990; 29:777–779.
15. Miyamoto T, Miyayi S, Hariuchi Y. Gold therapy in bronchial asthma—special emphasis upon blood levels of gold and its teratogenicity. J Jap Soc Intern Med 1974; 63:1190–1197.
16. Rynes RI. Antimalarial drugs. In: Kelley WN, Harris ED, Ruddy S, Sledge CB, eds. Textbook of Rheumatology, 4th ed. Philadelphia: Saunders, 1993: 731–742.
17. Esdaile JM. The efficacy of antimalarials in systemic lupus erythematosus. Lupus 1993; 2(Suppl. 1):S3–S8.
18. Gladman DD, Blake R, Brubacher B, Farewell VT. Chloroquine therapy in psoriatic arthritis. J Rheumatol 1992; 19:1724–1726.
19. Hart CW, Nauton RF. The ototoxicity of chloroquine phosphate. Arch Otolaryngol 1964; 80:497–512.
20. Tozman ECS, Urowitz MB, Gladman DD. Systemic lupus erythematosus and pregnancy. J Rheumatol 1980; 7:624–632.
21. Levy M, Buskila D, Gladman DD, et al. Pregnancy outcome following first trimester exposure to chloroquine. Am J Perinatol 1991; 8:174–177.
22. Nation RL, Hacektt LP, Dusci LJ, Ilett KF. Excretion of hydroxychloroquine in human mild. Br J Clin Pharmacol 1984; 17:368–369.
23. Jaffe IA. Penicillamine. In: Kelley WN, Harris ED, Ruddy S, Sledge CB, eds. Textbook of Rheumatology, 4th ed. Philadelphia: Saunders, 1993:760–766.
24. Roux H, Schiano AA, Maestracci D, et al. Notre Experience du traitement du rheumatisme psoriatique par la D-Penicillamine. Rev Rhum 1979; 46:631–633.
25. Lyle WH. Penicillamine in pregnancy. Lancet 1984; 1:606–607.
26. Schneiberg IH, Sternlieb I. Pregnancy in penicillamine treated patients with Wilson's disease. N Engl J Med 1975; 293:1300–1302.
27. Endres W. D-Penicillamine in pregnancy—to ban or not to ban? Klin Wochenschr 1981; 59:535–537.
28. Day RO. Sulphasalazine. In: Kelley WN, Harris ED, Ruddy S, Sledge CB, eds. Textbook of Rheumatology, 4th ed. Philadelphia: Saunders, 1993:692–699.
29. Bosi Ferraz M, Tugwell P, Goldsmith CH, et al. Meta-analysis of sulfasalazine in ankylosing spondylitis. J Rheumatol 1990; 17:1482–1486.
30. Zwillich SH, Comer SS, Lee E, et al. Treatment of the seronegative spondyloarthropathies with sulphasalazine. J Rheumatol 1988; 15(Suppl. 1):33–39.
31. Farr M, Kitas GD, Waterhouse L, et al. Sulphasalazine in psoriatic arthritis: a double-blind placebo-controlled study. Br J Rheumatol 1990; 29:46–49.
32. Miller JP. Inflammatory bowel disease in pregnancy: a review. J R Soc Med 1986; 79:221–225.

33. Jarnerol G, Into-Maimberg MB. Sulphasalazine treatment during breast feeding. Scand J Gastroenterol 1979; 14:869–871.
34. Schmid BP. Monitoring of organ formation in rat embryos after in vitro exposure to azathioprine, mercaptopurine, methotrexate or cyclosporin A. Toxicology 1984; 31:9–21.
35. Alstead EM, Ritchie JK, Lennard-Jones JE, et al. Safety of azathioprine in pregnancy in inflammatory bowel disease. Gastroenterology 1990; 99:443–446.
36. Sharon E, Jones J, Diamond H, et al. Pregnancy and azathioprine in systemic lupus erythematosus. Am J Obstet Gynecol 1974; 118:25–28.
37. Sztejnbok J, Stuart A, Diamond H, et al. Azathioprine in the treatment of systemic lupus erythematosus. Arthritis Rheum 1971; 14:639.
38. Ramsay-Goldman R, Mientus JM, Kutzer JE, et al. Pregnancy outcome in women with systemic lupus erythematosus treated with immunosuppressive drugs. J Rheumatol 1993; 20:1152–1157.
39. Ostrer H, Stamberg J, Perinchief P. Two chromosomal aberrations in the child of a woman with systemic lupus erythematosus treated with azathioprine and prednisone. Am J Med Genet 1984; 17:627–632.
40. Hayes E, Symington G, Mackay IR. Maternal immunosuppression and cytomegalovirus infection of the fetus. Aust NZ J Med 1979; 9:430–433.
41. Schordein F: Chemically Induced Birth Defects, 2nd ed. New York: Marcel Dekker, 1993:464–486.
42. Black RL, O'Brien WM, Van Scott EJ, et al. Methotrexate therapy in psoriatic arthritis. Double blind study on 21 patients. JAMA 1964; 189:743–747.
43. Weinblatt ME. Methotrexate. In: Kelley WN, Harris ED, Ruddy S, Sledge CB, eds. Textbook of Rheumatology, 4th ed. Philadelphia: Saunders, 1993:767–778.
44. Walz-LeBlanc BA, Dagenais P, Urowitz MB, Gladman DD. Methotrexate in systemic lupus erythematosus. J Rheumatol 1994; 21:836–838.
45. Hausknecht RU: Methotrexate and misoprostal to terminate early pregnancy. N Engl J Med 1995; 333:537–540.
46. Kozlowski RD, Steinbrunner JV, Mackenzie AH, et al. Outcome of first trimester exposure to low-dose methotrexate in eight patients with rheumatic diseases. Am J Med 1990; 88:589–592.
47. Feldkamp M, Carey JC. Clinical teratology counselling and consultation case report: low dose methotrexate exposure in the early weeks of pregnancy. Teratology 1993; 47:533–539.
48. Donnenfeld AC, Palusza KA, Salfokk Noah J, Schick B, et al. Methotrexate exposure prior to and during pregnancy. Teratology 1994; 491:79–81.
49. Johns DG, Rutherford LD, Leighton PC, Vogel CL. Secretion of methotrexate into human milk. Am J Obstet Gynecol 1972; 112:978–980.
50. Yocum DE, Klippel JH, Wilder RL, et al. Cyclosporin in severe, treatment-refractory rheumatoid arthritis: a randomized study. Ann Intern Med 1988; 109:863–869.
51. Gupta AK, Matteson EI, Ellis CN, et al. Cyclosporin in the treatment of psoriatic arthritis. Arch Dermatol 1989; 125:507–510.
52. Fauci AS, Young KR: Immunoregulatory agents. In: Kelley WN, Harris ED, Ruddy S, Sledge CB, eds. Textbook of Rheumatology, 4th ed. Philadelphia: Saunders, 1993:797–821.
53. Cockburn I, Krupp P, Mouka C. Present experience of Sandimmun in pregnancy. Transplant Proc 1989; 21:3720–3732.
54. Wright S, Glover M, Baker H. Psoriasis, cyclosporin and pregnancy [letter]. Arch Dermatol 1991; 127:436.
55. Doria A, Di Lenardo L, Vario S, et al. Cyclosporin A in a pregnant patient affected with systemic lupus erythematosus. Rheumatol Int 1992; 12:77–78.

56. Fauci AS, Young KR: Immunoregulatory agents. In: Kelley WN, Harris ED, Ruddy S, Sledge CB, eds. Textbook of Rheumatology, 4th ed. Philadelphia: Saunders, 1993:797–821.
57. Zemlickis D, Lishner M, Erlich R, Koren G. Teratogenicity and carcinogenicity in a twin exposed in utero to cyclophosphamide. Teratog Carcinogen Mutagen 1993; 13:139–143.

35
Cytotoxic Drugs and the Risk for Malignancies

Grant W. Cannon
Veterans Affairs Medical Center, and University of Utah
Salt Lake City, Utah

I. INTRODUCTION

Cytotoxic drugs have provided a major advance in the treatment of many rheumatic diseases. Convincing data in patients with rheumatoid arthritis (RA) [1–10], systemic lupus erythematosus (SLE) [11–13], and vasculitis [14–16] have suggested that both morbidity and/or mortality can be improved with these agents. Despite these well-recognized benefits, concerns have developed about long-term toxicities with these therapeutic regimens. These concerns have been particularly focused on the increased incidence of malignancies following the use of cytotoxic drugs [17–75]. These two observations—definite therapeutic benefit and clear risk for malignancy—provide a significant dilemma for the physician recommending such treatment.

Clearly, when a rheumatic disease can be treated with either cytotoxic drugs or an equally efficacious alternative program with less toxicity, the less toxic therapeutic regimen should be selected. However, when cytotoxic drugs are indicated, a risk/benefit estimate must be made by the clinician. The majority of this book describes a variety of therapeutic options, including cytotoxic drugs, for the treatment of rheumatic diseases. These chapters present information which will allow the clinician to estimate the benefits and relative efficacy of the possible therapies. In this chapter, the data are presented which will allow an assessment of the malignancy risk associated with the use of cytotoxic drugs in rheumatic diseases. The physician must then balance the available information concerning the known natural history of the rheumatic disease being treated, the potential benefits for cytotoxic drugs, and the possible risk for malignancy. The clinician can then discuss this information with the patient to allow an informed decision on the appropriate treatment course.

II. GENERAL PRINCIPLES CONCERNING THE CARCINOGENSIS OF CYTOTOXIC DRUGS

A. Secondary Malignancies Associated with Cytotoxic Drug Therapy for Cancer

Although an increase in malignancies has been seen in patients with rheumatic diseases treated with cytotoxic drugs, the majority of the research on the carcinogenic potential of these agents has been determined during their use in malignancies. Large population studies in cancer patients have provided excellent clinical epidemiology data to establish an increase in secondary malignancies and to classify agents as to their relative potential to induce malignancies [21]. These data have required comparative studies and multivariant analysis, because frequently these drugs are given in combination. When combinations of agents are used, the potential for synergistic effects could be anticipated; however, little data are available to support the concept of more than additive effects of these agents.

These data have shown that the use of alkylating agents, including cyclophosphamide [21,27,64] and chlorambucil [21,19,30], are associated with the development of secondary malignancies. This observation is true both for when these drugs are used alone and in combination. In contrast, there is little evidence on the review of a large experience from the use of methotrexate in malignant disease to suggest that this drug is associated with an increased risk for the development of cancer [28,54].

One difficulty with the many epidemiological studies is the lack of appropriate control populations. The development of a relative risk and quantitative estimates of this risk requires a simultaneous evaluation of an appropriate control population, which is often not available for the evaluation of many studies. The potential of "overdetection" of malignancies in a population under close follow-up because of the primary disease is another concern in studies evaluating secondary malignancies. However, this overdetection should only effect the detection but not mortality unless early detection is associated with an improved survival. Despite these limitations, data from the study of cytotoxic drugs in malignancies provide some important information and observations which can be applies to the evaluation of these agents in rheumatic diseases.

B. Malignancy in Rheumatic Diseases

The development of malignancies during the use of a cytotoxic drug in a rheumatic diseases must be reviewed in the context of the known information about the baseline rate of malignancies in these disorders. The use of appropriate controlled studies must be utilized to establish that an increased rate of malignancy exists rather than relying only on case reports or comparisons to the general population. As will be reviewed below, significant information is being developed to determine and establish the rate of malignancies in rheumatic diseases.

1. Rheumatoid Arthritis

The rate of hematological malignancies may be increased in patients with rheumatoid arthritis (RA) [76–79]. A large study in Finland with 46,101 subjects evaluated for a total of 213,911 patient years reported a 2.7 relative risk for lymphoma in RA patients when compared with the general population [76]. A British study of 489 RA patients showed a relative risk of 15 for the development of lymphoproliferative disorders [77].

In a prospective study, Fries et al. reported a relative risk of 3.5 for lymphoproliferative malignancies over a 12-year follow-up period [78]. Another prospective study of 100 RA patients suggested a relative risk of 5 for lymphoproliferative malignancies in RA patients in an 11-year follow-up [79].

Other studies have not suggested an increase in malignancy in RA patients [80–83]. Allebeck et al. did not report an increased incidence of malignancy despite an increase in total mortality in 1165 RA patents evaluated in Stockholm [80]. Vandenbroucke et al. did not show an increase in malignancies in 209 RA patients followed in a 25-year prospective study despite an increase in overall mortality rate [81]. Mitchell found no increased incidence of malignancy in 805 RA patients followed prospectively for an average of 12 years [82]. Mutru et al. suggested an increased mortality but not an increased mortality from malignancies in 1000 RA patients observed over 10 years [83]. In all of these studies, the overall mortality for RA was increased in comparison to the general population, but the mortality from malignant diseases was not increased.

The observation that the frequency of malignancies may be increased in RA patients has complicated the evaluation of the association between cytotoxic drug therapy and the induction of malignancies. The data suggesting that malignancies and particularly hematological and lymphoproliferative malignancies [76–79] are increased in RA has raised concern that the propensity to develop a malignancy during RA may increase in proportion to the disease severity and disease duration. Because cytotoxic drugs are most generally reserved for the most severe RA patients, the possibility that the observed increased prevalence of malignancies in RA patients associated with cytotoxic drug therapy may be an indirect measurement of disease severity and duration rather than a direct effect of the cytotoxic drug. This possibility has not been completely excluded, but it seems unlikely in view of the increased prevalence of malignancies associated with the use of cytotoxic drug in other diseases [21] and the increased prevalence of malignancies associated with cytotoxic drug therapy in RA patients during studies which have controlled for RA disease duration and severity [18,22].

2. *Systemic Lupus Erythematosus*

Lewis et al. reported a chart review of hospitalized patients with RA and systemic lupus erythematosus (SLE) which suggested a slight increase in malignancies in RA patients (0.6%) ($P < .005$) but a larger increased prevalence of malignancies in SLE patients (4%) ($P < .0005$) [84]. The treatment with cytotoxic drugs was not specifically mentioned nor analyzed in this study. No firm data support the concept that malignancies may be increase in SLE [56], although there are case reports suggesting a possible association [20,32,39,85].

3. *Systemic Sclerosis*

Multiple case reports have suggested an association between systemic sclerosis and lung cancer [86–90] and breast cancer [31,53,91–93]. A large survey not specifically designed for epidemiological purposes reported malignancies in 2141 patients with scleroderma. This study did not clearly identify an increase in lung cancer in systemic sclerosis patients [31]; however, a subsequent study with 262 patients suggested an increased incidence of lung cancer in systemic sclerosis patients with a prevalence rate of 5% with a relative risk of 4.4, which was statistically significantly different than controls [93]. The incidence of breast cancer does not appear to be higher than that observed in the general population [53]. No data are available to determine if cytotoxic drug therapy increases the malignancy rate in systemic sclerosis patients.

4. *Inflammatory Muscle Disease*

The association of malignancies with inflammatory muscle disease, and particularly dermatomyositis, is well established [94–99], with the prevalence of cancer ranging from 15.1 to 24% [94]. Malignancies most commonly associated with dermatomyositis/polymyositis are breast, lung, ovary, stomach, uterine, and colon [94–96]. No studies have specifically evaluated the possible effects of cytotoxic drugs used to treat inflammatory muscle disease and the subsequent development of malignancies.

5. *Other Rheumatic Diseases*

The association between Sjögren's syndrome and lymphoma is quite well established [100-102]. In Sjögren's syndrome patients, the risk for malignancy appeared to increase more after irradiation therapy than after chemotherapy [102].

6. *Summary*

As described above, questions still remain as to what effect the underlying rheumatic disease has on the propensity to develop malignancies during cytotoxic drug therapy. Question remains as to whether RA patients are more likely to develop malignancies than the general population. However, most data would suggest that both the incidence of lymphoproliferative malignancies is increased in RA patients without cytotoxic drug therapy, and that this risk for cancer is further enhanced in RA patients treated with cytotoxic drugs, particularly alkylating agents.

III. ALKYLATING AGENTS

A. General Concepts

Cancer chemotherapy evaluations have provide much useful data on the risk of secondary malignancies after the use of alkylating agents. The risk for leukemia after chemotherapy for Hodgkin's disease is increased in patients treated with chemotherapy in comparison with the general population and Hodgkin's disease patients receiving radiation therapy alone [49]. The estimated range for this increase is in the order of 10- to 100-fold over the baseline rate [21]. The highest rates are associated with combination chemotherapy, including nitrogen mustard, vincristine, procarbazine, and prednisone (MOPP) [21]. In addition to studies of patients with Hodgkin's disease, an increase in leukemia has been suggested in patients receiving chemotherapy for multiple other malignancies including non-Hodgkin's lymphoma, multiple myeloma, and solid tumors such as carcinomas of the ovary, breast, lung, and gastrointestinal tract [21]. In addition to leukemia, many of the patients will also experience a myelodysplastic syndrome related to leukemia. Leukemias induced by alkylating agents are often myelogenous or "acute nonlymphocytic leukemias." The risk for chemotherapy-induced leukemia appears to be increased for several years after the initiation of chemotherapy, with the peak of this risk occurring about 8 years after therapy is initiated [21].

Solid tumors and non-Hodgkin's lymphoma are also noted to increase following treatment of Hodgkin's disease [21]. The role of chemotherapy versus radiation therapy in these patients has been somewhat controversial and the numbers of secondary malignancies is probably still insufficient to reach a definite conclusion. Solid tumors developing after the treatment of Hodgkin's disease include lung, breast, stomach, melanoma, thyroid, and bone [21].

B. Cyclophosphamide

1. Oral Cyclophosphamide Treatment

A long-term case control study of RA patients treated with cyclophosphamide compared with RA patients not treated with cyclophosphamide showed an increase in malignancies in patients receiving cyclophosphamide [17]. In this study, long-term follow-up was conducted on 130 RA patients enrolled in an investigational protocol of cyclophosphamide in RA. One hundred and nineteen patients were available for follow-up. These patients were matched with control RA patients from the same practice group not treated with cyclophosphamide of similar sex, age, disease duration, and American Rheumatism Association functional class at the time of entry. Clinic and hospital records were reviewed and telephone contacts made with either the patients or surviving family members. These reviews and interviews determined the patient's race, primary occupation, family history of malignancy, history of tobacco and alcohol use, serum rheumatoid factor, concurrent use of other antirheumatic drugs, durations and total doses of cyclophosphamide, adverse effects potentially attributable to cyclophosphamide, diagnosis and specific cell type of malignancy, current survival status, cause of death, and the presence of concomitant medical problems.

The two study groups were comparable for matched variables, including sex, age, disease duration, and functional class. The mean follow-up duration was 10.8 years in the cyclophosphamide group and 11.8 years in the control group. The mortality at the end of follow-up was statistically significantly higher (51%) in the cyclophosphamide group in comparison with the mortality in the control group (35%) ($P < .025$). Thirty-seven malignancies developed in 29 of the 119 patients treated with cyclophosphamide and 16 malignancies developed in 16 of the control RA patients not treated with cyclophosphamide. The rate of malignancies was statistically significantly higher (24%) in the cyclophosphamide group in comparison with the control group (13%) ($P < .05$). Reviewing the cell type of the different malignancies showed that 6 bladder malignancies and 10 skin cancers were detected in the cyclophosphamide group, whereas no bladder tumors or skin cancers were reported in the control group ($P < .05$). With respect to hematological malignancies, two cases of leukemia, two cases of non-Hodgkin's lymphoma, and one myeloma were detected in the cyclophosphamide group, whereas only one case of chronic lymphocytic leukemia was detected in the control group. The prevalence of solid tumors (lung, stomach, colon, breast, endometrium ovary, cervix, prostate, larynx, and oropharyngeal) appeared equally distributed between the cyclophosphamide and control groups. An evaluation of the interval between the initiation of cyclophosphamide treatment to the development of malignancy for the cyclophosphamide group and the similar follow-up period for the matched control patients showed that malignancies were diagnosed at a significantly increased rate following the sixth year after the beginning of cyclophosphamide administration in the cyclophosphamide treated patients ($P < .01$). An evaluation for current risk factors related to malignancies did not show an association with family history for malignancy, occupation history, rheumatoid factor status, or other concurrent or previous antirheumatic drug treatment. The use of alcohol was more prevalent in cyclophosphamide-treated patients developing malignancies than in cyclophosphamide-treated patients who did not develop malignancies; however, this difference was not statistically significant. In contrast, tobacco use was increased in cyclophosphamide-treated patients who developed bladder cancer ($P < .01$).

Although the mean daily dose of cyclophosphamide was similar in cyclophosphamide-treated patients who did and did not develop cancer, the duration of treatment and total dose of cyclophosphamide was higher in the cyclophosphamide patients who developed malignancies ($P < .01$) (Table 1). Of all the risk factors studied, the total dose of cyclophosphamide was determined to be the most important risk factor for the development of malignancies (Table 1). A previous history of hemorrhagic cystitis was also associated with a higher prevalence of bladder cancer in cyclophosphamide treated patients ($P < .005$)

Although an increased mortality rate and increased malignancy rate was seen in the cyclophosphamide-treated patients, the slight increase in mortality rate of 10.7 versus 6.8% was not statistically significantly different between the cyclophosphamide treated and control patients. In both groups, atherosclerotic cardiovascular disease was the most common cause of death.

Another large study of RA patients treated with cyclophosphamide was completed by Baltus [18] (see Table 1). In this study, 81 patients with RA were compared with 81 control RA patients not treated with cyclophosphamide matched for age and sex. Fifteen malignancies were detected in the patients treated with cyclophosphamide while only four malignancies were detected in the RA controls ($P < .01$). An analysis of the total dose of cyclophosphamide and the duration of cyclophosphamide therapy suggested a trend for an association of larger doses of cyclophosphamide and a longer duration of treatment in patients developing malignancies, but these differences were not statistically significant.

Bladder cancer was also increased in patients receiving cyclophosphamide with a relative risk of 6.8 in a large population follow-up from Denmark [49]. Acrolein, a cyclophosphamide metabolite, [27] and immunosuppression [64] are suspected as an important factors in the development of bladder cancer.

Kinlen et al. reported a follow-up of 1349 patients treated with cytotoxic agents for nonmalignant diseases including patients with RA and SLE [44]. Azathioprine, cyclophosphamide, and chlorambucil were the cytotoxic drugs studied, and the cohorts of patients treated with each agent were not analyzed individually. In the combined treatment groups, the incidence of non-Hodgkin's lymphoma ($P < .001$), squamous carcinoma of the skin ($P=.06$), and the tumors other than skin cancer ($P < .01$) were significantly increased in relationship to the expected observations predicted from normal populations studies.

Although these data, in addition to the information available from cancer chemotherapy studies, provide firm support for the concept that malignancies are increased during treatment of RA patients with cyclophosphamide, other studies have suggested no increase in malignancy with cyclophosphamide treatment of RA [22,36].

In addition to observations in RA, SLE patients have been noted to develop malignancies during the use of oral cyclophosphamide [62,69]. The limited numbers of SLE patients receiving cyclophosphamide have precluded the large controlled studies which have been performed in RA patients. The prevalence of malignancies in SLE patients treated with cyclophosphamide would appear to be similar to that seen in RA patients with comparable therapy. The most common malignancies are hematological malignancies, including leukemia. Also, bladder cancer appears to be increased in SLE patients treated with daily oral cyclophosphamide [51], including a report of a bladder leiomyosarcoma [62].

Table 1 Risk for Development of Cancer in RA Patients Treated With Cyclophosphamide. Comparison of Dose and Duration of Therapy in RA Patients With and Without Subsequent Malignancies After Cyclophosphamide Treatment

	Developed cancer (n = 29)	No cancer (n = 90)	Statistical significance
Baker et al. [17]			
follow-up (years)	10.8	11.8	NS
mean daily dose (mg/kg/day)	0.81	0.85	NS
mean duration (months)	43.8	28.1	$P < .01$
mean total dose (grams)	74.9	45.8	$P < .01$
Baltus et al. [18]			
mean duration (months)	54	43	$P < .229$
mean total dose (grams)	82	61	$P < .054$

NS, not significant.

2. *Intravenous Pulse Cyclophosphamide Therapy*

Recently, intravenous pulse cyclophosphamide has been studied in rheumatic diseases with a particular emphasis on its use in lupus nephritis. This treatment has been shown to have a significant potential for the increase of renal survival and has been associated with a lower incidence of hemorrhagic cystitis [10] and ovarian failure [11]. These observations have provided hope that the associated bladder tumors and hematological malignancies may also be reduced in these patients. Despite these hopes, acute nonlymphocytic leukemia has been reported following intermittent pulse intravenous cyclophosphamide for SLE [38,63]. Many years of follow-up will be needed to determine if pulse intravenous cyclophosphamide is associated with the same incidence of malignancies that is seen inpatients treated with oral daily cyclophosphamide.

C. Chlorambucil

Chlorambucil is an alkylating agent which has been used in the treatment of RA [5,8,9,24], juvenile rheumatoid arthritis [23,45], and other rheumatic and immunological diseases [96]. The majority of the clinically experience with the drug has been in Europe, particularly France. Although clearly effective in the above disorders, significant reservations about the appropriateness of its use in rheumatic diseases remain; primarily because of the documented potential for this agent to induce malignancies. The studies involving chlorambucil are not as extensive as those with cyclophosphamide, but they clearly support an increase in hematological malignancies, particularly lymphomas [24] and leukemia [19,30,73,74]. The possibility that chlorambucil may induce solid tumors is also suggested from other data.

The relative toxicity of chlorambucil in comparison with other cytotoxic drugs is not currently possible, because no clinical studies have been performed which directly compare these agents. However, the clinical data available would suggest that hemorrhagic cystitis and the subsequent bladder tumors are only seen with cyclophosphamide treatment and not increased in patients receiving chlorambucil [72]. One study comparing the oncogenicity of chlorambucil and azathioprine in RA patients reported an increased incidence of malignancy in patients receiving chlorambucil in comparison with patients receiving azathioprine ($P < .03$) [48].

A comparison of the potential for different alkylating agents to induce leukemia has not been performed in patients receiving different chemotherapeutic protocols for similar malignancies. One study, however, suggested more induced chromosome damage with cyclophosphamide than with chlorambucil [103–105).

D. Summary

Cyclophosphamide has been used to treat a large number of rheumatic diseases. Most of the original literature reports the use of oral daily cyclophosphamide. These protocols have generally demonstrated significant clinical benefit associated with this treatment; however, significant side effects were also noted. These concerns have focused on hematological toxicity, hemorrhagic cystitis, and secondary malignancies. These data provide evidence that hematological malignancies are increased during the treatment of RA with alkylating agents. In view of the increased malignancies induced by these agents, most patients with RA would probably best be treated with programs other than alkylating agents if other agents are available.

Intravenous pulse cyclophosphamide has been used in an effort to reduce the incidence of toxic side effects seen with oral cyclophosphamide and may potentially result in a reduced incidence of secondary malignancies. However, data to date have not firmly established that this treatment will produce a lower incidence of induced cancer than that seen with oral cyclophosphamide.

IV. AZATHIOPRINE

A follow-up of 530 RA patients in a long-term study of the effects of disease-modifying antirheumatic drugs (DMARDs) included both past and present users of azathioprine. Criteria for enrollment were an established diagnosis of RA, treatment with at least one DMARD, and no history of previous malignancy or "premalignant condition" [105]. A report of the patients with at least 1 year of follow-up showed 185 patients with at least 2 weeks of exposure to azathioprine. Twenty-five malignant or premalignant conditions were diagnosed in 24 patients during the initial 7 years of the study registry. Four cancers were nonmelanotic skin cancers, with one patient developing both a basal cell skin cancer and actinic keratosis. Four lymphoproliferative or leukemic malignancies were identified and 16 solid tumors. The most common solid tumors were lung tumors. The smoking history appeared to be the strongest correlate for the development of lung cancer in this population. A comparison of RA patients exposed to azathioprine and similar patients not treated with azathioprine did not suggest an increase in malignancy rate associated with azathioprine; however, the relatively short length of follow-up in this cohort has not allowed sufficient time for definite conclusions. This registry is continuing to monitor RA patients treated with DMARDs. Because of the larger numbers of patients in this cohort treated with azathioprine, the longitudinal follow-up of these patients will help determine if the treatment of RA with azathioprine is associated with an increased incidence of malignancy.

Silman reported on 202 RA patients treated with azathioprine who were compared with 202 RA patients not treated with azathioprine [67]. Controls were matched for age, year of diagnosis, sex, and rheumatoid factor status. Both groups were followed for similar periods indexed for 10 years after starting azathioprine and compared with the general population. Four lymphoproliferative malignancies were detected in the azathioprine-treated groups and two similar neoplasms in the RA control group. This analysis suggested a 4.8-fold increase in lymphoma rate in the RA control group and a 10-fold increase in the RA group treated with azathioprine when compared with the general population. In addition to the increased rate of lymphoproliferative cancers in patients treated with azathioprine, the nonlymphoproliferative cancer rates were 13.4 versus 8.3 per 1000 patient years for the azathioprine-treated and control populations, respectively. ($P < .05$). The duration or arthritis or maximum daily azathioprine dose did not correlated with the rate of malignancy; however, a statistically significant correlation between the rate of malignancy and total azathioprine dose was identified ($P < .05$).

A large postmarketing surveillance of 393 RA patients treated with azathioprine did not suggest an increase in cancer in these patients [61]. Ten patients continuing to receive azathioprine replied positively to the question, "In the past 6 months, have you been told that you have any kind of cancer?" A follow-up of these respondents identified three hospitalizations for cancer (hypernephroma, bladder tumor, lung carcinoma). The other respondents reported ovarian cancer, four skin cancers, and two cases of benign breast lumps. No cases of lymphoma or leukemia were identified in these patients [60]. Although these results are encouraging, the study was limited to patients who were continuing to receive azathioprine at the time of the study, and the duration of follow-up (mean 21 months) may not have been sufficient to detect long-term effects.

Lewis et al. evaluated 311 RA patients of whom 303 were treated with azathioprine and 52 received either cyclophosphamide or chlorambucil [46]. In this group, the mortality rate was increased in comparison with the general population, but the majority of deaths were related to ischemic heart disease. The rate of neoplasms was not increased in comparison with the general population.

An evaluation of 755 patients treated with azathioprine for inflammatory bowel disease did not show an increase in malignancy in these patients in comparison with the general population [69].

Prolonged azathioprine therapy has been associated with chromosomal abnormalities [73,106], and malignancies have occurred in several RA patients during treatment with this drug [51].

Overall, the data available do not suggest a strong association between azathioprine treatment of rheumatic diseases and an increased incidence of malignancies. The information from the transplantation literature suggests that azathioprine does increase the tendency to develop malignancies, particularly when used in association with other immunosuppressive agents (particularly cyclosporin and corticosteroids). This information would suggest a slight risk for the induction of cancer with the use of azathioprine in rheumatic diseases, but this risk appears to be much less than the risk seen with the use of alkylating agents in similar conditions.

V. METHOTREXATE

Although not considered a classic cytotoxic agent, the predominant and increasing use of methotrexate in rheumatic diseases warrants some discussion of the malignancy potential of this agent. A recent analysis of 16,263 RA patient treated with methotrexate did not identify any increase in malignancies in this population [107]. In support of this finding, no increase in malignancy was seen in 205 psoriasis patients treated with methotrexate in a review of Cleveland Clinic patients. [75]. Review of the oncology literature have failed to identify an increase in secondary malignancies in patient after treatment with methotrexate [21,54]. An evaluation of the long-term follow-up of patients treated with high doses of methotrexate for gestational trophoblastic tumors did not show an increase in malignancies [54]. A review of the use of methotrexate in malignant diseases suggested a very low association of methotrexate with the development of secondary malignancies [21].

Reversible lymphomas are reported in patients with rheumatic diseases receiving methotrexate [33,43,108–110]. These cases are similar to posttransplant lymphoproliferative disorders [111], which are frequently associated with Epstein-Barr virus (EBV) infection [112] and may be associated with impaired immune regulation in response to this infection [113,114]. The characteristics of lymphoproliferative lesions are described in a series of 18 patients with RA or dermatomyositis, 11 of whom were taking methotrexate at the time of diagnosis [110]. These patients tend to have longstanding seropositive RA. The tumors are extranodal in 56% of patients, with locations including salivary gland, soft tissue, skin, small or large bowel, and lung. One half were large cell lymphomas histologically, and one third contained the EBV genome and membrane protein. Three of the cases had all four characteristics of immunosuppression-associated lymphomas with large or polymorphous histology, areas of necrosis, the presence of EBV, and an extranodal location of the tumor.

The treatment of methotrexate-associated lymphoproliferative disorders includes a discontinuation of methotrexate and close clinical follow-up with treatment initiated or withheld dependent on the patient's clinical course. Kamel and coworkers reported that 5 of the 18 patients with RA or dermatomyositis died of their lymphoma 1–7 months after diagnosis, 2 were alive with evidence of lymphoma, and the remaining patients were alive without evidence of disease [110]. Other reported cases have shown a rapid regression of the tumors after cessation of methotrexate without additional therapy [108].

Several other cases of malignancies have been reported during the treatment of methotrexate for RA. These cancers include non-Hodgkin's lymphoma [28,33,34,57, 61,65,68], acute myeloid leukemia [52], cholangiocarcinoma of the common hepatic duct [55], anaplastic squamous cell carcinoma [40], and thymoma [26]. The role of methotrexate in these cases in unclear, and in view of the developing epidemological data, methotrexate does not appear to be a significant carcinogen.

In summary, the only malignancy which appears to be related to the treatment of rheumatic diseases with methotrexate is EBV-associated B-cell lymphomas which appear reversible after the discontinuation of methotrexate. The incidence of other hematological malignancies or other tumors does not appear increased during or following the treatment of rheumatic diseases or cancer.

VI. COMBINATION THERAPY

Csuka et al. reported the development of four malignancies in 31 RA patients treated with a combination of cyclophosphamide, azathioprine, and hydroxychloroquine [3]. The observed cancers were one colon, one endometrial, one lung, and one erythroleukemia. Three of the patients (colon, endometrial, and erythroleukemia) died rapidly after the malignancies were detected. In this report, the investigators suggested that the malignancy potential was most likely attributable to the use of cyclophosphamide. This group has subsequently changed from advocating the above combination therapy to their currently preferred combination of methotrexate, azathioprine, and hydroxychloroquine for RA patients with refractory disease [115].

VII. APPROACH TO RHEUMATIC DISEASE PATIENTS RECEIVING CYTOTOXIC DRUGS

In approaching patients considered for the use of cytotoxic drugs, the following steps should be taken. The clinician should remember that in the United States, the Food and Drug Administration (FDA) has not approved the use of any alkylating agents for the treatment of rheumatic diseases and has only approved the use of azathioprine and methotrexate for use in RA. Thus, the use of cytotoxic drugs in other situations must be considered as being "unapproved" therapy despite the firm clinical evidence of their efficacy in many situations. All patients who receive these agents should be thoroughly evaluated and counseled. The patient's informed agreement with the clinical treatment program should be well documented in the medical record before cytotoxic drugs are initiated (Table 2).

A. The Diagnosis Should Be Firmly Established

Although the etiology of most rheumatic diseases is unknown, an analysis of the clinical features and associated laboratory finding can often establish a clinical diagnosis. Without a specific rheumatic diagnosis, cytotoxic drugs should generally be withheld. The only exception to this concept would be when a specific diagnosis cannot be established, but a pathological finding of a significant clinical importance—such as necrotizing vasculitis with end organ damage—is identified.

B. A High Probability of a Significant Increase in Morbidity and/or Mortality Without Therapy Should Be Expected

When a diagnosis is established, the natural history and prognosis of the condition should be reviewed. For example, significant data suggest a significant increase in both morbidity and morality for severe RA patients. Despite this observation and the data showing an improvement of clinical features in RA with alkylating agents, most rheumatologists would not recommend the use of these drugs in RA patients because of the increased risk for malignancies. In contrast, because of the much more significant increase in mortality with necrotizing vasculitis, alkylating agents are the drugs of choice.

C. Previous Reported Experience Must Support a Benefit for the Use of the Drug in the Diagnosed Condition

As discussed in other chapters of this book and the medical literature, cytotoxic drugs are an effective treatment for many rheumatic diseases. However, not all conditions are responsive to these agents. For example, despite some suggestions of improvement in uncontrolled studies, recent double-blind placebo-controlled studies have failed to demonstrate clinical improvements in systemic sclerosis patients treated with chlorambucil

Table 2 Approach to Rheumatic Disease Patients Receiving Cytotoxic Drugs

1. The diagnosis should be firmly established.
2. A high probability of a significant increase in morbidity and/or mortality without therapy should be expected.
3. Previous reported experience must support a benefit for the use of the drug in the diagnosed condition.
4. Active and/or reversible disease should be present.
5. No contraindications to the specific agent should be present.
6. Clear goals and endpoints should be established prior to the initiation of therapy.
7. Informed consent and understanding of potential risk and benefits of therapy, including the risks for malignancy.
8. Willingness to comply with the needed follow-up and monitoring during therapy.

[116]. The clinician must be aware of the literature to assure that the underlying condition has the potential to respond to the cytotoxic therapy under consideration.

D. Active and/or Reversible Disease Should Be Present

Although many conditions may respond to cytotoxic drug therapy, the potential response of each patient must be evaluated. For example, although SLE, particularly lupus nephritis, is frequently responsive to cyclophosphamide, patients with end-stage renal disease will have little benefit from this agent after the renal lesions are sufficiently advanced. In a similar situation, a patient with "burned out" RA with minimal synovial inflammation will be unlikely to respond to azathioprine or other cytotoxic drug therapy despite the well-documented response of active synovitis to azathioprine in other RA patients.

E. No Contraindications to the Specific Agent Should Be Present

Potential contraindications to the cytotoxic drugs must be reviewed and the patient screened for these potential concerns. A hematological assessment is essential prior to the initiation of cytotoxic drug therapy and throughout treatment. Other specific concerns must be evaluated on the basis of the individual agents selected. For example, azathioprine would be considered to be contraindicated in most patients concurrently receiving allopurinol.

F. Clear Goals and Endpoints Should Be Established Prior to the Initiation of Therapy

Because the malignancy potential of cytotoxic drugs appears to be dependent on the total dose and duration of therapy, a decision to continue cytotoxic agents for a prolonged period of time must be based on objective data that the continued therapy is beneficial and necessary. If predetermined goals are not achieved, the use of cytotoxic drugs should be reevaluated and these agents should not be continued. Efforts should then be directed to explore other potential treatments which could benefit the patients.

G. Informed Consent and Understanding of Potential Risk and Benefits of Therapy Including the Risks for Malignancy

As discussed above, in most rheumatic diseases, cytotoxic drugs are not FDA approved. The liability of using any agent which has not received formal approval should always be considered by the physician as he or she approaches the patient about the use of this therapy. A thorough explanation of the associated risks and benefits, discussion of the "unapproved" nature of the therapy, and documentation of the patient's understand and willingness to procede with therapy are essential. Although this process is time consuming, the potential liabilities make these discussions and their associated documentation well worthwhile.

H. Willness to Comply with the Needed Follow-up and Monitoring During Therapy

Regular follow-up with clinical and laboratory monitoring in essential to avoid significant toxicity and assure optimal clinical benefit. Evaluations should generally be performed at least monthly and monitoring be directed by the specific agent be utilized.

VIII. SUMMARY

Cytotoxic drugs have provided a significant advance in the treatment of rheumatic diseases. A major concern with their continued and potentially expanded use has been the potential to induce malignancies. Available data strongly suggest that the use of the alkylating agents cyclophosphamide and chlorambucil are both associated with an increased risk for malignancy. The risk increases with both the duration and total dose of medication used. The data concerning azathioprine treatment are incomplete, and most information would suggest no or little risk for an increase in malignancies with this treatment. Methotrexate treatment does not appear to increase the risk for malignancies except for relatively rare B-cell EBV-associated lymphomas which often regress after the discontinuation of methotrexate. When considering the use of cytotoxic drug in a rheumatic disease, the clinician must carefully assess the risks and benefits of the therapy with the patient and document the patient's acceptance and willingness to participate in the proposed treatment plan before initiating therapy.

REFERENCES

1. Williams HJ, Reading JC, Ward JR, et al. Comparison of high and low dose cyclophosphamide therapy in rheumatoid arthritis. Arthritis Rheum 1980; 23:521–527.
2. Townes AS, Sowa JM, Schulman LE. Controlled trial of cyclophosphamide in rheumatoid arthritis. Arthritis Rheum 1976; 19:563–573.
3. Csuka M, Carrera GF, McCarty DJ. Treatment of intractable rheumatoid arthritis with combined cyclophosphamide, azathioprine, and hydroxychloroquine. A follow-up study. JAMA 1986; 255:2315–2319.
4. Hunter T, Urowitz MD, Gordon DA, et al. Azathioprine in rheumatoid arthritis. A long-term follow-up study. Arthritis Rheum 1975; 18:15–20.
5. Kahn MF, Bedorseau M, Six B, et al. Chlorambucil in rheumatoid arthritis. Rev Rhum Mal Osteoartic 1971; 38:741–748.
6. Renier JC, Deschayes P, Hondent G, et al. Le traitement de la polyarthrite rhumatoide par le chlorambucil. Etude de 113 observations. Arch Med de l'Ouest 1971; 1:47–58.
7. Smith CJ, Bartholomew BA, Mills DM, et al. Cyclophosphamide therapy for rheumatoid arthritis. Arch Intern Med 1975; 135:789–793.
8. Thorpe P, Hassall MB, York JR. Rheumatoid arthritis treated with chlorambucil: a five-year follow-up. Med J Aust 1976; 2:197–199, 1976.
9. Cayla J, Rondier J. The treatment of 67 cases of rheumatoid arthritis with chlorambucil drugs. Rev Rhum Mal Oseoartic 1971; 38:765–770.
10. Austin HA III, Klippel JH, Balow JE, et al. Therapy of lupus nephritis. Controlled trial of prednisone and cytotoxic drugs. N Engl J Med 1986; 314:614–619.
11. Balow JE, Austin HA, Tsokas GC, et al. Lupus nephritis. Ann Intern Med 1987; 106:79–94.

12. McCune WJ, Golbus J, Zeldes W, et al. Clinical and immunologic effects of monthly administration of intravenous cyclophosphamide in severe systemic lupus erythematosus. N Engl J Med 1988; 318:1423–1431.
13. Arundell FD, Wilkinson RD, Haserick JR. Dermatomyositis and malignant neoplasms in adults. A survey of twenty years' experience. Arch Dermatol 1960; 82:772–775.
14. Fort JG, Abruzzo JL. Reversal of progressive necrotizing vasculitis with intravenous pulse cyclophosphamide and methylprednisolone. Arthritis Rheum 1988; 31:1194–1198.
15. Guillevin L, Jarrousse B, Lok C, et al. Longterm followup after treatment of polyarteritis nodosa and Churg-Strauss angiitis with comparison of steriods, plasma exchange and cyclophosphamide to steroids and plasma exchange. A prospective randomized trial of 71 patients. J Rheumatol 1991; 18:567–574.
16. Chapman PT, O'Donnell JL. Respiratory failure in Wegener's granulomatosis: response to pulse intravenous methylprednisolone and cyclophosphamide. J Rheumatol 1993; 20:504–506.
17. Baker GL, Kahl LE, Zee BC, et al. Malignancy following treatment of rheumatoid arthritis with cyclophosphamide. Am J Med 1987; 83:1–9.
18. Baltus JAM, Boersma JW, Hartman AP, et al. The occurrence of malignancies in patients with rheumatoid arthritis treated with cyclophosphamide: a controlled retrospective follow-up. Ann Rheum Dis 1983; 42:368–373.
19. Berk PD, Goldberg JD, Silverstein MN, et al. Increased incidence of acute leukemia in polycythemia vera associated with chlorambucil therapy. N Engl J Med 1981; 304:441–447.
20. Berliner J, Shoenfeld Y, Sidi Y, et al. Systemic lupus erythematosus and lymphoma. Scand J Rheumatol 1983; 12:310–314.
21. Boffetta P, Kaldor JM. Secondary malignancies following cancer chemotherapy. Acta Oncol 1994; 33:591–598.
22. Boyle DJ. Incidence of malignancy 10 years following cyclophosphamide use for rheumatoid arthritis [abstr]. Arthritis Rheum 1981; 27:71.
23. Buriot D, Prieur AM, Lebranchu Y, et al. Leucemie aigue chez trois enfants atteints d'arthrite chronique juvenille traites par le chlorambucil. Arch Fr Pediatr 1979; 36:592–598.
24. Cannon GW, Jackson CG, Samuelson CO Jr, et al. Chlorambucil therapy in rheumatoid arthritis: clinical experience in 28 patients and literature review. Semin Arthritis Rheum 1985; 15:106–118.
25. Cash JM, Klippel JH. Rheumatic diseases and cancer. Clin Exp Rheumatol 1991; 9:109–112.
26. Colburn KK, Cao JD. Thymoma associated with rheumatoid arthritis in a patient taking methotrexate. J Rheumatol 1986; 13:437–439.
27. Cox PJ. Cyclophosphamide cystitis and bladder cancer; a hypothesis. Eur J Cancer Clin Oncol 1979; 15:1071–1072.
28. Craig SR, Rosenberg EW. Methotrexate-induced carcinoma? Arch Derm 1971; 103:505–506.
29. Cras P, Franckx C, Martin JJ. Primary intracerebral lymphoma in systemic lupus erythematosus treated with immunosuppressives. Clin Neuropathol 1989; 8:200–205.
30. Dumont J, Thiery JP, Mazabraud A, et al. Acute myeloid leukemia following non's lymphoma. Danger of prolonged use of chlorambucil as maintenance therapy. Nouv Rev Fr Hematol 1980; 22:391–404.
31. Duncan SC, Winkelman RR. Cancer and scleroderma. Arch Dermatol 1979; 115:950–955.
32. Efremidis A, Eiser AR, Grishman E, et al. Hodgkin's lymphoma in an adolscent with systemic lupus erythematosus. Cancer 1984; 53:142–146.
33. Ellman MH. Non-hodgkin's lymphoma, rheumatoid arthritis and methotrexate. J Rheumatol 1993; 20:200–202.

34. Ellman MH, Hurwitz H, Thomas C, et al. Lymphoma developing in a patient with rheumatoid arthritis taking low dose weekly methotrexate. J Rheumatol 1991; 18:1741–1743.
35. Escalante A, Kaufman RL, Beardmore TD. Acute myelocytic leukemia after the use of cyclophosphamide in the treatment of polyarteritis nodosa. J Rheumatol 1989; 16:1147–1149.
36. Farber SJ. Incidence of malignant disease in patients receiving cytotoxic therapy for rheumatoid arthritis [abstr]. Arthritis Rheum 1979; 22:608.
37. Fiere D, Felman P, Vu Van H, et al. Leucemies aigues myeloids apres administration de chlorambucil. Deux observations. Lett Nouv Presse Med 1977:756.
38. Gibbons RB, Westerman E. Acute nonlymphocytic leukemia following short-term intermittent, intravenous cyclophosphamide treatment of lupus nephritis. Arthritis Rheum 1988; 31:1552–1554.
39. Green JA, Dawson AA, Walker W. Systemic lupus erythematosus and lymphoma. Lancet 1978; 2:753–755.
40. Harris CC. Malignancy during methotrexate and steroid therapy for psoriasis. Arch Dermatol 1971; 103:501–504.
41. Hornbaker JH, Foster EA, Williams GS, et al. Sjögren's syndrome and nodular reticulum-cell sarcoma. Arch Int Med 1966; 118:449–452.
42. Kahn MF, Arlet J, Bloch-Michel H, et al. Acute leukemia after treatment using cytotoxic agents for rheumatologic purposes. 19 cases among 2006 patients. Nouv Presse Med 1979; 8:1393–1397.
43. Kamel OW, Van de Rijn M, Weiss LM, et al. Brief Report: Reversible lymphomas associated with Epstein-Barr virus occurring during methotrexate therapy for rheumatoid arthritis and dermatomyositis. New Engl J Med 1993; 328:1317–1321.
44. Kinlen LJ, Sheil AGR, Peto J, et al. Collaborative United Kingdom–Australian study of cancer in patients treated with immunosuppressive drugs. Br Med J 1979; 2:1461–1466.
45. Lebranchu Y, Drucker J, Nivet H, et al. Acute monoblastic leukaemia in child receiving chlorambucil for juvenile rheumatoid arthritis [letter]. Lancet 1980; 1:649.
46. Lewis P, Hazleman BL, Hanka R, et al. Cause of death in patients with rheumatoid arthritis with particular reference to azathioprine. Ann Rheum Dis 1980; 39:457–461.
47. Morris CR, Morris AJ. Localized lymphoma in a patient with rheumatoid arthritis treated with parenteral methotrexate. J Rheumatol 1993; 20:2172–2173.
48. Patapanian H, Graham S, Sambrook PN, et al. The oncogenicity of chlorambucil in rheumatoid arthritis. Br J Rheumatol 1988; 27:44–47.
49. Pedersen-Bjergaard J, Olesen Larsen S, Struck J, et al. Risk of therapy-related leukaemia and preleukaemia after Hodgkin's disease: relation to age, cumulative dose of alkylating agents, and time from chemotherapy. Lancet 1987; 2:83–88.
50. Pitt PI, Sultan AH, Malone M, et al. Association between azathioprine therapy and lymphoma in rheumatoid disease. J R Soc Med 1987; 80:428–429.
51. Plotz PH, Lkippel JH, Decker JL, et al. Bladder complications in patients receiving cyclophosphamide for systemic lupus erythematosus or rheumatoid arthritis. Ann Intern Med 1979; 91:221–223.
52. Pointud P. Prudat M, Peron J. Acute leukemia after low dose methotrexate therapy in a patient with rheumatoid arthritis. J Rheumatol 1993; 20:1215–1216.
53. Roumm AD, Medsger TA. Cancer and systemic sclerosis. Arthritis Rheum 1985; 28:1336–1340.
54. Rustin GJS, Rustin F, Dent J, et al. No increase in second tumors after cytotoxic chemotherapy for gestational trophoblastic tumors. N Engl J Med 1983; 308:473–476.
55. Sanders KM. Low-dose methotrexate and cholangiocarcinoma of the common hepatic duct. Arthritis Rheum 1991; 34:498.
56. Schuermann H. Maligne tumoren bei dermatomyositis and progressive sklerodermie. Arch Dermatol Syph 1951; 192:575–582.

57. Seidenfeld AM, Smythe HA, Ogryzlo MA, et al. Acute leukemia in rheumatoid arthritis treated with cytotoxic agents. J Rheumatol 1976; 3:295–304.
58. Seidenfeld AM, Smythe HA, Ogryzlo MA, et al. Acute leukemia in rheumatoid arthritis treated with cytotoxic agents. J Rheumatol 1984; 11:586–587.
59. Sela O, Shoenfeld Y. Cancer in autoimmune diseases. Semin Arthritis Rheum 1988; 18:77–87.
60. Singh G, Fries JF, Spitz P, et al. Toxic effects of azathioprine in rheumatoid arthritis. A national post-marketing perspective. Arthritis Rheum 1989; 32:837–843.
61. Taillan B, Garnier G, Ferrari E, et al. Malignant lymphoma in a patient with rheumatoid arthritis treated with low-dose methotrexate. Rev Rhum 1993; 60:214–216.
62. Thrasher JB, Miller GJ, Wettlaufer JN. Bladder leiomyosarcoma following cyclophosphamide therapy for lupus nephritis. J Urol 1990; 143:119–121.
63. Vasquez S, Kavanaugh AF, Schneider NR, et al. Acute nonlymphocytic leukemia after treatment of systemic lupus erythematosus with immunosuppressive agents. J Rheumatol 1992; 19:1625–1627.
64. Wall RL, Clausen KP. Carcinoma of the urinary bladder in patients receiving cyclophosphamide. N Engl J Med 1975; 293:271–273.
65. Zimmer-Galler I and Lie JT. Choroidal infiltrates as the initial manifestation of lymphoma in rheumatoid arthritis after treatment with low-dose methotrexate. Mayo Clin Proc 1994; 69:258–261.
66. Zittoun R, Debre P, Gardais J, et al. Small intestine lymphosarcoma after treatment of rheumatoid arthritis by chlorambucil. Nouv Presse Med 1972; 1:2477–2479.
67. Silman AJ, Petrie J, Hazleman B, et al. Lymphoproliferative cancer and other malignancy in patients with rheumatoid arthritis treated with azathioprine: a 20 year follow up study. Ann Rheum Dis 1988; 47:988–992.
68. Kingsmore SF, Hall BD, Allen NB, et al. Association of methotrexate, rheumatoid arthritis and lymphoma: report of 2 cases and literature review. J Rheumatol 1992; 19:1462–1465.
69. Connell WR, Kamm MA, Dickson M. Long-term neoplasia risk after azathioprine treatment in inflammatory bowel disease. Lancet 1994; 343:1249–1252.
70. Ortiz A, Gonzalez-Parra E, Alvarez-Costa G. Bladder cancer after cyclophosphamide therapy for lupus nephritis [letter]. Nephron 1992; 60:378–379.
71. Anderson LG, Talal N. The spectrum of benign to malignant proliferation in Sjögren's syndrome. Clin Exp Immunol 1972; 10:199–218.
72. deVries C, Freiha FS. Hemorrhagic cystitis: a review. J Urol 1990; 143:1–9.
73. Aymard JP, Frustin J, Witz F, et al. Acute leukemia after prolonged chlorambucil treatment for non-malignant disease: report of a new case and literature survey. Acta Haematol 1980; 63:283–285.
74. Aymard JP, Lederlin P, Witz F, et al. Acute leukemia following prolonged chlorambucil treatment of non-neoplastic disease—a study of two cases and literature review. Acta Clin Belg 1983;38:228–235.
75. Bailin PL, Tindall JP, Roenigk HH, et al. Is methotrexate therapy for psoriasis carcinogenic? JAMA 1975; 232:359–362.
76. Isomaki HA, Hakulinen T, Joutsenlahti V. Excess risk of lymphomas, leukemia, and myeloma in patients with rheumatoid arthritis. J Chronic Dis 1978; 31:691–696.
77. Prior P, Symmons PM, Hawkins CF, et al. Cancer morbidity in rheumatoid arthritis. Ann Rheum Dis 1984; 43:128–131.
78. Fries JT, Bloch D, Spitz P, et al. Cancer in rheumatoid arthritis: A prospective long-term study of mortality. Am J Med 1985; 78:56–59.
79. Laakso M, Mutru O, Isomaki H, et al. Cancer mortality in patients with rheumatoid arthritis. J Rheumatol 1986; 13:522–526.

80. Allebeck P. Increased mortality in rheumatoid arthritis. Scand J Rheumatol 1982; 11:81–86.
81. Vandenbroucke JP, Hazevoet HM, Cats A. Survival and cause of death in rheumatoid arthritis: A 25-year prospective followup. J Rheumatol 1984; 11:158–161.
82. Mitchell DM, Spitz PW, Young DY, et al. Survival, prognosis, and causes of death in rheumatoid arthritis. Arthritis Rheum 1986; 29:706–714.
83. Mutru O, Laakso M, Isomäki H, et al. Ten year mortality and causes of death in patients with rheumatoid arthritis. Br Med J 1985; 290:1797–1799.
84. Lewis RB, Castor CW, Knisley RE, et al. Frequency of neoplasia in systemic lupus erythematosus and rheumatoid arthritis. Arthritis Rheum 1976; 19:1256–1260.
85. Wyburn-Mason R. SLE and lymphoma. Lancet 1979; 1:156.
86. Zatuchini J, Campbell WN, Zarafonetis CJD. Pulmonary fibrosis and terminal bronchiolar ("alveolar cell") carcinoma in scleroderma. Cancer 1953; 6:1147–1158.
87. Haddad R, Massaro D. Idiopathic diffuse interstitial pulmonary fibrosis (fibrosing alveolitis), atypical epithelial proliferation and lung cancer. Am J Med 1968; 45:211–219.
88. Fox B, Risdon RA. Carcinoma of the lung and diffuse interstitial pulmonary fibrosis. J Clin Pathol 1968; 21:486–491.
89. Jones AW. Alveolar cell carcinoma occurring in ideopathic interstitial pulmonary fibrosis. Br J Dis Chest 1970; 64:78–84.
90. Fraire AE, Greenberg SD. Carcinoma and diffuse interstitial fibrosis of lung. Cancer 1973; 31:1078–1086.
91. Talbott JH, Barrocas M. Carcinoma of the lung in progressive systemic sclerosis: a tabular review of the literature and a detailed report of the roentgenographic changes in two cases. Semin Arthritis Rheum 1980; 9:191–216.
92. Medsger TA, Masi AT. The epidemiology of systemic sclerosis (scleroderma) among male US veterans. J Chronic Dis 1978; 31:73–85.
93. Peters-Golden M, Wise RA, Hochberg M, et al. Incidence of lung cancer in systemic sclerosis. J Rhematol 1985; 12:1136–1139.
94. Williams RC. Dermatomyositis and malignancy—a review of the literature. Ann Intern Med 1959; 50:1174–1181.
95. Barnes BE. Dermatomyositis and malignancy—a review of the literature. Ann Intern Med 1976; 84:68–76.
96. Callen JP. Dermatomyositis and malignancy. Clin Rheum Dis 1982; 8:369–387.
97. Christianson HB, Brunspry LA, Perry HO. Dermatoymyositis: Unusual features, complications and treatment. Arch Dermatol 1956; 74:581–589.
98. Pearson CM. Polymyositis and related disorders. In: Walton JN, ed. Disorders of Voluntery Muscle, 2nd ed. Boston: Little, Brown, 1969:501–539.
99. Curtis AC, Blaylock HC, Harrel ER Jr. Malignant lesions associated with dermatomyositis. JAMA 1952; 150:844–846.
100. Talal N, Bunim JJ. Development of malignant lymphoma in the course of Sjögren's syndrome. Am J Med 1964; 36:529–540.
101. Talal N, Sokoloff L, Barth WF. Extra salivary lymphoid abnormalities in Sjögren's syndrome (reticulum cell sarcoma, "pseudolymphoma" macroglobulinemia). Am J Med 1967; 43:50–65.
102. Kassan SS, Thomas TL, Moutsopoulus HM, et al. Increased risk of lymphoma in sicca syndrome. Ann Intern Med 1978; 89:888–892.
103. O'Duffy TD, Robertson DM, Goldstein NP. Chlorambucil in the treatment of ureitis and meningoencephalitis of Behçet's disease. Am J Med 1984; 76:75–84.
104. Palmer RG, Dore CJ,Denman AM. Cyclophosphamide induces more chromosome damage than chlorambucil in patients with connective tissue diseases. Q J Med 1986; 59:395–400.

105. Matteson EL, Hickey AR, Maguire L, et al. Occurrence of neoplasia in patients with rheumatoid arthritis enrolled in a DMARD registry. J Rheumatol 1991; 18:809–814.
106. Leb DE, Weisskopf B, Kanovitz, BS. Chromosome aberrations in the child of a kidney transplant recipient. Arch Intern Med 1971; 128:441-444.
107. Moder KG, Tefferi A, Cohen MD, et al. Hematologic malignancies and the use of methotrexate in rheumatoid arthritis: a retrospective study. Am J Med 1995; 99:276–281.
108. Bachman TR, Sawitzke AD, Perkins SL, et al. Reversible lymphoma in rheumatoid arthritis patients treated with methotrexate: A report of two cases. Arthritis Rheum 1996; 39:325-329.
109. Shiroky J, Frost A, Skelton J, et al. Complications of immunosuppression associated with weekly low dose methotrexate. J Rheumatol 1991; 18:1172–1175.
110. Kamel O, Van de Rijn M, LeBrun D, et al. Lymphoid neoplasms in patients with rheumatoid arthritis and dermatomyositis: frequency of Epstein-Barr virus and other features associated with immunosuppression. Hum Pathol 1994; 25:638-643.
111. Nalesnik M, Makowka L, Starzl T. The diagnosis and treatment of posttransplant lymphoproliferative disorders. Curr Probl Surg 1988; 25:365–472.
112. Ho M, Miller G, Atchison RW, et al. Epstein-Barr Virus infections and DNA hybridization studies in posttransplantation lymphoma and lymphoproliferative lesions: the role of primary infection. J Infect Dis 1985; 152:876–886.
113. Tosato G, Steinberg A, Yarchoan R, et al. Abnormally elevated frequency of Epstein-Barr virus–infected B cells in the blood of patients with rheumatoid arthritis. J Clin Invest 1984; 73:1789–1795.
114. Depper J, Bluestein H, Zvaifler N. Impaired regulation of Epstein-Barr virus–induced lymphocyte proliferation in rheumatoid arthritis is due to a T cell defect. J Immunol 1981; 127:1899-1902.
115. McCarty, D.J.: Suppress rheumatoid inflammation early and lave the pyramid to the Egyptians. J Rheumatol 1990; 17:115–118.
116. Furst, D.E., Clements, P.J., Hillis, S., et al. Immunosuppression with chlorambucil, versus placebo, for scleroderma; results of a three-year, parallel, randomized, double-blind study. Arthritis Rheum 1989; 32:584–593.

Index

About the Editors

LEO B. A. VAN DE PUTTE is Professor of Rheumatology at University Hospital, Nijmegen, The Netherlands. The author of several key professional papers on clinical and experimental rheumatology, clinical immunology, nephrology, and pharmacology, he is a member of the Dutch Association of Rheumatology and is the 1995–1997 President of the European League Against Rheumatism. Dr. van de Putte received the M.D. degree (1967) from the University of Leiden, The Netherlands.

DANIEL E. FURST is Director of the Arthritis Clinical Research Unit at Virginia Mason Medical Center, Seattle, Washington, and Clinical Professor of Medicine and Rheumatology at the University of Washington, Seattle. The author or coauthor of more than 200 publications, he is the editor of the *Inflammatory Disease and Therapy Series* and coeditor of the books *Nonsteroidal AntiInflammatory Drugs: Mechanisms and Clinical Uses, Second Edition*; *Second-Line Agents in the Treatment of Arthritis*; and *Immunomodulators in the Rheumatic Diseases* (all titles, Marcel Dekker, Inc.). Dr. Furst received the M.D. degree (1968) from The Johns Hopkins University, Baltimore, Maryland.

H. JAMES WILLIAMS is Professor, Associate Chairman of the Department of Internal Medicine, and Chief of the Division of Rheumatology at the University of Utah, Salt Lake City. The author or coauthor of over 100 professional papers and book chapters, he is a Fellow of the American College of Physicians and the American College of Rheumatology. He holds the Thomas E. and Rebecca D. Jeremy Presidential Endowed Chair for Arthritis Research. Dr. Williams received the M.D. degree (1969) from the University of Utah, Salt Lake City.

PIET L. C. M. VAN RIEL is Professor, Vice Chairman of the Department of Rheumatology and Director of the Clinical Research Unit at the University Hospital, Nijmegen, The Netherlands. The author or coauthor of numerous publications, he is a member of the American College of Rheumatology, the Dutch Society for Rheumatology, and the British Society for Rheumatology. Dr. van Riel received the M.D. degree (1978) and the Ph.D. degree (1983) in rheumatology from the University of Nijmegen, The Netherlands.